NEUROLOGY
for the Speech-Language Pathologist

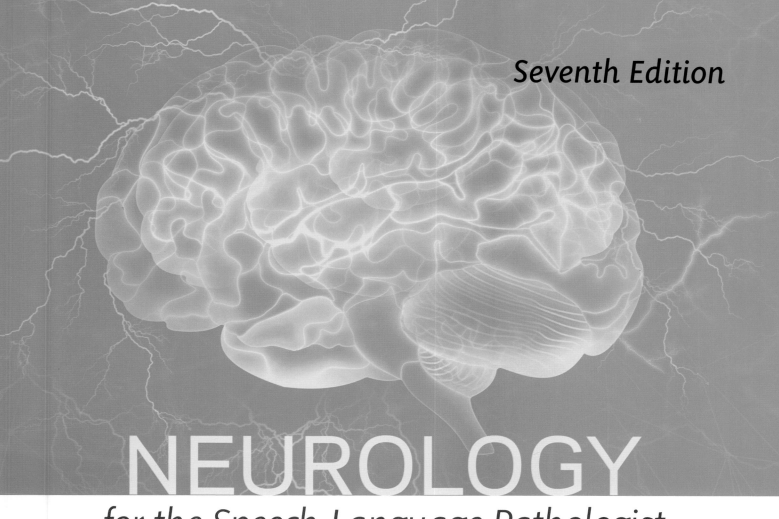

Seventh Edition

NEUROLOGY
for the Speech-Language Pathologist

RIMA ABOU-KHALIL, PHD, CCC-SLP
Clinical Assistant Professor/Speech-Language Pathologist
Vanderbilt University School of Medicine
Vanderbilt Bill Wilkerson Center
Nashville, Tennessee, United States

WANDA G. WEBB, PHD, CCC-SLP
Assistant Professor
Department of Hearing and Speech Sciences
School of Medicine
Vanderbilt University
Nashville, Tennessee, United States

ELSEVIER

Elsevier
3251 Riverport Lane
St. Louis, Missouri 63043

NEUROLOGY FOR THE SPEECH-LANGUAGE PATHOLOGIST, SEVENTH EDITION.   ISBN: 978-0-323-83098-0

Previous editions copyrighted 2017, 2008, 2001, 1996, 1991, and 1986.

Senior Content Strategist: Lauren Willis
Senior Content Development Specialist: Priyadarshini Pandey
Publishing Services Manager: Deepthi Unni
Project Manager: Thoufiq Mohammed
Design Direction: Brian Salisbury

Printed in India

Last digit is the print number: 9   8   7   6   5   4   3   2   1

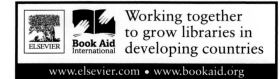

This text is dedicated to the many patients with neurologic cognitive-communicative disorders who have trusted us with their rehabilitation. We have learned numerous lessons from them, most importantly about perseverance in the face of adversity and the brain's ability to adapt and relearn. We are grateful to each and every one of you.

ACKNOWLEDGMENTS

I have led a magical life, filled with supportive people who have guided and nurtured me. Foremost among them is my family with their willingness to allow me to explore various projects and to grow both professionally and personally. My husband and best friend, Bassel Abou-Khalil, has been an unwitting mentor, with his strong work ethics and dedication to his profession yet his willingness to put work aside when a compassionate ear is called for. My two lovely daughters, May and Lena, have continuously inspired me with their cheerfulness, sweetness, and intelligence, and their helpfulness when needed.

No accomplishments can occur in a vacuum, and I owe so much of my career to my professor, mentor, colleague, and friend, Dr. Wanda Webb. She has guided and nudged me throughout my long association with her, and I continue to learn from her on a daily basis.

Two of my colleagues read chapters as they were revised and offered suggestions and wisdom: my good friends Dr. Barbara Jacobson and Dr. Antje Mefferd. Their time and effort were provided despite their hectic schedules and myriad commitments. I am so grateful to them for their time and expertise.

Lastly, I learn every day by my association with my colleagues, my students, and the patients I serve. Colleagues have answered my many questions and provided generous insights and wisdom. Students have posed thought-provoking questions over the years, enabling me to think more deeply about anatomic relationships or clinical correlations. Any interaction with a patient has the potential to teach me about fortitude and compassion. May the lessons never stop.

Rima Abou-Khalil

I first want to acknowledge and express my enormous gratitude to the new senior author of this text, Dr. Rima Abou-Khalil. Rima is a former student of mine when she was working on her master's degree at Vanderbilt, was my teaching assistant for 1 year, and has become a cherished friend. I was hesitant to ask anyone I actually know to take over this text as I retire from it because it is a great deal of work to revise and update a text. It is especially difficult with one in its seventh edition, having been authored by other people in the previous six editions; however, it was important to me to ask someone I trust and whose knowledge, teaching skill, and clinical expertise I know and admire. I was delighted when Rima agreed to do it and was happy to help with the four chapters she asked me to do. I am so proud to be her colleague and am so very grateful to her for agreeing to make such a sacrifice of time and energy to revise this text.

In addition, I want to acknowledge the contribution of my colleagues in the professions of speech-language pathology and neurology/neuroscience. Without their clinical and research expertise and dedication, a text like this would never be possible. There is an explosion of excellence in our field and dedication to finding answers for the patients we treat. I am proud to be a conduit of information provided by their work.

Finally, to my friends and family who did not abandon me when I agreed to contribute to the textbook this time after saying I would NOT work on another edition. You know who you are, and I hope you know how much I appreciate your patience and understanding and unwavering support! You are the best!

Wanda G. Webb

FOREWORD

SPEECH PATHOLOGY AND NEUROLOGY: INTERSECTING SPECIALTIES

Neurology is the study of the effects of disease in the nervous system—brain, spinal cord, cerebellum, nerves, and muscles—on human behavior. The neurologist examines specific functions—including higher cortical functions; cranial nerve functions; and motor, sensory, and cerebellar functions—to localize disorders to specific areas of the nervous system. These lesion localizations, along with the clinical history of how the deficit developed, allow for a precise diagnosis of the disease process. Laboratory and brain imaging tests may help to confirm the diagnosis, but the process should always start with localization and disease diagnosis in a clinical neurologic evaluation.

Speech and communication are among the most complicated functions of the human brain, involving myriad interactions among personality, cognitive processes, imagination, language, emotion, and lower sensory and motor systems necessary for articulation and comprehension. These functions involve brain pathways and mechanisms, some well understood and others only beginning to be conceptualized. The brain mechanisms underlying higher functions such as language are known largely through neurologic studies of human patients with acquired brain lesions. Animal models have shed only limited light on these complex disorders.

Stroke has historically been a great source of information because this so-called experiment of nature damages one brain area while leaving the rest of the nervous system intact. For more than a century, patients with strokes and other brain diseases have been studied in life, and the clinical syndromes have then been correlated with brain lesions found at autopsy. New methods of brain imaging have made possible the simultaneous study of a lesion in the brain and a deficit of communication in the same patient. These advances in brain imaging, including computed tomography, magnetic resonance imaging (MRI), and positron emission tomography (PET), have brought about a burgeoning of knowledge in this area. Functional brain imaging modalities such as functional MRI and PET scanning now permit the visualization of brain activation in normal subjects during language tasks, and these studies have contributed further to our knowledge of the organization of language in the brain.

In this book, the factual groundwork has been laid for the understanding of the nervous system in terms of the organization of the brain, descending motor and ascending sensory pathways, and cranial nerves and muscles. Understanding these anatomic systems makes possible the understanding and classification of the syndromes of aphasia, alexia, dysarthria, and dysphonia, as well as the effects of specific, localized disease processes on human speech and communication. All these subjects are clearly and accurately reviewed. The speech-language pathologist who studies this book should have a much improved comprehension of the brain mechanisms disrupted in speech-impaired and language-impaired patients, and thereby a greater understanding of the disorders of speech and language themselves.

Perhaps the most important by-product of this book should be a closer interaction between neurologists and speech-language pathologists. Neurologists understand the anatomic relationships of the brain and its connections, but they often fail to use speech and language to their full limits in assessing the function of specific parts of the nervous system. A careful analysis of speech and language functions can supplement the more cursory portions of the standard neurologic examination devoted to these functions. Thus detailed aphasia testing supplements the neurologist's bedside mental status examination, and close observation of palatal, lingual, and facial motion during articulation supplements the neurologist's cranial nerve examination. The neurologist's diagnosis of the patient's disorder, on the other hand, should aid the speech-language pathologist in understanding the nature and prognosis of the speech and language disorder. The neurologist and speech-language pathologist should ideally function as a team, complementing each other. For this teamwork to occur, however, each specialist must comprehend the other's language. To this end, these authors have made the language of the neurologist understandable to the speech-language pathologist. As a neurologist who worked closely with Drs. Webb and Love, I applaud this important accomplishment. I also welcome Dr. Rima Abou-Khalil to this edition. She, too, has worked closely with neurologists and has contributed to aphasia research.

I would like to end with a personal statement about Dr. Russell Love, one of the two original authors of this book. Dr. Love was an inspiring scientist and colleague who personified the relationship between speech-language pathologist and neurologist. In his long career, he taught generations of speech-language pathologists and neurologists. To the end, he was always gracious, optimistic, and informative in every interaction.

Howard S. Kirshner
Professor and Vice-Chair, Department of Neurology,
Vanderbilt University Medical Center, Nashville, Tennessee

INTRODUCTION

It is indeed rare to find a speech-language pathologist in practice today who does not interact with the medical profession. The person practicing in hospitals, rehabilitation settings, nursing homes, or home health settings obviously will be a part of a medical team, whether formal or informal. The person practicing in the school systems, where the majority of speech-language pathologists and many educational audiologists are employed, also frequently will need to interact in some way with the medical profession, as will persons in private practice. In both of these settings, medically fragile children and adults are treated who have a communication disorder associated with a medical condition. This evolution in patient population has made it critical for the speech-language pathologist and audiologist to be well versed concerning anatomy and physiology of body systems related to speech, language, and hearing. Arguably the most important system is the nervous system—the foundation of all movement and thought associated with speech and language.

BACKGROUND

The idea for this text was first conceived by Dr. Russell Love and Dr. Wanda Webb, both speech-language pathologists, out of a frustration that there was, at that time (1986), no textbook written by speech-language pathologists for that profession that was devoted strictly to the neurology of "the human communication nervous system." Over the years, there have been several textbooks published that are devoted to this topic and written by practicing speech-language pathologists. However, most of these texts only emphasize the anatomy and physiology of the nervous system underlying normal communication. *Neurology for the Speech-Language Pathologist* is dedicated not only to the study of the normal system function but also to an introduction to the disorders that occur when the nervous system is developmentally abnormal or becomes diseased or damaged.

AUDIENCE

The targeted audience for this book is, of course, students preparing to become practicing speech-language pathologists. Students intending to enter the profession of audiology frequently will be enrolled in a class on neurology of human communication. Although this text does not go into the depth of the auditory system that students will need later, they will find it useful for their future endeavors. The text is also written to serve as a reference for speech and hearing professionals already in practice who wish to update themselves in neurology or who may not have had a specific curriculum regarding the neurologic foundation of communication and its disorders.

CONCEPT AND IMPORTANCE TO THE PROFESSION

As Dr. Howard Kirshner states in the foreword to this book, the speech-language pathologist and the neurologist can work together more successfully for the patient's benefit when they "speak the same language." This was one of the initial thrusts of the creation of this textbook. Ultimate benefit is also achieved when speech-language pathologists can understand the terminology and the concerns of other professions involved in the habilitation and rehabilitation of patients. Thus the content has evolved over the years to help the speech-language pathologist obtain a better understanding of nervous system function in related systems often treated by other professionals, such as those in physical therapy, occupational therapy, and neuropsychology.

In this new century, there is a demand for evidence-based practice, meaning that there is a demand that the speech-language pathologist design and use diagnostic and treatment methodologies based on sound theory and research-based evidence that supports that theory and practice. Knowledge about nervous system function and how the brain develops, initiates, and maintains movement; learns and remembers; and recovers or changes after injury is critical to successful practice. This book is dedicated to enhancing that knowledge.

ORGANIZATION

The seventh edition includes a few new sections. In Chapter 4, a discussion about mRNA is included in the discussion of cellular functions, a topic of significance following the COVID-19 pandemic and the development of the vaccine that uses this structure. Similarly, in Chapter 10, there is a short discussion about cognitive-communicative impairments following long COVID infection, an emerging concern to our field. New sections on genetics as well as speech and language development in premature infants are included in Chapters 11 and 13. In regard to organization and content of the entire text, the introductory chapter discusses the intertwining histories of the professions of speech-language pathology and neurology. Chapters 2 and 3 are foundation chapters, providing an overview of the anatomy of the central and peripheral nervous systems. Chapter 3 also includes a section on some of the more popular neurodiagnostic studies that are becoming increasingly important in our profession's research and clinical literature. Chapters 4 and 5 describe anatomy and physiology of neuronal function and the sensory systems of vision, hearing, and touch. Chapters 6 through 8 are devoted to anatomy and physiology of normal motor function, the cranial nerves, and the motor speech disorders that result from damage or disease affecting oral-motor function. Chapter 9 explores the neuroanatomy and neurophysiology underlying language and learning. Chapter 10 discusses various language and cognitive disorders in adults with neurologic damage. Chapter 11 is the new chapter reviewing the development of the human brain from conception through the early postnatal period. Chapter 12 provides information on pediatric disorders of speech, and Chapter 13 examines pediatric language disorders.

The first four chapters provide the reader with anatomic terms and location and function of structures in an overview of the entire nervous system without getting too much into the details of the specific systems. The idea is to have a mental concept of the entire nervous system and the structural and functional relationships before studying in depth the systems most relevant to communication and related disorders.

DISTINCTIVE FEATURES

- The text combines information concerning both neuro-anatomy and neurophysiology with information about speech and language disorders associated with nervous system dysfunction.
- The disorder section of the text includes separate chapters on speech and language, which are further divided into pediatric and adult disorders.
- Included in the text is information designed to help the reader understand related disorders, such as disorders of visual processing and hearing and limb movement, that are treated by other members of the habilitation or rehabilitation team.
- The text also includes a description of a neurologist's typical bedside examination and assessment for adults and pediatric patients.

LEARNING AIDS

- There are 115 photos, scans, illustrations, and diagrams, many of them highlighted with the second color for clarity, that depict anatomic structure and function within the nervous system as well as characteristics of neurologic disease or injury.
- Detailed vocabulary listings are provided on the first page of each chapter, highlighted within the chapter discussion, and defined in the back-of-book glossary.
- Certain chapters contain a case history and description of a patient with a condition pertinent to the system or disorder discussed within that chapter. Cases are followed by questions for consideration and discussion.

- Detailed summary and application boxes appear at the end of each chapter and organize the information into bulleted listings for ease of reference.
- Appendices provide a listing and brief description of medical conditions related to communication disorders, an outline of a bedside neurologic examination, and a screening neurologic examination—all invaluable references for student clinicians and practitioners.

ANCILLARY MATERIALS

An Evolve website has been created specifically to accompany this seventh edition of *Neurology for the Speech-Language Pathologist*. Resources are available free of cost to all students via the URL http://evolve.elsevier.com/Abou-Khalil/neurology/. Instructor resources are available to all adopting instructors, who can register for free access via their sales representative. Following is a summary of the resources available online:

FOR INSTRUCTORS

- A **test bank** features over 400 objective-style questions—multiple choice, true/false, and fill in the blank—each with an accompanying rationale for the correct answer and a page-number reference to direct the reader to the exact textbook page where that content is discussed.
- An **image collection** featuring artwork from the textbook—two-color renderings, photographs, and brain-imaging scans—is available for download into PowerPoint or other presentations.

FOR STUDENTS

- **Flashcards** reproduce the book's glossary into a fun and interactive tool that helps readers practice terminology and ensure content mastery. The flashcards are excellent resources for examination preparation.
- **Answers to case study questions** are included to help readers test their knowledge and understand chapter content as it applies to realistic patient situations.
- **Animations** are also included, providing amazing views of various neuroanatomy and neurophysiology structures, concepts, and diseases and disorders.

Rima N. Abou-Khalil
Wanda G. Webb

CONTENTS

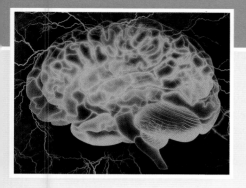

Introduction to Speech-Language Neurology

We must admit that the divine banquet of the brain was, and still is, a feast with dishes that remain elusive in their blending, and with sauces whose ingredients are even now a secret.

MacDonald Critchley, The Divine Banquet of the Brain, 1979

KEY TERMS

ADA
agnosias
anterior
aphasia
apraxias
association fiber tracts
asymmetry
Carl Wernicke
cephalic
clinical neurology

dorsal
dysarthrias
fMRI
IDEA
IDT
inferior
localization of function
Noam Chomsky
Norman Geschwind
Pierre Paul Broca

plasticity
posterior
rostral
SPECT
superior
traumatic brain injury (TBI)
ventral
videofluoroscopy

WHY NEUROLOGY?

The 1990s were labeled by the US Congress as the decade of the brain. Likewise, 1990 was the year of the Americans with Disabilities Act (**ADA**). In 2006 American Speech-Language-Hearing Association (ASHA) members learned about the reauthorization of the Individuals with Disabilities Education Act (**IDEA**). Since the inception of the federal laws to help and protect Americans who have a variety of disabilities, including communication and hearing disorders, ASHA academic and clinical standards have undergone major changes as well. A tremendous expansion of knowledge has occurred in the neurosciences, including increased complexities of the types and severity of disorders treated by all speech-language pathologists (SLPs), from the school-based SLP and educational audiologist to the hospital-based certified SLP professional. ASHA has recognized these advances in neuroscience

by realizing that an SLP or audiologist must have an expanded knowledge of neuroanatomy and physiology to remain a viable member of either the individualized education plan (IEP) or the interdisciplinary team (**IDT**). That is why academic and clinical standards for all SLPs and audiologists underwent a major change in the early 21st century.

For the student of speech-language pathology and audiology, these governmental reform acts and advances in neuroscience have played a significant role in forming the current academic and clinical standards used by ASHA. The new certification standards required as of July 2004 mandate particular knowledge and skills for students to be prepared to serve a variety of communication and hearing disorders in children and adults. From an undergraduate's general education, which is now required to include biologic and physical sciences, to the graduate student's in-depth study of stroke, traumatic brain injury (TBI), or autism, academic programs have had to increase neuroscience offerings. The work of the linguist, the cognitive psychologist, and the neuroscientist, as well as the SLP and audiologist, has brought to the field of communication sciences and disorders an accelerated knowledge of the specialized brain mechanisms that underlie speech, language, and hearing and their disorders. Specialists now possess the knowledge and skills to understand, implement, analyze, and synthesize the neurologic bases of speech, language, and hearing, as well as the skills required to meet ADA, IDEA, and ASHA standards.

Widespread interest in the study of neurogenic issues has increased among speech and language students as opportunities for clinical experiences and employment in schools, hospitals, rehabilitation centers, and other health care agencies continue to increase. Increased longevity of human beings has caused a greater incidence of hearing, speech, and language disorders such as presbycusis, dementia, **aphasia**, dysarthria, and apraxia. With improving medical technology, traumatically brain-injured infants, children, and adults are now saved from death much more frequently than in the past. The speech and language disorders of these survivors present new and greater challenges to the SLP and audiologist.

In 1986, when the first edition of this text appeared, only half of undergraduate and graduate training programs in communication disorders offered specific coursework in neurology with an emphasis on speech and language mechanisms. As of this new edition, 36 years later, the majority of the 300 programs (www.asha.org) in the field provide such coursework. In 2004 Adler[1] surveyed all accredited ASHA programs in *Speech-Language Pathology and Audiology*. The survey consisted of questions asking academic programs to give information about the anatomy and physiology (A&P) and neuroanatomy and physiology (N&P) courses required in their undergraduate and master's degree course sequences. Results indicated that the A&P course is offered in every program, and more than 70% of the accredited programs offered N&P courses. Respondents to other surveys made it clear that the N&P course is quite relevant and should be required for all students to meet the standards and prepare students for challenging SLP positions.[18]

Accompanying a growing interest among neurologists in communication sciences and disorders has been a parallel increase in the number of practicing SLPs. In the past 4 decades, membership in ASHA has risen from 2203 in 1952 to more than 173,000 members and affiliates in 2013 (www. asha.org). Although not all of these individuals are interested in neurologic disorders, many are, and for those who wish to study and specialize in neurologic speech and language disorders, a certification body, the Academy of Neurologic Communication Disorders and Sciences, accepts qualified members. Specialization in adult neurologic impairment, child neurologic impairment, or both is possible. In the past 5 to 10 years, ASHA special interest divisions have begun the process of specialization certifications in many areas, including child language, swallowing, fluency, and intraoperative monitoring. Most SLPs and audiologists work in schools, hospitals, or medical center or university clinics. All settings currently use an IDT approach and call the team a variety of names, including IDT, IEP team, clinical rounds team, or interdisciplinary management team (IMT). Regardless of name, the main function is to assess the client, discuss results from all disciplines, write a treatment plan that includes goals and objectives, and ensure that all goals and objectives have one outcome—the improvement of speech and language functioning for that client. The client might be seen in a school setting, a hospital, an outpatient clinic, a developmental center, through a home health agency, in a rehabilitation center, a university clinic, or in an office of a private practice. The SLP provides important information to what is usually a team of educational or medical professionals regarding a person's speech and language deficits and assets as related to brain functioning.

HISTORIC ROOTS: DEVELOPMENT OF SPEECH-LANGUAGE PATHOLOGY AS A BRAIN SCIENCE

Speech-language pathology traces many of its roots to clinical neurology. In 1861 French physician **Pierre Paul Broca** (1824–1880) studied the brains of two patients who had sustained language loss and motor speech disorders.[3] This study allowed him to localize human language to a definite circumscribed area of the left hemisphere, thereby laying the foundation for a brain science of speech and language. Broca's discovery went far beyond the now-classic description of an interesting brain disorder called aphasia. Possibly foremost among his conclusions were the assertions that the two hemispheres of the brain are asymmetric in function and that the left cerebral hemisphere contains the language center in most human beings. Important implications of brain **asymmetry** are even now coming to light some 130 years later. Asymmetry of function is more pervasive than originally thought. It extends well beyond language to other brain areas and their functions.

Another conclusion that has had lasting importance for neurology since Broca's death is that specific behavioral functions appear to be associated with clearly localized sites in the brain. The corollary of this observation is that behavioral dysfunction can point to lesions at specific sites in the nervous system. The concept of **localization of function** in the nervous system has been repeatedly demonstrated by clinical and research methods since Broca first articulated it more than a century ago. This observation was so profound that it became a significant historic force in the establishment of the medical discipline of **clinical neurology**. Much of clinical neurology depends on the physician's ability to lateralize and localize a lesion in the nervous system.

An important fact for speech-language pathology was that Broca's discovery stimulated a period of intensive search for a workable explanation of the brain mechanisms of speech and language. Probably no period in the history of neurologic science has so advanced the understanding of communication

BOX 1.1   The Work of Pierre Paul Broca (1824–1880)

- Touchstone study in 1861 allowed Broca to localize human language to a specific region of the left hemisphere, suggesting that the two hemispheres of the brain are asymmetric in function
- First to identify the brain disorder aphasia
- Articulated localization of function, leading to the establishment of the medical discipline of clinical neurology
- Stimulated intensive research into a workable explanation of the brain mechanisms of speech and language

and its disorders as those years between Broca's discovery and World War I. An overview of Broca's life work can be found in Box 1.1.

One of the first and foremost outcomes of this intensive study of speech-language brain mechanisms was the establishment of neurologic substrata for modalities of language deficit other than the expressive oral language described by Broca. In 1867 William Ogle published a case that demonstrated a cerebral writing center was independent of Broca's center for oral language.[19] In 1874 **Carl Wernicke** (1848–1905) identified an auditory speech center in the temporal lobe associated with comprehension of speech, as opposed to Broca's area in the frontal lobe that was an expressive speech center.[26] In the terminology of that time, lesions in Broca's area produced a *motor* aphasia, and one in Wernicke's area produced a *sensory* aphasia. These terms are no longer used in medical terminology. The very general descriptor terms now used are *expressive* (motor) and *receptive* (sensory) aphasia. In 1892 Joseph Dejerine identified mechanisms underlying reading disorders.[10] Disorders of cortical sensory recognition, or the **agnosias**, were named by Sigmund Freud in 1891,[11] and in 1900 Hugo Liepmann comprehensively analyzed the **apraxias**, disorders of executing motor acts resulting from brain lesions.[17]

Early Language Models

Of the many neurologic models of the cerebral language mechanisms generated soon after Broca's great discovery, Wernicke's 1874 model has best withstood the test of time. Wernicke stressed the importance of cortical language centers associated with the various language modalities, but he also emphasized the importance of **association fiber tracts** connecting areas or centers. In addition, Wernicke organized the symptoms of language disturbance in such a way that they could be used diagnostically to predict the lesion site in either connective pathways or centers in the language system. Ironically, the Wernicke model was eclipsed until the last half of the 20th century, when it was revitalized and expanded by neurologist **Norman Geschwind** (1926–1984) and his followers.[13]

Neurologic speech mechanisms, as opposed to language mechanisms, also received attention in the late 19th century. In 1871 French neurologist Jean Charcot (1825–1893) described the "scanning speech" that he associated with

"disseminated sclerosis," now known as multiple sclerosis.[6] The term *scanning*, probably inappropriate, has also been widely used to describe speech with cerebellar or cerebellar pathway lesions (see Chapter 8). In 1888 English neurologist William Gowers (1845–1915) surveyed the neurologic speech disorders known as dysarthrias in his book *A Manual of Diseases of the Nervous System*.[14]

World War I

World War I had a profound influence on the study of speech and language mechanisms resulting from neurologic insult. With a large population of head-injured young men with penetrating skull wounds, some neurologists felt an urgency for treatment. A handful of dedicated neurologists provided therapy for these traumatic language disorders because the profession of speech pathology was not yet born. Not until the next decade did the profession really begin. Lee Edward Travis (1896–1987) has the distinction of being the first individual in the United States to specialize in the field of speech-language disorders at the doctoral level. In 1927 he became the first director of the speech clinic at the University of Iowa. His special interest was in stuttering, which he began to study in a neurologic context. Travis researched the hypothesis that stuttering was the result of brain dysfunction,[23] specifically an imbalance or competition between the two cerebral hemispheres to control the normal bilateral functioning of the speech musculature. This hypothesis of dysfunctional neural control of the speech musculature has generally been discredited, but the hemisphere competition theory of stuttering still surfaces from time to time in different guises to explain certain communication disorders.

Although several of the founders of speech-language pathology in the United States believed that psychological explanations were more rewarding for understanding speech and language problems, notable exceptions existed. In particular, Harold Westlake of Northwestern University; Robert West of the University of Wisconsin; Jon Eisenson, formerly of California State University; and Joseph Wepman of the University of Chicago were all advocates of neurologic principles in communication disorders.

The 20th Century

During World War II, which brought in its wake thousands of injured soldiers and other military personnel with traumatic aphasia, neurologists, psychologists, and SLPs were used in treatment programs for the first time. This effort produced a series of books and articles on aphasia rehabilitation; perhaps the most notable for the neurologically oriented SLP was Wepman's *Recovery from Aphasia* (1951).[25] It served as a textbook of language disorders for the growing number of students in the field and often served as their first introduction to the study of a major neurologic communication disorder.

The study of neurologic speech mechanisms was greatly advanced after World War II by the work of Wilder G. Penfield (1891–1976) and his colleagues in Canada. Penfield, a neurosurgeon, used the technique of electrical cortical stimulation to map cortical areas directly, particularly speech and language centers. In 1959 in *Speech and Brain Mechanisms*[20] (written with Lamar Roberts), he documented his observations on cerebral control of speech-language function and wrote on the concepts of subcortical speech mechanisms and infantile cerebral **plasticity**.

The 1960s and 1970s were marked by several advances of neurologic concepts in communication and its disorders. Newer linguistic theory, particularly that proposed by **Noam Chomsky**,[7] emphasized the universal features and innate mechanisms reflected in language. The biologic aspects of language and speech were highlighted by linguist and psychologist Eric Lenneberg, who specifically placed language acquisition in the context of developmental neurology.[16] The split-brain studies reported by Roger Sperry and his colleagues,[22] in which the commissural tracts between the hemispheres were severed, indicated specific functions of the right hemisphere were different from the left.

Major anatomic differences in the right and left language centers were also demonstrated in the human brain. Most significant for SLPs and audiologists are larger areas in the left temporal lobe in the fetus, infant, and adult.[13,24,27] These differences suggest an anatomic basis for cerebral dominance for language and appear to contradict a theory of progressive lateralization of speech centers.

Throughout the 1960s and 1970s considerable attention was paid to neurologic speech disorders. Neurologists and SLPs in the Mayo Clinic Neurology Department[8,9] documented the acoustic-perceptual characteristics of the major **dysarthrias** in a viable classification scheme. This work has stimulated widespread study of the various adult dysarthrias in speech science laboratories around the country. Geschwind almost single-handedly resurrected the early neurologic literature of Europe focusing on language disorders and related deficits. Geschwind brought this body of knowledge to the attention of the American medical audience when interest in aphasia and related disorders was waning. He particularly highlighted the value of identifying lesions in the connective pathways of the brain, as well as diagnosing lesions in the traditional localized cortical areas of the brain.[12] His collaboration with SLPs in the Boston medical community resulted in the development of several tests and treatment methods for aphasia and other acquired speech-language disorders, many of which continue to be used daily in clinical practice.

The 1980s found researchers talking about the importance of early stimulation and experience for brain and language development[15] and brought further advances in diagnostic testing for neurogenic disorders, including, for the first time, a standardized assessment tool for language and communication problems caused by dementia.

The 1990s saw significant advances in knowledge about language development and the brain with publication of *The Language Instinct*.[21] In 1997 Martha Taylor Sarno completed a 5-year study funded by National Institutes of Health on the effects of aphasia secondary to stroke on the quality of life in middle-aged and older people. Findings indicated that age was not a major factor in the recovery and quality of life of individuals with aphasia.[23] During the 1990s, research into the incidence, prevalence, and rehabilitation needs of persons with TBI proliferated, and in 1999 a congressional report highlighted the need for further research and rehabilitation funding for persons affected by TBI.[9]

Modern Times

Research and treatment have taken giant steps forward into the 21st century, where we now find ourselves. In 2018 a congressional report highlighted the need for research and funding for pediatric TBI patients, recognizing the previously unacknowledged trauma sometimes resulting from participation in sports TBI.[2,4,5,7] Research in pediatric disorders such as autism and the problems often associated with prematurity has burgeoned. Collaboration by SLPs with neurologists and radiologists utilizing advanced technology such as functional magnetic resonance imaging (**fMRI**), single photon emission computed tomography (**SPECT**), **videofluoroscopy**, and fiberscopic endoscopy is rapidly expanding our knowledge of how neurodevelopmental problems, disease, or acquired brain damage alters language, speech, and/or swallowing. Thus, the study of brain anatomy and function is more important than ever, allowing the SLP to understand the literature and evaluate the efficacy of diagnostic and treatment methods to provide the best service to children and adults with neurogenic speech-language disorders.

DIRECTIONS AND PLANES

This text uses many drawings and photographs to aid in visualization. The human body itself may be defined in terms of a standard anatomic position, one in which the body is erect and the head, eyes, and toes are pointed forward. The limbs are at the side of the body, and the palms face forward (Fig. 1.1). When viewing drawings in texts or creating anatomic sketches, constantly orient yourself in terms of the standard anatomic positions and planes. From this fundamental position, other positions, planes, and directions are defined (Fig. 1.2). Box 1.2 summarizes the major planes or sections used in anatomic drawings to orient the reader to the view that was used. The orienting directional terms that may be used when navigating around an illustration of the brain may be slightly different because the brain itself is tilted inside the skull. Fig. 1.3 illustrates the anatomic planes of the brain.

To understand what you are reading as well as the drawings and pictures you will be seeing when studying neuroanatomy, it is imperative that you understand the directional terms and the different planes in which the views may be pictured. Conventional textbooks are only two dimensional, and thus it is of excellent benefit to the student to use websites that are designed to picture anatomic structures with three-dimensional reconstruction technique.

Several terms are used to designate direction in neuroanatomy (see Figs. 1.1 and 1.2). Some of these terms are used synonymously. **Anterior** and **ventral** mean toward the front or in front of when any part of the body (including

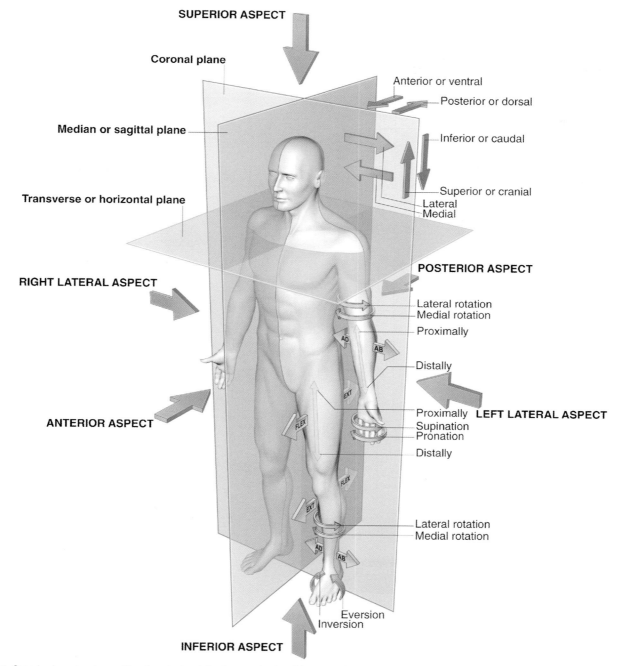

SUPERIOR ASPECT

Coronal plane

Median or sagittal plane

Transverse or horizontal plane

RIGHT LATERAL ASPECT

ANTERIOR ASPECT

Anterior or ventral
Posterior or dorsal
Inferior or caudal
Superior or cranial
Lateral
Medial

POSTERIOR ASPECT

Lateral rotation
Medial rotation
Proximally

Distally

Proximally   **LEFT LATERAL ASPECT**
Supination
Pronation
Distally

Lateral rotation
Medial rotation

Eversion
Inversion

INFERIOR ASPECT

Fig. 1.1 Standard anatomic position for study of the human body with anatomic planes and terms for type or direction of movement included. (From Standring, S. [2016]. *Gray's anatomy: The anatomical basis of clinical practice* [41st ed.]. Churchill Livingstone.)

the spinal cord) except the brain is illustrated. However, note in Fig. 1.3 that if it is the brain that is being discussed or illustrated, ventral means **inferior**. When orienting in the brain, **rostral** is the synonymous term for anterior (see Fig. 1.3). **Posterior** or **dorsal** indicates toward the back or behind for both. **Superior** refers to above or upward in both; inferior means below or downward in both but is synonymous with ventral in the brain. The terms *cranial* and **cephalic** can be used in place of superior when orienting direction in the body.

HOW TO STUDY

Most students in speech-language pathology receive a limited introduction to the neurosciences in their undergraduate careers. The majority of students are enrolled in courses designed to acquaint them with the anatomy and physiology of speech, but these courses usually focus on speech musculature. Students often do not receive an adequate introduction to neuroanatomy and neurophysiology of speech and language. It is assumed that students will learn these details in courses

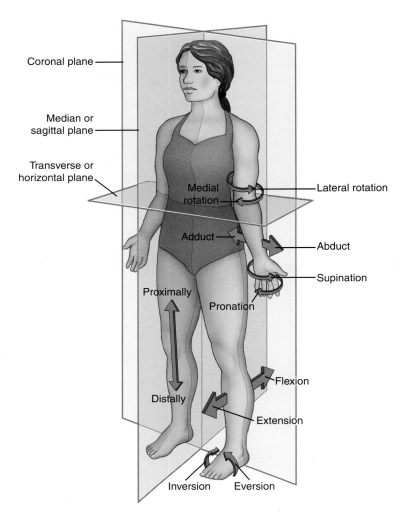

Fig. 1.2 Directional references for the human body. (Reprinted from Blaussen.com staff. Blaussen gallery 2014. *Wikiversity Journal of Medicine.* https://en.wikiversity.org/wiki/Wikiversity_Journal_of_Medicine/Blausen_gallery_2014#Other_anatomy)

BOX 1.2 Standard Anatomic Positions and Planes

- The median plane, or section, passes longitudinally through the brain and divides the right hemisphere from the left hemisphere.
- The sagittal plane divides the brain vertically at any point and parallels the medial plane.
- A coronal, or frontal, section is any vertical cut that separates the brain into front and back halves.
- A horizontal plane divides the brain into upper and lower halves and is at right angles to the median and coronal planes.
- A transverse cut is any section at right angles to the longitudinal axis of the structure.

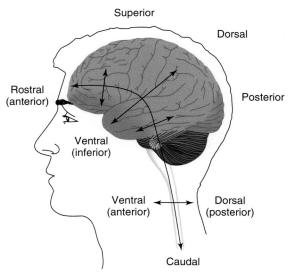

Fig. 1.3 Axes of the human brain. (Reprinted from Martin, J. G. [1989]. *Neuroanatomy.* Elsevier.)

in aphasia, adult dysarthria, and rehabilitation of speech in cerebral palsy. Students find that neuroscience courses taken as advanced undergraduates or beginning graduate students are difficult.

Students often say that neurology courses are difficult because they believe they must learn the technical term for

each hill and valley in the complex anatomy of the brain. In addition, the technical terms are unfamiliar, usually derived from Greek and Roman word roots. This text concentrates on crucial terminology for an understanding of speech and language and the diseases and conditions that result in communication disorders. The number of terms believed to be important has increased over the various editions of this text as the scope of practice for SLPs has expanded. Because of the crucial role that SLPs now play on many medical, rehabilitation, and educational teams, they also must be familiar with terminology used by other health professionals when discussing the client's condition. A glossary is provided at the end of the text.

Part of the strategy in mastering any text in the biologic sciences is to give the study of drawings, diagrams, and tables in the text as much time as the narrative sections. If the reader can come away from a study of this text with a set of working mental images of the structures and pathways of the nervous system that are important to communication and can recall them at critical times, then one of the purposes of the authors will be realized. With an emphasis on imagery as one of the better ways to learn neurology, it should be no surprise that the authors urge readers to use as a teaching aid their own drawings of structures and pathways. Even crude sketches, carefully labeled, teach the necessary anatomic relations and fix pathways, structures, and names in the mind. Students (and instructors!) are also encouraged to use the vast resource of the Internet. There are now literally thousands of photos, illustrations, and videos dealing with neuroanatomy, neuroscience, and neurology on various websites sponsored by universities, government agencies, and research institutes. We encourage you to be careful; choose sites that are well established in terms of the credentials for providing such technical information. Because of the precipitous manner in which websites and the information contained on them change, only a few sites are recommended or referenced in these chapters. Your instructor is likely to recommend or help you find valuable sites to assist your exploration of the nervous system.

Chapters 2 and 3 provide an overview of the nervous system in total. Subsequent chapters often refer back to certain sections of these chapters to review the written information and the illustrations that provide a beginning foundation of knowledge regarding the neurologic characteristics of the communicative nervous system. Chapters 4 through 6 expand teaching on the structure and physiology of neurons; the sensory systems of touch, vision, and hearing; and the motor system. Chapters 7 and 8 discuss cranial nerves and the disorders of speech production that SLPs commonly assess and treat in adults. Chapter 9 deals with the anatomy and physiology of the parts of the nervous system primarily concerned with language and learning, and Chapter 10 discusses acquired language disorders in adults. The last three chapters of this text are dedicated to learning how the brain develops from birth (Chapter 11), to pediatric speech (Chapter 12), and pediatric language disorders (Chapter 13).

A synopsis of facts and clinical applications important to the SLP are presented at the end of each chapter. Students should be aware that these are not the only important facts in the chapter! This synopsis should not be the only thing you study for your examinations because your task is not to memorize a lot of facts with little understanding as to how they relate to the human communication nervous system.

Chapters 5 through 8, 10, 12, and 13 also provide case studies, that is, a description of a patient and the signs and symptoms of the patient's disorder. Questions are provided to consider regarding the patient's symptoms. Answers can be found on the Evolve website.

The reader is encouraged to attempt to integrate verbal material with eidetic imagery, as well as with thoughtful consideration of what patients with these conditions experience. Students must call on all their brainpower, bringing into play the special capacities of both the right and left hemispheres of the brain. The left hemisphere is specialized for its capacities of verbal analysis and reasoning, whereas the right hemisphere is specialized for its visual-spatial functions. However, it will become clear to you that, though this specialization exists, the right and the left hemispheres are integrated in communication and cognition. Both hemispheres also use subcortical areas to retrieve memories and empathize with others. Therefore, readers will use their whole brain to learn about the whole brain!

SYNOPSIS OF CLINICAL INFORMATION AND APPLICATIONS FOR THE SLP

- Brain: source of all speech and language behavior
- 1990: Americans with Disabilities Act
- 2004: New ASHA clinical and academic standards
- 2005: IDEA was reauthorized
- 2008: Revised ASHA clinical and academic standards
- ASHA membership, 2013 = more than 173,000
- Geschwind: first neurologist to outline the literature focusing on language disorders and related deficits; influenced linguistics, psychology, and philosophy
- Chomsky: first international linguist to correlate language and speech with brain functioning; states language is innate and implies a biologic, neurologic, and genetic basis for language
- Lenneberg: wrote *The Biological Foundations of Language*
- Broca: first to localize human language to the left hemisphere; states behavioral functions are attributed to specific sites in the brain
- Ogle: identified a writing center in the brain independent of Broca area
- Wernicke: identified an auditory center for speech associated with comprehension of speech, opposing Broca, who identified the expressive center
- The temporal lobe has become identified with language and speech comprehension and the frontal lobe with language and speech expression
- Freud: first to identify cortical sensory areas or agnosias
- Liepmann: first to identify the apraxias of motor execution

Continued

SYNOPSIS OF CLINICAL INFORMATION AND APPLICATIONS FOR THE SLP—cont'd

- Travis: first identified stuttering to be the result of brain dysfunction, specifically the imbalance between the two hemispheres
- Neurologic aspects of communication disorders by Westlake, Wepman, West, and Eisenson
- Wepman's *Recovery from Aphasia* served as the first textbook of language disorders in the field of speech pathology
- Penfield: first to use cortical mapping for identifying areas of language and speech functions in the brain

- Importance of environment, parental input, quality of social interaction begins to be recognized for children and adults with communication disorders
- Professional advocacy for children and adults experiencing cognitive and communication deficits post TBI
- Directions and planes help orient to identify structures and sites of lesions and injuries

REFERENCES

1. Adler, R. K. (2004). *The anatomy and physiology of speech and the neuroanatomy and physiology of speech courses*. Chicago: State of the art. ASHA Convention.
2. Bayles, K., & Tomoeda, C. (1993). *Arizona battery for communication disorders of dementia*. Pro-Ed.
3. Broca, P. (1861). *Remarques sur le siége de la faculté du langage articulé, suivies d'une observation d'aphémie (perte de la parole)*. Société: Bulletin.
4. Centers for Disease Control and Prevention. (2018). *Report to Congress: The management of traumatic brain injury in children*. National Center for Injury Prevention and Control; Division of Unintentional Injury Prevention.
5. Centers for Disease Control and Prevention. Traumatic brain injury in the United States: A report to Congress. https://www.cdc.gov/traumaticbraininjury/pubs/tbi_report_to_congress.html.
6. Charcot, J. M. (1890). *Oeuvres complète de J. M. Charcot*. Lecrosnier et Babe.
7. Chomsky, N. (1975). *Reflections on language*. Pantheon Books.
8. Darley, F. L., Aronson, A. E., & Brown, J. R. (1969). Clusters of deviant speech dimensions in the dysarthrias. *Journal of Speech and Hearing Research, 12*(3), 462–496.
9. Darley, F. L., Aronson, A. E., & Brown, J. R. (1969). Differential diagnostic patterns of dysarthria. *Journal of Speech and Hearing Research, 12*(2), 246–269.
10. Dejerine, J. (1892). Contribution a etude anatomopathologique et clinique des differentes varietes de cectie verbal. *Mémoires de la Société de Biologie, 4*, 61–90.
11. Freud, S. (1953). On aphasia: A critical study. In F. Stengel (Ed.), *International Universities Press*.
12. Geschwind, N. (1965). Disconnexion syndromes in animals and man. *Brain*, 237–294 (I); 585–644 (II).
13. Geschwind, N. (1974). *Selected papers on language and the brain*. D. Reidel.
14. Gowers, W. R. (1888). *A manual of diseases of the nervous system*. Blakiston.
15. Greenough, W. T., Black, J. E., & Wallace, C. S. (1987). Experience and brain development. *Child Development, 58*(3),186–216.
16. Lenneberg, E. (1967). *Biological foundations of language*. Wiley.
17. Liepmann, H. (1900). Das Krankheitsbild der apraxie ("motorischen asymbolie"). *Monatsschrift fur Psychiatrie und Neurologie, 8*, 15–44.
18. Martin, K., Bessell, N. J., & Scholten, I. (2014). The perceived importance of anatomy and neuroanatomy in the practice of speech-language pathology. *Anatomical Sciences Education, 7*(1), 28–37. https://doi.org/10.1002/ase.1377. Epub ahead of print. PMID: 23775941.
19. Ogle, W. (1867). Aphasia and agraphia. *St. George's Hospital Reports, 2*, 83–122.
20. Penfield, W., & Roberts, L. (1959). *Speech and brain mechanisms*. Princeton University Press.
21. Pinker, S. (1994). *The language instinct*. William Morrow.
22. Sperry, R. W., Gazzaniga, M. S., & Bogen, J. E. (1969). Interhemispheric relationships: The neocortical commissures; syndromes of hemispheric disconnection. In P. J. Vinken & G. W. Bruyn (Eds.), *Handbook of clinical neurology* (vol. 4). North Holland.
23. Taylor-Sarno, M. (1997). Quality of life in the first post-stroke year. *Aphasiology, 11*(7), 665–679.
24. Wada, J. A., Clark, R., & Hamm, A. (1975). Cerebral asymmetry in humans. *Archives of Neurology, 32*(4), 239–246.
25. Wepman, J. (1951). *Recovery from aphasia*. The Ronald Press.
26. Wernicke, C. (1874). *Der aphasische symptomenkomplex*. Cohn and Weigert. Translated in Eggert, G. H. (1977). *Wernicke's works on aphasia. A sourcebook and review*. Mouton.
27. Whitelson, S. F., & Pallie, W. (1973). Left hemisphere specialization for language in the newborn: Neuroanatomical evidence of asymmetry. *Brain, 96*(3), 641–646.

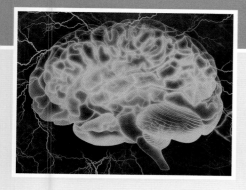

Organization of the Nervous System I

The brain is the organ of destiny. It holds within its humming mechanism secrets that will determine the future of the human race.

Wilder Graves Penfield, The Second Career, 1963

CHAPTER OUTLINE

KEY TERMS

angular gyrus
arcuate fasciculus
association cortex
astrocytes
ATP
axon
axon hillock
axoplasm
basal ganglia
blood-brain barrier
boutons
brainstem
Broca area
cell respiration
CNS
cerebellum
cerebrum
choroid plexuses
cingulate gyrus
colliculi
corpus callosum
corpus striatum
dendrites
dendritic spines
diencephalon
ependymal cells

fasciculus
fissure
ganglia
glial
gray matter
Heschl gyrus
homunculus
hypothalamus
innervate
insula
internal capsule
lentiform (lenticular) nucleus
limbic system
medulla oblongata
mesencephalon
microglia
midbrain
myelin
neuroglial cells
neuron
neurotransmitters
nucleolus
occipital lobe
oligodendrocytes
parahippocampal gyrus
paralimbic areas

parietal lobe
perisylvian zone
PNS
pons
premotor area
primary cortical areas
reflex arc
Schwann cells
somatosensory
striatum
substantia nigra
subthalamus
sulcus
supplementary (secondary) motor
   area
supramarginal gyrus
synapse
tectum
temporal lobe
thalamus
uncus
Wernicke aphasia
Wernicke area
white matter

HUMAN COMMUNICATION NERVOUS SYSTEM

The nervous system is the source of all communication in human beings. Our highly advanced system of oral and gestural language identifies us as unique in the animal kingdom. This facility is the result of an aggregate of intricate nervous system mechanisms that have developed in the human brain through a series of dramatic evolutionary changes. Over thousands of years, a novel representation and organization of neural structures and processes has been created in the human brain that results in what may be called the human communication nervous system. How does this nervous system differ from the communication nervous system of other animals? A clear answer to this question began to emerge from attempts to teach the great apes, particularly chimpanzees, different types of communication systems; attempts to teach *oral* speech to chimpanzees were notably unsuccessful. Only human beings have the specialized vocal tract enabling the potential for producing the complex acoustic signal known as speech or oral language. On the other hand, attempts to teach chimpanzees by using visual and gestural representations of human language have been somewhat successful. Chimpanzees have been taught to use colored plastic chips to represent morphemes and in other cases have learned to use some signs taken from American Sign Language to the extent that they can communicate adequately, and even creatively, in a rudimentary manner. Whether these nonverbal languages are characteristically human is open to question, but human beings and chimpanzees share some characteristics of communication. The chimpanzee most likely uses cortical structures of the brain to master visual and gestural components of human language.

Some have suggested that overall brain size, which reflects the total volume of the cerebral cortex, the total number of nerve cells in the brain, and the degree of dendrite growth or proliferation of the processes of the nerve cell, is crucial to information processing and communication processing. Considering these factors, what are the differences between the human brain and that of the chimpanzee?

The chimpanzee's impressive but limited gestural language is reflected by its average brain weight of 450 g compared with an average weight of 1350 g for the human brain. Generally, a lack of uniqueness has been found in the parietal, occipital, and temporal lobes of both chimpanzees and human beings. In the frontal lobe of the brain, however, human beings are distinguished by an area of cortex that has been named Broca area. This specialized cortical area has been associated with the control of expressive language. With the exception of Broca area, the primary difference between the human and chimpanzee cortex is quantitative, with the temporal lobe, inferior parietal lobe, and frontal lobe anterior to Broca area being larger in human beings. These areas, as detailed in later chapters, are portions of the cerebral cortex that make an advanced language system possible. These species-specific brain structures, plus the human being's special vocal tract and the significant increase in the size of the information- and communication-processing cortex, account for the exceptional capability for communication.[24]

Foundations of the Nervous System

This chapter and Chapter 3 provide an overview of the anatomy and physiology of the human nervous system. This text takes a top-down approach to the gross anatomy, beginning with the cortex and ending with the spinal cord. This organization was chosen because as human beings, cortical processing and control are vital to all but the most basic motor, cognitive, and emotional functions. It is not your ears that hear; it is really your brain. Your thoughts are initiated through cortical networks. Your memories and their associated emotions are stored in your brain. Therefore, it seems appropriate to start with the "boss" and work our way down the organizational ladder of the nervous system to understand it better.

Before we begin looking more closely at the individual structures of the brain and spinal cord, however, a study of the microstructure and foundation of this miraculous nervous system of ours will be helpful for understanding the complex function of the larger structures.

The Neuron

The nervous system is composed of highly specialized tissues, with the **neuron** as its basic building block. The function of the nervous system is to communicate, and it does so by transmitting messages from one neuron to another, from one neuron to a muscle, or from a sensory receptor (e.g., receptors mediating vision or hearing) to other neural structures.

In addition to neurons, the nervous system contains neuroglial, or glial cells. Recent research[2,13] found approximately 86 billion neurons with an almost equal number of **neuroglial cells** making up the human nervous system. Originally considered to provide only structural support to neurons, glia do much more, as demonstrated by recent research; they also maintain homeostasis, clean up waste, form myelin, and influence nervous system development.[1]

The Chemical Makeup of Nerve Cells

Although cells are the building blocks on which the human body is structured, they themselves are also composed of smaller units. These units are organelles, functional units within the cytoplasm that have their own bilipid membrane. Breaking down the organelles, we see that they, like all living matter, are composed of molecules. As is typical in living matter, nerve cells have four major classes of molecules: lipids, proteins, carbohydrates, and nucleic acid. There are two types of nucleic acid within each cell, deoxyribonucleic acid (DNA) and ribonucleic acid (RNA).

All cells contain an organelle called the nucleus. The nucleus contains most of the DNA of the cell and is bound by a bilipid membrane that has several openings or pores in it. DNA carries the genetic code of each living organism. It is helpful when studying genetic-based disorders in children to know at least basic facts about DNA, RNA, and the chromosomes that each carry a copy of the genetic code of a person.

The code stored in our DNA is made up of four chemical bases with the four chemicals typically referred to by the first letter: A, adenine; G, guanine; C, cytosine; and T, thymine. Each chemical base is attached to a complex molecule made up of a two-sugar molecule and a one-phosphate molecule. This combination of sugar molecules and phosphate molecule is referred to as a nucleotide. The nucleotide and its attached chemical base will pair up with another such structure and form a unit called a base pair; base pair units are formed by the pairing of A with T and the pairing of C with G. DNA is arranged in two long strands that form a spiral called a double helix. This double helix looks somewhat like a ladder with the base pairs forming the ladder's rungs and the sugar and phosphate molecules forming the vertical sides of the ladder (Fig. 2.1). In human beings, the human genome (the entire genetic set) is found in the 46 chromosomes duplicated in each cell of the body. This is possible because the DNA can make copies of itself. Within the double helix, each strand can duplicate the pattern and sequence of the bases. This allows for exact copies of the DNA in the cell to be present in the new cell when cell division takes place in the embryo.

The genetic information contained in the DNA is encoded into proteins. Proteins are the "worker bees" of the cell, performing most of the various cellular reactions that constitute life. The other nucleic acid molecule in the cell, RNA, serves both storage and transcoder functions as an intermediary between the DNA and a targeted protein. The nucleus of the cell contains at least one prominent dense area, the **nucleolus**, where RNA is synthesized. RNA is only single stranded and is made up of four bases as well, but there is no thymine base; rather the chemical uracil (U) is present instead. There are different types of RNA in a cell: messenger (mRNA), ribosomal (rRNA), and transfer (tRNA). rRNA is the most abundant and works with proteins to form the ribosomes (discussed later in the chapter) of a cell. mRNA leaves the cell, moving to the cytoplasm where proteins are synthesized. In protein synthesis, the base sequence carried in the genetic code on the RNA is "read" by the ribosome and translated

into corresponding amino acids. Cellular proteins are formed by the chemical linking of two or more amino acids, forming peptides. These peptides are then linked in a series becoming polypeptides. One or more polypeptides make up all cellular proteins. The tRNA transfers a particular amino acid to the polypeptide chain during protein synthesis.

As alluded to earlier, surrounding the nucleus is a mass of cytoplasm containing organelles that serve to synthesize proteins and maintain cellular metabolic balance. Found in this cytoplasm are rough and smooth endoplasmic reticulum, free ribosomes, Golgi apparatus, lysosomes, and mitochondria. The endoplasmic reticulum and the ribosomes are in abundance in neuronal cell bodies because of their key participation in lipid and protein synthesis, which is constantly needed for optimal nervous system function. Vesicles, which are little transporter membrane sacs, "bud" off from the endoplasmic reticulum and help deliver the proteins and lipids to the Golgi apparatus organelles. The Golgi apparatus organelle sorts the substances, and the vesicles eventually deliver them to the plasma membrane where they may fuse with the membrane delivering proteins to it or shed their contents to the outside of the cell. The vesicles may also carry digestive enzymes and become the organelles called lysosomes.[17]

Mitochondria are the power source of the cell, providing the energy a cell needs to function by converting the energy from food into a usable form for cellular function. The mitochondria produce adenosine triphosphate (**ATP**), the cell's main energy source. Cells in the nervous system have the highest metabolic rate of any cells in the human body and therefore must continually renew their energy source. Our bodies, through the action of ATP, convert energy from the sun into a usable form for cellular function. A process called **cell respiration**, which is driven by enzymes in the body, regenerates ATP constantly. Only about 250 g of ATP are available at any one time in the body (about as much energy as provided by a AA battery), and this small amount is being used persistently in healthy cells.[14] Therefore, it must be reproduced repetitively by the cells.

Although most of your DNA is contained in chromosomes within the cell's nucleus, mitochondria have a small amount of their own DNA (37 genes) that is vital for normal mitochondria cell functioning. The mitochondrial DNA is, except in rare cases, inherited from maternal lineage, being provided by the egg rather than by the sperm. Thus, this DNA changes much more slowly through the generations than nuclear DNA.

Because lipids do not dissolve in water, the bilipid membrane surrounding the nerve cell body forms a barrier between what is inside the cell (the intracellular material) and what surrounds it on the outside (the extracellular material). This membrane is also studded with globular proteins that serve as channels that allow molecules of certain chemicals (**neurotransmitters**) to pass through when the membrane is appropriately stimulated. These channels are usually specific to one type of molecule, barring others from entering the cell. Understanding the function of the channels becomes important when we study how neural impulses are generated and how neurons communicate within networks.

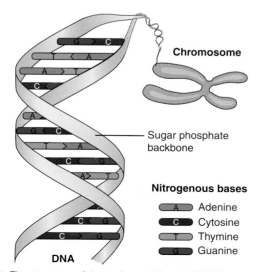

Fig. 2.1 The structure of deoxyribonucleic acid *(DNA)*.

The Structure and Function of Neurons

Like other cells in your body, both neurons and neuroglial cells consist of a cell body, also known as a soma or perikaryon. Also, as with other cells in the body, cells of the nervous system maintain their defined structure with a cytoskeleton. A cytoskeleton is composed of microtubules, intermediate filaments (neurofilaments), and microfilaments. Neurons can also be seen microscopically to have processes extending from them; these processes include one **axon** per neuron and many **dendrites**. The axon and the dendrites are critical to neuronal communication between different parts of the nervous system. The cytoskeleton of these appendages provides scaffolding for transport of molecules along these structures. Cytoskeleton dysfunction has been linked to disorders affecting the human nervous system, such as neurofibromatosis and type 2 and Duchenne muscular dystrophy.

Fig. 2.2 shows a multipolar neuron or nerve cell. Neurons are specialized to receive, conduct, and transmit nerve impulses. This transmission may be to or from a muscle, gland, or another nerve cell. Although nerve cells vary widely in terms of size and shape, they all have certain characteristics in common. They all have two types of processes extending from the cell body. The processes specialized to receive the impulses moving *toward* the cell are dendrites. They have a broad base, taper away from the cell body, and branch somewhere in the vicinity of the cell body. Most neurons are multipolar and have several dendrites extending from the cell body. Effectively, these dendrites expand the area of the neuron available for contact by other neurons, thus allowing *convergence* of neural impulses onto one neuron from many other neurons. Small protrusions, called **dendritic spines**, help expand the area of contact even farther. These dendritic spines appear as small hairlike or bulbous structures on the dendrite's membrane.

The other type of process extending from a neuron conducts the impulse *away from* the cell and is called the *axon*.

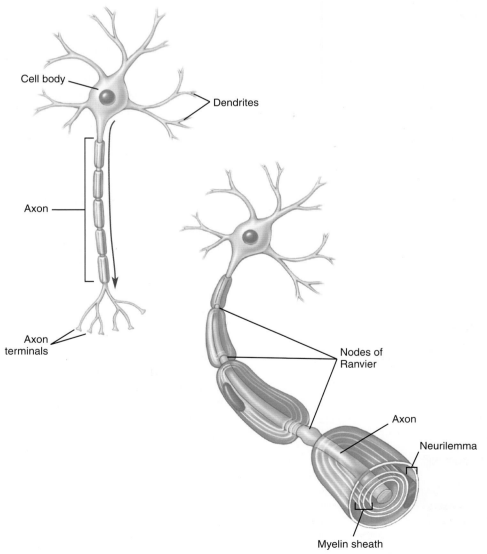

Fig. 2.2 Structure of a neuron. (From Herlihy, B. [2007]. *The human body in health and illness* [3rd ed.]. Saunders.)

Each neuron has only one axon, and it connects with the body of the neuron at a site called the **axon hillock**. Collateral branches, however, are frequently found coming off the axon itself. Because the axon carries all the neural information out of the cell, this branching increases the opportunity for *divergence* in the nervous system.

The cytoplasm of an axon contains structural elements called microtubules and neurofilaments that help maintain its cytoskeleton. These elements also help transport organelles and metabolic substances along the axon. Axons come in different diameters and lengths. The thicker axons conduct impulses more rapidly than thinner ones because they are usually myelinated (i.e., covered by a white, glistening lipoprotein sheath called the myelin sheath). This fatty sheath of **myelin** insulates the axon and allows more rapid propagation of the impulse along the axon. Most axons (and some dendrites) are well myelinated, although some thinner axons are either unmyelinated or thinly myelinated. Fig. 2.3 shows a longitudinal cut of a myelinated axon.

The axon loses its myelin sheath at its destination and divides into several small terminal branches. At the end of these branches there are usually swellings, referred to as axon terminals or **boutons**. The bouton establishes contact with another neuron or the cells of a muscle or gland. The site of this contact is a **synapse** or a synaptic junction. The synapse is the primary means by which the neuron elicits responses in target cells, typically by a release of a chemical known as a neurotransmitter. Chapter 4 provides a more in-depth discussion of the synapse.

Aside from the movement of neural impulses down an axon, proteins and other organelles move along the axon in its protoplasm (known as **axoplasm**), a process called axoplasmic transport. This helps maintain the structural and functional integrity of the axon. This transport may be anterograde, from the cell body distally, and retrograde, back toward the cell body from the axon terminal. The retrograde transport mediates the movement of substances providing *trophic*, or nutritional, support for the neuron. An example of trophic support is a substance known as nerve growth factor.

Clusters of interconnected neurons with specific functions can be found throughout the nervous system. These groups are called neuronal pools (see Chapter 4).

Neuroglia

Composing roughly half the cells in the nervous system are the **glial**, or neuroglial, cells. Our nervous system contains four types of neuroglial cells: astrocytes, microglia, ependyma, and the glia that form myelin around axons, which in the central nervous system (**CNS**) are called oligodendrocytes and in the peripheral nervous system (**PNS**) are called **Schwann cells**.

Glial cells do not propagate neural impulses but provide extremely important supportive and facilitative functions to the nervous system. Although we spend a majority of our study looking at signals generated by the neurons and the ensuing activations (or lack thereof), you must understand that neuroglia make it possible for neurons to function optimally. Many of the disorders you will study result from a breakdown in the neuroglial support for the nervous system. Brain tumors often form in the neuroglial cells (e.g., astrocytoma); diseases that affect children (e.g., mitochondrial disease) and adults (e.g., multiple sclerosis) involve neuroglia and affect CNS and/or PNS functioning with consequent effect on speech and language. The following neuroglia are critical to optimal nervous system function.

Astrocytes provide the structural matrix surrounding neuron cell bodies in the CNS and modulate neuronal activity locally and regionally. Astrocytes of the CNS also play a major role in maintaining the extracellular environment around the neuron. Astrocytes are responsive to and may have specific receptors for certain neurotransmitters. They are now thought to take an active role in modulating neuronal activity and synaptic plasticity.[20]

In many tissues of the body, solutes can pass rather freely from the blood into the cells of that tissue by diffusing through gaps between the endothelial cells, those cells that line the interior surface of blood and lymphatic vessels. In the CNS, however, the astrocytes cause the walls of the capillaries to form tight endothelial junctions, forming what is called the **blood-brain barrier**. Therefore, most solutes passing into neural tissue must go through the endothelial cells themselves. Water, gases, and small lipid-soluble molecules may pass easily across the endothelial cells, but most other substances must be carried across by transport systems. Consequently, the passage of substances into neural tissue from the blood is not always easily accomplished. Dysfunction of the astroglial cells or the complex surrounding particular neuronal networks is receiving more and more attention in research into neurogenerative diseases as a possible etiology or major contributor to the disease process. The astroglia are also being studied due to possibly serving a neuroprotective role.[23]

Microglia are numerous and perform "scavenger" functions. They may migrate to the site of injury in the brain, multiply, and become brain macrophages, cleaning out debris after neural cell death. They are sometimes referred to as

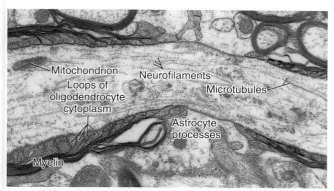

Fig. 2.3 Longitudinal view of a myelinated axon in the central nervous system. (Reprinted from Haines, D. [2006]. *Fundamental neuroscience* [3rd ed.]. Churchill Livingstone.)

the brain's immune system because the microglia mediate immune response to injury or infection.

Ependymal cells provide nourishment and possibly metabolic support, and they may play an important role in containing fluid fluxes within the ventricles. Ventricles are cavities within the brain through which cerebrospinal fluid circulates. The spinal cord also contains a central cavity, called the central canal, though which this cerebrospinal fluid flows. Ependymal cells line these cavities in the brain and spinal cord. Specialized ependymal cells form structures called **choroid plexuses**, which are found in each ventricle of the brain. The choroidal epithelial cells on the surface of the choroid plexus structures are responsible for the manufacture of cerebrospinal fluid. Dysfunction of ependymal adhesion can cause hydrocephalus, which is a condition where fluid accumulates in the brain. In infants, hydrocephalus can enlarge the head and may result in brain damage.[6]

Oligodendrocytes are found within the CNS; here they form and maintain myelin, the white fatty sheath covering on the CNS axons. In the PNS, Schwann cells perform this function for nerves and nerve roots.

In the PNS, glial cells called satellite cells are present, which form thin sheaths around individual **ganglia** associated with sensory, sympathetic, and parasympathetic nerves. These cells surround the cell bodies, and although their specific physiologic role is not well understood, some current theories suggest that they may have a significant role in maintaining the microenvironment of the ganglion cells.

Beyond the function stated previously for glial cells, they are also important in the early development of the CNS. Study of the embryology of the nervous system indicates that glia serve to guide developing neurons in their migration to the correct location. Box 2.1 outlines the basic structure of neuroglial cells in the human nervous system.

Gray and White Matter. Some areas of the brain and spinal cord appear gray, and others appear white. The white areas, called white matter, contain many myelinated axons, with the pearly white myelin covering responsible for the color of the area. The cortex is the superficial covering of gray matter found over the cerebral hemispheres and in the cerebellum. **Gray matter** contains aggregations of nerve cell bodies embedded in delicate nerve processes. The gray matter seen in the *interior* of the brain consists of large groups of nerve cell bodies; these are called subcortical nuclei. The thalamus and the structures making up the basal nuclei (also known as the basal ganglia) are composed of subcortical nuclei. Gray matter is also found in the spinal cord; the cell bodies aggregate as columns in the spinal cord and form the H-shaped midportion of the cord.

The cells of the cerebral cortex are horizontally organized into six cell layers. The organization of these layers is known as the cytoarchitecture of the brain. Each layer contains a different type of cell, with the pyramidal cells, the largest cells in the brain, found in layer 5. The cortex is organized vertically as well as horizontally. Vertical columns of interconnected neurons each hold a functional unit of cells that share a related purpose and a related location of the stimulus that

drives their function (e.g., the visual cortex has visual orientation columns).

Organization

To comprehend the human communicative nervous system thoroughly, a basic understanding of the organization of the system as a whole is required. The nervous system should be thought of as separate from the other tissues and structures of the body. Imagine the major parts of the nervous system as if they were displayed on a dissection table spread out for study. On the table would be an oval-shaped brain with a tail-like appendage, called the spinal cord, hanging from its base. The cranial nerves, which we will study in the most depth, are attached to the base of the brain. Another set of nerves, the spinal nerves, project from both sides of the spinal cord (Fig. 2.4). Of all these parts—the brain, cord, and nerves—the brain is by far the most important for communication. Within the brain, evolutionary neural mechanisms of the communication nervous system are developed.

The nerves that exit the brain merely transmit sensory or motor information to and from the brain to control the speech, language, and hearing mechanisms. The nerves attached to the spinal cord innervate, or send nerve impulses to, muscles of the neck, trunk, and limbs and bring sensation from these parts to the brain.

BOX 2.1 Summary of Glial (Neuroglial) Cells

- Provide supportive functions in the nervous system
- Do not propagate neural impulses
- Serve in early development of central nervous system (CNS), guiding developing neurons to their correct locations

Astrocytes
- Provide structural matrix for cell bodies in the CNS
- Cause capillary walls to form tight endothelial junctions to ensure that most solutes must pass through endothelial cells
- Help maintain appropriate environment for neuronal function
- Allow for neural plasticity and help brain adapt to injury

Oligodendrocytes
- Form and maintain myelin

Microglia
- Perform scavenger functions such as cleaning out debris after neural cell damage and forming brain macrophages
- Mediate immune response after injury or infection to the brain

Ependyma
- Line ventricles in the brain and spinal cord
- Specialized types form choroid plexus, which manufactures cerebrospinal fluid

Satellite Cells
- Found in CNS and peripheral nervous system
- Surround neuron bodies but function unknown

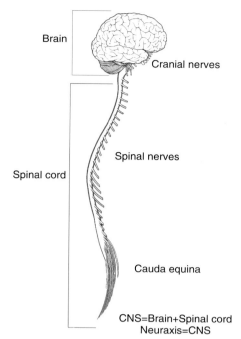

Fig. 2.4 The central nervous system *(CNS)*, including the brain and spinal cord. The CNS is synonymous with the term *neuraxis*.

From this oversimplified first mental image of the structure and function of the communication nervous system, a more precise and complex picture will be developed of the aspects of anatomy, physiology, and diagnosis of neurogenic speech, language, and hearing disorders. This chapter and the next take an in-depth look at the two major divisions of your nervous system, beginning with the CNS. Chapter 3 deals with the anatomy of the PNS and will also discuss a third system important to both the CNS and the PNS, called the autonomic nervous system. Chapter 3 also introduces you to the anatomic structures and the processes that nourish and protect these systems.

CENTRAL NERVOUS SYSTEM

Anatomically, the human nervous system has two major divisions: the CNS and the PNS. The CNS, also called the neuraxis, consists of the brain and spinal cord, with the brain being contained within the bones of the skull and the spinal cord within the vertebral column.

The nerves of the PNS connect the brain and spinal cord with peripheral structures such as muscles, glands, and organs. Both divisions of the nervous system contain somatic parts that control bodily movements and **innervate** sensory organs as well as autonomic parts that innervate visceral organs.

The brain is gray, oval shaped, and slightly soft to the touch. The average brain weighs approximately 1350 g (~3 pounds). The brain is housed in the bony skull area called the cranium. A synonym for brain is encephalon. The largest mass of brain tissue is identified as the **cerebrum**. The human cerebrum has evolved to include three parts: the cerebral hemispheres,

limbic system (in earlier terminology, rhinencephalon), and basal nuclei (aka, basal ganglia).

The cerebral hemispheres are the two readily discernible large halves of the brain. The cerebral hemispheres are connected by a mass of white matter called the **corpus callosum**. During embryologic development the cerebral hemispheres become enormously enlarged and overhang the structures deep in the brain called the diencephalon and brainstem. The cerebral hemispheres are crucial for communication, particularly the left hemisphere, where the major neurologic mechanisms of speech and language are found.

Cortical Divisions

The cerebral hemispheres are almost identical twins in looks, but the functions of their parts dramatically differ. Each cortical mantle, or cover, of a hemisphere is anatomically divided into four different principal lobes: frontal, temporal, parietal, and occipital. These lobes can be located on the brain's outer and medial (between the hemispheres) surfaces by using certain landmarks, the gyri and sulci. A gyrus is formed from the enfolding of the cortex during development; a gyrus appears as a slight elevation on the surface. A **sulcus** is a groovelike depression that separates the gyri. A sulcus that separates lobes within a hemisphere is called a fissure. Another name for sulcus is **fissure**. The gyri and sulci that serve as important landmarks are highlighted in Figs. 2.4 and 2.5.

The fissure that separates the two hemispheres is called the cerebral longitudinal fissure. Alternate names for this fissure include the superior longitudinal fissure or the interhemispheric fissure. The lateral sulcus, also called the sylvian fissure, separates the temporal lobe from the other lobes. The central sulcus, also known as the Rolandic sulcus or Rolandic fissure, separates the frontal and parietal lobes. This sulcus is easy to find, as it is a deep groove running from the cerebral longitudinal fissure to the lateral sulcus.

Cortical Localization Maps

For more than a century, neuroanatomists have divided and classified the human cortex into different areas. These tireless attempts to fractionate the cortex followed the unparalleled achievement of Paul Broca. In 1861 Broca demonstrated that different cortical regions were associated with different mental functions, one of which was expression of speech.[5] The localization systems that followed have most frequently been based on cell study of the cortex made by histologic methods. This allows the development of cytoarchitectural diagrams or maps based on the varied cell structures of the cortex. The most popular map, developed by German neurologist Korbinian Brodmann (1868–1918), is represented in Figs. 2.5 and 2.6. Note that each area of the cortex is numbered, providing a much more convenient way to specify a cortical site than by a complex description of gyri and sulci. Brodmann's map is open to criticism on the grounds that it chops the cortex into innumerable specific centers, implying that cortical areas have sharply defined limits, but it is a convenient tool in clinical practice for indicating cortical localization. Brodmann's

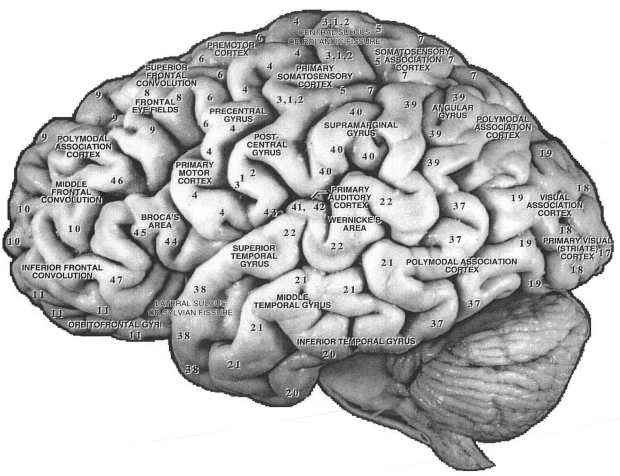

Fig. 2.5 Superior view of the cerebral hemispheres with cortical binding, according to Brodmann. (Reprinted from Werner, J. J. [2001]. *Atlas of neuroanatomy*. Butterworth-Heinemann.)

classification numbers are sometimes provided in this text to orient the reader to Figs. 2.5 and 2.6.

Cerebral Lobes

Why is this important for speech-language pathology? Contemporary practice in speech-language pathology, regardless of where one practices, often requires medical record review and understanding. The cerebral hemispheres contain networks for information processing and contain the **primary cortical areas** that activate muscles and initially receive sensory input. When these mechanisms are underdeveloped or disrupted by disease or injury, speech, swallowing, hearing, and/or language deficits as well as cognitive deficits may occur. It is important as a practitioner to know the location in the cerebral hemispheres of the primary areas and to know the key processing functions thought to be associated with each of the principal lobes. We often recommend that in the beginning you tag the lobes in your memory as containing certain structures and performing certain critical functions for speech, language, or hearing (e.g., temporal lobe = Heschl gyrus, Wernicke area, hearing, auditory comprehension).

The cortex contains regions of primary activity as well as areas devoted to processing and integrating information from the primary areas. Primary areas activate muscles and receive sensory input. The motor strip of the frontal lobe is an example of a primary area, as is Heschl gyrus in the temporal lobe, and the primary area for vision, located in the occipital lobe.

The secondary areas, also called association areas, comprise much (~80%) of the cortex. These association areas receive inputs from the primary areas close to them, allowing for processing of multiple-input processing. For this reason, they are considered the highest order of processing in the cerebral cortex. Both types of areas will be discussed in the chapter as part of their location within the cortex.

Frontal lobe. The frontal lobe is bounded anteriorly by the lateral sulcus, or sylvian fissure, and posteriorly by the central sulcus, or Rolandic fissure. The frontal lobe accounts for approximately one-third of the hemisphere's surface. In the frontal lobe is a long gyrus immediately anterior to the central sulcus. This prominent gyrus is called the precentral gyrus, and it comprises the majority of what is known as the *primary* motor cortex (area 4). The term *motor strip* is also used for this area. Nerve fibers composing a large motor pathway called the pyramidal tract descend into the brain and spinal cord from starting points in the primary motor area. The cells in this area are responsible for voluntary control of skeletal

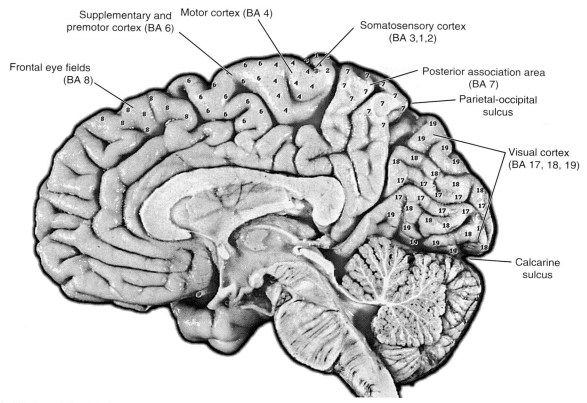

Fig. 2.6 Medial view of the right hemisphere. (Reprinted from Werner, J. J. [2001]. *Atlas of neuroanatomy.* Butterworth-Heinemann.)

muscles on the opposite, or contralateral, side of the body. This fact has important clinical significance, which is discussed later in the chapter.

The connections between the controlling area on the primary motor cortex and the voluntary muscles served are arranged so that a map of motor control can be drawn on the cerebral cortex to show the pattern of cortical innervation (Fig. 2.7B). This map is referred to as a **homunculus**, which is Latin for "little man." The areas are represented in an almost upside-down or inverted fashion. The area of cortical representation given to a particular part does not appear to be strongly related to the size of that part of the body because the leg and arm are given a smaller area of cortical tissue than the hand or mouth. Rather, the body parts that require the most precision in motor control are apportioned the larger cortical areas. Shown in Fig. 2.7A is the cortical sensory map or sensory homunculus, which is a mirror image of the motor map and represents the pattern of sensory input from the body to the somatosensory cortex on the post central gyrus, which is located not in the frontal but in the parietal lobe.

Immediately anterior to the primary motor area are the premotor cortex and another area with motor assignment, the supplementary motor area. These ancillary motor areas (area 6) are important in motor learning and in the performance of routine and less-practiced motor sequences.

In the frontal lobe of the left hemisphere is an important region known as **Broca area** (areas 44 and 45). Located in the inferior (third) frontal gyrus of the lobe (2–4), Broca area

in most people appears to be important to produce fluent, well-articulated speech. The left hemisphere is the dominant hemisphere in most persons, meaning that this hemisphere controls language functions. Approximately 90% of the population is right handed with left hemisphere dominance for language. Even the majority of persons who are left handed show left dominance for language. If damage to Broca area occurs in adults who are left hemisphere-dominant for language, a characteristic breakdown usually occurs in the normally fluent production of verbal language; if the damage is limited to Broca area specifically, this breakdown is usually transient. If the damage results from a larger lesion that includes Broca area but also surrounding cortical tissue in what is known as the **perisylvian zone**, a classic syndrome of acquired language disorders or *aphasia*, called Broca aphasia, may be diagnosed (discussed further in Chapter 10). Ablation of the area in the nondominant hemisphere corresponding to Broca area affects language in only a small percentage of the population.

Another part of the frontal lobe concerned with initiation of movement is the area devoted to control of the eyes. The frontal eye fields (area 8) lie just anterior to the premotor cortical area. These areas are involved in initiating rapid eye movements and directing attention.

The rest of the frontal lobe is composed of **association cortex**, a different type of cortical tissue with less-defined functional assignment. This frontal area is often referred to as the prefrontal cortex (areas 9–11, 46, and 47) and contains the

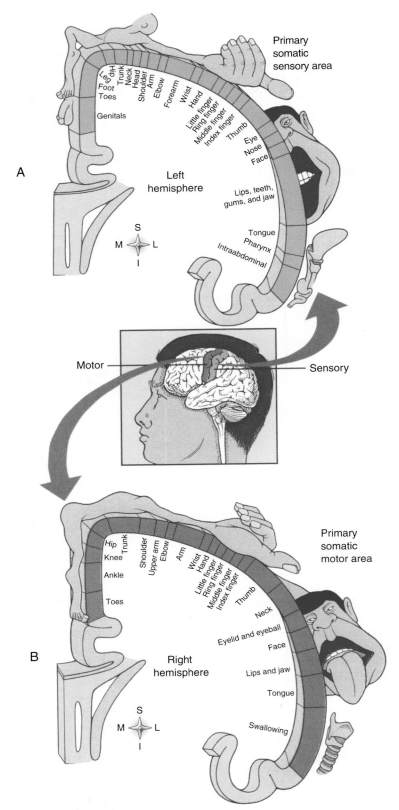

Fig. 2.7 Primary somatic sensory (A) and motor (B) areas of the cortex. The illustrations show which parts of the body are mapped to specific areas of the postcentral (sensory) and precentral (motor) gyri. The exaggerated face indicates that more cortical area is devoted to processing information to and from the face than, for example, the leg or arm. This disparity is due to the precision of motor control and distinct sensory processing needed for speech and swallowing. (Reprinted from Thibodeau, G., & Patton, K. [2006]. *Anatomy & physiology* [6th ed.]. Mosby.)

frontal association areas. Frontal association areas are vital to successful executive functioning. Appropriate and well-developed executive functioning allows the execution of non-routine processes that require planning, analysis, feedback, self-regulation, and so forth. The ability to participate successfully in school, work, family, and social settings depends on these frontal association areas.

Parietal lobe. The **parietal lobe** is bounded anteriorly by the central sulcus, inferiorly by the posterior end of the lateral sulcus, and posteriorly by an imaginary borderline. The primary sensory, also known as somatosensory or somesthetic cortex, is found in the parietal lobe (areas 1–3), the major portion of which is the postcentral gyrus (see Fig. 2.5). It is also known as the sensory strip, but it is helpful to use the term **somatosensory** to help remember that bodily sensations, as opposed to visual and auditory sensations, are processed here. This gyrus lies directly posterior to the central sulcus, or Rolandic fissure. On this sensory cortex can be mapped the sensory control of various parts of the body. Somesthetic sensations (e.g., pain, temperature, touch) are sent to the sensory cortex from the opposite side of the body. This arrangement is a mirror image of the motor strip (see Fig. 2.7).

Two gyri in the parietal lobe are important to locate and become familiar with in regard to language, and they are both contained in the inferior parietal lobule (Brodmann area 40). The first is the **supramarginal gyrus** (area 40), which curves around the posterior end of the lateral sylvian fissure. The second, the **angular gyrus** (area 39), lies directly posterior to the supramarginal gyrus. It curves around the end of a prominent sulcus in the temporal lobe, the superior temporal sulcus (see Fig. 2.5). The supramarginal gyrus is important for phonologic processing, while the angular gyrus is important for semantic processing of auditorily presented language.[16] Damage to the angular gyrus in the dominant left hemisphere may cause word-finding problems (anomia), reading and writing deficits (alexia with agraphia), as well as left-right disorientation, finger agnosia (inability to identify the fingers), and difficulty with arithmetic (acalculia).

The postcentral gyrus (somatosensory cortex) is a *primary* cortical area, whereas most of the remaining parietal lobe cortex is composed of association cortex, primarily concerned with somatosensory and visual association function. The parietal lobe has been characterized as the "association area of association areas" because of the multimodal processing that takes place there. As a whole, the parietal lobes may be the most lateralized in function of all the lobes in the cerebrum, although the specialization is not complete. Language functions tend to be concentrated in the left parietal lobe around the gyri just discussed. In the nondominant hemisphere, the parietal lobe association cortex primarily processes spatial information and related selective attention. Damage here may result in difficulty attending to or a complete neglect of the contralateral side of space. Visuospatial and constructional deficits (such as in drawing, building small models, and so on) may be found on testing the patient with right-hemisphere parietal lobe damage.

Temporal lobe. The **temporal lobe** is the seat of auditory processing in the brain. It is bounded superiorly by the sylvian fissure and posteriorly by an imaginary line that forms the anterior border of the occipital lobe. Two gyri of the temporal lobe are prominent on the lateral surface of the brain: the superior and middle temporal gyri. The third important gyrus, the inferior gyrus, can be seen on the lateral surface but continues onto the interior surface of the lobe as well (see Fig. 2.5). Less visible on the lateral surface are the transverse temporal gyri (areas 41 and 42), which can be found on the upper edge of the temporal lobe, extending deep in the medial surface of the brain. The transverse gyrus of Heschl (most commonly called **Heschl gyrus**, area 41) forms the primary auditory cortex, representing the cortical center for hearing in each hemisphere. There is bilateral representation of the auditory signal, though more fibers terminate in the gyrus of the contralateral hemisphere than will terminate on the ipsilateral side of the brain. The ability to detect the presence of sound is a function of the peripheral hearing mechanism and the auditory nerves. The cortical area is the site of conscious processing of those impulses as "sound," allowing us to perceive these signals as sound and do what we call "hear."

Area 42 is adjacent to Heschl gyrus and is an auditory association area, although it is frequently presented as part of the primary cortical area of hearing. It has been found to participate in the processing of harmonic and rhythmic patterns. Unilateral damage in areas 41 and/or 42 of the auditory cortex does not cause deafness in one ear but may result in difficulty interpreting a sound or locating a sound in space. Bilateral lesions in the auditory cortex cause cortical deafness (see Chapter 5).

The posterior part of the superior temporal gyrus in the left temporal lobe is the auditory association area, best known as **Wernicke area** (area 22), which is important to the development and use of language. Damage to Wernicke area may result in a particular classification of acquired language disorder called **Wernicke aphasia** (see Chapter 10).

On the medial aspect of the temporal lobes, near the sagittal plane between the two hemispheres, one can locate several important deep brain areas important to memory. These include the hippocampal region and the parahippocampal gyrus. On the parahippocampal gyrus can be found subcortical areas known as the perirhinal, parahippocampal, and entorhinal cortices.

If the two borders of the lateral (sylvian) fissure are pulled apart, a cortical structure called the **insula**, or the island of Reil, may be seen hidden under the area where the temporal, parietal, and frontal lobes come together. It includes some of the oldest cortical tissue in the brain. The insula is not part of the temporal lobe or any of the four major lobes but is considered a lobe unto itself. Fiber connections to the insula are not well defined, and the functions are not well understood, but the insula is thought to receive input regarding pain and viscerosensory input. As discussed in Chapter 10, lesions involving the insula in the dominant hemisphere may also contribute to difficulty producing well-articulated, fluent speech.

Occipital lobe. The **occipital lobe** occupies the small area behind the parietal lobe and is marked on the lateral surface by imaginary lines rather than prominent sulci. Two sulci that can be found on the medial surface of the brain that help locate the occipital lobe are the parietal-occipital sulcus and the calcarine sulcus (see Fig. 2.6). The occipital lobe is concerned with vision, with the primary visual area (area 17) located in gyri that border the calcarine sulcus.

Primary Cortical Areas

The primary motor projection cortices are found in the frontal lobes on the precentral gyri, the bilateral cortical strips from which voluntary movement patterns are initiated. The motor strip serves as a source of descending motor pathways, projecting to lower levels of the nervous system.

The primary sensory reception areas register sensory impulses relayed from the periphery to the thalamus and upward to the cortex. The pathways from thalamus to cortex are called thalamic radiations. The primary sensory reception areas of the cortex are (1) the primary auditory cortex (areas 41 and 42), located in Heschl's gyrus in the temporal lobes; (2) the primary somatosensory cortex in the postcentral gyri of the parietal lobes (areas 1, 2, and 3); and (3) the primary visual cortex (area 17) in the occipital lobes.

Primary Motor Projection Cortex

The primary motor projection cortex is known as the motor area, or motor strip. In Brodmann's system, it is area 4. The motor area is located on the anterior wall of the central sulcus and the adjacent precentral gyrus. Fig. 2.6 shows the areas devoted to the motor control of the different parts of the body. Recall that this area allows contralateral motor control of the limbs. Some of the muscles of the oral mechanism have contralateral control, but many are bilaterally innervated. The inverted arrangement of motor control areas on the bilateral motor cortices reveals that cortical control for the muscles and functions of the speech mechanism is represented at the lower end of the motor area on the lateral wall of the cerebrum. The large areas given over to motor control of the oral mechanism contribute to the coordination of its rapid and precise movements during talking, singing, and changing facial expression.

Anterior to the motor area is the **premotor area** (area 6), considered a supplement to the primary motor projection cortex and related to the extrapyramidal system. If areas 4 and 6 are ablated, spasticity in the limbs results. A third motor area, discovered by neurosurgeon Wilder G. Penfield (1891–1976), is found on the ventral surface of the precentral and postcentral gyri. It is called the **supplementary**, or **secondary motor area**.

In more recent years the supplementary motor area has received considerable attention. One of its primary functions appears to work in conjunction with other structures in the control of sequential movements, and speech production is a prime example of sequential movement. Research is also finding support for the supplementary area's involvement in the timing of speech for fluent speech production.[8]

Primary Somatosensory Cortex

The primary somatosensory cortex (areas 1–3) is on the postcentral gyrus and is a primary receptor of general bodily sensation. Thalamic radiations relay sensory data from skin, muscles, tendons, and joints of the body to the primary somatosensory cortex. Lesions of this cortex produce partial sensory loss (paresthesia); rarely does complete sensory loss (anesthesia) occur. A lesion causes numbness and tingling in the opposite side of the body. Widespread destructive lesions produce gross sensory loss with an inability to localize sensation.

Primary Auditory Receptor Cortex

Heschl gyrus (areas 41 and 42), as previously described, is the primary auditory receptor cortex. The area is found in each temporal lobe, but the left Heschl area appears to be somewhat larger in most individuals. The significance of this neuroanatomic difference is not completely clear, but it may be related to language dominance.

Primary Visual Receptor Cortex

The primary visual receptor cortex is in the occipital lobe along the calcarine fissure, which can be seen from the medial surface of the hemisphere and is not obvious on the outside of the brain. The area, 17 in the Brodmann scheme, is also known as the striate area. It receives fibers from the optic tract. Lesions of the optic pathways cause various degrees of blindness. This partial blindness is considered a visual field defect.

Primary Olfactory Receptor Cortex

The cortical area that allows appreciation of smell is deep in the temporal lobe and is called the primary olfactory receptor cortex (area 28, medial surface). It includes an area called the **uncus** and the nearby parts of the parahippocampal gyri of the temporal lobe. The olfactory nerves, the end organs for smell, lie in a bony structure in the nose. The nerves end in the olfactory bulb, which is an extension of brain tissue in the nasal area. The bulbs are supported by an olfactory stalk. Destruction of the olfactory system causes anosmia, or lack of smell. Irritative lesions produce olfactory hallucinations or uncinate fits.

Perisylvian Zone

The cortex surrounding the sylvian fissure in the dominant temporal lobe, which is the left for most people, is identified as the perisylvian zone, where the major neurologic components for understanding and producing language are found. These components include Broca area, Wernicke area, the supramarginal and angular gyri, as well as major long association tracts that connect the components (Fig. 2.8). The central language mechanism and its disorders are discussed in depth in Chapters 9 and 10.

Cerebral Connections

The surface structures already discussed are composed mainly of the cell bodies of neurons, the gray matter (see earlier). The myelinated axons, the white matter, allow for communication between neurons. Myelinated axons come in three basic types: projection, association, and commissural; these permit specialized communication between cortical areas.

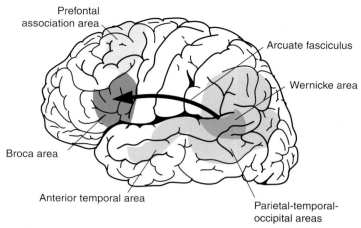

Fig. 2.8 Primary language and association areas of the cortex.

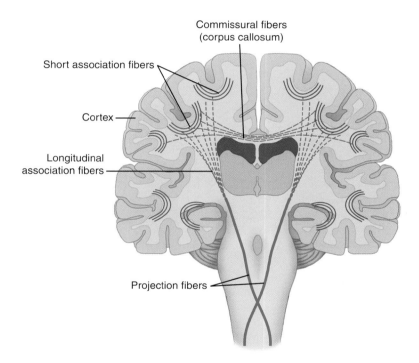

Fig. 2.9 Schematic representation of the types of connective fibers in the central nervous system.

Why is this important for speech-language pathology? *We have acknowledged that the cerebrum is the boss of the nervous system. This must mean that the connections between and within the cerebral hemispheres and with lower structures are a vital part of how the nervous system works. Knowledge of the nervous system must include the types of fibers found in these areas. This eventually leads you to an understanding of how the various structures are connected and form pathways for neural impulses to traverse.* Fig. 2.9 *schematically depicts the different types of fibers discussed later in the chapter.*

Projection Fibers

Projection fibers are long axons of neurons that send impulses to a distant structure in the CNS. The most notable projection fibers are the corticospinal fibers, which project from the

primary motor cortex down to the spinal cord, and the corticobulbar fibers, which project from the primary motor cortex down to the cranial nerve nuclei. Corticopontine fibers are also projection fibers, projecting from the motor areas to the brainstem down to the cerebellum.

Association Fibers

Association fibers form association tracts, connecting areas within the hemisphere. Short association tracts connect neurons of one gyrus to the next, while long association tracts connect neurons between lobes within their own hemisphere. **Fasciculus**, meaning "little bundle," is the type of name given to many of these tracts important to language and speech. Fig. 2.10A is a graphic depiction of some of these fiber tracts.

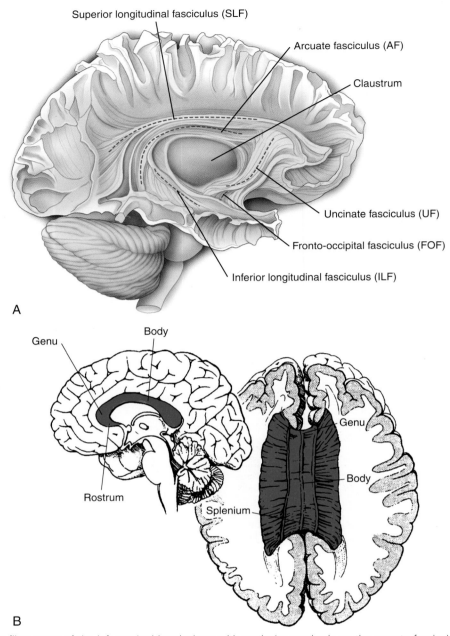

Fig. 2.10 (A) Association fiber tracts of the left cerebral hemisphere with particular emphasis on the arcuate fasciculus and the uncinate fasciculus. (B) The corpus callosum in a medial view and transverse section. It is the largest of the commissures connecting the two hemispheres.

One important association tract is the **arcuate fasciculus** (AF). The AF is important to language because many of its fibers travel from the posterior temporal lobe forward by way of another set of fibers, the superior longitudinal fasciculus (SLF), to the motor association cortex in the frontal lobe. Lesions near the arcuate fasciculus may cause a major syndrome of aphasia (an acquired language disorder caused by brain damage) called conduction aphasia. There are also indirect AF fiber connections between Broca area and the parietal lobe as well as connecting the parietal lobe with Wernicke area.[7]

The uncinate fasciculus (UF) gathers fibers from the temporal pole, uncus, hippocampal gyrus, and amygdala in the rostral portion of the temporal lobe. The UF follows a complicated path and eventually extends into the orbitofrontal cortex and prefrontal cortex. Thus, it links areas of the temporal lobe important for sound recognition, object recognition, and recognition memory with areas of the frontal lobe involved in emotion, inhibition, and self-regulation.[22] The functional significance of this pathway is not totally understood, although it has been suggested that it allows the reward/punishment biased association memories stored in the orbitofrontal cortex to access mnemonic associations (e.g., names, facial features, voice) stored in the temporal lobe, thus perhaps influencing decisions, learning, and memory as well as social behavior.[21]

TABLE 2.1   White Matter Association Pathways, Location, and Function

Association Fibers	Main Pathway(s)	Function
Superior longitudinal fasciculus	Posterior arm fanning out into parietal, occipital, and posterior temporal lobes; anterior arm recurves to the anterior temporal lobe	Interconnects frontal with the other three lobes Significant for initiation of motor activity, spatial attention, gesture, and orofacial memory
Arcuate fasciculus	Connects Wernicke area with Broca area; different segments connect inferior parietal lobule with those two areas; connects Broca with middle frontal and precentral gyri; connects Wernicke with middle temporal gyrus	Ability to recognize language and respond to it appropriately
Uncinate fasciculus	Complex pathway from rostral temporal lobe (temporal pole, uncus, hippocampal gyrus, amygdala) to the white matter of the orbitofrontal cortex (may ascend and reach prefrontal areas)	Ventral limbic path; significant for processing novel information, self-regulation, and positive/negative evaluation of emotional information; may be important for visual learning
Superior fronto-occipital fasciculus	Fibers from occipital and parietal lobes join and run horizontal and forward to prefrontal and premotor cortex	Significant for peripheral vision, visual motion perception, and visuospatial processing
Inferior fronto-occipital fasciculus	Superior parietal, posterior temporal, and inferior occipital fibers follow complex dorsal and ventral paths to frontal and prefrontal cortical areas	May be important to object recognition and discrimination, semantic processing, and emotional-cognitive interaction
Inferior longitudinal fasciculus	From extrastriate visual association areas in occipital lobe to anterior temporal lobe, uncus, parahippocampal gyrus, and amygdala	Significant for its role in object recognition, visual discrimination, and memory; may link visual object recognition to lexical label
Cingulum bundle	Forms most of white matter of the cingulate gyrus; longer fibers connect multiple areas around corpus callosum	Major component of dorsal limbic pathway; involved in motivation and emotion as well as spatial working memory

From Nadich, T. P., Krayenbuhl, N., Kollias, S., Bou-Haidar, P., Bluestone, A. Y., & Carpenter D. M. (2010). White matter. In T. P. Nadich, M. Castillo, S. Cha, & J. G. Smirniotopoulos (Eds.), *Imaging of the brain* (pp. 205–244). Elsevier Saunders.

The inferior longitudinal fasciculus (ILF) runs along with and lateral to a fasciculus known as the inferior fronto-occipital fasciculus (FOF), whose fibers eventually enter the frontal lobe. The ILF has vertical fibers arising in the occipital lobe outside the striate cortex (in extrastriate cortical areas). There are also horizontal fibers that run along the length of the temporal lobe, terminating in the anterior temporal region. The ILF appears to have a role in object recognition as well as memory and visual discrimination. Table 2.1 describes some of the important fasciculi in the cerebral hemispheres.

Forkel and colleagues[10] present a helpful and colorful depiction of these association tracts. The visual depiction is helpful, and we recommend you follow the listed link in the References section.

Commissural Fibers

These fibers connect an area in one hemisphere with an area in the opposite hemisphere. The corpus callosum is the largest set of commissural fibers in the brain and is a pathway of crucial importance to speech-language functions (see Fig. 2.10 B). The corpus callosum serves as the major connection between the hemispheres and conveys neural information from one hemisphere to the other. The corpus callosum is the largest of the side-to-side interconnections between the two hemispheres and, in general, connects analogous areas in the two hemispheres.

The anterior and posterior commissures are other small bundles of interhemispheric fibers, located anteriorly and posteriorly to the corpus callosum. The anterior commissure connects the olfactory bulbs, amygdaloid nuclei, and medial and inferior temporal lobes. The posterior commissure fibers connect areas in the occipital lobes, primarily areas concerned with pupillary response and eye movement control.

Split-Brain Research

The corpus callosum and its role in the transfer of information from one hemisphere to another attracted wide attention when split-brain operations were first performed on human beings in the 1960s.[17] This large bundle of commissural fibers may be cleanly and completely severed surgically without damage to other tissue. This operation, called a commissurotomy, has been performed on patients plagued by chronic and severe epileptic seizures that could not be controlled by massive doses of anticonvulsive medication. A seizure that begins in one cerebral hemisphere may easily travel across the corpus callosum to the other hemisphere, producing a bilateral generalized seizure. Neurosurgeons reasoned that sectioning the corpus callosum would contain the seizure to one hemisphere.

Results of the early commissurotomies were even more beneficial than had been anticipated. Not only did the surgery contain seizures to a single hemisphere, but it also reduced seizures overall because of the severing of apparent reciprocal actions between the hemispheres.

The surgery also provided information on the differing psychological functions of each hemisphere and on the role of the corpus callosum in the brain mechanisms for speech and language. The split-brain patients clearly showed asymmetry for speech and language functions, indicating that the corpus callosum plays a decisive role in transmitting language received at the right primary auditory area and heard in the right ear to the left hemisphere, where it is processed by the major mechanisms for speech and language.

Experiments on patients who underwent the split-brain procedure suggested that the right hemisphere was responsible for spatial, tactile, and constructional tasks. These experiments led to speculations that the two hemispheres function in different ways, each having its own cognitive style. The left hemisphere was characterized as logical, analytic, and verbal; the right as intuitive, holistic, and perceptual/spatial. However, as will become increasingly clear to you, they are unquestionably integrated in intact brain function.

Association Cortex
Cortical Motor Speech Association Areas

Surrounding the foot of the motor and premotor cortices are areas considered motor association areas. These areas are numbered 44 through 47 in the Brodmann system. They are called the opercular gyri. Areas 44 and 45 include the pars opercularis, the pars triangularis, and the pars orbitalis. Areas 44 and 45 in the left hemisphere are sometimes called the frontal operculum. Area 44 is known best as Broca area. Although its function is controversial, Broca area usually is associated with the formation of motor speech plans for oral expression. In 2015 using electrocorticographic (ECoG) recordings directly from the surface of the cortex, researchers suggested that Broca area is important in coordinating information from other cortical sites during speech production.[9]

The cytoarchitecture of Broca area is similar in both right and left hemispheres, but traditional theory maintains that only the left is involved with verbal formulation. Regional cerebral blood flow and metabolic rate studies have suggested that right cortical areas may also be activated during some speech and language activities.

Sensory association areas. The sensory association areas, where elaboration of sensation occurs, can best be considered as extensions of the primary sensory receptor areas. They are also known as secondary association areas or unimodal association areas because only one type of sensory input is processed there. Their margins are necessarily vague, and the exact functions of certain areas are controversial. The sensory association areas are richly connected to the receptor areas by a host of association fibers, but these association fibers are often difficult to follow because of the vast number of relays in the cortical association system. Areas 5 and 7 in the parietal lobe are related to general somesthetic sensation.

Areas 42 (part of Heschl gyrus) and 22 (Wernicke area) are related to language comprehension. Areas 18 and 19 in the occipital lobe are visual association areas, important for visual perception and for some visual reflexes such as visual fixation. Lesions in this area may cause visual hallucinatory symptoms.

The function of the sensory association areas is that of gnosis ("knowing"). A deficit in the sensory association function is known as agnosia, a perceptual-cognitive deficit presumed to follow a destructive cerebral lesion; agnosia means lack of recognition. Lesions in auditory association areas affecting the appreciation of incoming sound produce language disorders. Areas surrounding Heschl gyrus are involved in adding meaning to sound and providing comprehension of language. Lesions in area 42 destroy the ability to appreciate the meaning of sound, and lesions in area 22 compromise the ability to understand spoken language. Lesions of visual association areas may cause different types of visual agnosia in which the patient cannot, through the visual modality alone, recognize certain visual patterns (e.g., objects or faces).

Categories of association cortex. The cytoarchitecture of association cortex is different for different areas and determines what kind of neural information can be processed by those cells. Generally, the association areas adjacent to primary motor and sensory areas are unimodal; that is, only one type of information is processed by those cells. These association areas elaborate on the information received at the specific primary motor and sensory areas to which they are adjacent.

Further removed from the primary motor or sensory cortical areas, other types of association cortices are found, termed polymodal and supramodal. Polymodal is sometimes referred to as multimodal, and supramodal may be referred to as heteromodal in some texts.

Polymodal association areas are found somewhat close to the unimodal areas near the primary reception cortex. Polymodal association cortex is linked to processing of two or more sensory modalities. For example, polymodal association cortex, processing both auditory and visual information, can be found in the temporal lobe and in the occipital lobe. The **parahippocampal gyrus** receives input from all areas of the cerebral cortex, processing several types of sensory information.

The association areas add meaning and significance to the sensory or motor information received in the primary motor or sensory areas. The matching of present sensory information with past sensory information drawn from memory probably takes place in the polymodal association areas, which are linked to several sensory modalities. Motor association areas are sites where motor plans, programs, and commands are formulated with input from auditory and somatosensory processing, particularly touch, as well as other modalities.

Certain sensory association areas blend and mingle sensory information from several association areas to establish a higher level of cortical sensory information. This type of processing results in a complex level of awareness that is above and beyond mere recognition of sensory data. This level of sensory awareness is known as perception, which is defined as the mental process of becoming aware of or recognizing an object or idea. The processes are primarily cognitive rather than affective or conative, although all three aspects are manifested.[20] For example, if someone places a door key in your hand in the dark, you must recognize its shape and judge its size, weight, texture, and metallic surface to match this information with memories and concepts of keys. This is called stereognostic perception. Only when you can identify your perception of the key can you name the key and relate its function if asked. The everyday sensory recognition of objects relies on complex sensory integration of multiple sensations enhanced by memory and conceptual knowledge of objects with similar qualities. This complex activity of knowing is called gnosis. Other common kinds of perception are such skills as depth perception and visuospatial perception. Intuition can be thought of as a type of perception.

The highest level of processing is carried on in association areas best described as supramodal, meaning that these cortical areas are concerned with neural processing that is not directly linked to sensory or motor functions. This kind of association cortex and cortical function can be found primarily in the following areas:

- The prefrontal area, for higher executive function
- Perisylvian cortex, subserving language
- Limbic lobe, subserving emotion and motivation

The prefrontal cortex and the perisylvian cortical area and function were previously outlined and are discussed in depth in Chapter 9. The limbic lobe, its structures, and probable association functions are examined next. A summary of categories of the association cortex is provided in Box 2.2.

The Limbic System

Why is this important for speech-language pathology?

Speech-language pathologists (SLPs) will encounter disorders that have caused dysfunction of deeper structures of the cerebral hemispheres. This is especially true with more diffuse

---

BOX 2.2 Categories of the Association Cortex

Unimodal
- Only one type of information is processed by the cells in these areas
- Areas elaborate on information received at adjacent primary motor and sensory areas
- Information can be related to either motor or sensory input

Polymodal
- Found in close proximity to unimodal areas, near the primary reception cortex
- Linked to processing two or more kinds of sensory information (e.g., auditory and visual information)
- Matches present sensory information with past sensory information

Supramodal
- Highest level of processing
- Areas concerned with neural processing not linked directly with sensory or motor functions
- Found primarily in prefrontal area, perisylvian cortex, and limbic lobe

---

brain damage caused by a traumatic brain injury. A critical cognitive skill, memory, is often affected with damage to these structures, resulting in major alterations to the treatment plan. Emotional processing is an important function of some of these structures, and the client's emotional state impacts the treatment plan and the success of therapy. The SLP should be familiar with these structures and their functions so that this may be anticipated in planning.

Cortical-Like Tissue

The associative function of the structures of the limbic system have been discussed and supported by Mesulam[16] and Benson.[3] They indicate that these areas of the brain are architecturally considered cortical areas, although not named as part of the cortex in most instances. As most other anatomists do, these authors include in their overviews of association cortex what Mesulam calls heteromodal cortex, which is composed of the six-layer formation accepted as cortical tissue. These associative areas include the supramodal cortex previously discussed. This cortex has the six-layer formation found in 90% of cortex, including the primary motor and sensory areas as well as the multimodal and supramodal association areas. The six-cell-layer cortex is called neocortex or isocortex.

Cortical regions with tissue composed of fewer than six cell layers are functionally associated with the limbic system and are classified as allocortex. Allocortex can also be broken down into different types or regions. Cortical structures with three to five cellular layers are classified as paleocortex, whereas structures with only three cellular layers are classified as archicortex.

Mesulam's and Benson's discussions of these other types of associative cortices focus on patterns formed by regions sharing common functions. Beyond the primary association areas and the secondary motor and sensory association areas previously discussed, neuroanatomists of this school point to the higher-level associative functions of the more primitive cortex found deep to the neocortex and best seen on the medial surface of the brain (Fig. 2.11). The cytoarchitecture of these structures reveals a composition of primarily three layers, rather than six layers, with some structures showing transition between the six- and three-layer formation. Thus, these structures are cortical-like in nature because true cortex has six layers.

Parahippocampal and Hippocampal Gyri

The parahippocampal gyrus (see Fig. 2.11) is a transitional architecture representing a six-layer formation laterally with a change to a three-layer formation more medially. Folded within the parahippocampal gyrus is the hippocampus. The hippocampal gyrus is part of the hippocampal formation, which is a curved, rolled-in-and-under area of cortex bulging into the floor of the temporal (inferior) horn of the lateral ventricle. The hippocampal formation consists of the dentate gyrus, hippocampal gyrus, and **white matter**, called fimbria, that issues from this area and eventually forms the crus (leg) of the fornix. Traditionally included as part of the limbic

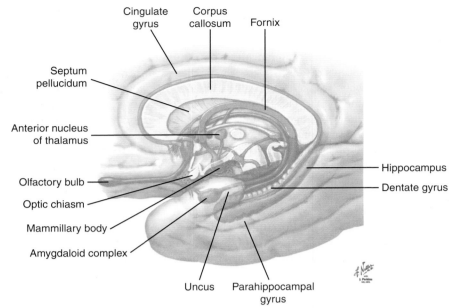

Fig. 2.11 The limbic system with limbic and paralimbic structures. (Netter illustrations from www.netterimages.com © Elsevier, Inc., All Rights Reserved.)

system, most anatomists now separate these hippocampal structures from the limbic system because of their involvement in encoding new memories. However, the parahippocampal cortex plays a role in memory as well. In a recent study, Bohbot et al.,[4] found a correlation between lesions to the parahippocampal region and spatial memory. For the sake of discussion of anatomic location, the hippocampal formation will be discussed with the limbic system here.

Limbic and Paralimbic Structures

The **limbic system** or limbic lobe (see Fig. 2.11) was named by Pierre Paul Broca, who thought of it as the fifth lobe of the brain. It is occasionally referred to as Broca lobe because of this. The "lobe" is on the medial surfaces of the two hemispheres. An archlike pattern of cortex surrounding the non-convoluted central portions of the brain can be observed on the medial surfaces of the hemispheres with the brainstem removed. This internal circular arch is called the limbic lobe (or limbic system or formation). The limbic system includes the oldest or most primitive cortex, the rhinencephalon, also called the "smell brain." The prefix *rhino-* means "nose"; the functions of the old animal brain dealt primarily with the sense of olfaction (smell). Because smell is a much more crucial sense for animals in their adaptation to the environment than it is to human beings, the old brain is relatively large in animals, and the cerebral hemispheres are less well developed.

The histologic makeup of the rest of the limbic system is phylogenetically old in relation to the cerebral hemispheres (neocortex), but not as old as the olfactory brain tissue. The limbic system structures have many connections among themselves as well as connections to the hypothalamus (see Diencephalon later in this chapter) and to neocortical structures. In the evolution of the human brain, the older parts have come under the direction of the newer cortical systems, creating a hierarchy.

Autonomic and hormonal responses caused by hypothalamic action are under the direction of the limbic structures, which in turn are under the direction of the higher cortical structures. Through these connections, the limbic area helps shape behavioral reaction to sensory input through analysis, reaction, and remembrance of stimuli, situations, reactions, and results. Heimer[12] asserts that the anatomic and functional characteristics of some of the structures of this area are distinct enough to be considered apart from the others, and therefore questions the concept of a limbic system. For example, the amygdala is the key structure in emotional behavior, and the hippocampus and related structures are of primary importance when discussing memory (see Chapter 9).

Mesulam[16] conceives of the limbic system as being formed by several smaller structures, including the subcallosal gyrus, cingulate gyrus, isthmus, hippocampal gyrus, and uncus. A medial view of the left hemisphere indicates some of these structures (see Fig. 2.11). The **cingulate gyrus** (gyrus cinguli) arches over the corpus callosum, beginning at the anterior subcallosal area and arching back to the junction with the parahippocampal gyrus. This juncture is called the isthmus. The *uncus* is the knob or hooklike area of the parahippocampal gyrus. Mesulam includes in the limbic system structures that are cortical-like in archetype. Cortical-like refers to the fact that their formations are part cortical and part subcortical nuclear in architecture. These structures are the amygdala (or amygdaloid body), substantia innominata, and septal area. They are formed by the simplest and most undifferentiated type of cortex in the forebrain.

A second associative area of cortex is composed of the **paralimbic areas** (see Fig. 2.11). Although some neuroanatomists include these areas as part of the limbic system rather than refer to them as paralimbic, Mesulam[16] points out that gradual increases in complexity of the cortex can be found in these areas when compared with the previously mentioned limbic system formations. These structures form an uninterrupted girdle around the medial and basal aspects of the cerebral hemispheres. The paralimbic areas include the caudal orbitofrontal cortex, insula, temporal pole, parahippocampal gyrus (proper), and cingulate complex. The caudal orbitofrontal cortex includes Brodmann areas 10, 11, and 47[15] (see Fig. 2.5). The cingulate complex includes the tissue of the anterior cingulate and middle cingulate cortex. Studies of these areas have shown different functional connections for these anatomically close areas. Strong connections with limbic and autonomic functional areas have been traced for the anterior cingulate cortex. The middle cingulate cortex connections are primarily with cognitive processing and sensorimotor processing areas.[19]

The parahippocampal gyrus completes the C shape of the "limbic lobe." Most of the rostral part of the parahippocampal gyrus is occupied by an area known as the entorhinal area, which can be identified by its irregular surface (similar to an orange peel). The entorhinal cortex is closely related to the hippocampus.

If the premise is accepted that cortical functioning is hierarchical and a vast network of interrelated functional systems have different, but similar, neuroanatomic substrates, then the study of the functional systems (such as language, memory, emotion) and their disorders must be tempered with the knowledge that brain function is highly complex, with interdependent systems throughout, and only partially understood. While functional subunits of brain operations are studied, attempts to analyze and synthesize the integration of the neural systems that control human behavior continue at a rapid pace.

Other Structures of the CNS

Cell bodies of other structures are amassed into nuclei below the level of the cortex and appear gray in fresh dissection, although a large number of white matter tracts pass through these areas. The structures or areas of the CNS discussed in this section are the diencephalon (thalamus and related structures), basal ganglia, cerebellum, brainstem, and spinal cord.

Why is this important for speech-language pathology? The functions of the following structures are primarily associated with sensory and motor processing rather than information processing. SLPs diagnose and treat several conditions in which information processing remains intact but sensory and/or motor systems are impaired affecting speech, voice, hearing, and swallowing. As discussion of these structures continues in this text, it also will be pointed out that connections with cortical and limbic areas that do contribute to cognitive and emotional processing are also found in these areas. Discussion of these important structures begins with the diencephalon and takes you down to the spinal cord.

Diencephalon

Buried deep within the cerebral hemispheres is a group of structures known collectively as the **diencephalon** (Fig. 2.12). This region is composed of the following four primary structures:

- Thalamus
- Hypothalamus

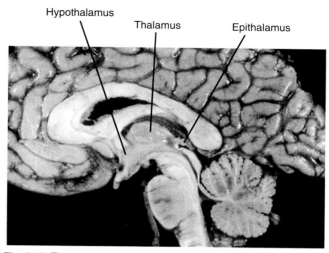

Fig. 2.12 The structures of the diencephalon. (Modified from Lundy-Ekman, L. [2013]. *Neuroscience: Fundamentals for rehabilitation* [4th ed., fig. 1–12, p. 11]. Saunders.)

- Epithalamus
- Subthalamus

The pituitary gland is also considered part of the diencephalon.

Thalamus. The **thalamus** is located ventrally (toward the belly), and the hypothalamus is located dorsally (toward the back). The thalamus is a large, rounded structure consisting of gray matter. It is made up of two egglike masses that lie on either side of the third ventricle, one of the large openings in the brain through which cerebrospinal fluid flows. The posterior end of the thalamus expands in a large swelling, the pulvinar. Penfield (mentioned earlier) was the first to ascribe special subcortical speech and language functions to this structure.

The thalamus integrates sensation in the nervous system. It brings together and organizes sensation from all the classic sensory systems except olfaction. Anatomists usually divide the thalamus into regions and discuss the important nuclei in a particular region. These nuclei act as thalamic relays, sending sensory information upward to sensory areas of the cerebral cortex. The to-and-fro sensory pathways between the thalamus and cerebral cortex are so numerous, and the two structures so interdependent, that assigning a sensory deficit to the thalamus versus the sensory cortical areas of the cerebrum is sometimes difficult. Relays from the cerebellar, limbic, and basal ganglia pathways are also found in the thalamus, subserving motor and autonomic functions as well. The thalamus in the left hemisphere may also play a role in speech and language (see Chapters 6 and 9).

Hypothalamus. The lower part of the lateral wall and the floor of the third ventricle make up the **hypothalamus** (see Fig. 2.12). Also on the floor of the third ventricle are two nipple-shaped protuberances called the mammillary bodies (see Fig. 2.11), which contain nuclei important to hypothalamic function. The hypothalamus is a critical structure to autonomic and endocrine function (see Chapter 3). It controls several aspects of emotional behavior, such as rage and aggression, as well as escape behavior. In addition, it helps regulate body temperature, food and water intake, and sexual and sleep behavior. The hypothalamus exerts neural control over the pituitary gland, which releases hormones involved in many bodily functions.

Epithalamus and subthalamus. The epithalamus is a small region of the diencephalon consisting of the pineal gland, habenular nuclei, and stria medullaris thalami. The pineal gland contains no true neurons, only glial cells. Through a complicated process involving the hormone melatonin, it participates in regulation of the body's circadian (24-hour) rhythms. The stria medullaris connects fibers from the habenular nuclei with the limbic system. The specific function of the habenular nuclei in human beings is unclear.

The **subthalamus** consists of a large subthalamic nucleus that is functionally considered a part of the basal ganglia, as discussed in the next section. The subthalamus also consists of a caudal area called the zona incerta. Fibers from neurons in the zona incerta project to many areas, including the cerebral cortex, and may exert an inhibitory effect on the motor pathways.

Basal Ganglia

The **basal ganglia**, or basal nuclei as some texts use, are large masses of gray matter deep within the cerebrum below its outer surface or cerebral cortex. The division of the structures known as basal ganglia has been confusing in the literature because various anatomists have categorized the structures differently. A review of current literature indicates that most neuroanatomists include the following structures as basal ganglia (or basal nuclei):

- Caudate nucleus
- Putamen
- Globus pallidus
- Substantia nigra
- Subthalamic nucleus

The putamen and globus pallidus are sometimes grouped and called the **lentiform** or **lenticular nucleus**. The caudate and the putamen grouped together are called the **striatum** (or neostriatum in some texts). These three main parts—caudate, putamen, and globus pallidus—when grouped together are referred to as the **corpus striatum**. Fig. 2.13 illustrates the basal ganglia as seen in a coronal section, and Fig. 2.14 represents a medial view of the nuclei.

Squire et al.,[18] also include nuclei that are not traditionally included as basal ganglia structures but which, they point out, are analogous to those traditionally discussed. This set of nuclei consists of the nucleus accumbens (see Fig. 2.14) and the olfactory tubercle, which they refer to collectively as the ventral striatum (as opposed to the neostriatum). Other nuclei corresponding to the globus pallidus are termed the ventral pallidum by these authors. These nuclei are mentioned because you may see these structures included in the basal ganglia in other texts or in articles. This text will not discuss the function of these structures as part of the basal ganglia. Research literature, particularly on motivation and emotion, may present you with more discussion on these structures and their relation to the basal ganglia.

Striatum. Making up the striatum (or neostriatum) are the caudate nucleus and the putamen. The term striatum resulted from the striped appearance of the area due to the many axon fibers passing through it. The caudate nucleus is a C-shaped formation. Because of the C shape, a coronal view of the basal ganglia will reveal only a small portion of the caudate and may show part of the head, the body, or the tail. The head of the caudate is enlarged, and the structure tapers into a narrow tail. It lies close to the thalamus and adjacent to the wall of the lateral ventricle. The caudate is connected to

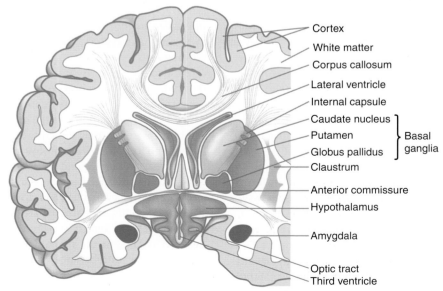

Cortex
White matter
Corpus callosum
Lateral ventricle
Internal capsule
Caudate nucleus ⎫
Putamen   ⎬ Basal ganglia
Globus pallidus ⎭
Claustrum
Anterior commissure
Hypothalamus
Amygdala
Optic tract
Third ventricle

Fig. 2.13 The structures of the basal ganglia illustrated in a horizontal section through the cerebrum. (Redrawn from Guyton, A. C. [1991]. *Basic neuroscience: Anatomy and physiology* [2nd ed.]. Saunders. In Drain, C. B. [2009]. *Perianesthesia nursing: A critical care approach* [5th ed.]. Saunders.)

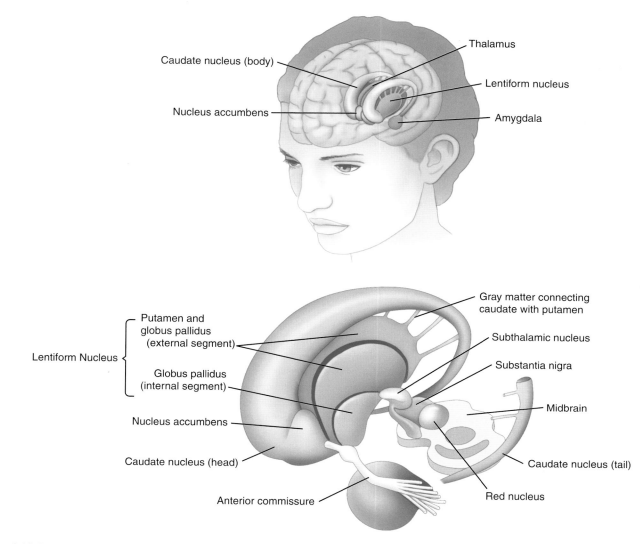

Fig. 2.14 Basal ganglia. Illustration of dissection allowing a medial view of the nuclei of the basal ganglia.

the putamen by strands of gray matter but is separated physically from it by the anterior portion of the large white band of descending axons called the **internal capsule**. The striatum receives most of the excitatory input that is provided to the basal ganglia from the cortex. In turn, the striatum transmits inhibitory impulses to the globus pallidus and the substantia nigra using the neurotransmitter GABA (gamma-aminobutyric acid).

Substantia nigra. The **substantia nigra** ("black substance" in Latin) is a long nucleus located in the midbrain but considered functionally a part of the basal ganglia because of its reciprocal connections with other brainstem nuclei. It consists of two components, the pars compacta and the pars reticulata, which have different connections and use different neurotransmitters. Degeneration of the pars compacta of the substantia nigra results in the reduction of the availability of the neurotransmitter dopamine. This lack of dopaminergic innervation to the striatum results in disorders associated with hypokinesia or reduced motor movements. Parkinson

disease is a result of reduced functioning of the substantia nigra.

Subthalamic nucleus. The subthalamic nucleus is the large nucleus of the subthalamus, which is anatomically part of the diencephalon. The subthalamic nucleus itself, however, is functionally considered part of the basal ganglia. It receives projections from the globus pallidus, the cerebral cortex, the substantia nigra, and the reticular formation of the pons. The subthalamic nucleus sends projections to the globus pallidus and the substantia nigra. The neurons of this nucleus use an excitatory neurotransmitter, glutamate. The neurons of the subthalamic nucleus are, in normal motor function, usually inhibited from firing by thalamic override. When damage occurs to the basal ganglia pathways and subthalamic or related neurons are not inhibited from firing (i.e., disinhibition occurs), an abnormal increase in involuntary motor movements is seen. This results in disorders associated with hyperkinesia or increased motor movements, such as Huntington chorea.

Input to the basal ganglia is generally considered to be through the caudate nucleus and the putamen (i.e., the striatum). Received here are afferents from all four lobes of the cortex, thalamic nuclei, and part of the substantia nigra (the pars compacta). The output fibers of the basal ganglia usually are from the globus pallidus and another part of the substantia nigra (the pars reticulata). The output of these structures usually is projected to certain thalamic nuclei, the brainstem reticular formation, the superior colliculus, and cortical motor areas in the frontal lobe.

Cerebellum and Brainstem

The brain contains two other quickly identifiable parts in addition to the large cerebrum: the cerebellum and the brainstem. Both structures are extremely important to an understanding of the neurology of speech.

Cerebellum. The word **cerebellum** means "little brain," and the cerebellum is indeed a much smaller structure than the cerebrum, weighing approximately one-eighth as much. The cerebellum is located at the rear of the brain, below and at the base of the cerebrum (Fig. 2.15). It resembles a small orange that is wedged in the juncture of the attachment of the spinal cord to the melon-shaped cerebrum. The cerebellum as it is understood is a relatively recent evolutionary addition to the nervous system. Initially, it was found in fish and was almost solely related to vestibular functioning. As movement on four legs evolved, the cerebellum developed a rich mass of connections to the spinal cord. As upright posture developed and human beings continued to learn new physical skills, the cerebellum, particularly the posterior lobes, developed many linkages with the cerebrum.

Like the cerebrum, the cerebellum consists of two hemispheres. Each is primarily concerned with coordination of movements ipsilaterally, providing fine coordination of movement. The cerebellum plays an important role in postural stability and fixation, as well as in learning a novel motor

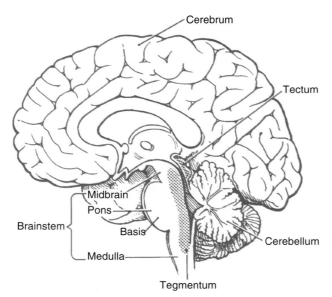

Fig. 2.15 Medial view of the right cerebrum, brainstem, and cerebellum.

act. Coordination of the extremely rapid and precise movements of normal articulation of speech also depends on intact cerebellar functioning. Damage may result in a particular type of motor speech disorder, one of the classic dysarthria types called ataxic dysarthria (see Chapter 8). The cerebellum may also have a role in cognitive processing with linkages found with the lateral prefrontal cortex. Cerebellar anatomy and function are discussed in Chapter 6.

Brainstem and Its Internal Anatomy

The fourth major part of the brain is the **brainstem** (see Fig. 2.15). The brainstem and its subdivisions cannot be directly viewed unless the cerebral hemispheres are cut away to reveal the internal structures of the brain. The brainstem appears as a series of structures that seem to be an upward extension of the spinal cord, thrust upward into the brain between the cerebral hemispheres. Often, the parts of the brainstem are depicted as extending as vertical segments one above the other, but the parts of the brainstem actually do not sit in a vertical plane. The upper structures are crowded together to fit within the cranium. In some texts, the diencephalon is included as part of the brainstem. Contemporary neuroanatomy teaching separates the diencephalon and includes only three structures. Moving from the rostral (head) to the caudal (tail) segments, the three brainstem structures are as follows (Figs. 2.16 and 2.17):

- Mesencephalon (midbrain)
- Pons
- Medulla oblongata

The brainstem also has internal regions, with the presence and function of these regions depending on which structure is being examined. The midbrain has three regions: the **tectum**, tegmentum, and basis. The pons has a tegmentum and a basis. The tegmental regions are always found in the dorsal (posterior) aspect of the structures, whereas the basilar areas are on the anterior (ventral) aspect. The medulla is not considered to have a tegmental or basilar region as such, but the function of the areas of the medulla that are continuous with the tegmentum and the basis of the other two structures are quite similar in nature. Thus, they are referred to as being contiguous areas with the tegmentum and the basilar regions of the midbrain and pons. Basically, the tegmental areas of the brainstem contain cranial nerve nuclei from which the axons of the cranial nerves exit the brain and become part of the PNS. The basilar areas of the brainstem structures all contain ascending and descending sensory and motor fibers. These regions are illustrated in Figs. 2.15 and 2.17.

Midbrain. The **midbrain** (see Fig. 2.17), located immediately below the thalamus and hypothalamus, is also called the **mesencephalon**. The midbrain is the narrowest part of the brainstem and contains the tectum, or roof, one of the three longitudinal divisions of the brainstem. On the tectum are four swellings called **colliculi** ("little hills"): two inferior colliculi and two superior colliculi. The tectum and the four colliculi are known collectively as the corpus quadrigemina. The inferior colliculi serve as waystations in the central auditory nervous system, and the superior colliculi are waystations in the visual nervous system.

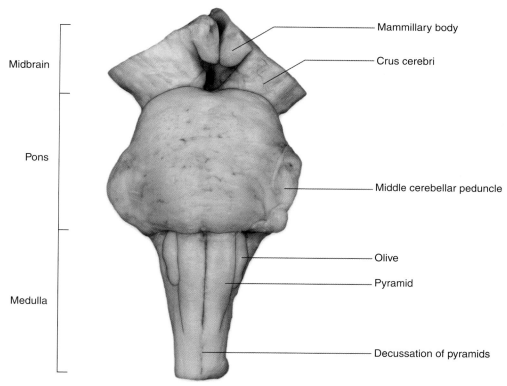

Fig. 2.16 Ventral aspect of the brainstem. (From Crossman, A., & Neary, D. [2015]. *Neuroanatomy* [5th ed.]. Churchill Livingstone.)

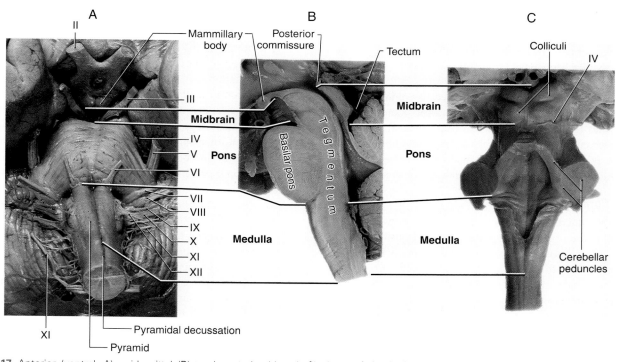

Fig. 2.17 Anterior (ventral; A), midsagittal (B), and posterior (dorsal; C) views of the brainstem, with cranial nerves referenced by Roman numerals. In (C), the cerebellum is removed to expose the posterior surface of the brainstem and fourth ventricle. (Reprinted from Haines, D. [2006]. *Fundamental neuroscience* [3rd ed.]. Churchill Livingstone.)

The crus cerebri is a massive fiber bundle found at the base of the midbrain. It includes fibers descending to the spine (corticospinal), the medulla (corticobulbar), and the pons (corticopontine). The tegmentum of the midbrain contains all the ascending and many of the descending systems of the spinal cord or lower brainstem. The term *cerebral peduncles* is often used interchangeably with the term *crus cerebri*, but according to Haines,[11] cerebral peduncle should be used to represent the area of the entire midbrain below the tectum. The base of the midbrain also contains the substantia nigra, which, as explained earlier, is a basal ganglia structure.

Pons. Just below the midbrain in the neuraxis is the **pons**, a massive and rounded structure that serves in part as a connection to the hemispheres of the cerebellum (see Fig. 2.17). The connections to the cerebellum are made by numerous transverse fibers on the anterior surface of the pons, forming the cerebellar peduncles. The pons is aptly named; the Latin word for "bridge" is *pons*, and the pons is a bridge to the cerebellum. Several cranial nerves exit the brain from the pons, including three that are important to speech and hearing: cranial nerves V (trigeminal), VII (facial), and VIII (vestibulocochlear).

Medulla oblongata. The **medulla oblongata** is the most caudal brainstem structure. Older terminology identified it as the bulb. It is a rounded bulge that is an enlargement of the upper spinal cord (see Fig. 2.17). A median fissure (furrow) is present on the anterior surface. On either side of this fissure are landmark swellings called pyramids. The pyramids arise from the basilar pons and extend caudally to an area known as the pyramidal decussation. This area is formed by the decussation (crossing to the opposite side) of motor fibers traveling from the precentral gyrus in the frontal lobe to the spinal cord (corticospinal fibers of the pyramidal tract). Posterior to the pyramids are oval elevations, called olives, produced by the olivary nuclei. The olives are important waystations on the pathways of the auditory nervous system. The inferior cerebellar peduncles are also found on the medulla. The peduncles connect the cerebellum to the brainstem at the level of the medulla. The nuclei of several cranial nerves important to speech production can be found in the medulla, with their axons exiting the brain at this level. Because older terminology for the medulla was bulb, these motor fibers of cranial nerves that terminate in nuclei in brainstem structures are often referred to as corticobulbar fibers. These fibers are also sometimes referred to as corticonuclear fibers because their destination in the brainstem is the nuclei of the cranial nerves.

Spinal Cord

Recall a mental image of the dissection of the nervous system. Looking at the brain, a long pigtail of flesh is visible hanging from its base; this is the spinal cord. It is normally found in an opening running through the center of the bony vertebral column. The spinal cord is strictly defined. It is caudal to the large opening at the base of the skull called the magnum foramen; the nervous tissue encased in the skull proper is the brain.

The spinal cord is divided into five regions. Each of these regions is named for a section of the 31 spinal vertebrae that surround the spinal cord itself; these regions of the cord are cervical, thoracic, lumbar, sacral, and coccygeal. The spinal cord does not extend the complete length of the vertebral column. In the adult it terminates at the level of the lower border of the first lumbar vertebra. In the child it is longer, ending at the upper border of the third lumbar vertebra. Fig. 2.18 shows the segmental spinal nerve and the comparable vertebral levels.

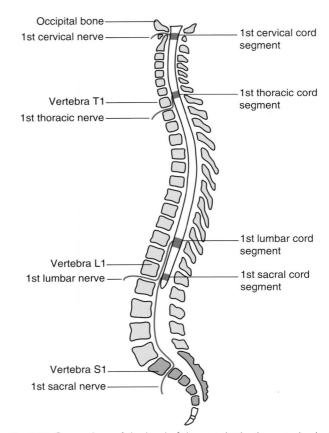

Fig. 2.18 Comparison of the level of the vertebral column and spinal cord. Spinal nerves C1–C7 emerge above the corresponding vertebrae, whereas the remaining nerves emerge below. (Reprinted from FitzGerald, M. J. T., & Folan-Curran, J. [2002]. *Clinical neuroanatomy and related neuroscience* [4th ed.]. Saunders.)

A cross section of the spinal cord (Fig. 2.19) reveals an H-shaped mass of gray matter in the center of the spinal segment. As in other parts of the CNS, the gray matter contains neuronal and glial cell bodies and their dendrites. Laminar organization is present in the gray matter, with 10 layers identified. Each layer is composed of neurons that respond to different sensory stimuli or innervate different muscle fibers.

The ventral, or anterior, portion of the cord mediates motor output. The anterior horn cell of the ventral gray matter is the point of synapse of the descending motor tracts (corticospinal) with the ventral roots of the spinal cord. The dorsal, or posterior, portion of the cord mediates sensory input coming into the spinal cord through the dorsal root of the spinal nerves.

Each lateral half of the spinal cord also has white matter columns: a dorsal or posterior column, a ventral or anterior column, and a lateral column. This white matter is composed of myelinated and unmyelinated nerve fibers as well as glial cells. The myelinated fibers form bundles or fasciculi that rapidly conduct nerve impulses that ascend or descend for varying distances. Bundles of white matter with a common function are called tracts. Major anatomic landmarks of a cross section of the spinal cord are shown in Fig. 2.19. Refer often to this drawing when studying sensory and motor pathways.

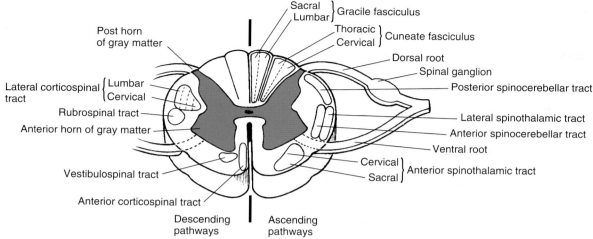

Fig. 2.19 Cross section of the spinal cord.

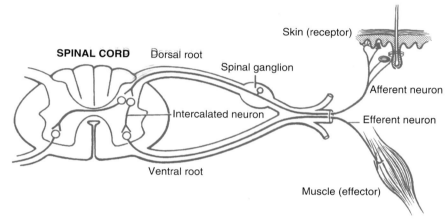

Fig. 2.20 A simple reflex arc.

Close inspection of the form and quantity of gray versus white matter reveals variations at the different levels of the spinal cord. The proportion of gray to white is greatest in the lumbar and cervical regions where the major motor and sensory neurons for the arms and legs are found. In the cervical regions the dorsal column (mediating sensory input) is somewhat narrow, and the ventral column (mediating motor output) is broad and expansive. Both columns are broad and expansive in the lumbar region, and in the thoracic region both are narrow.

Combined with a careful sensory examination, testing of muscle functions can be most valuable to the physician in assessing the extent of a lesion. Most muscles are innervated by axons from several adjacent spinal roots. This peripheral nerve innervation pattern is discussed in Chapter 3.

Reflexes

Reflexes are subconscious automatic stimulus response mechanisms. In human beings, as in all vertebrates, reflexes are basic defense mechanisms to painful or potentially damaging sensory stimulation. If, for instance, you accidentally touch a hot stove, the sensation of pain does not need to be sent up the sensory tracts to the cortex. Motor commands from the cortex need not be sent down motor tracts to allow movement. The rapid response to noxious stimuli is processed quickly at the spinal level by a mechanism called the simple **reflex arc**. The reflex arc contains a receptor and an afferent neuron, which transmits an impulse along the peripheral nerve to the CNS, where the nerve synapses through an intercalated neuron with a lower motor or efferent neuron. From this point an impulse is sent to an efferent nerve, and then an efferent impulse passes outward in the nerve, which moves the effector (i.e., the muscle or gland). A response is then elicited—you simply suddenly withdraw your finger (Fig. 2.20).

There are several types of reflexes: superficial or skin reflexes, deep tendon or myotactic reflexes, visceral reflexes, and pathologic reflexes. Reflexes occur at different levels in the nervous system: spinal level, bulbar level, midbrain level, and cerebellar level. Reflex assessment is a vital tool for assessing the intactness of various sensory motor systems. Reflexes are discussed in more detail in Chapters 6 and 11.

SYNOPSIS OF CLINICAL INFORMATION AND APPLICATIONS FOR THE SLP

- The uniqueness of Broca area, a specialized vocal tract, and the expanse of information and communication processing areas give humans their exceptional ability to communicate.
- The human communication nervous system consists of the CNS and PNS. The autonomic nervous system is subsumed under both.
- Neurons are composed of organelles, which are composed of molecules. The four major classes of molecules in cells are lipids, proteins, carbohydrates, and nucleic acid.
- A bilipid layer surrounds the cell body of a neuron. The neuron has one axon, which typically carries impulses away from the cell body and may have many dendrites that carry information toward the cell body.
- Retrograde transport up the axon mediates movement of trophic substances, which provide nourishment for the cell.
- Astrocytes, oligodendrocytes, microglia, and ependyma cells are the main types of neuroglial cells. Each has its own specific purpose, primarily providing the structural support and environmental maintenance for the work of the neurons. For example, after cerebral injury, microglia clean up the debris caused by cellular deterioration.
- Gray-appearing areas of the brain contain the nuclei of cell bodies. White-appearing areas signal the presence of myelinated fiber tracts.
- The cortex is organized into six horizontal layers. The most recent (phylogenetically) cortical tissue is called neocortex. Cortical-like tissue with three to five layers is found in paralimbic and limbic system structures.
- The brain is divided into two hemispheres, left and right, with communication between the two primarily occurring through the commissural fiber pathway called the corpus callosum. In most people the left hemisphere is the dominant hemisphere for language.
- Gyri (elevations) and sulci (depressions) on the lateral and medial surfaces of the brain provide important landmarks for delineating the four lobes: frontal, temporal, parietal, and occipital. Particular types of language and other types of neurobehavioral disorders may result from developmental interruption or acquired injury to these areas.
- Important functional areas located in the frontal lobe are primary motor cortex, premotor cortex, supplementary motor area, Broca area, and the prefrontal association cortex.
- Important functional areas in the temporal lobes are Heschl gyrus (primary auditory cortex) and Wernicke area.
- Important functional areas of the parietal lobe are the primary sensory cortex, angular gyrus, and supramarginal gyrus.
- Important functional areas in the occipital lobes are the primary visual cortex and visual association cortex.
- The insula is an older area of cortex located deep to the sylvian fissure. It may have a role in motor programming for speech.
- The perisylvian area in the dominant hemisphere is the major area for understanding and producing language.
- Cerebral connections are made by projection fibers (to distant structures), association fibers (intrahemispheric), and commissural fibers (interhemispheric).
- Approximately 86% of cortex is categorized as association cortex. Some association areas are unimodal (process only one type of information), and some are polymodal (processing two or more types of information). The highest level of processing is carried on in supramodal association areas, which are not associated with any particular type of information. The prefrontal association area, perisylvian area, and the limbic areas have supramodal capability.
- Allocortex is composed of fewer than six layers, is inferior to the cortical mantle, and can be found in paralimbic and limbic system structures. Some of the limbic system structures are the rhinencephalon, cingulate gyrus, isthmus, hippocampal gyrus, and uncus. Paralimbic structures include the temporal pole, parahippocampal gyrus, and cingulate complex. These paralimbic and limbic areas are primarily involved with emotion and memory.
- The diencephalon is composed of the thalamus, hypothalamus, epithalamus, and subthalamus, as well as the pituitary gland. The thalamus is the main relay structure of the brain. The hypothalamus is concerned with autonomic and endocrine functions.
- The brainstem consists of three divisions: midbrain, pons, and medulla. The tectum, tegmentum, and basis are longitudinal divisions of the three structures. The brainstem contains the nuclei of most of the cranial nerves, which control the sensory input and motor output of the oral and facial musculature.
- The basal ganglia or basal nuclei are groups of subcortical nuclei found deep within the brain. The structures of the basal ganglia are the caudate nucleus, putamen, globus pallidus, and substantia nigra. These function in regulation and control of motor movement, muscle tone, and planning for movement. Damage may result in hypokinesia or hyperkinesia and characteristic motor speech disorders.
- The cerebellum has two hemispheres and is located at the base of the cerebrum, connected through peduncles primarily to the pons. It plays an important part in postural stability and fixation and in learning a novel motor act. A specific motor speech disorder may follow damage to the cerebellum.
- The spinal cord is divided into five regions, each named for a section of the spinal vertebrae surrounding the cord: cervical, thoracic, lumbar, sacral, and coccygeal.
- The center of the spinal cord consists of gray matter. The ventral portion contains motor nuclei, and the anterior contains horn cells. The dorsal part mediates sensation through the dorsal nuclei. White matter tracts ascend from and descend to the spinal cord, mediating motor output and sensation to the limbs and trunk.

REFERENCES

1. Allen, N. J., & Lyons, D. A. (2018). Glia as architects of central nervous system formation and function. *Science, 362*(6411), 181–185.
2. Azevedo, F. A., Carvalho, L. R., Grinberg, L. T., Farfel, J. M., Ferretti, R. E., Leite, R. E., Jacob Filho, W., Lent, R.,

Herculano-Houzel, S. (2009). Equal numbers of neuronal and nonneuronal cells make the human brain an isometrically scaled-up primate brain. *J Comp Neurol, 2009 Apr 10; 513*(5), 532–41. https://doi.org/10.1002/cne.21974. PMID: 19226510.
3. Benson, D. F. (1994). *The neurology of thinking.* Oxford University Press.

4. Bohbot, V. D., Allen, J. J. B., Dagher, A., Dumoulin, S. O., Evans, A. C., Petrides, M., Kalina, M., Stepankova, K., & Nadel, L. (2015). Role of the parahippocampal cortex in memory for the configuration but not the identity of objects: Converging evidence from patients with selective thermal lesions and fMRI. *Frontiers in Human Neuroscience*, 9. https://www.frontiersin.org/articles/10.3389/fnhum.2015.00431/full.

5. Broca, P. (1861). Remarques sur le siège de la faculté du langage articulé, suivis d'une observation d'aphemie. *Bulletin de la Société* Anatomique, 6, 330–357.

6. Del Bigio, M. R., (1993). Neuropathological changes caused by hydrocephalus. *Acta Neuropathologica*, 85, 573–585.

7. Dick, A. S., & Tremblay, P. (2012). Beyond the arcuate fasciculus: Consensus and controversy in the connectional anatomy of language. *Brain*, 135, 3529–3550.

8. Etchell, A. C., Johnson, B. W., & Sowman, P. F. (2014). Behavioral and multimodal neuroimaging evidence for a deficit in brain timing networks in stuttering: A hypothesis and theory. *Frontiers in Human Neuroscience*, 8, 1–10.

9. Flinker, A., Korzeniewska, A., Shestyuk, A., Franaszczuk, P. J., Dronkers, N. F., Knight, R. T., & Crone, N. E. (2015). Redefining the role of Broca's area in speech. *Proceedings of the National Academy of Sciences of the United States of America*, 112(9), 2871–2875.

10. Forkel, S. J., Friedrich, P., Thiebaut de Schotten, M., & Howells, H. (2022). White matter variability, cognition, and disorders: A systematic review. *Brain Structure and Function*, 227(2), 529–544. https://doi.org/10.1007/s00429-021-02382-w.

11. Haines, D. (2006). *Fundamental neuroscience for basic and clinical applications* (3rd ed.). Churchill Livingstone.

12. Heimer, L., & Van Hoesen, G. W. (2006). The limbic lobe and its output channels: Implications for emotional functions and adaptive behavior. *Neuroscience & Biobehavioral Reviews*, 30(2), 126–147.

13. Herculano-Houzel, S. (2014). The glia/neuron ratio: How it varies uniformly across brain structures and species and what that means for brain physiology and evolution. *Glia*, 62(9), 1377–1391.

14. Johnson, T. A., Jinnah, H. A., & Kamatani, N. (2019). Shortage of cellular ATP as a cause of disease and strategies to enhance ATP. *Frontiers in Pharmacology*, 19. https://www.frontiersin.org/articles/10.3389/fphar.2019.00098/full.

15. Kringelbach, M. L., & Rapuano, K. M. (2016). Time in the orbitofrontal cortex. *Brain*, 139, 1010–1013.

16. Mesulam, M. M. (1985). *Principles of behavioral neurology*. F. A. Davis.

17. Singh-Cundy, A., & Shin, G. (2012). *Discover biology* (5th ed.). Sinauer Associates, W. W. Norton.

18. Squire, L. R., Berg, D., Bloom, F. E., du Lac, S., Ghosh, A., & Spitzer, N. C. (2013). *Fundamental neuroscience* (4th ed.). Elsevier Academic Press.

19. Stevens, F. L., Hurley, R. A., & Taber, K. H. (2011). Anterior cingulate cortex: Unique role in cognition and emotion. *Journal of Neuropsychiatry and Clinical Neurosciences*, 23(2), 121–125.

20. Taber, K. H., & Hurley, R. A. (2008). Astroglia: not just glue. *Journal of Neuropsychiatry and Clinical Neurosciences*, 20(2). iv–129.

21. University of Leeds. (2010). "Nature's batteries" may have helped power early lifeforms. *Science Daily*. http://www.sciencedaily.com/releases/2010/05/100525094906.htm.

22. Verkhratsky, A., Rodríguez, J. J., & Parpura, V. (2013). Astroglia in neurological diseases. *Future Neurology*, 8(2), 149–158.

23. Von Der Heide, R. J., Skipper, L. M., Klobusicky, E., & Olson, I. R. (2013). Dissecting the uncinate fasciculus: Disorders, controversies and a hypothesis. *Brain*, 136(6), 1692–1707. https://doi.org/10.1093/brain/awt094.

24. Wallman, J. (2009). *Aping language*. Cambridge University Press.

3

Organization of the Nervous System II

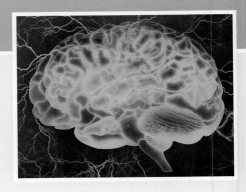

The charm of neurology . . . lies in the way it forces us into daily contact with principles. A knowledge of the structure and function of the nervous system is necessary to explain the simplest phenomena of disease, and it can only be attained by thinking scientifically.

Henry Head

CHAPTER OUTLINE

KEY TERMS

afferent
afferent fibers
anterior (ventral) horn cells
aqueduct of Sylvius
arachnoid granulations
arachnoid mater
autonomic nervous system
bilateral
Broca (expressive) aphasia
cerebrospinal fluid (CSF)
choroid plexus
circle of Willis
constructional disturbances
contralateral
cranial nerves
diaphragma sella
dura mater
efferent fibers

encephalitis
enteric nervous system
falx cerebelli
falx cerebri
foramen
foramina
hemorrhage
homeostasis
internal carotid arteries
intervertebral foramina
ipsilateral
ischemia
lesion
meninges
motor fibers
nucleus solitaries
parasympathetic divisions
peripheral nervous system (PNS)

phrenic nerves
pia mater
postganglionic
preganglionic
sensory fibers
septa
somites
spinal peripheral nerves
subarachnoid space
sympathetic divisions
tentorium cerebelli
unilateral
venous sinuses
ventricular system
vertebral artery
Wernicke (receptive) aphasia
x-ray

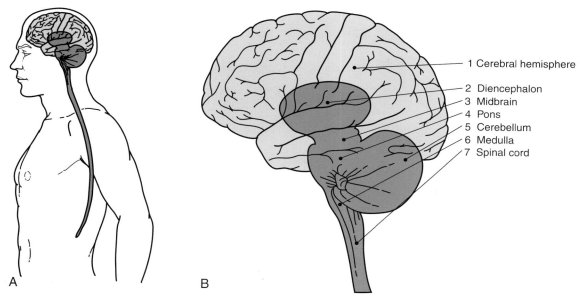

Fig. 3.1 (A) Location of the central nervous system (CNS) in the body. (B) Seven major divisions of the CNS: (1) cerebral hemisphere, (2) diencephalon, (3) midbrain, (4) pons, (5) cerebellum, (6) medulla, and (7) spinal cord. The midbrain, pons, and medulla comprise the brainstem. (Reprinted from Martin, J. H. [1996]. *Neuroanatomy text and atlas* [2nd ed.]. McGraw-Hill.)

The central nervous system (CNS) with its vast network of neurons and neural connections is the controlling influence in the human communication nervous system. Glial cells reside within the CNS and provide structure and metabolic support for the neurons. The CNS, however, would not be functional, or necessary, without the lower-level structures reviewed in this chapter. The nervous system consists of separate peripheral and central components organized into two parts—not independent from each other, but interdependent on each other. This chapter outlines the functions of the peripheral nervous system that allow this interdependence with the CNS (Fig. 3.1).

PERIPHERAL NERVOUS SYSTEM

The **peripheral nervous system** (**PNS**) includes (1) the cranial nerves with their roots and rami (branches), (2) the peripheral (spinal) nerves, and (3) the peripheral parts of the autonomic nervous system. The peripheral ganglia are groups of nerve cell bodies located outside the CNS forming an enlargement on a nerve or on two or more nerves at their junction. They are primarily sensory in nature, although motor ganglia are found particularly in the autonomic nervous system.

The cranial nerves exit from the neuraxis at various levels of the brainstem and the uppermost part of the spinal cord. When we use the term *peripheral nerves*, we are typically referring to the spinal nerves plus their branches.

Cranial nerves V (the trigeminal nerve), VII (the facial nerve), IX (the glossopharyngeal nerve), and X (the vagus nerve) have dedicated sensory ganglia originating from the neural crest during embryonic development. They contain pseudounipolar cell bodies. These sensory ganglia are classified as the trigeminal or semilunar ganglion (cranial nerve V); the geniculate ganglion of cranial nerve VII; the superior and inferior ganglia of cranial nerve IX, or the glossopharyngeal nerve; and the jugular and nodose ganglia of cranial nerve X, or the vagus nerve. The jugular and nodose ganglia are often referred to as the superior and inferior ganglia of the vagus nerve. Cranial nerve VIII, the vestibulocochlear nerve, primarily arises from the otic placodes. Fig. 3.2 illustrates the cranial nerve nuclei and their juxtaposition within the brainstem.

Spinal Nerves

Spinal peripheral nerves are described as mixed nerves, meaning they carry both sensory and motor fibers. Each spinal nerve is connected to the spinal cord by two roots: the anterior root and the posterior root. The anterior root of the spinal nerve consists of bundles of nerve fibers that transmit nerve impulses away from the CNS. These nerve fibers are called **efferent fibers**. Efferent fibers that go to the muscles and make them contract are also called **motor fibers**. The motor fibers of the spinal nerves originate from a group of cells or motor nuclei in the spinal cord called the **anterior (ventral) horn cells**. The anterior horn cells are the point of synapse, or connection, with the spinal nerves as they leave the neuraxis. When nerve impulses have left the neuraxis, they have reached what British neurophysiologist Charles Sherrington (1857–1952) called "the final common pathway," or the terminal route of all neural impulses acting on the muscles.

The posterior root of the spinal nerve consists of **afferent fibers** that carry information about the sensations of touch, pain, temperature, and vibration into the CNS via the spinal cord. They are also called **sensory fibers**. The cell bodies of

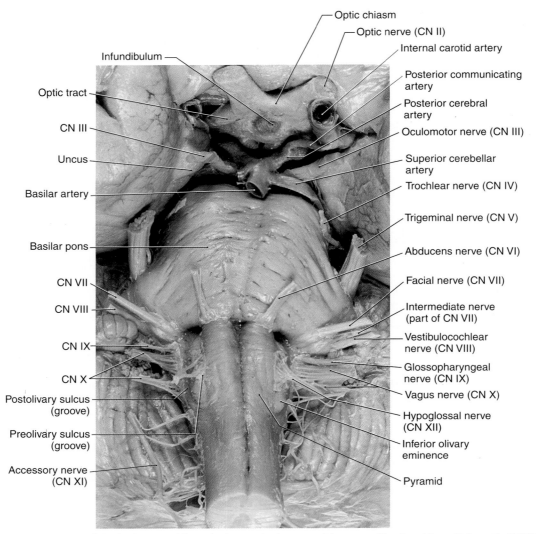

Optic chiasm
Optic nerve (CN II)
Internal carotid artery
Infundibulum
Posterior communicating artery
Optic tract
Posterior cerebral artery
CN III
Oculomotor nerve (CN III)
Uncus
Superior cerebellar artery
Basilar artery
Trochlear nerve (CN IV)
Trigeminal nerve (CN V)
Basilar pons
Abducens nerve (CN VI)
CN VII
Facial nerve (CN VII)
CN VIII
Intermediate nerve (part of CN VII)
CN IX
Vestibulocochlear nerve (CN VIII)
CN X
Glossopharyngeal nerve (CN IX)
Postolivary sulcus (groove)
Vagus nerve (CN X)
Preolivary sulcus (groove)
Hypoglossal nerve (CN XII)
Inferior olivary eminence
Accessory nerve (CN XI)
Pyramid

Fig. 3.2 An interior (ventral) view of the brainstem with particular emphasis on cranial nerves. (Reprinted from Haines, D. [2006]. *Fundamental neuroscience* [3rd ed.]. Churchill Livingstone.)

the sensory fibers are a swelling on the posterior root of the spinal nerve called the posterior root ganglion.

The motor and sensory roots leave and enter the spinal cord at the **intervertebral foramina**, where the roots unite to form a spinal nerve. At this point the motor and sensory fibers mix together.

Clinical principles have been developed based on the organization of the spinal roots that can be used when damage occurs to the spinal cord or spinal nerves. First, recall that a generalization can be made that the anterior, or ventral, half of the spinal cord is devoted to motor or efferent activity, and the posterior, or dorsal, half is devoted to sensory or **afferent** activity. Which motor and sensory activities are impaired depends on the specific site of lesion in the spinal cord. A **lesion**, or damaged area, impairs motor and/or sensory activities at and below that cord level depending on the specific site of the lesion and the particular tracks interrupted. Naturally, large lesions in the spinal cord impair both sensory and motor functions.

As discussed later in this text, in early embryologic development, paired structures called **somites** are formed on the embryo. These somites differentiate into nonneural tissue (e.g., muscle, bone, and connective tissue). This somitic differentiation results in segmentally distributed zones called dermatomes. The dermatome region of each somite gives rise to a myotome, which is a muscle-forming body, and a skin plate, which is involved in formation of dermal tissue. The sensory component of each spinal nerve is distributed to a dermatome. Fig. 3.3 shows the segmental distribution of cutaneous innervation, showing on the left side of the figure which area of skin is supplied by which spinal nerve. The peripheral nerve field illustration on the right refers to an area of skin that is supplied by a particular peripheral nerve in that spinal nerve's distribution. Myotomes generally follow the same distribution as the dermatome, although there is more overlap of control. Box 3.1 lists the general myotome distribution for muscle innervation of upper and lower limbs by spinal nerves.

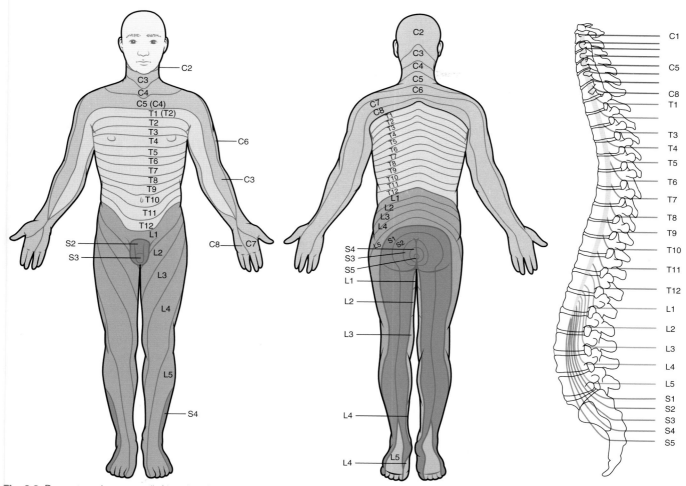

Fig. 3.3 Dermatomal patterns *(left)* and peripheral nerve fields *(right)*. (https://azneuromod.com/dermatomes-link-to-pain/.)

BOX 3.1 Myotome Distributions of the Upper and Lower Extremity

C1/C2: neck flexion/extension
C3: neck lateral flexion
C4: shoulder elevation
C5: shoulder abduction
C6: elbow flexion/wrist extension
C7: elbow extension/wrist flexion
C8: finger flexion
T1: finger abduction
L2: hip flexion
L3: knee extension
L4: ankle dorsiflexion
L5: great toe extension
S1: ankle plantar flexion/ankle eversion/hip extension
S2: knee flexion
S3–S4: perineal reflex

From Magee, D. J. (2009). *Orthopaedic physical assessment* (4th ed., pp. 467–566). Elsevier.

If there is a high spinal cord injury or lesion at the level of the cervical vertebrae, speech production may be affected because the respiratory muscles are controlled by spinal nerves exiting from the intervertebral foramina of the cervical and thoracic regions. The **phrenic nerves**, which supply motor signals to the diaphragm, originate mainly from C4, but contributions are also from C3 and C5. If respiration is stopped, death may follow with a lesion above the third, fourth, and fifth cervical nerves. Spinal cord injuries involving the caudal portion of the cord do not affect speech production but are of interest to the speech-language pathologist (SLP), who may work with spinal cord–injured patients on language or other related problems. These injuries are instructive in understanding the effect of lesions at various levels of the nervous system. Injuries in the spinal cord may produce partial or complete loss of function at the level of the lesion. Function is also completely or partially impaired below the level of the lesion. Spinal cord injuries must be considered very serious because they impair functions beyond those directly controlled at the lesion point.

Cranial Nerves

The **cranial nerves**, in contrast to the spinal nerves, are of more significance to the SLP because most of the cranial nerves have some relation to the speech, language, and hearing process and 7 of the 12 nerves are directly related to speech production and hearing.

On dissection, the 12 pairs of cranial nerves look like thin, gray-white cords. They consist of nerve fiber bundles surrounded by connective tissue. Like the spinal nerves, they are relatively unprotected and may be damaged by trauma. The cranial nerves leave the brain and pass through **foramina** of the skull to reach the sense organs or muscles of the head and neck with which they are associated. Some are associated with special senses such as vision, olfaction, and hearing. Cranial nerves innervate the muscles of the jaw, face, pharynx, larynx, tongue, and neck.

Unlike the spinal nerves, which attach to the cord at regular intervals, the cranial nerves are attached to the brain at irregular intervals. They do not all have dorsal (sensory) and ventral (motor) roots. Some have motor functions, some have sensory functions, and some have mixed functions. Their origin, distribution, brain and brainstem connections, functions, and evolution are complicated. (The cranial nerves are discussed in detail in Chapter 7.) They are traditionally designated by Roman numerals: cranial nerve I, olfactory; cranial nerve II, optic; cranial nerve III, oculomotor; cranial nerve IV, trochlear; cranial nerve V, trigeminal; cranial nerve VI, abducens; cranial nerve VII, facial; cranial nerve VIII,

acoustic-vestibular; cranial nerve IX, glossopharyngeal; cranial nerve X, vagus; cranial nerve XI, spinal accessory; and cranial nerve XII, hypoglossal.

The cranial nerves from the brainstem are explicitly illustrated in Fig. 3.2 and further outlined in Fig. 3.4 regarding their location in the anterior (ventral) view and the anterolateral (ventrolateral) view of the brainstem.

AUTONOMIC NERVOUS SYSTEM

The innervation of involuntary structures such as the heart, smooth muscles, and glands is accomplished through the **autonomic nervous system**. Although this system has primarily indirect effects on speech, language, and hearing, the speech-language pathology and audiology student must be familiar with its contribution to total body function to understand how involuntary but vital functions such as hormonal secretions, visual reflexes, and blood pressure are controlled within the nervous system.

The autonomic nervous system is distributed throughout both the CNS and the PNS. The **enteric nervous system**, which is formed by neuronal plexus in the gastrointestinal tract, is considered a division of the autonomic nervous system. Enteric functioning has a direct effect on the deglutition and digestion of food.

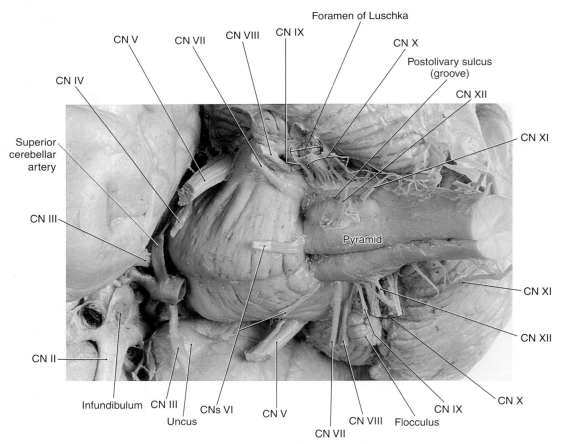

Fig. 3.4 An anterolateral (ventrolateral) view of the brainstem with special emphasis on cranial nerves. Note the position and relations of the foramen of Luschka. (Reprinted from Haines, D. [2006]. *Fundamental neuroscience* [3rd ed.]. Churchill Livingstone.)

Aside from the enteric system that deals directly with swallowing and digestion, the major divisions of the autonomic nervous system are the **sympathetic** and **parasympathetic divisions**, which have almost antagonistic functions. The sympathetic system is the body's alerting system, sometimes referred to as the fight-or-flight system. This part of the autonomic nervous system is responsible for such preparatory measures as accelerating the heart rate, causing constriction of the peripheral blood vessels, raising the blood pressure, and redistributing the blood so that it leaves the skin and intestines to be used in the brain, heart, and skeletal muscles if needed. It serves to raise the eyelids and dilate the pupils. The sympathetic part also decreases peristalsis (the propelling contractions of the intestine) and closes the sphincters.

The parasympathetic part of the autonomic nervous system has an almost opposite calming effect on bodily function. It serves to conserve and restore energy by slowing the heart rate, increasing intestinal peristalsis, and opening the sphincters. As a result of parasympathetic action, other functions, such as increased salivation and increased secretion of the glands of the gastrointestinal tract, may take place.

The autonomic nervous system is composed of both efferent (conducting away from the CNS) and afferent (conducting toward the CNS) nerve fibers. Several similarities and differences exist between the neural control of skeletal muscle and control of visceral effectors, also known as involuntary or smooth muscles. Lower motor neurons function as the final common pathway linking the CNS to skeletal muscle fibers. Similarly, the sympathetic and parasympathetic outflows serve as the final, but often dual, common neural pathway from the CNS to visceral effectors. However, unlike the somatic nervous system, the peripheral visceral motor pathway consists of two neurons. The first is the **preganglionic** neuron, which has its cell body in either the brainstem or the spinal cord. Its axons project as a thinly myelinated preganglionic fiber to an autonomic ganglion. The second, the **postganglionic** neuron, has its cell body in the ganglion and sends unmyelinated axon (postganglionic fiber) to visceral effector cells, such as smooth muscle. Typically, parasympathetic ganglia are close to the effector tissue, and sympathetic ganglia are close to the CNS. Consequently, parasympathetic pathways typically have long preganglionic fibers and short postganglionic fibers, whereas sympathetic pathways more often have short preganglionic and long postganglionic fibers.

The autonomic system also provides neural control of smooth muscle, cardiac muscle, glandular secretory cells, or a combination of these. For example, the gut wall is composed of smooth muscle and glandular epithelium. The sympathetic and parasympathetic systems have overlapping and, as stated previously, antagonistic influences on those viscera located in body cavities and on some structures of the head such as the iris. Visceral targets are also present in the body wall and limbs. These are found in skeletal muscle (blood vessels) and in the skin (blood vessels and sweat glands). Visceral structures of the body wall and extremities are generally regulated by the sympathetic division alone. Thus the sympathetic outflow has a global distribution in that it innervates visceral structures in all parts of the body, whereas the parasympathetic outflow serves only the head and body cavities.

Rarely is autonomic activity solely sympathetic or parasympathetic. Both parts work together in the autonomic nervous system along with the endocrine system to maintain the stability of the body's internal environment or **homeostasis**. The endocrine system is a group of glands and other structures that release internal secretions called hormones into the circulatory system. These hormones influence metabolism and other body processes. The endocrine system includes such organs as the pancreas, pineal gland, pituitary gland, gonads, thyroid, and adrenal glands. These work more slowly than the autonomic nervous system.

The integration of the autonomic activity with endocrine and somatic responses, allowing homeostasis to be maintained, is regulated by the hypothalamus. Evidence exists for a network of central neuronal circuits that includes the hypothalamus and the insula, the amygdala, and an area in the midbrain called the periaqueductal gray matter. These structures receive input from the **nucleus solitarius**, a prominent nucleus of the medulla that receives input from all visceral organs. Input is also received from other nuclei in the brainstem and spinal cord. This network is referred to as the central autonomic network and is probably responsible for adjustments to basic cardiovascular and respiratory functions as they relate to a wide range of body activities, such as food intake, emotional behavior, and mental activity.[15]

As stated earlier, the autonomic nervous system is of importance to the SLP because of its indirect effect on communication functioning. A good example of the power of the autonomic nervous system is the sweaty palms, dry mouth, blushing, and upset stomach some people experience before delivering a speech. Those indirect effects may make a great deal of difference in how well one communicates.

PROTECTION AND NOURISHMENT OF THE BRAIN

The brain and the spinal cord, which make up part of the CNS, PNS, and autonomic nervous system and house most of their mechanisms, must be protected and nourished to continue to function. Following is a discussion of the protection and nourishment of these structures.

Meninges

The spinal cord and brain are the major coordinating and integrating structures for all physical and mental activities of the body and are fortunately well protected. The brain and spinal cord are covered by layers of tissue called the **meninges**. Within certain layers of these meninges is a cushioning layer of clear, colorless fluid called **cerebrospinal fluid** (**CSF**). The meninges are composed of three membranes; moving from the outermost to the innermost covering, they are the **dura mater** ("tough mother" in Latin), the **arachnoid mater**, and the **pia mater**.

The dura mater of the spinal cord is continuous with that of the brain through the opening in the skull called the **foramen** magnum. It consists of two layers that are closely united except where, in certain spots, they separate. In some parts of the dura mater of the brain they separate to form the **venous sinuses** (Fig. 3.5). In other parts of the brain, the inner layer also separates from the outer layer to reflect inward and form partitions, described as complex folds that divide the contents of the cranial cavity into different cerebral subdivisions. These infoldings or **septa** of the dura join with those formed in the opposite hemisphere to create three different double-layered partitions: the falx cerebri, the tentorium cerebelli, and the falx cerebelli (Fig. 3.6).

The **falx cerebri** develops first as two portions that become a single continuous structure later. It reflects downward between the hemispheres, attaching anteriorly and laterally to points on the skull and posteriorly to another partition, the tentorium cerebelli (also known simply as the tentorium). The falx cerebri creates a barrier between the two cerebral hemispheres.

The **falx cerebelli** is located below the tentorium cerebelli on the middle of the occipital bone. This small dural infolding extends into the space between the cerebellar hemispheres, attaching to the occipital crest of the skull and the posterior portion of the tentorium. Part of it encloses the occipital venous sinuses. The falx cerebelli creates a barrier between the two cerebellar hemispheres.

The **tentorium cerebelli** is the second largest of the dural folds. It attaches to bony walls of the skull in the temporal, occipital, and parietal regions. The tentorium cerebelli is the infolding found between the cerebral hemispheres above and the cerebellar hemispheres below. It is only found in mammals and birds, being absent in fish, amphibians, and reptiles. The tentorium separates the cerebrum from the cerebellum.

There is another very small infolding of the dura, the **diaphragma sella**, which forms the roof of the sella turcica, the structure that encloses the pituitary gland. There is a tiny hole in the center of it, allowing the stalk (or infundibulum) of the pituitary to pass through. The anterior and posterior intercavernous sinuses are found in their respective edges of the diaphragma sella. These infoldings are illustrated in Figs. 3.6 and 3.7. They are pictured as they appear on a magnetic resonance imaging (MRI) scan.

When you consider the placement of these sturdy partitions being under and between the cerebral hemispheres as well as over and between the cerebellar hemispheres, it is fairly easy to understand how the dural infoldings brace the brain against rotary displacement.

There is no subdural space between the dura mater and the next layer of the meninges. When there is subdural space identified, it means that tissue damage has occurred to the

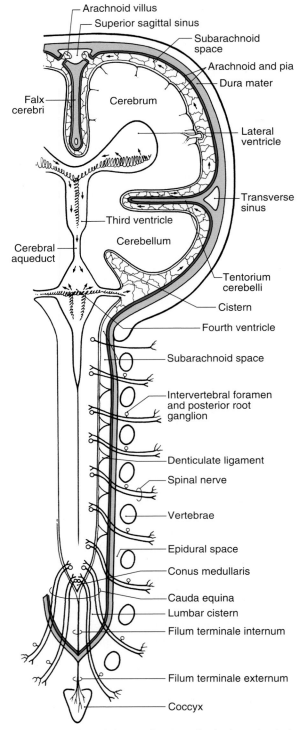

Fig. 3.5 The relation of the meninges to the brain and spinal cord and to their surrounding bony structures. The dura is represented in light green, the arachnoid in dark green. (Reprinted from Haines, D. E. [2000]. *Neuroanatomy: An atlas of structures, sections, and systems* [5th ed.]. Lippincott Williams & Wilkins.)

deepest layer, creating a space. Because there is no normal subdural space, the next meningeal layer can be found immediately below the dura. This second layer is the arachnoid mater, so named because it resembles a spiderweb. This

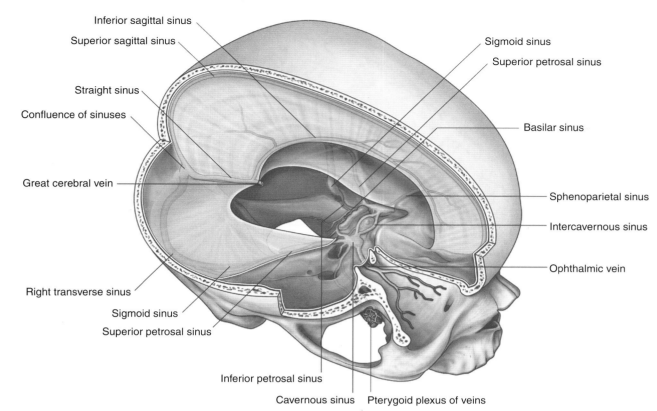

Inferior sagittal sinus

Superior sagittal sinus

Straight sinus

Confluence of sinuses

Great cerebral vein

Right transverse sinus

Sigmoid sinus

Superior petrosal sinus

Inferior petrosal sinus

Cavernous sinus   Pterygoid plexus of veins

Sigmoid sinus

Superior petrosal sinus

Basilar sinus

Sphenoparietal sinus

Intercavernous sinus

Ophthalmic vein

Fig. 3.6 Veins, meninges, and dural sinuses. (Reprinted from Drake, R., Vogl, W., & Mitchell [2006]. *Gray's anatomy for students* [2nd ed.]. Churchill Livingstone.)

membrane bridges over the sulci or folds of the brain. In some areas it projects into the venous sinuses to form arachnoid villi. The arachnoid villi aggregate to form the **arachnoid granulations**. From this location the CSF diffuses into the bloodstream.

Beneath the arachnoid mater layer is a space called the **subarachnoid space**, which is filled with CSF. All cerebral arteries and veins, as well as the cranial nerves, pass through this space. This is why you often hear of subarachnoid hemorrhage or bleed because damage to the brain has resulted in artery or vein tears, and blood is released into this subarachnoid space.

The third meningeal layer, the pia mater, closely adheres to the surface of the brain, covering the gyri (ridges) and going down into the sulci. The pia mater also fuses with the ependyma (a cellular membrane lining the ventricles) to form the choroid plexus of the ventricles. Fig. 3.8 illustrates the meningeal layers.[7]

Ventricular System

The **ventricular system** of the brain has three parts: the lateral ventricles, the third ventricle, and the fourth ventricle. These actually are small cavities within the brain joined to each other by small ducts and canals. Each ventricle contains a tuftlike structure called the **choroid plexus**, which mainly is concerned with the production of CSF.

Fig. 3.9 is an example of a midsagittal view of the brain showing the third and fourth ventricles in relation to the cerebral aqueduct and nearby structures.

The lateral ventricles are paired, one in each hemisphere. Each is a C-shaped cavity and can be divided into a body, located in the parietal lobe, and anterior, posterior, and inferior or temporal horns, extending into the frontal, occipital, and temporal lobes, respectively. The lateral ventricle is connected to the third ventricle by an opening called the intraventricular foramen, or the foramen of Munro. The choroid plexus of the lateral ventricle projects into the cavity on its medial aspect (see Fig. 3.9).

The third ventricle is a small slit between the thalami. It also is connected to the fourth ventricle through the cerebral aqueduct or the **aqueduct of Sylvius**. The choroid plexus is situated above the roof of the ventricle.

The fourth ventricle sits anterior to the cerebellum and posterior to the pons and the superior half of the medulla. It is continuous superiorly with the cerebral aqueduct and the central canal below. The fourth ventricle has a tent-shaped roof, two lateral walls, and a floor (see Fig. 3.9). It contains three small openings: the two lateral foramina of Luschka and the median foramen of Magendie. Through these openings the CSF enters the subarachnoid space. The ventricular system serves as a pathway for the circulation of the CSF. The choroid plexus of the ventricles appears to secrete CSF

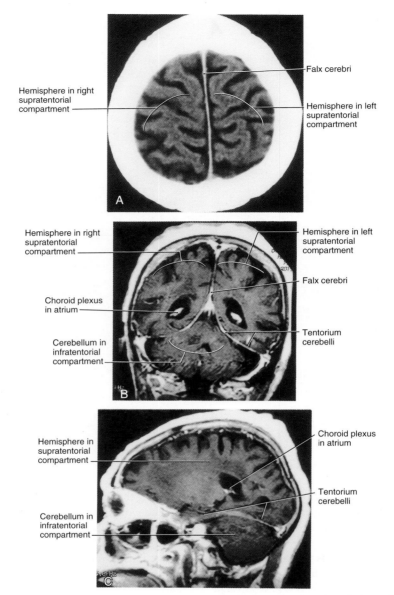

Fig. 3.7 Axial (A), coronal (B), and sagittal (C) T1-weighted magnetic resonance images showing the relations of the falx cerebri (A, B) and the tentorium cerebelli (B, C). Note the positions of the right and left supratentorial compartments and the infratentorial compartment in relation to these large dural reflections in all three planes. (Reprinted from Haines, D. [2006]. *Fundamental neuroscience* [3rd ed.]. Churchill Livingstone.)

actively, although some of the fluid may originate as tissue fluid formed in the brain substance.

Cerebrospinal Fluid

The brain and the spinal cord are suspended in CSF, which serves as a cushion between the CNS and the surrounding bones, thereby protecting the brain against direct trauma. This fluid aids in regulation of intracranial pressure, nourishment of the nervous tissue, and removal of waste products.

The path of circulation of the CSF is illustrated in Fig. 3.10. It flows from the lateral ventricles into the third ventricle, to the fourth ventricle, and into the subarachnoid space. It then travels to reach the inferior surface of the cerebrum and moves superiorly over the lateral aspect of each hemisphere. Some of it moves into the subarachnoid space around the spinal cord.

The CSF produced by the choroid plexus passes through the ventricular system to exit the fourth ventricle through the foramina of Luschka and Magendie. At this point, the CSF enters the subarachnoid space, which is continuous around the brain and spinal cord. The CSF in this subarachnoid space provides the buoyancy necessary to prevent the weight of the brain from crushing nerve roots and blood vessels against the internal surface of the skull. The weight of the brain (~1400 g in air) is reduced to 45 g when suspended in CSF. Consequently, the tethers formed by delicate connective tissue strands traversing the subarachnoid space, the arachnoid trabeculae (see Fig. 3.8), are adequate to maintain the brain in a stable position.

The movement of the CSF through the ventricular system and the subarachnoid space is influenced by two major

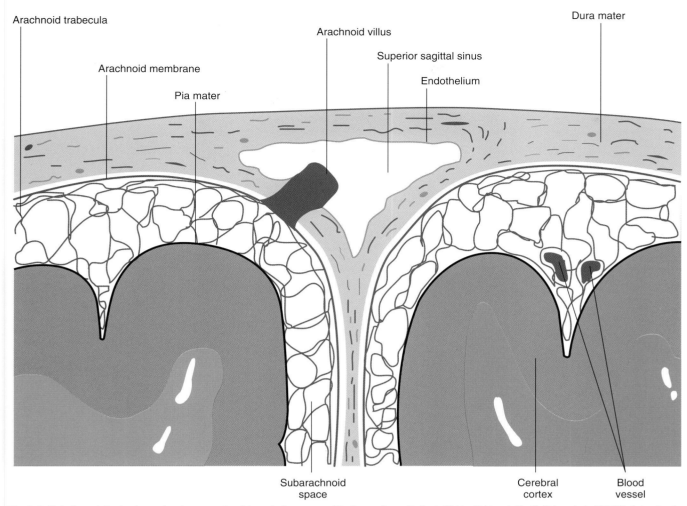

Fig. 3.8 Relation of the brain to the dura, arachnoid, and pia maters. (Redrawn from Bullock, T. H., Orkland, R., & Grinnel, A. [1977]. *Introduction to the nervous system*. W. H. Freeman.)

factors. A subtle pressure gradient exists between the points of production of CSF (the choroid plexus in the cerebral ventricles) and the points of transfer into the venous system (arachnoid villi). Because CSF is not compressible, it tends to move along this gradient. It also moves into the subarachnoid space by purely mechanical means, including gentle movements of the brain on its arachnoid trabecular tethers during normal activities and the pulsations of the numerous arteries found in the subarachnoid space.

Blockage of the CSF movement or a failure of the absorption mechanism results in the accumulation of fluid in the ventricles or around the brain tissue (Fig. 3.11). This results in hydrocephalus and is characterized by an increase in CSF volume enlargement of one or more of the ventricles, and usually an increase in CSF pressure.

The CSF is important in medical diagnostic procedures. The pressure of the fluid can be measured; if it is abnormally high, intracranial tumor, **hemorrhage**, hydrocephalus, meningitis, or **encephalitis** may be suspected. Chemical and cell studies may be made on CSF that is drawn out of the nervous system through a procedure called a lumbar puncture or spinal tap. This route also may be used to inject drugs to combat

infection or induce anesthesia. Circulation of the CSF is illustrated in Fig. 3.10.

Blood Supply of the Brain

The blood serves the brain much as food serves the body; it nourishes it by supplying its most important element, oxygen. The brain uses ~20% of the blood in the body at any given time and requires ~25% of the body's oxygen to function maximally. Initially blood is delivered to the brain through four main arteries. Two large internal carotid arteries are on either side of the neck; these are a result of bifurcation, or splitting, of the common carotid artery from the heart. The other two main arteries supplying the brain are the vertebral arteries (Fig. 3.12).

Internal Carotid Arteries and Their Branches

The **internal carotid arteries** ascend in the neck and pass through the base of the skull at the carotid canal of the temporal bone. Each artery then runs horizontally forward and perforates the dura mater. After entering the subarachnoid space, the artery turns posteriorly and, at the medial end of the lateral sulcus, divides into the anterior and middle

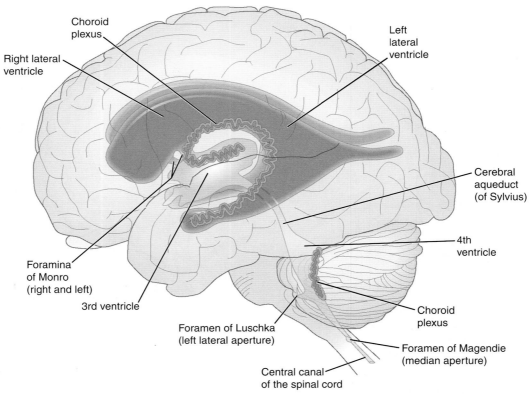

Fig. 3.9 The brain ventricles and the cerebrospinal fluid. This is a transparent view, looking from the left side of the brain. The two lateral ventricles communicate with the third ventricle, which in turn communicates with the fourth ventricle. (Modified from Boron, W., & Boulpaep, E. [2009]. *Medical physiology* [2nd ed.]. Elsevier.)

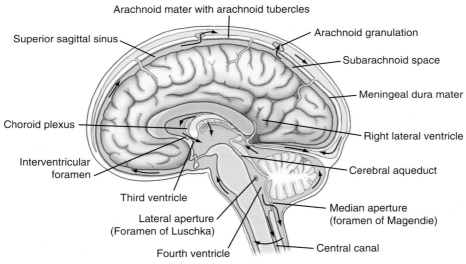

Fig. 3.10 Cerebrospinal fluid circulation.

cerebral arteries. Other cerebral arteries are also given off by the internal carotid artery. The ophthalmic artery supplies the eye, the frontal area of the scalp, the dorsum of the nose, and the ethmoid and frontal sinuses. The posterior communicating artery runs posteriorly above the oculomotor nerve and joins the posterior cerebral artery, forming part of the circle of Willis. The anterior communicating artery joins the

two anterior cerebral arteries together in the circle of Willis (Fig. 3.13).

Through these cortical branches, the internal carotid artery provides the blood supply to a large portion of the cerebral hemisphere. The anterior cerebral artery supplies the medial surface of the cortex as far back as the parietal-temporal-occipital sulcus. It also supplies the so-called leg

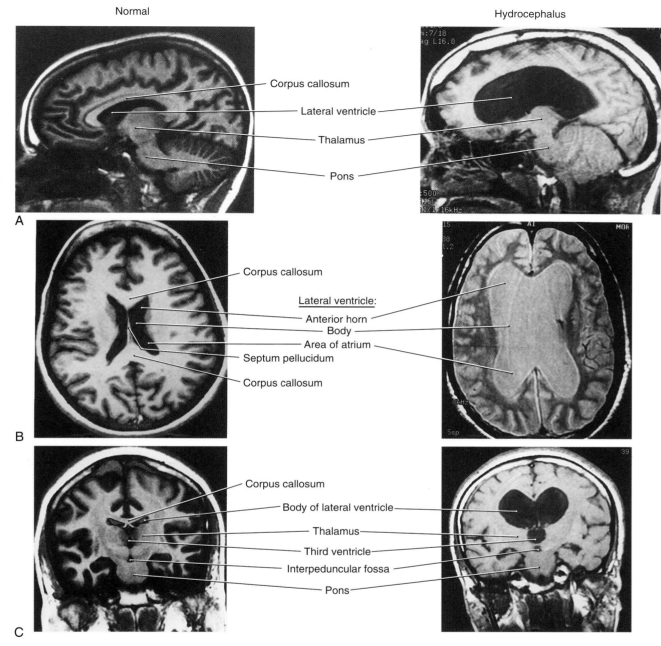

Normal   Hydrocephalus

Fig. 3.11 Comparison of normal and hydrocephalic brains in sagittal (A), axial (B), and coronal (C) planes as seen on magnetic resonance images. (Reprinted from Haines, D. [2006]. *Fundamental neuroscience* [3rd ed.]. Churchill Livingstone.)

areas of the motor strip. Branches of this artery supply a small portion of the caudate nucleus, lentiform nucleus, and internal capsule. Following is a summary of the internal carotid artery branches (see Fig. 3.12):

- The ophthalmic artery gives rise to the central artery of the retina; damage to this artery (including ophthalmic aneurysms) causes ipsilateral visual loss.
- The posterior communicating artery joins the posterior cerebral artery and the anterior choroidal artery and follows along the optic tract.
- The anterior cerebral artery passes superiorly over the optic chiasm and is joined by its counterpart the anterior

communicating artery; it supplies blood to the hypothalamus and the optic chiasm.
- The middle cerebral artery usually is the larger of the two terminal branches of the internal carotid artery (Fig. 3.14). The middle cerebral artery is the largest branch of the internal carotid. Its branches supply the entire lateral surface of the hemisphere except for the small area of the motor strip supplied by the anterior cerebral artery, the occipital pole, and the inferolateral surface of the hemisphere, which is supplied by the posterior cerebral artery. The middle cerebral artery's central branches also provide the primary blood supply to the lentiform and caudate nuclei and the internal capsule.

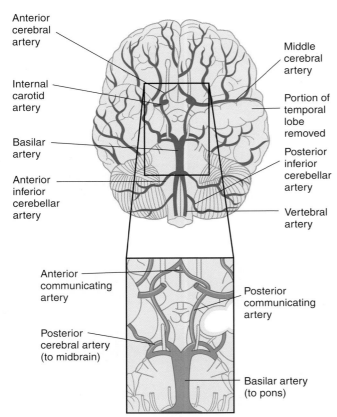

Anterior cerebral artery

Internal carotid artery

Basilar artery

Anterior inferior cerebellar artery

Middle cerebral artery

Portion of temporal lobe removed

Posterior inferior cerebellar artery

Vertebral artery

Anterior communicating artery

Posterior communicating artery

Posterior cerebral artery (to midbrain)

Basilar artery (to pons)

Fig. 3.12 The major arteries of the brain. Ventral view: the enlargement of the boxed area showing the circle of Willis. (From Aitken, L., Marshall, A., & Chaboyer, W. [2012]. *ACCCN's critical care nursing* [2nd ed.]. Mosby Australia.)

Vertebral Artery and Its Branches

The **vertebral artery** passes through the foramina in the upper six cervical vertebrae and enters the skull through the foramen magnum. It passes upward and forward along the medulla and at the lower border of the pons and joins the vertebral artery from the opposite side to form the basilar artery. Before the formulation of the basilar artery, several branches are given off, including the following:

- The meningeal branches, which supply the bone and dura of the posterior cranial fossa
- The posterior spinal artery, which supplies the posterior third of the spinal cord
- The anterior spinal artery, which supplies the anterior two-thirds of the spinal cord
- The posterior inferior cerebellar artery, which supplies part of the cerebellum, the medulla, and the choroid plexus of the fourth ventricle
- The medullary arteries, which are distributed to the medulla
  After the basilar artery is formed by the union of the opposite vertebral arteries, it ascends and then divides at the upper border of the pons into the two posterior cerebral arteries. These arteries supply the inferolateral surface of the temporal lobe and the lateral and medial surfaces of the occipital lobe (i.e., the visual cortex). They also supply parts of the thalamus and other internal structures (see Fig. 3.13).

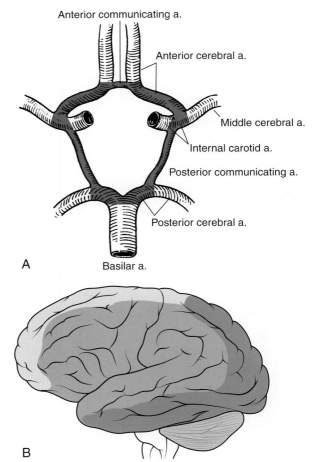

Anterior communicating a.

Anterior cerebral a.

Middle cerebral a.

Internal carotid a.

Posterior communicating a.

Posterior cerebral a.

A   Basilar a.

B

Fig. 3.13 The cerebral arterial circle (circle of Willis; (A) The circle of Willis. (B) Dark blue area shows Posterior Cerebral Artery circulation; Light blue area shows Middle Cerebral Artery circulation; White area shows Anterior Cerebral Artery circulation. (A, From Nolte, J. [2010]. *Essentials of the human brain.* Mosby; B, from Lundy-Eckman, L. [2013]. *Neuroscience* [4th ed.]. Saunders.)

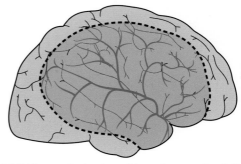

Fig. 3.14 Middle cerebral artery. (From Kenyon, K., & Kenyon, J. [2010]. *The physiotherapist's pocket book* [2nd ed.]. Elsevier.)

Other branches of the basilar artery include the following (see Fig. 3.12):

- The pontine arteries, which enter the pons
- The labyrinthine artery, which supplies the internal ear
- The anterior inferior cerebellar artery, which supplies the anterior and inferior parts of the cerebellum
- The superior cerebellar artery, which supplies the superior portion of the cerebellum

Circle of Willis

The **circle of Willis**, or the circulus arteriosus, is formed by the anastomosis of the two internal carotid arteries with the two vertebral arteries. The anterior communicating, anterior cerebral, internal carotid, posterior communicating, posterior cerebral, and basilar arteries are all part of the circle of Willis (see Fig. 3.13). This formation of arteries allows distribution of the blood entering from the internal carotid artery or vertebral artery to any part of both hemispheres. Cortical and central branches arise from the circle and further supply the brain.

The bloodstreams from the internal carotid artery and vertebral artery on both sides come together at a certain point in the posterior communicating artery. At that point the pressure is equal, and they do not mix. Should, however, the internal carotid artery or the vertebral artery be occluded or blocked, the blood will pass forward or backward across that point to compensate for the reduced flow. The circle of Willis also allows blood to flow across the midline of the brain if an artery on one side is occluded. The circle of Willis thereby serves a safety valve function for the brain, allowing collateral circulation (or flow of blood through an alternate route) to take place if the flow is reduced to one area. The state of a person's collateral circulation helps determine the outcome after a vascular insult, such as a stroke, occurs and affects blood flow to the brain.

GENERAL PRINCIPLES OF NEUROLOGIC ORGANIZATION

Certain fundamental principles of neurologic organization are particularly crucial to the understanding and diagnosis of communication disorders. The following principles will also be built on in later chapters.

Contralateral Motor Control

The first principle to remember is that major movement patterns in human beings have **contralateral** neurologic control in the brain. The arms and legs are represented in the motor strip of the cerebral cortex in a contralateral fashion. In other words, the cerebral hemisphere on one side of the body controls movements of the arm and leg on the other side of the body. This contralateral motor control is brought about by the crossing of the major voluntary motor pathway at the level of the lower brainstem. Auditory and visual sensory systems also have some contralateral organization, a fact that will become clinically important (see Chapters 5 and 6). The cranial nerves, as discussed subsequently, have mixed control; thus to know the innervation pattern, you must know which cranial nerve and/or muscle group is involved.

If a patient sent to the SLP has a severe language disorder and some paralysis of the right arm and leg, these symptoms suggest that the brain lesion causing this motor deficit is probably in the left cerebral hemisphere (Fig. 3.15). The severe language disturbance accompanying the right limb paralysis serves as a confirming sign of left-sided brain lesion because in the majority of the population language dominance is located in the left hemisphere. Why the nervous system provides contralateral motor control of the limbs is not completely known,

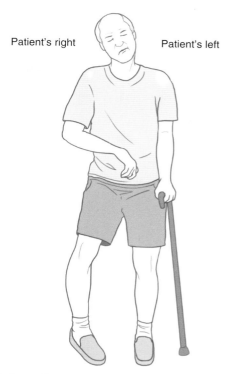

Patient's right   Patient's left

Fig. 3.15 Patient with a lesion of the internal capsule on the left side. This man exhibits a right hemiparesis, drooping of the lower part of the face on the right, and slight turning of the head to the left (weak left sternocleidomastoid muscle).

but the fact illustrates that knowledge of principles of neurologic organization can be used to posit the location of causative lesions seen in neurology and speech pathology.

Ipsilateral Motor Control

If a lesion occurs in the nervous system below the crossing of the major descending motor pathways, the effect is observed below the level of the lesion on the same side of the body where the lesion occurs. In many spinal cord injuries, paralysis and sensory loss occur below the point of injury. Thus a second important principle is to determine whether effects of lesions are **ipsilateral** or contralateral. An illustration of how the tongue might deviate ipsilateral to a lesion is shown in Fig. 3.16. In this figure, the tongue is paralyzed on the left side from surgery to remove a lymph node from the left side of the neck, resulting in damage to the ipsilateral hypoglossal nerve fibers.

Bilateral Speech Motor Control

For the most part, the midline muscles of the body in the head, neck, and trunk tend to be represented bilaterally, and the nerve fibers supplying these regions, with certain exceptions, descend from both cerebral hemispheres. This **bilateral** neural control provides smooth, symmetric movement for those muscles used in speaking: the lips, tongue, soft palate, jaw, abdominal muscles, and diaphragm. The principle of bilateral control of speech muscles suggests that serious involvement of the speech muscles usually results from diseases that affect

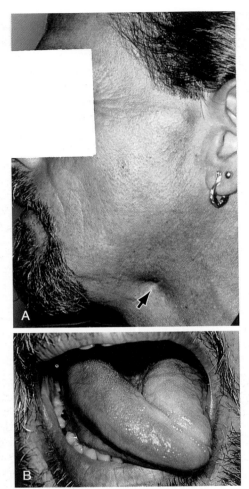

Fig. 3.16 Paralysis of the tongue on the left side. Removal of a lymph node from the left side of the neck (A, *arrow*) inadvertently resulted in damage to peripheral fibers of the hypoglossal nerve on that side. The tongue deviates to the left (side of the lesion) on protrusion (B). (Reprinted from Haines, D. [2006]. *Fundamental neuroscience* [3rd ed.]. Churchill Livingstone.)

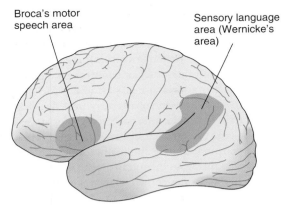

Fig. 3.17 Motor and sensory language areas. (Reprinted from Castro, A., Merchut, M. P., Neafsey, E. J., & Wurster, R. D. [2002]. *Neuroscience: An outline approach.* Mosby.)

bilateral neurologic mechanisms. With **unilateral** damage to the nervous system, effects on speech are generally less serious, and compensatory mechanisms are made available from the other side of the midline speech system.

Representation of the body is found in an inverted fashion on the motor areas of the cerebral cortex. Pathways concerned with movements of the lower limbs originate in the upper parts of the motor strip, whereas movements of the head and neck originate at the lower end of the motor strip, just above the sylvian fissure. The area surrounding the left sylvian fissure contains major areas for language processing. The anatomic relations of motor speech areas and language suggest that speech and language disturbances may commonly coexist because of the close proximity of their control areas on the cortex.[10]

An example of bilateral damage effects of motor speech lesions may be seen in spastic dysarthria. When damage to the upper motor neurons (the neurons that originate in the brain) occurs, spasticity results. With spasticity,

affected muscles (in this case, those dealing with articulation, respiration, and phonation) show an increased resistance to passive movements or movement manipulation. The more rapidly the individual tries to move the articulators (or even an upper or lower extremity, as in cerebral palsy), the greater is the resistance to the movement. In spastic dysarthria, bilateral damage to the upper motor neurons usually is caused by stroke, head trauma, or a degenerative disease (see Chapter 8). The bilateral damage is within both direct activation pathways (corticobulbar and corticospinal tracts) and indirect pathways (extrapyramidal tract).

Unilateral Language Mechanisms

An impressive facet of cerebral asymmetry is that language mechanisms, for the most part, are unilaterally controlled in the brain, in contrast to the bilateral speech muscle mechanism. Language dominance the world over is primarily in the left brain. Handedness usually appears between 18 and 48 months of age. Among the adult population, more than 95% of right-handed people have their language mechanisms in the left cerebral hemisphere. Left-handed people are more variable. Some are right brained for language; others have bilateral representation of language. Fig. 3.17 illustrates the left hemisphere and its relation to the motor and sensory (receptive) language areas. The obvious clinical principle suggested by these facts is that major language disturbance is a neurologic sign of left cerebral injury and that the left hemisphere has special anatomic properties for language.[8]

Scheme of Cortical Organization

Students and clinicians should have in mind a general scheme of organization of the cortex because it is the site of most language functions. Although any such scheme is oversimplified and exaggerated, it nevertheless provides a crude but workable framework for conceptualizing functional localization. Later chapters in this text detail the specifics of cortical localization.

The right and left hemispheres may be designated as nonverbal and verbal, and the anterior and posterior portions may be characterized as motor and sensory areas. The central sulcus divides the cerebral hemispheres into anterior and posterior regions. Fig. 3.18 provides a lateral view of the cerebral hemisphere, showing lobes and the sensory and motor cortices. In human beings, approximately half of the volume of the cerebral cortex is taken up by the frontal cortex. The frontal lobe contains the primary motor cortex, the premotor cortex, and Broca area (the primary motor speech association area). In the anterior portion of the frontal lobes are the prefrontal areas, which are generally concerned with behavioral control of both cognitive and emotional functions.

Szczapanski et al.[13] investigated the role of the prefrontal cortex using imaging and concluded that this brain region controls "different aspects of executive function and, in turn, make different contributions to goal-directed behaviors." Lesions to the prefrontal cortex may affect attention, memory, planning and problem solving, mental flexibility, and language skills. Mental shifts become difficult, and perseveration and rigidity are observed, as are a lack of self-awareness and a tendency toward concreteness. In brief, the frontal lobe appears to excel in the control, integration, and regulation of emotional and cognitive behavior. Cortical areas of the left

hemisphere that mediate the processing of language are shown in Fig. 3.19. Lesions in the inferior frontal lobe may result in **Broca**, or **expressive**, **aphasia**, whereas damage to the angular gyrus, the supramarginal gyrus, and the superior temporal gyrus may result in **Wernicke**, or **receptive**, **aphasia**.

In contrast, the posterior cortex appears to dominate the control, integration, and regulation of sensory behavior. The defects arising from the posterior cortex are related to the specific sensory association areas implicated by a lesion.

The occipital lobe, as previously noted, contains the primary visual cortex and visual association areas. Deficits in the primary cortex result in blind spots in the visual field, and total destruction of the cortex produces complete blindness. Visual imperception and agnosias (see Chapter 5) are associated with the visual association areas.

The left parietal lobe is associated with **constructional disturbances** and visuospatial defects. Disorders of recognition, called agnosias, are common. The inferior parietal lobe is concerned with language association tasks, and lesions there cause defects in reading and writing. Contralateral neglect is associated with hemispheric lesions of the nondominant parietal association cortex. Such patients usually neglect stimuli on their left (Fig. 3.20). In extreme cases patients do not recognize the left side of their own body, a condition termed *asomatognosia*. An example is when a patient has a left neglect and ignores the left side when getting dressed or grooming.

The temporal lobe on the left is concerned with hearing and related functions. It contains the primary auditory and auditory association areas. Auditory memory storage and complex auditory perception are among the functions of the temporal lobe. An area known as the speech zone surrounds the sylvian fissure and appears to contain the major components of the language mechanism. Damage in the speech zone produces Wernicke aphasia (see Fig. 3.19).

With a clinical knowledge of primary sensory and related association areas and behavioral correlates to these areas, the SLP is able to infer the approximate location of a lesion from the patient's behavioral symptoms and to recognize the well-known speech-language syndromes associated with cortical dysfunction. The general clinical principle is that specific cortical deficits can be associated with specific behavioral syndromes. A major exception to this is difficulty with word-finding or naming, which is typically a nonlocalizable symptom.

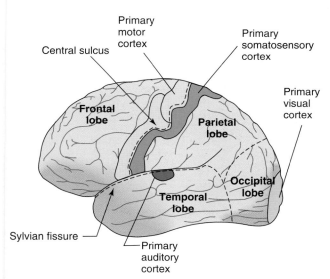

Fig. 3.18 Lateral view of the cerebral hemisphere. *Dashed lines demarcate major lobes.* (Reprinted from Castro, A., Merchut, M. P., Neafsey, E. J., & Wurster, R. D. [2002]. *Neuroscience: An outline approach.* Mosby.)

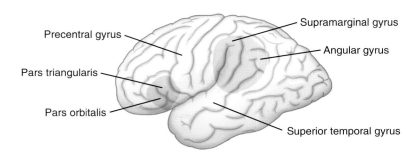

Fig. 3.19 Cortical areas that mediate the processing of language. Lesions in the pars orbitalis and pars triangularis of the inferior frontal lobe result in Broca aphasia, whereas damage in the supramarginal and angular gyri and adjacent superior temporal gyrus results in Wernicke aphasia.

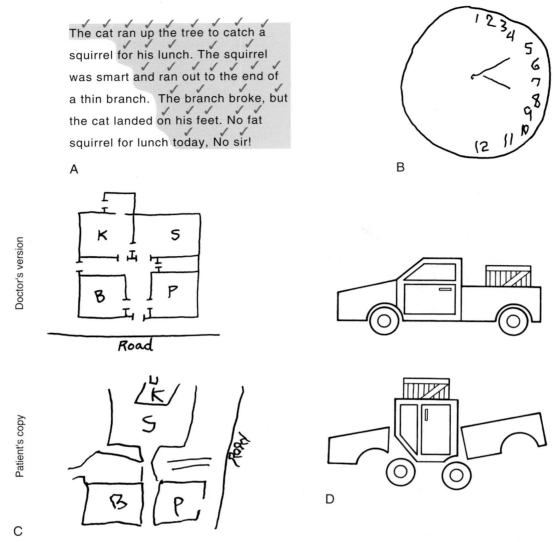

A

B

Doctor's version

Patient's copy

C

D

Fig. 3.20 Signs (A–D) of damage to the nondominant parietal association cortex. (Reprinted from Haines, D. [2006]. *Fundamental neuroscience* [3rd ed.]. Churchill Livingstone.)

NEURODIAGNOSTIC STUDIES IN SPEECH AND LANGUAGE

The structures of the brain believed to be critical for speech and language function have been established by the clinico-pathologic method in neurology. Developed into a powerful technique by French neurologist Jean Charcot, this method establishes a relation between the site of a lesion and the behavioral functions that are lost or modified. The underlying assumption is that the area of lesion is related to the lost or disordered function. This simple logic is important in clinical neurology; it forms the basis of neurologic diagnosis and is the foundation of the historically traditional neurologic examination. Some of these neurobehavioral signs have been discussed in Chapter 2 and in this chapter.

Fortunately for the evolution of medical science and clinical treatment, the field of neurology has been advanced through the years by technology that has vastly clarified

the actual sites of lesions and made diagnoses more valid and reliable, now through relatively noninvasive means. Objective neurodiagnostic tests, such as computed tomography (CT), MRI, electroencephalography (EEG), and evoked related potentials (ERPs) as well as other clinical neurodiagnostic tests, have established the value of the clinicopathologic method in medicine yet dramatically enhanced the identification and treatment of neurologic disorders, including those impacting communication. SLPs are expected to be somewhat familiar with these types of studies and use the reported information (if available) to plan diagnostic and treatment procedures. Use of the information provided by these studies can also help the SLP to identify inconsistencies between the behaviorally based diagnostic findings and the findings of the reported study. Speech and language function is quite vulnerable to neurologic changes; the results of the imaging or electrophysiologic study may not be consistent, perhaps warranting more exploration by one or both. Therefore, as we come to the end of our overview of the communicative nervous system, a brief discussion of some of the more commonly used neurodiagnostic methodologies that the SLP might find reported in the medical record or research articles seems fitting to include at this point.

Static Brain Imaging

CT and MRI were the foundation tools of early neurologic imaging, permitting study of the structure of the human brain with a degree of detail that is occasionally comparable with the detail revealed by postmortem examination. In fact, MRI, which generates fine cross sections of brain structure without penetrating radiation, may even go beyond postmortem examination because it allows views of multiple slices of the brain.

The CT scan yields a three-dimensional representation of the brain (Fig. 3.21), unlike the conventional radiograph, which provides a two-dimensional projection of a three-dimensional object. On a radiograph, the body appears on **x-ray** films as overlapping structures that are sometimes difficult to distinguish. The CT scanner uses an x-ray beam that is passed through the brain from one side of the head, and the radiation not absorbed by the intervening tissue is absorbed by a series of detectors revolving around the subject's head. The data from the radiation detectors allow a calculation of

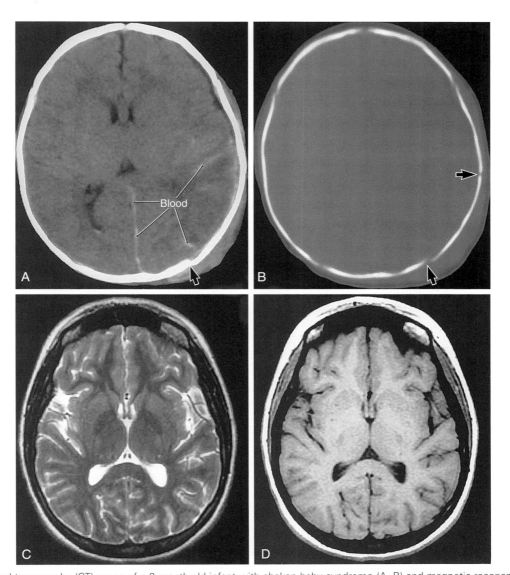

Fig. 3.21 Computed tomography (CT) scans of a 2-month-old infant with shaken baby syndrome (A, B) and magnetic resonance imaging (MRI) of a normal 20-year-old woman (C, D). On the CT study, note that the brain detail is less than on the MRI but that the presence of blood (A, in the interhemispheric fissure between the hemisphere and the brain substance) is obvious. In the same patient, the bone window (B) clearly illustrates the outline of the skull but also clearly shows skull fractures (*arrows* in A, B). In this infant, the ventricles on the left are largely compressed, and the gyri have largely disappeared because of pressure from bleeding into the hemisphere. The pressure results in the effacement of the sulci and gyri on the left side. In the T2-weighted image (C), cerebrospinal fluid is white, internal brain structures are seen in excellent detail, and vessels are obvious. In the T1-weighted image (D), cerebrospinal fluid is dark and internal structures of the brain are somewhat less obvious. (Reprinted from Haines, D. [2006]. *Fundamental neuroscience* [3rd ed.]. Churchill Livingstone.)

the density of tissue in a particular slice of brain. A computer then reconstructs a two-dimensional cross-sectional picture of the brain observed by the camera. Several cross sections may be printed corresponding to different planes through the head. Contrast substances are sometimes injected in the patient to increase the density of damaged tissue. This enhancement technique allows clearer visualization and more accurate diagnosis. Spiral CT, in which the x-ray tube rotates continuously around the patients while the table moves, was developed in the early 1990s along with a computational method that would eliminate the motion artifact this introduced. Spiral CT allowed much more flexible and rapid study. Because CT studies are quicker and less expensive to perform than MRI, the technology is more widely available in general medical settings. CT is frequently used in the emergency department and other acute settings. It is more sensitive to skull fracture and can detect the presence of foreign bodies, such as glass and metal, that are radiopaque. It can reveal the presence of blood in the linings and parenchyma of the brain and, therefore, is the first study of choice in a vascular event of unknown etiology so that hemorrhage could be ruled out first. Because MRI uses a magnetic field, CT is the study that would be chosen for patients with pacemakers, defibrillators, and other such devices.

MRI, probably the most widely used diagnostic imaging technique in neurology, generates cross-sectional images by using radio waves, a strong magnetic field, and gradient coils to detect the distribution of water molecules in living tissue (Figs. 3.22 and 3.23). The technique allows accurate assessment of brain tissue densities, and an excellent pictorial image can be generated by the computer. The explanation of the technology is beyond the scope of this text, but it is helpful to know what tissue weighting, which you will see as T1, T2, or proton density (PDW), does for an image. These parameters determine the contrast between tissues, allowing certain tissues to be more easily seen in an image. A T1-weighted image highlights tissues such as fat (like white matter) and proteins, whereas CSF will appear dark. A T2-weighted image makes CSF lighter and fat appears darker, which may make this weighting more useful for identifying pathologies. If the contrast between these T1 tissues and CSF is not what is of interest, a PDW will be used, which will highlight differences in the proton densities of the two tissues with the denser tissue emphasized in the image and gray matter appearing brighter than white matter.[9]

Generally, MRI is more sensitive to abnormalities than CT. However, it is significantly more expensive to generate the image, and it is more time consuming. In acute situations, CT scans may be preferable. The major drawback of CT is exposure to radiation. Vymazal et al.[16] found that either technology can provide good diagnostic information when used by experienced personnel and good quality scanners.

Diffusion-weighted imaging (DWI) is another way of enhancing the usefulness of MRI in some cases. DWI allows the imaging of molecular motion or diffusion of water protons within tissue. DWI, which highlights reduced diffusion, has been found to be very useful to rapidly identify acute cerebral ischemia or loss of blood flow to an area. MRI study using DWI can be positive for reduced diffusion in these cases as early as 30 minutes after onset.[11] Fig. 3.24 shows the usefulness of DWI in identifying axonal shearing, which has been typically difficult to verify in traumatic injury.

Another advance in imaging to better see the white and gray matter in the brain is through voxel-based morphometry (VBM). This is primarily a research tool in which statistical methods originally applied to positron emission tomography (PET) scans are used on MRI scans. A voxel is the basic unit of CT measurement, and the term comes from a combination of the words *volume* and *pixel*. It is essentially an imaged "slab" of tissue that has been divided into small volume elements called voxels, with each voxel having an *x*, *y*, and *z* dimension on which statistical and other manipulations can be studied.[1] VBM has been used to study changes in gray matter volume in normal development, aging, and disease, including speech-language disorders.[11] Studies on normal subjects have focused on the impact of learning and practice on brain structures. For example, the brain changes in response to learning a second language or a complex motor task such as juggling. Comparing the images of MRI, functional MRI (fMRI), and VBM has made it possible for advances in VBM for future research and clinical assessment.

Dynamic or Functional Brain Imaging

CT and MRI are unable to detect certain forms of cellular and subcellular brain pathology directly. Dynamic neuroimaging procedures that use emission tomography (PET and single-photon emission CT [SPECT]) are helpful in cases in which imaging of brain structures alone is not decisive. For instance, in some cases of early dementia, CT and MRI scans appear normal, but language and neuropsychological testing reveals serious cerebral dysfunction.

fMRI uses an MRI scanner to measure regional blood flow, cerebral blood volume, and change in blood oxygenation. fMRI study results in inferences about the location of brain activity. The most common fMRI study is a blood oxygenation level–dependent (BOLD) contrast study. This study tracks the hemodynamic response to neural activity. This means that changes in blood flow and blood oxygenation are traced. fMRI has begun to be a popular technology for research by SLPs in collaboration with neurology and radiology. Brain activity in such areas as acquired language disorders, autism, and other communication disorders has been investigated with BOLD MRI.[4,5,9]

PET is a visual technique in which the subject is given a radioactively labeled form of glucose, which is metabolized by the brain. The radioactivity is later recorded by a special detector. Unlike CT and MRI scans, a PET scan measures metabolic activity in different brain areas. More active areas metabolize more glucose, focusing more radioactivity in these areas. Thus regional three-dimensional quantification of glucose and oxygen metabolism or blood flow in the human brain is achieved. This technique is advantageous in that glucose metabolism is a more direct measure of the function of neural tissue than is cerebral blood flow,

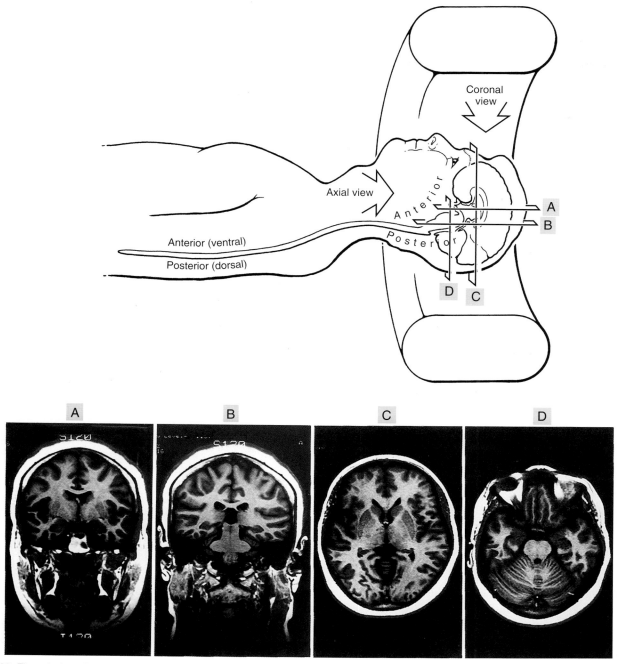

Fig. 3.22 The relation of imaging planes to the brain. The diagram shows the usual orientation of a patient in a magnetic resonance imaging machine and the planes of the four scans (T1-weighted images) that are shown. (A, B) Coronal scans; (C, D) axial scans. (Reprinted from Haines, D. [2006]. *Fundamental neuroscience* [3rd ed.]. Churchill Livingstone.)

particularly in patients whose regulatory vascular mechanisms are affected by cerebral injury or disease. PET scan studies have been used to research higher mental functions during different cognitive and language tasks and appear to offer an excellent tool for the study of language in the human brain. This technology is expensive because it requires a cyclotron or atomic accelerator. Because of the color limitations of this text, an example PET scan cannot be displayed, but many can be found through a search of web images. One interesting example is found from the Berkeley Labs site *(www.lbl.gov)*.

SPECT uses the mechanism of CT scan reconstruction, but instead of detecting x-rays, the instrument detects single photons emitted from an external tracer. Radioactive compounds that emit gamma rays are injected into the subject. As these biochemicals reach the brain, emissions are picked up that are converted into patterns of metabolism or blood flow in three-dimensional cross sections of the brain. SPECT has somewhat better temporal resolution than PET, but its spatial resolution is less than PET or MRI and it is more invasive. The equipment is less expensive because a cyclotron is not required, and it therefore may be used at small medical centers.

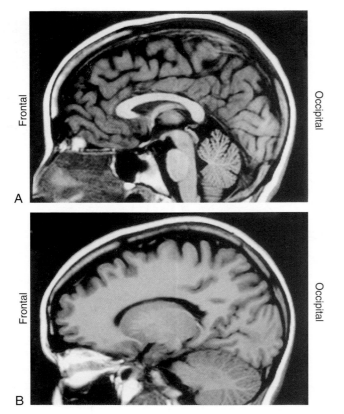

Fig. 3.23 Magnetic resonance imaging of the brain in the median sagittal plane (A) and in the sagittal plane but off the midline (B). The frontal lobe is to the left, and the occipital lobe is to the right. (Reprinted from Haines, D. [2006]. *Fundamental neuroscience* [3rd ed.]. Churchill Livingstone.)

Measures of Neural Connectivity

Diffusion tensor imaging (DTI) is the preferred method used to study white matter, as is VBM for gray matter. DTI is a recently developed technique that is an extended version of DWI. It can measure neuronal activity and, in particular, the white matter neuronal cell networks (including the directionality of the actual tracts). Diffusion of water can be described as isotropic, which means that diffusion occurs in the same degree in all directions, or anisotropic, meaning that diffusion pattern is dependent on the direction being viewed. Because diffusion of water molecules occurs in the brain much more easily along lines that are parallel to axon bundles rather than perpendicular to them, the diffusion is anisotropic. Therefore this diffusion in the brain tissue must be assessed in multiple directions, with the resulting images then combined into an isotropic map, imaging the integrity of white matter tracts. DTI considers three factors in constructing the final image. One factor is the fractional anisotropy (FA); this results in essentially a gray scale representing the degree of variation of fiber direction at any point. The other two factors considered are the mean diffusivity (MD), or overall displacement of the molecules in that voxel, and the direction of greatest water mobility, or the principal eigenvector (PE). FA values have been established for the normal brain, which will allow differentiation between gray and white matter. Intensity (FA)

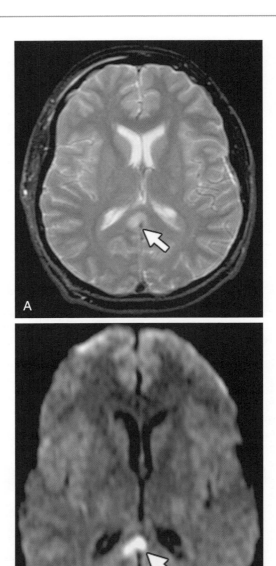

Fig. 3.24 Axonal shearing injury. (A) Axial T2-weighted image shows a subtle area of reduced diffusion within the right paramedian corpus callosum *(arrow)*. (B) Axial diffusion-weighted image more clearly demonstrates abnormal reduced diffusion within the callosal lesion *(arrow)*. (From Nadich, T.P., Krayenbuhl, N., Kollias, S., et al. [2013]. White matter. In T. P. Nadich, M. Castillo, S. Cha, & Smirniotopoulos [Eds.], *Imaging of the brain*. Elsevier/Saunders.)

and directionality (PE) data can be combined into spectacular images called DTI color maps. In these maps, red signifies diffusion in a left-right direction, blue predominantly in a superior-inferior direction, and green represents diffusion in the anterior-posterior plane. Diffusion tensor tractography uses the data from DTI to construct a three-dimensional image of axon bundles. The Human Connectome Project is a large, National Institutes of Health–funded research project to map the human brain. It was begun in 1990 and completed in 2003. Breathtaking images made from DTI studies can be found at the project's website gallery.[8]

A promising recent functional imaging technique that has been put to use both clinically and in research protocols is that of optical imaging, which uses the technology called near infrared spectroscopy (NIRS)[14] to assess response to brain activation. It is similar to fMRI in its objective, but unlike fMRI, which measures changes in deoxygenated hemoglobin, NIRS can monitor changes in deoxygenated and oxygenated hemoglobin plus changes in localized blood volume. Optical imaging is based on measuring the light absorption of different tissue properties through use of various infrared sources and detectors. It is noninvasive and can be done during motor, sensory, and cognitive tasks. Zeller et al.[17] used optical imaging in a visual-spatial task with patients with Alzheimer disease and found decreased activation in the parietal lobe compared with control subjects.

Measures of Timing of Neural Activity

It is well known that neurons emit small currents of electrical activity. In 1924, Hans Berger developed the first method to capture this activity. Other methods evolved from his early invention of the EEG.

Electroencephalography

An older diagnostic technique, EEG has been used for decades to diagnose lesions of the brain and help clarify their nature. EEG measures voltage fluctuations resulting from ionic currents between neurons in the brain. It measures these changes with the use of noninvasive scalp electrodes. EEG is used to study seizure activity and diagnose epilepsy and its subtypes. The temporal resolution of EEG is excellent, but the limitation is that it is not correlated with any specific brain activity.

Another current use of EEG technology is the prediction of outcomes from patients with coma-related injuries. According to Boccagni et al.,[2,3] standard EEG has been proven to be a predictor of recovery of cognitive functioning in patients after coma caused by cerebral anoxia.

Evoked Potentials

Measurement of ERP is a derivative of EEG. Rather than measuring spontaneous potentials detected from nervous system activity, this study reveals specific electrical potentials evoked and time-locked to the presentation of a known stimulus. The stimuli used are usually sensory (visual, auditory, somatosensory). If a stimulus is repeated enough times and each repetition produces a circumscribed electrical response, computer averaging can establish the onset of a response and its termination. ERP measurement involves using an averaging computer to separate the electrical activity surrounding more complex processing events from the ongoing electrical background activity of the brain. It may be a response to internal or external stimulation of the nervous system. ERPs are often used in cognitive research. Although this technique has been used widely by some speech and psychological researchers, it is not without problems. Both its validity and reliability can be questioned. Whether an electrical potential that occurs after a stimulus is of cerebral origin or is brought about by a motor act is not always certain. When a language stimulus evokes a cerebral potential, brain activity is not always present, and the absence of an electrical potential to a language stimulus does not mean no electrical activity occurred. Many electrical currents simply do not reach the surface electrodes; some are too small and erratic. In addition, the waveforms derived from stimulation are highly complex; therefore determining which section of the waveform that was generated in response to the language stimulus has psychological meaning is sometimes difficult.

Despite these limitations, ERP has the capacity to measure events in the brain millisecond by millisecond. A research paradigm frequently used in language studies yields a readiness potential. The subject is asked to repeat a word or phrase or speak freely with pauses of 3 or 4 seconds between portions of an utterance. The continuous EEG recording that precedes the onset of speech is analyzed by averaging waveforms across several utterances to discover the readiness potential.

Audiology has made good use of ERP with the auditory brainstem response (ABR) study or brainstem auditory evoked response (BAER). For this study, electrodes are placed on the scalp, and electrical activity is recorded in response to click stimuli. The recordings from an ABR are displayed in vertical waves, and waves I through V can be used to evaluate the integrity of the brainstem's response following the response from the cranial nerve to the upper brainstem.

Magnetoencephalography

Those electrical currents inside the head also produce magnetic field oscillations around active neurons. The strength and orientation of these magnetic fields can be detected from above the scalp by use of a magnetometer (MEG), which marks spontaneous or event-related activity (event-related magnetic fields [ERFs]). The MEG locates sources of the neural activity, and the locations are superimposed on anatomic images such as MRI. MEG has been used to map the brain prior to surgical intervention, such as for epilepsy, and can be a useful research tool for mapping language.[6,18]

Vascular Imaging

Noncontrast CT, contrast-enhanced CT, and MRI are the most frequently used studies at this time to identify the presence and extent of vascular infarction or disease. For the acute stroke, the most important task of the physician is to exclude hemorrhage. Hemorrhage would be a contraindication to any procedure introducing blood thinners or to the use of thrombolytic drugs or so-called clot busters to perfuse an area of the brain deprived of blood flow by the presence of a thrombus or an embolus. The noncontrast CT is the most frequently used study for this purpose if the patient is seen early in the progression of the stroke. If it is available and there are no contraindications, MRI is somewhat superior to CT for the acute-stage studies. Contrast-enhanced CT presents more risk to the patient but may better identify lesions.

It may be important for the physician to know the patency of the vascular system of a patient with suspected neurologic disease or injury. Once it is determined by a functional study that there is reduced blood flow to an area, it will be necessary to determine where the vascular perfusion has been interrupted or which vasculature is at risk of future occlusion, hemorrhage, or spasm.

Transcranial Doppler

A transcranial Doppler study is a noninvasive procedure done by passing inaudible low-frequency sound waves to the base of the brain. This is done by placing the probes over areas where thin bones are located: above the cheekbone, beneath the jaw, at the orbit of the eyes, or at the back of the head. It depends on where the best signal is found. The Doppler analyzes reflected sound waves coming from the major blood vessels. It can reveal disruption of blood flow and identify the affected vessels. Doppler studies of the carotid arteries are often done after a transient ischemic attack to assess the patency of the major vessel from the heart to the brain.

Cerebral Angiography and Magnetic Resonance Angiography

Conventional cerebral angiography is an invasive procedure because it involves the injection of a contrast media into the carotid artery. Once this dye is injected, a radiographic study is done while it works its way through the circulation paths of the brain, providing a radiographic picture of the vascular distribution to the brain. The risks of this procedure, especially in the acute stages of possible vascular compromise, are obvious. A plaque on the wall of the artery could be dislodged by the catheter carrying the dye resulting in an embolism, causing further deprivation of blood to the brain. In addition, allergic reaction to the contrast is possible. Therefore conventional angiography is used now only in selected patients and has been replaced, especially in the case of cerebrovascular accident, with magnetic resonance angiography.

Summary of Neuroimaging

As pointed out in the beginning of this section, it is clinically useful for the practicing SLP to have knowledge of different types of neuroimaging studies that may be used by physicians in the care of their patient. This familiarity will also be quite useful in reading research in speech-language pathology and audiology. Increasing collaboration is seen between SLPs and medical researchers using the various neuroimaging methods to understand normal brain function underlying communication and to identify brain differences related to acquired or developmental problems with communication. In addition to the techniques discussed in this section, additional neuroimaging methods are briefly described in Box 3.2.

Overview of the Human Communication Nervous System

The organization of the human communication nervous system is fundamental to understand and recall. In the first three chapters of this text, you have been introduced to the history of the interaction between neurology and speech-language pathology, to structural anatomy and functionality of the main components of the CNS and PNS, and to some typical methods of imaging those structures in static images and in functional studies. From this point on, we further explore various aspects of this complex nervous system of

---

BOX 3.2   Additional Neuroimaging Technologies

Type	Description
Magnetic resonance microscopy	Uses high-field scanners and specific scanning technique to display information about internal composition of the cortex: differing thickness of the cortical layers, definition of the layers (agranular vs granular), variation in myelination of regions of brain
Computed tomography perfusion (CTP)	CT study using intervenous injection of a contrast agent, cinefluoroscopy, and rapid temporal sampling methodology; higher spatial resolution than MRP but limited by spatial issues
Magnetic resonance perfusion (MRP)	MR study using a paramagnetic contrast agent (gadolinium); yields information about vascularity of a region of interest; vulnerable to patient motion and leakage across blood-brain barrier
Arterial spin labeling (ASL)	A noninvasive magnetic resonance imaging (MRI) study quantifying cereval blood flow without the use of an exogenous agent; uses tagging of endogenous arterial spinning through a complicated poststudy comparison technique; study largely limited to large research centers at present
Magnetization transfer imaging	MRI technique sensitive to the exchange of magnetization between a liquid pool of free protons and a semisolid pool of restricted protons; a magnetization transfer ratio will quantify transfer between free and restricted water molecules; used to study white matter and gray matter; has been found to be useful in studies of patients with multiple sclerosis and other progressive diseases where brain tissue may appear normal in other studies

---

ours. We will look at how neurons communicate with each other, briefly explore sensory systems intimately involved in communication (touch and vision), and then, in more depth, explore the structures and their function that are primarily responsible for our miraculous ability to hear, speak, and process information in order to communicate with each other efficiently and effectively. The outline in Appendix 3.1 is a summary figure of the levels and an outline of the most important structures of the CNS. You may wish to quiz yourself at this point and, if necessary, review the preliminary information from this and the previous chapter on these structures. We go into more depth about them and the disorders associated with breakdown in their various systems in later chapters, and at times you will be reminded to review some of the information in these chapters.

SYNOPSIS OF CLINICAL INFORMATION OR APPLICATIONS FOR THE SLP

- The CNS is the controlling influence for the human communication nervous system.
- The PNS is composed of the cranial nerves, peripheral nerves, and peripheral parts of the autonomic nervous system.
- Mixed nerves carry both sensory and motor fibers.
- Sensory and motor nerves exit at the intervertebral foramina.
- Roots unite to form a spinal nerve, whereas sensory and motor fibers mix.
- A lesion is a damaged area in the brain.
- Injury at the cervical cord (C1–C8) could affect speech production because of respiratory weakness.
- Cranial nerves have some relation to the speech, language, and hearing process.
- Seven of the 12 cranial nerves are directly related to speech production.
- Cranial nerves are unprotected and are vulnerable to trauma damage due to their point of exit from the brainstem.
- Some cranial nerves are motor, some are sensory, and some are mixed:
  - Cranial nerve I, olfactory: sensory/afferent; smell
  - Cranial nerve II, optic: sensory/afferent; vision
  - Cranial nerve III, oculomotor: motor/efferent; eye movement
  - Cranial nerve IV, trochlear: motor/efferent; eye
  - Cranial nerve V, trigeminal: mixed; pharynx, mastication, mandible, maxillary, eye, teeth, upper lip, scalp
  - Cranial nerve VI, abducens: motor/efferent; eye
  - Cranial nerve VII, facial: mixed; tongue/taste, oral cavity, facial movement, expression, salivary glands, Bell palsy
  - Cranial nerve VIII, vestibulocochlear: sensory/afferent; hearing and balance
  - Cranial nerve IX, glossopharyngeal: mixed; gag reflex, swallowing, taste, external ear
  - Cranial nerve X, vagus: mixed; larynx, pharynx, taste buds, heart
  - Cranial nerve XI, spinal, accessory: motor/efferent; sternocleidomastoid muscles, trapezius muscles
  - Cranial nerve XII, hypoglossal: motor/efferent; intrinsic muscles of the tongue, movement, fasciculations, fibrillations of tongue
- The enteric nervous system is part of the autonomic nervous system and controls digestion and deglutition.
- The autonomic nervous system is composed of the sympathetic (fight-or-flight reaction) and parasympathetic (calming effect of bodily functions) systems.
- The autonomic nervous system involves neural control of smooth and cardiac muscles and gland secretions.
- The autonomic nervous system allows homeostasis to be maintained.
- The brain and spinal cord are protected and covered by meninges and a cushioning layer of tissue from CSF.
- Dura mater is the outermost layer of protection for the brain from rotary displacement.
- Arachnoid mater and subarachnoid space compose the middle layer in the meninges; all cranial nerves and cerebral arteries and veins pass through this space.
- Pia mater is the most internal layer of meninges; it adheres to the surface of the brain and contains blood supply.
- The brain has a three-part ventricle system: the lateral (two), third, and fourth ventricles.
- The ventricles are connected by small ducts and canals.
- Each ventricle contains a choroid plexus, which is responsible for the production of CSF.
- CSF is a clear, colorless fluid that cushions the CNS from the surrounding bones and protects against direct trauma.
- CSF helps regulate intracranial pressure, remove waste products, and nourish the nervous tissues.
- Hydrocephalus is a blockage of CSF or failure to absorb CSF.
- Elevated intracranial pressure may also be indicative of a tumor, hemorrhage, meningitis, or encephalitis.
- The brain requires ~25% of the body's oxygen.
- Two large internal carotid arteries and two vertebral arteries are the main suppliers of blood to the brain.
- The internal carotid divides into the anterior and middle cerebral arteries.
- The internal carotid also divides into the ophthalmic artery, posterior communicating artery, and posterior cerebral artery, which are part of the circle of Willis.
- The anterior communicating artery joins anterior cerebral arteries at the circle of Willis.
- The internal carotid supplies much of the cerebral hemisphere.
- The middle cerebral artery is the largest branch of the internal carotid.
- The vertebral artery divides into the meningeal branch, posterior spinal branch, anterior spinal branch, posterior inferior cerebellar artery, and medullary branches.
- The basilar artery divides in the pontine arteries, labyrinthine artery, anterior inferior cerebellar artery, and superior cerebellar artery.
- The circle of Willis is formed by the anastomosis of the two internal carotids with the two vertebral arteries and its branches.
- Contralateral refers to a lesion affecting the opposite side of the body.
- Ipsilateral refers to a lesion affecting the same side of the body.
- Major movements in human beings have contralateral neurologic control because of fiber decussation (crossing) at the medullary location.
- Left cerebrovascular accident (stroke) results in contralateral (right side) paralysis or paresis (weakness).
- Right cerebrovascular accident (stroke) results in contralateral (left side) paralysis or paresis (weakness).
- If a lesion occurs after decussation, the affected side is ipsilateral.
- Bilateral damage to cortical areas (upper motor neurons) controlling speech musculature results in spastic dysarthria.
- In general, the right hemisphere of the brain governs nonverbal activity, and the left hemisphere of the brain governs verbal activity.
- In general, the anterior portions of the brain govern motor activity, and posterior portions of the brain govern sensory activity.
- Neuroimaging studies are used frequently in current practice with the most common being variations of CT, MRI, and ERP.

REFERENCES

1. Avin, R. I., Bitar, R., Letourneau-Guillion, L., Young, R., Symons, S. P., & Fox, A. J. (2013). Atherosclerosis and the chronology of infarction. In T. P. Nadich, M. Castillo, S. Cha, & J. G. Smirniotopoulos (Eds.), *Imaging of the brain* (pp. 399–450). Elsevier Saunders.
2. Bagbati, S., Boccagni, C., Sant'Angelo, A., Prestandrea, C., & Mazzilli, R. (2015). EEG predictors of outcome in patients with disorders of consciousness admitted for intensive rehabilitation. *Clinical Neurophysiology, 126,* 959–966.
3. Boccagni, C., Bagnato, S. S. A., Prestandrea, C., & Galardi, G. (2011). Usefulness of standard EEG in predicting the outcome of patients with disorders of consciousness after anoxic coma. *Journal of Clinical Neurophysiology, 28,* 489–492.
4. Bonakdarpour, B., Beeson, P. M., DeMarco, A. T., & Rapcsak, S. Z. (2015). Variability in blood oxygen level dependent (BOLD) signal in patients with stroke-induced and primary progressive aphasia. *Neuroimage Clinical, 8,* 87–94.
5. Castro, A. J., Merchut, M. P., Neafsey, E. J., & Wurster, R. D. (2002). *Neuroscience: An outline approach.* Mosby.
6. Frye, R. E., Rezaie, R., & Papanicolaou, A. C. (2009). Functional neuroimaging of language using magnetoencephalography. *Physics of Life Reviews, 6,* 1–10.
7. Galper, M. W., Nadich, T. P., Kleinman, G. M., Stein, E.,G., & Lento, P. A. (2013). Cranial meninges. In T. P. Nadich, M. Castillo, S. Cha, & J. G. Smirniotopoulos (Eds.), *Imaging of the brain* (pp. 101–125). Elsevier Saunders.
8. Human Connectome Project (n.d.). Gallery. Retrieved from www.humanconnectomeproject.org/gallery
9. Kim, J. J., & Mukherjee, P. (2013). . Static anatomic techniques. In T. P. Nadich, M. Castillo, S. Cha, & J. G. Smirniotopoulos (Eds.), *Imaging of the brain* (pp. 3–22). Elsevier Saunders.
10. Knecht, S., Frager, B., Deppe, M., Bobe, L., Lohmann, H., Floel, A., Ringelstein, E. B., & Henningsen, H. (2000). Handedness and hemispheric language dominance in healthy humans. *Brain, 123,* 2512–2518.
11. Mechelli, A., Price, C. J., Friston, K., & Wellcom, J. A. (2005). *Voxel-based morphometry of the human brain: Methods and applications.* Bentham Science Publishers Ltd.
12. Mummery, C. J., Patterson, K., Price, C. J., Ashburner, J., Frackowiak, R. S. J., & Hodges, J. R. (2000). A voxel-based morphometry study of semantic dementia: Relationship between temporal lobe atrophy and semantic memory. *Annals of Neurology, 47,* 36–45.
13. Szczapanski, S. M., & Knight, R. T. (2014). Insights into human behavior from lesions to the prefrontal cortex. *Neuron, 83,* 1002–1018.
14. Taber, K.H., Hillman, E.M., & Hurley, R.A. Optical imaging: A new window to the adult brain. *Journal of Neuropsychiatry and Clinical Neuroscience, 22,* 4.
15. Valenza, G., Sclocco, R., Duggento, A., Passamonti, V., Napadow, R., Barbieri, N., & Toschi, P., II (2019). The central autonomic network at rest: Uncovering functional MRI correlates of time-varying autonomic outflow. *Neuroimage* https://doi.org/10.1016/j.neuroimage.2019.04.075.
16. Vymazal, J., Rulseh, A. M., Keller, J., & Janouskova, L. (2012). Comparison of CT and MR imaging in ischemic stroke. *Insights into Imaging, 3,* 619–627.
17. Zeller, J. B., Herrmann, M. J., Ehlis, A. C., Polak, T., & Fallgatter, A. J. (2010). Altered parietal brain oxygenation in Alzheimer's disease as assessed with near infrared spectroscopy. *American Journal of Geriatric Psychiatry, 18,* 433–441.
18. Bowyer, S., Zillgitt, A., Greenwald, M., & Lajiness-O'Neill, R. (2020). Language mapping with magnetoencephalography: An update on the current state of clinical research and practice with considerations for clinical practice guidelines. *Journal of Clinical Neurophysiology, 37,* 554–563. https://doi.org/10.1097/WNP.0000000000000489.

APPENDIX 3.1

A vast amount of information is provided in Chapters 2 and 3. Fig. 3.25 is a summary drawing of the levels of the CNS to organize the information in Chapter 2. Referring to this figure while reading subsequent chapters will be helpful. An outline of the most important structures discussed in these chapters is also provided for review and organization. For each item, ask the following questions:

- What is it?
- Where is it?
- What does it do?

When appropriate, attempt to label drawings of some of the various structures for which illustrations were used. The effort put into doing this will be rewarded in understanding subsequent chapters.

I. The human nervous system
  A. Central nervous system
    1. Brain
  B. Cerebral hemispheres
    1. Four lobes
    2. Fissures
    3. Sulci
    4. Gyri
    5. Association cortex
    6. Connecting fibers
  C. Basal ganglia
    1. Corpus striatum
      a. Caudate nucleus
      b. Lentiform nucleus: putamen, globus pallidus
    2. Claustrum
  D. Limbic system
  E. Cerebellum
  F. Brainstem
    1. Medulla oblongata
      a. Pyramids
      b. Olives
      c. Peduncles

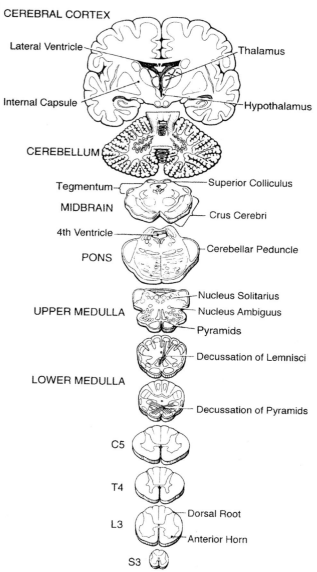

Fig. 3.25 Levels of the central nervous system.

Labels in figure:
CEREBRAL CORTEX
Lateral Ventricle
Internal Capsule
Thalamus
Hypothalamus
CEREBELLUM
Tegmentum — Superior Colliculus
MIDBRAIN — Crus Cerebri
4th Ventricle
PONS — Cerebellar Peduncle
UPPER MEDULLA — Nucleus Solitarius, Nucleus Ambiguus, Pyramids
LOWER MEDULLA — Decussation of Lemnisci
Decussation of Pyramids
C5
T4
L3 — Dorsal Root, Anterior Horn
S3

2. Pons
3. Mesencephalon
  a. Tectum
  b. Colliculi
4. Spinal cord
II. Spinal nerves
III. Peripheral nerves
IV. Five regions
  A. Meninges
V. Dura mater
VI. Arachnoid mater
VII. Pia mater
  A. Ventricles
VIII. Choroid plexus
IX. CSF
  A. Blood supply
X. Internal carotid artery and its branch
XI. Vertebral artery and its branches
XII. Circle of Willis
  A. PNS
    1. Spinal peripheral nerves
XIII. Anterior horn cell
XIV. Efferent fibers
XV. Afferent fibers
  A. Cranial nerves
XVI. Twelve pairs
  A. Autonomic nervous system
    1. Parasympathetic division
    2. Sympathetic division
    3. Enteric division (deglutition and peristalsis)
XVII. Clinical principles of neurologic organization
  A. Contralateral motor control
  B. Ipsilateral motor control
  C. Bilateral speech motor control
  D. Unilateral language mechanisms
  E. Scheme of cortical organization

4

Neuronal Function in the Nervous System

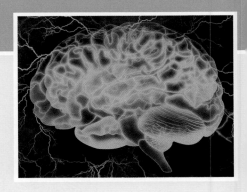

But strange that I was not told

That the brain can hold

In a tiny ivory cage

God's heaven and hell.

Oscar Wilde, Poems and Fairy Tales of Oscar Wilde, 1932

KEY TERMS

absolute refractory period
action potential (AP)
adequate stimulus
anastomosis
anion
anterograde
axon
axon hillock
axoplasm
bipolar cell
bouton
cations
cerebrovascular accident (CVA)
concentration gradient
convergence
dendrites
depolarization
distal
divergence
excitatory postsynaptic potential
  (EPSP)

graded potential
hyperpolarization
inhibitory postsynaptic potential
  (IPSP)
interstitial fluid
irritability
ligand sensitive
microtubules
motor endplate
multipolar cell
myasthenia gravis
myelin
necrose
neurofilaments
neuron
neurotransmitters
orthograde transneuronal atrophy
osmotic force
perikaryon
postsynaptic terminal (receptor
  membrane)

potential
presynaptic terminal
proximal
pseudounipolar cell
relative refractory period
resting potential
retrograde
retrograde transneuronal
  degeneration
saltatory transmission
selectivity
sodium-potassium pump
soma
spatial summation
summation
synapse
synaptic cleft
temporal summation

NEURONAL PHYSIOLOGY

Neuron: The Cell Body

The **neuron**, or nerve cell, is the basic anatomic and functional unit of the nervous system, underlying all neural behavior, including speech, language, and hearing. Each neuron consists of a cell body called a **soma**, or **perikaryon**. The structure of human cells is similar in all cells, and we should review the information from Chapter 2 and expand upon the structure of cells as we look closer at neuronal function. The anatomic division of the central nervous system (CNS) into cell bodies and their axons can be perceived visually by the human eye. The aggregate of axons leaving the neurons of the CNS appears white due to the white myelin sheathing most axons. The aggregate of neuronal cell bodies appears gray on dissection, though in living bodies appears more pinkish-gray due to the generous blood supply to the brain. This is why you will often hear the brain referred to as gray matter.

To review and expand on the makeup of the neuronal cell body, we are first reminded that each neuron has a bilipid membrane surrounding it and cytoplasm or cytosol inside. Inside the watery, potassium-rich cytosol are vital functional units called organelles, all having their own bilipid membrane. The cytosol also contains enzymes important to the metabolism of the cell.

The major organelles of the cell body are the cytoskeleton, nucleus, rough and smooth endoplasmic reticulum (ER), Golgi apparatus, and mitochondria. The cytoskeleton is a protein framework that maintains the structure of the cell and helps organize the microenvironment and activity inside the cell. The nucleus contains most of the deoxyribonucleic acid (DNA) of that cell. Within the nucleus is also a dense area called the nucleolus in which ribonucleic acid (RNA) is synthesized. Rough ER is studded with organelles called ribosomes and plays an important role in the synthesis and transport of proteins within and outside of the cell. The smooth ER serves to make and transport lipids. The Golgi apparatus is the organelle responsible for transporting and modifying specific proteins that leave the ER and are directed to other parts of the cell or are secreted into the extracellular space. Mitochondria organelles direct the energy production within the cell. The functions of the various organelles are summarized in Box 4.1.

Cellular Proteins

As in all cells of living matter, neuronal cells are made up of molecules, the major classes being lipids, proteins, carbohydrates, and nucleic acid. There are two major types of nucleic acid within cells, DNA and RNA. The nucleus of all cells contains most of the DNA because it contains the genes. The genes carry the basic information needed to structure the proteins characterizing that particular cell and its purpose in the body.

Though all of the molecules are important to cellular function, we are highlighting proteins here because these molecules enable major functions of the body to develop and continue throughout life. Importantly, medical science is also

---

BOX 4.1 Major Organelles of Cells and Summary of Their Function Within the Cell

Organelle	Summary of Makeup/Function
Cytoskeleton	Provides structure for the cell membrane
Nucleus	Contains the DNA, which contains the genes
Nucleolus	Dense area in the nucleus; mRNA synthesis here
Smooth endoplasmic reticulum (ER)	Synthesizes and stores lipids
Rough ER	Studded with ribosomes; involved in synthesis, modification, and transport of proteins
Golgi apparatus	Transports proteins out of the ER to lysomes or to the cellular membrane
Mitochondria	Directs the energy production within the cell

---

frequently targeting protein synthesis to alter cellular function allowing translation of function or cellular protection.

Proteins are built of amino acids chained together in a certain order and then folded into unique shapes as instructed by that cell's DNA. Since DNA does not leave the nucleus, a copy of the code is made and messenger RNA (mRNA) is synthesized within the nucleus to carry the particular code out into the cytosol. The mRNA is bound by ribosomes, which are the molecules responsible for making proteins. Though your DNA carries the original instructions on how to make proteins, the coding of instruction as carried in the mRNA cannot be understood by the ribosome mechanism unless translated. Francis Crick was the first scientist to theorize the existence of a molecule that would translate the coding in the mRNA into a viable protein code.[1] Other scientists later proved this theory with the discovery of transfer RNA (tRNA). Some proteins synthesized in the rough ER will remain there, while others will be transported through the Golgi apparatus and directed to lysosomes (which help with cellular cleanup) or to the cellular membrane. Others will be secreted outside the cell to perform various functions. Schubert et al.,[6] identified 197 different proteins secreted by nerve, astroglial, and/or neural precursor cells. They then identified and categorized the function of these proteins in the nervous system. Though as speech-language pathologists (SLPs) we do not need to know the chemical names of these proteins, the categorization of the various functions in the nervous system aids in the understanding of how vital they are to its normal performance. A summary of these categories can be seen in Box 4.2.

The importance of mRNA to medical science research in the 21st century cannot be overstated. It was the research on mRNA-based therapeutics through the years[2] that culminated in the rapidly produced lifesaving vaccine against severe acute respiratory syndrome coronavirus 2 (SARS-CoV-2), which caused the Covid-19 virus. Covid-19 triggered a global

---

BOX 4.2   Categorization of Functions Performed by Secreted Proteins in the Central Nervous System

Cell-to-cell interaction: enable the sending/receiving of signals between cells

Chaperone/redox: chaperone molecules help maintain homeostasis, assisting proteins to fold, stabilize, or degrade; redox refers to a cellular reaction, reduction-oxidation in which electrons are exchanged helping maintain certain functions

Metabolism: a complex chemical reaction, modifying one molecule into another to sustain/maintain the state of the cell; secreted proteins function in metabolism of proteins, amino acids, carbohydrates, nucleotides, lipids, neurotransmitters

Structural: help maintain cell shape

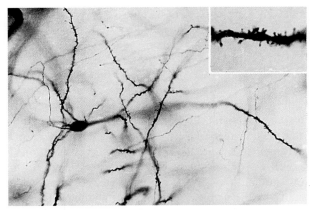

Fig. 4.1 Spiny neurons from the neostriatum with the detail inset showing the dendritic spines on the cells. (Reprinted from Ma, T. P., & Geyer, H. L. [2018]. The basal nuclei. In D. Haines, *Fundamental neuroscience for basic and clinical applications* [pp. 377–393.e1]. Elsevier.)

pandemic beginning in late 2019 and resulted in the deaths of millions of people globally with over 800,000 deaths in the United States alone. Expansion of this research and the use of mRNA-based therapeutics shows bright promise for the prevention and possible cure of many other diseases.

Neuron: Messaging Outside the Cell Body

Neurons vary greatly in size, but most of the billions of neurons of the CNS are small. Classifying on the basis of shape, three types of neurons may be identified: **multipolar, pseudounipolar,** and **bipolar cells.** Each nerve cell contains a nucleus and one to a dozen projections of varying length. These projections receive neural signals and conduct neural impulses. Those receiving neural stimuli are called **dendrites** and are the shorter and more numerous projections of the nerve cell. The dendrites of a neuron generally are no more than a few millimeters in length.

Dendrites usually branch extensively, giving an appearance similar to a tree branch configuration. The dendrites have specialized receptors through which they receive signals from other neurons at the synapse (the contact point with another neuron). Information travels from a **distal** to a **proximal** point along dendrites to the cell body.

Dendrites often display several thornlike protuberances, called dendritic spines (Fig. 4.1), usually on the most distal branches of the dendrite tree. They are most prolific in the CNS and are typically the sites of the synaptic contacts, forming an **anastomosis,** or connection.

The other process of a neuron is the **axon,** a longer single fiber that conducts nerve impulses away from the neuron to other parts of the nervous system, glands, or muscle. Axons arise from the cell body at an area called the axon initial segment or the **axon hillock.** Axons do not contain ribosomes, which is how scientists distinguish them from dendrites at the ultrastructural level. Axons range in length from several micrometers to more than 2 m. The diameter of individual axons varies greatly, and conduction velocity along the axon ranges from 2 to 100 m/s depending on the fiber size. The larger the diameter, the greater is the conduction velocity. In a physiologic sense, the term *axon* refers to a nerve fiber

that conducts impulses away from a nerve cell body. Any long nerve fiber, however, may be referred to as an axon regardless of the direction of the flow of nervous impulses.

The cytoplasm of the axon, called **axoplasm,** contains dense bundles of **microtubules** and **neurofilaments.** Each axon ends at a terminal button, or **bouton,** which is the point of contact with another neuron.

The site at which this bouton, or axon terminal, communicates with another neuron is called the **synapse.** The synapse is usually the point of contact between one neuron (typically the axon of that neuron) with another neuron's cell body, dendrites, dendritic spines, or axon. Axonal transport occurs either slowly or very fast. If the transport occurs from the cell body toward the axon terminal, it is known as **anterograde.** Transport up the axon from the terminal toward the cell is also possible and is called **retrograde.** Fig. 4.2 shows anterograde and retrograde axonal transport.

Neurons do the work of the nervous system by transmitting electrical signals or neural impulses to glands, muscles, and other neurons. Basically, the purpose of the neuron is to communicate, to send a "neural message." In the peripheral nervous system (PNS) many neuromuscular (i.e., neuron to muscle fiber) transmissions take place. In the brain itself, most of the neurons conduct neural impulses to other neurons, which are clustered quite close together, providing a high neuronal density in the cerebrum. This high density creates an almost unlimited capacity for complex neuronal activity. This neuronal activity, or brain activation, produces sensations, perceptions, and thoughts as well as nerve signals eventually resulting in voluntary muscle movement. Activation is the result of rapid biochemical and biophysical changes at the cellular level and in the neurons and glial cells of the brain.

In this chapter we examine this process very simplistically, looking at a basic communication process of neurons: the generation of an **action potential (AP)** for the types of neurons that conduct this straightforward type of firing pattern, an AP generated one spike at a time. We concentrate on learning the process through which this occurs. Once you understand the properties of neurons that enable this basic transmission, you

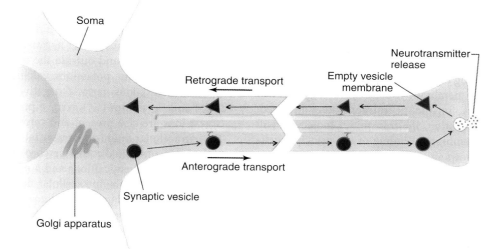

Fig. 4.2 Axoplasmic transport. Substances required by the axon are delivered from the soma via anterograde transport. Retrograde transport moves substances from the axon to the soma. The proteins that walk the vesicles along the microtubules are shown in blue. (Modified from Lundy-Eckman, L. [2013]. *Neuroscience* [4th ed.]. Saunders.)

will be better able to understand how other neurons may be different in their firing patterns. These other patterns are mentioned in this chapter, but further elucidation of these patterns is beyond the scope of this text. If you understand the cellular properties of neurons and how basic communication between neurons occurs, you will be on your way to exploring more advanced material should you choose to do so.

The Neural Transmission Process

To begin looking at this process, we need to step back and look at the macro level to answer the larger question: How does a neuron communicate with another cell? To begin the discussion, the process is first summarized and then broken down into details.

The neural message is a chemical or electrical signal sent to another neuron or another cell (such as a muscle cell). This neural message is most often chemical, though there are electrical-only transmissions in the brain as well. The following 10 steps summarize the generation of an AP (the neural impulse propagated down an axon) resulting in a basic chemical synaptic transmission. Following the summary, details of the process are discussed and illustrated, and an electrical transmission will also be described.

Steps in the neural transmission process (a summary):
1. Neurons contain fluid inside the cell (intracellular) and are bathed in fluid outside (extracellular fluid). These fluids are made up of water molecules and of chemicals that are ionic in nature—that is, they carry a positive or negative electrical charge.
2. The membrane surrounding the neuron and its extensions is a so-called excitable membrane. When inactive, or not firing, the neuron is at rest. This resting state is a result of the maintenance of a particular polarity or relative charge across that membrane. This resting polarity is obtained when the intracellular fluid surrounding the point of the axon hillock (initial segment of the axon) is

~70 mV more negative (–70 mV) than the fluid outside the cell membrane.
3. Due to this excitable state, the polarity at different points along the membrane is constantly being changed because there are neural signals being sent throughout your nervous system all the time. There is a certain threshold of change in polarity that will cause the neuron to fire or generate a neural electrical spike called an AP. An AP can be generated only at the axon hillock. However, most of the singular neural signals that reach the membrane of a neuron are not strong enough to generate movement around the membrane of the cell to the axon hillock to generate an AP. These signals do cause a change in polarity at a point on the cell membrane, resulting in what is called a **graded potential**. The changes in polarity can either depolarize (excitatory) or hyperpolarize (inhibitory) that section of the cell's membrane. Thus, neural firing (an AP) most often results not from a single transmission but from the summative effect of many signals resulting in a **spatial** and/or a **temporal summation** of signaling effects on the membrane. This summation will result in a strong enough change in polarity at the axon hillock to generate an AP.
4. The threshold for an AP is reached through a depolarization causing the intracellular fluid to become more positive (or less negative) relative to the outside. This occurs through an influx of sodium (Na$^+$) ions. At the point of the axon hillock, this threshold for depolarization is approximately –55 mV.
5. Once generated, an AP (in a healthy neuron with a normal axon) is propagated in an all-or-nothing fashion down the axon to the end of it, the terminal bouton (the presynaptic terminal).
6. The AP triggers calcium channels in the presynaptic terminal to open and release calcium. The calcium influx causes synaptic vesicles in the presynaptic terminal to

then bind with the newly inviting channel and are pumped through the opening and into the intracellular fluid. It is always a "3 Na⁺ out, then 2 K⁺ in" mechanism, thereby the excess of Na⁺ in the extracellular fluid is maintained. The concentration of sodium to potassium will also play an important part in the generation of chemical and electrical signals in the nervous system. An illustrated summary of membrane channels is shown in Fig. 4.3. An illustration of the mechanisms of the sodium-potassium pump is shown in Fig. 4.4.

Electrical Forces

Cellular Potential

Potential is defined as the relative amount of voltage in an electrical field. Think of the neuron as having two electrical fields, one outside and one inside the cell. At rest the electrical

charge within the nerve cell is negative (dominated by the presence of the protein anions) relative to the outside of the cell (dominated by sodium ions).

The importance of ions to nervous system functioning may be understood through a discussion of their electrical properties and movements. The major functions of neurons, including integration (i.e., cognition or thinking), always depend on their electrical properties and how the ions move, eventually resulting in the firing of neural impulses or the inhibition of neural firing. Because of their critical role in neural messaging, most of the energy consumed by the nervous system is used for ionic movement. Ion currents are responsible for the creation of electrical events in biologic systems. During stimulation of some part of the body (e.g., oral mechanism for speaking, brain cells for thinking), negative ions attract positive ions and

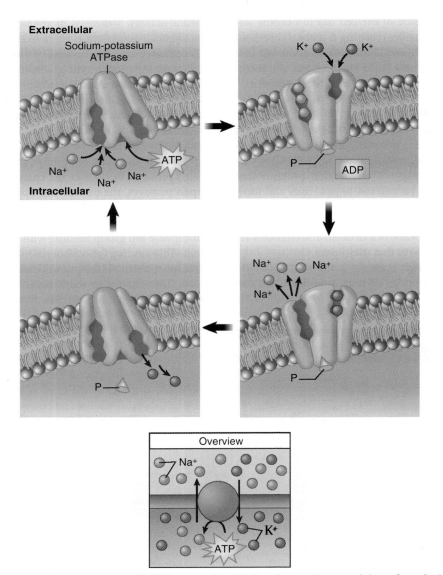

Fig. 4.4 Sodium-potassium pump. Three sodium ions (Na⁺) bind to sodium binding sites on the pump's inner face. At the same time, an energy-containing adenosine triphosphate *(ATP)* molecule produced by the cell's mitochondria binds to the pump. The ATP breaks apart, and its stored energy is transferred to the pump. The pump then changes shape, releases the three Na⁺ ions to the outside of the cell, and attracts two potassium ions (K⁺) to its potassium binding sites. The pump then returns to its original shape, and the two K⁺ ions and the remnant of the ATP molecule are released to the inside of the cell. The pump is now ready for another pumping cycle. The small inset is a simplified view of Na⁺-K⁺ pump activity. *ATPase*, Adenosine triphosphatase. (Adapted from McCance, K., & Huether, S. [2002]. *Pathophysiology* [4th ed.]. Mosby.)

repel other negative ions; the opposite occurs for a positive ion. Ions move because of voltage gradients (opposite ions attract and same ions repel), chemical gradients, and metabolic activity (sodium and potassium ions expending high-energy phosphates [ATP → adenosine diphosphate], thus producing what is known as metabolic energy).

The ionic difference across the membrane at steady state is called the cell's **resting potential**. At resting potential, the difference in potential, or the separation of electrical charge, across the cell membrane is calculated to be approximately –70 mV. This means that a probe inserted into the cytoplasm inside the cell would find its charge to be 70 mV more negative than the charge measured in the fluid outside the cell. The resting potential is one aspect of the cell's characteristic **irritability**, or ability to respond to outside influences. At the resting potential the cell is not responding to any outside influences, and it is not firing an impulse. An **adequate stimulus** is required, one that is capable of changing the cell's potential, to change the resting state. An adequate stimulus may be mechanical, thermal, electrical, or chemical in nature.

Neural Messaging

What an adequate stimulus may do to the membrane of a neuron is perturb it enough to (1) cause ion channels to open and (2) allow movement of the ions across the cell membrane, effecting a change in the relative charge, or polarization, across the membrane. An influx of the positively charged sodium ions causes a depolarization of the cell. **Depolarization** means that the inside of the cell has become less negative (or, if you prefer, more positive) relative to the outside of the cell. If that change in potential reaches a certain threshold (approximately –55 mV) at a certain point on the cell, the axon hillock, the generation of a neural impulse down the axon of the cell will begin. The neural impulse is in reality a trail of depolarization or spikes in electrical current traveling down the axon membrane. This brief spike is called the AP. There are few instances in which only one stimulation or neural signal to the membrane of a neuron will be of adequate strength to depolarize the membrane all on its own. This is why we must look at graded potentials before we get to the AP.

Graded Potentials

Graded potentials are primarily generated by sensory input, causing a change in the conductance of the membrane of the sensory receptor cell. Graded potentials also are those generated at a localized place on the cell membrane where an excitatory or inhibitory synapse has taken place. Graded potentials (also called local, or generator, potentials), which are excitatory in nature, are generated in the same way an AP is generated at the axon hillock, that is, by the influx of positively charged sodium ions into the intracellular fluid, decreasing the negativity of the charge inside relative to the outside of the cell. If this change in difference across the membrane reaches a certain threshold, a graded potential is generated at a segment of the cell membrane of the neuron or dendrite at which the stimulation occurred; that is, the change in the positive to negative ratio causes a local flow of current.

Unlike an AP, which is an all-or-nothing phenomenon, a graded potential is not likely to be fully propagated along the membrane; rather, the voltage will tend to decrease as the current spreads due to leakage of sodium ions through the resistance and capacitance of the membrane. The current may remain more localized, and potential may decrease in strength the further along the membrane it spreads. If the graded, or generator, potential initially is not strong enough to reach the threshold required to continue it to move along the membrane, it likely will decrease by the time it travels along the membrane to the axon hillock and an AP will not be generated at that time. Because of this decrement, graded potentials usually must summate either in time (a number of graded potentials occurring on the cell membrane at once) or in space (a number of graded potentials occurring at the same point on the membrane) to generate a signal strong enough to generate an AP.

Hyperpolarization

The ionic exchange that takes place as the cell's resting potential is changed may also result in a state called **hyperpolarization**. In this case the inside of the cell at the point of signaling to the membrane has become more negative relative to the outside of the cell. This occurs because of the influx of chloride anions.

Action Potential

APs are brief electrical transients visible when recorded as intracellular voltages or extracellular currents (Fig. 4.5). If a neural signal is independently strong enough or the temporal or spatial summation of electrical signals is strong enough to depolarize the receiving cell at the point called the axon hillock, the result will be this electrical impulse, or action current (the AP), sent down the axon of that cell.

APs occur throughout the body's tissues, regulating secretions of hormones and even signaling fertilization of the egg by the sperm. In a nervous system, APs serve to integrate neural messages sent to cell bodies from sense organs and from other parts of the nervous system.

Once an AP is initiated at the axon hillock, a series of these depolarizations along the cell membrane of the axon is begun. The action current is thus propagated along an axon for long distances without a change in the waveform and at a constant velocity. This means that all the neuronal signals of coded information transmitted along axons in the nervous system are conveyed by a series of uniformly sized impulses. The information transmitted is therefore signaled by the frequency of APs generated rather than by their amplitude. The AP functions in an all-or-nothing manner. A stimulus sets up either a full-sized impulse or nothing.

During the passage of an AP across a nerve cell membrane, that part of the membrane becomes briefly incapable of responding to another stimulus. This period of unresponsiveness is called an **absolute refractory period**. The absolute refractory period is relatively short, lasting approximately 0.8 ms. The absolute refractory period prevents an AP from traveling back up the axon, thus forcing the impulse down the fiber toward the terminal bouton of the axon. After the

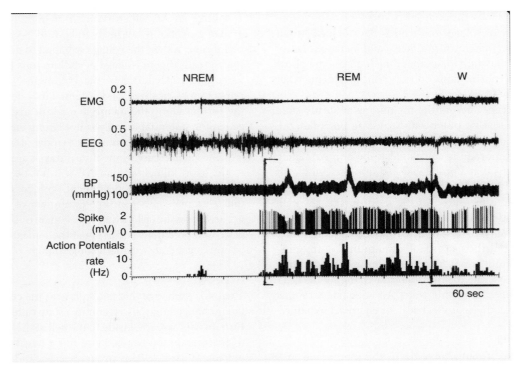

Fig. 4.5 An example of a cholinergic neuron in the laterodorsal tegmental nucleus whose firing during rapid eye movement *(REM)* sleep is correlated with fluctuations in blood pressure *(BP)*. *EEG*, Electroencephalogram; *EMG*, electromyogram (of neck muscle); *rate*, firing rate of the neuron; *spike*, trace of action potentials; *SWS*, slow wave sleep; *W*, wake. (From Séi, H. [2012]. Blood pressure surges in REM sleep: A mini review. *Pathophysiology, 19*[4], 233–241.)

absolute refractory period, there is a **relative refractory period** during which an AP may be produced by an intense stimulus and then by stimuli of less intensity (Fig. 4.6).

Myelin

Nerve fibers, or axons, may be classified as myelinated or unmyelinated. Large peripheral nerves and the large axons of the CNS acquire a white fatty sheath of wrapping as the brain develops. Layers of **myelin** are incorporated in the cells that produce myelin—oligodendrocytes in the CNS and Schwann cells in the PNS. Myelin is white, contrasting these nerves sharply with the gray unmyelinated nerves, and the myelin sheet is thick. It can be revealed by a special myelin stain. The thick insulation of myelin is interrupted at intervals by structures called the nodes of Ranvier. Because of how the myelin sheaths are designed, these nodes enhance rapid propagation of the electrical impulse along the nerve fiber. The APs necessary to propagate a signal down a myelinated axon develop only at these nodes (Fig. 4.7). The impulse is vastly increased in speed by hopping from node to node on a myelinated axon without any active contribution from the long internodal spaces.

This mode of transmission is extremely efficient compared with the slow gliding along of the nerve impulses on unmyelinated fibers. The type of transmission in myelinated fibers is called **saltatory transmission**. The efficiency of saltatory transmission is achieved because of the insulation that prevents current flow between nodes; in addition, little leakage of current from the fibers occurs. The conduction velocity of a myelinated fiber is directly proportional to the diameter of the fiber, whereas in an unmyelinated fiber the velocity is approximately proportional to the square root of the diameter. On average, transmission along a myelinated fiber is roughly 50 times as fast as one along an unmyelinated fiber.

Unmyelinated fibers are more common in the smaller nerve fibers of the PNS, although the cranial nerves, which are part of the PNS, are relatively large in diameter and are myelinated. Six of the cranial nerves innervate the speech muscles and provide neuromotor control for talking. The rapid muscular movements underlying speech would require the fastest mode of transmission of neural impulses.

Myelin Disorders

Certain diseases are in the category of demyelinating diseases. In your clinical practice you may treat patients with diseases in this category, particularly multiple sclerosis or Guillain-Barré syndrome. In demyelinating diseases, groups of oligodendrocytes and their myelin segments degenerate and are replaced by astrocytic plaques. This loss of myelin results in an interruption of the propagation of the AP. The axons that become demyelinized survive temporarily, and some may even regenerate. The particular variety of motor, visual, or general sensory losses that are found on examination reflect the location of the demyelization processes.

In multiple sclerosis the etiology is an autoimmune inflammatory response that damages the myelin sheath. If this inflammatory reaction is intense, the axons, too, may be damaged, producing irreversible neurologic deficits

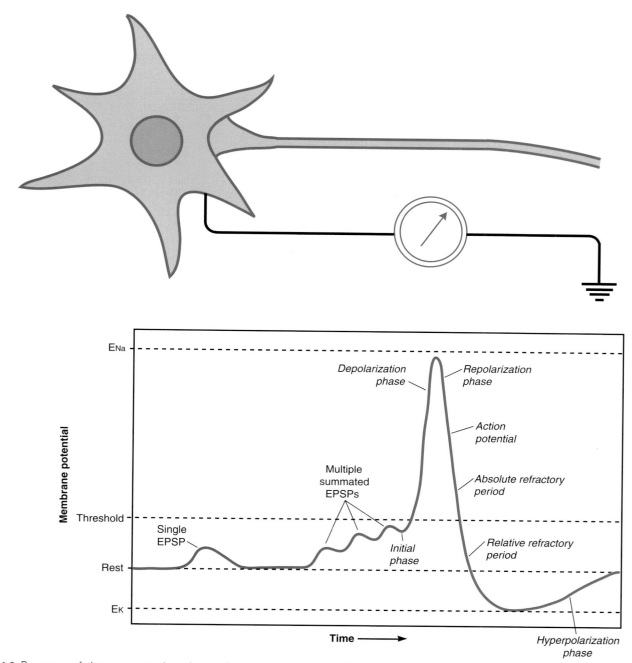

Fig. 4.6 Response of the neuron to the release of excitatory neurotransmitter by presynaptic neurons. The membrane potential (ordinate) becomes more positive as the binding of neurotransmitter released by firing of the presynaptic neuron increases sodium permeability through chemical-gated sodium channels, producing an EPSP. One EPSP of exaggerated amplitude is shown, after which sufficient EPSPs occur in quick succession to summate and elicit enough membrane depolarization to open up voltage-sensitive sodium channels. This reaches the threshold of depolarization necessary to generate an AP. The AP is terminated as the various sodium channels are inactivated, and voltage-sensitive potassium channels open and repolarize the membrane and, in this example, hyperpolarize it through efflux of potassium through opened potassium channels. (Reprinted from Nadeau, S., Ferguson, T. S., Valenstein, E., Vierck, C. J., Petruska, J. C., Streit, W. J., & Ritz, L. A. [2004]. *Medical neuroscience.* Saunders/Elsevier.)

that show irregular fluctuating periods of exacerbation and remission.

Impairment of speech is found in approximately half of the population afflicted with multiple sclerosis. A speech disorder resulting from involvement of the neuromuscular aspect of the nervous system is called dysarthria. Clinical symptoms of dysarthria are detailed in Chapter 8.

The Synapse

As the electrical nerve impulse, in the form of an AP, moves along an axon, it comes to a point where it must be transmitted to another neuron, a gland, or a muscle. This point is known as a synapse. Until the discovery that small junctures occur at the synapse, researchers assumed that neurons were

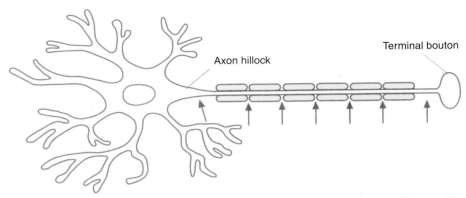

Fig. 4.7 A neuron with myelin sheathing of its axon. The interruptions in the myelin sheath are the nodes of Ranvier. The *arrows* indicate regions of high-density, voltage-sensitive sodium channels; current flow; and action potential generation. (Reprinted from Nadeau, S., Ferguson, T. S., Valenstein, E., Vierck, C. J., Petruska, J. C., Streit, W. J., & Ritz, L. A. [2004]. *Medical neuroscience.* Saunders.)

connected in one continuous network. Science now knows that between the membrane at the end of the axon (called the **presynaptic terminal**) and the membrane of the receiving cell (called the **postsynaptic terminal** or **receptor membrane**) is a small space called the **synaptic cleft**.

The transmission of a neural impulse across this synaptic juncture or gap is primarily a chemical process, sometimes an electrical process, and occasionally a combination of both. Electrical synapses will be discussed later in this chapter.

Most neural transmission is carried out through chemical messaging accomplished at the synapse. The transmission of nerve impulses to muscle in the PNS was the first well-established example of chemical synaptic transmission and remains the best understood. As recently as the 20th century, many neurophysiologists believed that the impulse transmission of one-thousandth of a second was too fast for any type of chemical mediation. An electrical nerve impulse was believed to excite the muscle fiber directly. The large electrical mismatch, however, between the tiny nerve fiber and the large muscle fiber indicated that an electrical explanation would be faulty by at least two orders of magnitude. In the 1930s researchers established that synaptic transmission in nerve-to-muscle synapses was entirely attributable to chemical mediation by a substance called acetylcholine.

When a neural impulse is generated down the axon by an AP, it travels to a point on the presynaptic membrane called the terminal bouton. At this point the AP causes opening of special voltage-gated calcium channels, allowing calcium to rush into the nerve terminal. This calcium release triggers synaptic vesicles in the axon to fuse with the presynaptic membrane and release chemicals called neurotransmitters, which have been synthesized and stored in those vesicles (see Fig. 4.7). These neurotransmitters are what determine whether the sending neuron is an excitatory neuron or an inhibitory neuron. Neurons are either one or the other, never both.

Looking through a powerful microscope, each neurotransmitter can be differentiated by molecular shape; no two are the same. Likewise, protein receptors dedicated to particular neurotransmitters also can be differentiated in the same

manner. At the synapse the released transmitter chemical diffuses across the synaptic cleft. Slightly protruding from the surface membrane of a receiving neuron will be a part of each receptor molecule associated with that neuron. This protruding part can sense the presence of its neurotransmitter and bind it to the membrane. This binding is described as similar to a key (the molecular shape of the neurotransmitter molecule) fitting into a lock (the matching shape of the receptor molecule). What happens after the binding to the receptor depends on the effect of that particular neurotransmitter and the type of receptor to which it binds.

Because the transmitter does effect a change in the target membrane, it must be rapidly inactivated so that too much is not released at one time. This inactivation may occur through action of an enzyme within the synaptic cleft (catabolism), a combination of enzyme action and reuptake, or a mix of diffusion out of the cleft and reuptake. The steps in neurotransmitter processing are shown in Fig. 4.8.

The most frequently used example of neurotransmitter action is that of a neurotransmitter such as glutamate, which is excitatory to the postsynaptic cell. In this kind of transmission (and in many others), the transmitter release changes the potential of the receptor membrane to a receptor potential by opening ionic channels. In an EPSP, the neurotransmitter binds to chemical-gated sodium channel receptors. The conductance of these channels is briefly increased, and sodium is allowed to flow into the cell. This partially depolarizes the membrane. If a sufficient number of EPSPs arrive at the membrane in a synchronous fashion, the depolarization is larger in strength. If strong enough, the threshold to open the voltage-gated sodium channels at the axon hillock is reached and an AP is generated. If the EPSP is not strong enough and does not summate with others, it decreases and an AP is not generated at that time.

A neurotransmitter such as gamma-aminobutyric acid (GABA), the primary inhibitory transmitter substance in the nervous system, has the opposite effect on the postsynaptic membrane. The binding of GABA with the membrane results in the influx of chloride ions or the efflux of potassium ions, either of which results in hyperpolarization of the membrane

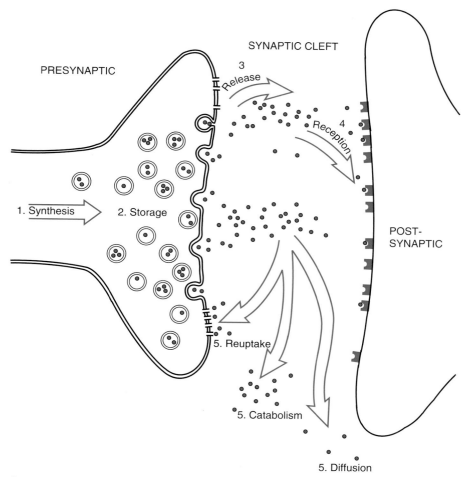

Fig. 4.8 The major steps in neurotransmitter processing. (Reprinted from Nadeau, S., Ferguson, T. S., Valenstein, E., Vierck, C. J., Petruska, J. C., Streit, W. J., & Ritz, L. A. [2004]. *Medical neuroscience.* Saunders/Elsevier.)

and an IPSP. With this, the receptor neuron becomes somewhat less likely to generate a neural impulse or spike.

It is the summation of all the EPSPs, the IPSPs, and the modulating effects of postsynaptic activity that will eventually determine whether neural firing occurs at that particular moment. The action of the protein receptors on the receiving neuron may make a great deal of difference as to how the neuron reacts to the signaling of a particular neuron or group of neurons. Receptor proteins can be classified into two broad categories.[3] Ionotropic receptors work to form ion channels or pores through which ions may easily move into the receptor neuron and alter the electric properties of the cell. Metabotropic receptors work by coupling with intracellular proteins called G-protein coupled receptors (GPCR). These G-proteins may have direct effects on the membrane ion channels or may regulate enzymes that work as second messenger molecules to alter cell properties. There are other postsynaptic actions that may occur, such as the influx of calcium through ion channels or the activation of receptors through membrane permeable substances such as nitric oxide.

In the next section we discuss some basic information about neurotransmitters. Elaboration on second messenger or other neuromodulation actions is beyond the scope of this text. It should be understood, however, that these events serve as neuromodulators and work with neurotransmitters, both natural and designed, to possibly alter properties of neurons and their synapses. These alterations might include changes in the firing rate, spike duration, ion channel selectivity, synaptic strength, and synaptic plasticity, to mention a few. Obviously, we have only scratched the surface of what is to be understood about how neurons communicate with each other, but the understanding of this basic information will enable you to explore further if you wish.

Neurotransmitters

Neurotransmitters are the fundamental basis for chemical action in the nervous system. Table 4.1 illustrates the criteria generally agreed on as necessary to define a substance as a neurotransmitter.

There are many different neurotransmitters in the nervous system. Squire et al.[9] classified them into three broad categories: classical, nonclassical, and unconventional neurotransmitters. Box 4.4 lists some of the neurotransmitters in each of these classifications. Early studies of neurons presented them as containing only one neurotransmitter, but it is now known that a single neuron usually contains

TABLE 4.1   What Makes a Chemical Substance a Neurotransmitter?

Production	A neurotransmitter must be synthesized by the neuron and released from the neuron. The presynaptic terminal should therefore contain the neurotransmitter and the enzymes necessary to synthesize it.
Identification	The substance should be released in a form that can be chemically or pharmacologically identified; therefore, it should be possible to isolate it and know its structure.
Reproduction capability	The events that occur on stimulation of the presynaptic terminal should be reproduced by the effect of this substance on the postsynaptic cell.
Blocking	The effects of the substance should be blocked by a competitive antagonist of the receptor in a dose-dependent manner. Treatments that inhibit the synthesis of the substance should block the effect of presynaptic stimulation as well.
Termination	There should be a mechanism that will terminate the action of the substance on the cell (uptake, enzymatic inactivation, etc.).

Modified from Squire, L. R., Berg, D., Bloom, F. E., du Lac, S., Ghosh, A., & Spitzer, N. C. (2013). *Fundamental neuroscience* (4th ed.). Academic Press.

BOX 4.4   Classical, Nonclassical, and Unconventional Neurotransmitters

Classical
GABA
Glycine
Glutamate
Aspartate
Homocysteine
Taurine
Acetylcholine
Monoamines
Catecholamines
Dopamine
Norepinephrine
Epinephrine
Serotonin
Adenosine
Adenosine triphosphate
Nitric oxide

Nonclassical: neuropeptides
Beta-endorphin
Dynorphin
Neoendorphin
Arginine vasopressin
Oxytocin
Substance P
Kassinin
Neurokinin A
Neurokinin B
Eledoisin
Vasoactive intestinal peptide
Glucagon
Secretin
Growth hormone-releasing hormone
Methionine enkephalin
Leucine enkephalin

Unconventional
Endocannabinoids
Nitric oxide

more than one and sometimes as many as three neurotransmitters.[4] Neurotransmitters carry information about and provide stimulation for changes in the functional state of a presynaptic or postsynaptic neuron. The effect on the postsynaptic membrane can be excitatory or inhibitory, but most serve to modulate the excitability of the neuron. For classification purposes, neurotransmitter specificity also can be used to describe neurons and their axons. For example, cells that contain the neurotransmitter dopamine are called dopaminergic neurons. If they contain glutamate, they are called glutamatergic.

SLPs and audiologists often are confronted with patients who are diagnosed with disorders of neurotransmitter metabolism. Parkinson disease results from a decrease in dopamine production in the substantia nigra. The decreased dopamine production accounts for the characteristic tremor and the inability to control movements. Research in Parkinson disease is striving to determine what triggers the rapid death of the dopaminergic cells.

The original treatment for Parkinson disease included administration of a form of L-dopa, a precursor of dopamine. This helped the nervous system increase dopamine synthesis, but it did not last long. More current pharmacologic therapy includes a combination of L-dopa with carbidopa because carbidopa cannot cross the blood-brain barrier (see Chapter 2). Carbidopa decreases L-dopa metabolism in the peripheral tissues, thus making it more readily available for the CNS to increase dopamine synthesis in the healthy neurons that are left.

Patients with seizures experience the effects of abnormal activity of glutamatergic neurons. Because it is an excitatory neurotransmitter, rapid and sustained firing of even a small group of these neurons in one area of the brain may lead to successive excitation of other similar neurons until a region, or in the case of a grand mal seizure, the entire brain, experiences a paroxysmal discharge, which is the seizure activity. Pharmacologic treatment is targeted toward utilization of GABA transmitters to inhibit neural firing. Drugs such as phenobarbital are used for long-term management of seizures.

Chemical Transmission in the Motor System

In peripheral nerve-to-muscle (neuromuscular) transmission, the nerve is known to be a structure on the muscle surface, making contact with the muscle fiber but not fusing with it. A special structural enlargement of the muscle fiber called the **motor endplate** is at the synaptic junction. In the PNS, electrical currents are generated by the flow of transmitter substance acetylcholine across the synapse to the postsynaptic membrane. In neuromuscular impulses, this membrane is the motor endplate. An impulse is then generated along the muscle fiber, which sets off a complex series of events for muscle contraction.

Myasthenia gravis is an unusual disorder of neurotransmitter relay in the motor system. With this neuromuscular disease, the patient shows muscle weakness on sustained effort. Neuromuscular transmission appears to fail after continuous muscle contraction as a result of reduced availability of acetylcholine at the synapse between nerve and muscle. Antibodies interfere with the transmission of the acetylcholine. These antibodies are an autoimmune disease reaction to the postsynaptic receptor protein, with an involvement of the postsynaptic membranes. In the earlier stages, if the muscle is allowed to rest, normal function is restored until further use again depletes the acetylcholine.

The primary symptom of weakness often affects the speech muscles. The nerves innervating the larynx and velum are sometimes the first to be affected by the disease. The weakened vocal folds do not close appropriately, and the voice becomes breathy and weak in intensity. A hypernasal voice quality may develop after sustained speaking because of weakness of the muscles of the soft palate. As the speech deteriorates, the tongue, lips, and respiratory muscles may be involved. Speech symptoms are discussed further in Chapter 8.

Certain drugs (e.g., neostigmine [Prostigmin] and edrophonium [Tensilon]) temporarily and promptly relieve the symptoms, and Tensilon was at one time used to help the neurologist diagnose the disease. However, in 2018 the US Food and Drug Administration discontinued edrophonium due to the high rate of false positives in testing for myasthenia. Serologic antibody testing is now performed in diagnosis. Neostigmine as well as current treatments with monoclonal antibodies (derived from cloning unique white blood cells) are used in treatment to reduce the antibodies blocking the acetylcholine transmission.

Electrical Synapses (Gap Junctions)

Although chemical synapses are by far the most common signaling mechanism in the nervous system, electrical synapses occur more frequently than once thought. In vertebrates, they occur often at sensory synapses (e.g., in the retina), in some nuclei of the thalamus, and in some cortico-cortical neuron transmissions. They allow more rapid signaling because there is no electrical-to-chemical-to-electrical transition necessary. Rather than occurring at the synaptic cleft, these transmissions occur primarily at gap junctions between dendrites or between two closely adjacent neuron cell bodies. Electrical synapses are excitatory only; there are no inhibitory electrical synapses. No neurotransmitter is involved, and no delay at the synapse occurs. Thus, no modulation of the transmission is possible. Electrical synapses occur to ensure that neurons that must participate in a common activity fire in synchrony. An example of this occurs in the medulla for synchronous discharge during inspiration.

PRINCIPLES OF NEURONAL OPERATION

The CNS is constantly bombarded by volleys of sensory nerve impulses. Both excitation and inhibition play a large role in the nervous system. The excitatory and inhibitory influences provide a process of **selectivity** of impulses for transmission at the level of the synapse. This selectivity of transmission of nerve impulse may be the basic function of the synapse. The synapse also allows transmission in an all-or-nothing manner. In other words, all that can be transmitted is either a full-sized response for the condition of the axon or nothing.

Furthermore, the CNS is characterized by the principle of **divergence**. Charles Sherrington[7] observed that within the human nervous system are numerous branchings of all axons. Axon branches, or collaterals, give rise to multiple terminals, thus resulting in numerous synaptic contacts. This results in great opportunity for wide dispersal of impulses because the impulses discharged by a neuron travel along those branches to activate all the associated synapses. Synaptic divergence means that an AP can trigger multiple EPSPs simultaneously, affecting many dendritic terminals at once. This amplifies the activity of a single axon. This kind of divergent synaptic action is found in the sensory afferents of the thalamus and is common in the cortical cells as well as in the cerebellum, which demonstrates great divergence. Thus, the CNS is composed of an almost infinite series of sources and routes for widespread or accessory neuronal activity. This accessory neuronal activity forms what may be considered neuronal pools of activity.

A complementary principle of **convergence** exists in the nervous system. This principle, also enumerated by Sherrington,[7] implies that all neurons receive synaptic information from many other neurons, some of an excitatory nature and some of an inhibitory nature. Synaptic convergence ensues when multiple synapses occur on one postsynaptic dendrite. The number of synapses on individual neurons is generally large, measured in hundreds or thousands, with the largest being approximately 80,000. When convergence occurs, two kinds of **summation**, or additive effects, may take place. Temporal summation may occur in which the effect of the neurotransmitters may be enhanced (e.g., if the additive effect of all synapses is excitatory). The convergence could also summate in time with the excitatory and inhibitory potentials canceling each other out, resulting in the resting potential being maintained. The integration of the excitatory and inhibitory synapses usually functions, however, to modulate action. With modulation, there is a change in potential, but it is not as great a change as it would have been without the convergence.

Another kind of convergence summation is spatial summation. During this, the varied sites of synapse along the dendritic surface of the neuron cause responses to rise in the different parts of the neuron (graded potentials). The summation may increase the possibility of more local mechanisms during activation from the site on one dendritic tree to another.

Principles of divergence and convergence also suggest that certain neuronal systems can act primarily as either excitatory or inhibitory mechanisms for effective overall neuronal functioning. An example is the large excitatory and inhibitory neuronal system in the reticular formation deep within the brain, which both activates and suppresses levels of consciousness during wakefulness and sleep, respectively. Box 4.5 summarizes the principles of divergence and convergence.

The complexity of the neuronal firings and synaptic connections, particularly on the surface of the brain called the cerebral cortex, provides an intricate weaving of impulses into complex spatial and temporal patterns. Sherrington[7] has compared this neuronal activity with the weaving of an enchanted loom. Today, in the age of technology, we tend to compare it with an extremely complex network. No doubt these ever-changing neuronal designs are the basis for the integrative activity of the nervous system and are the foundations of emotion, thought, language, and action, as well as that most human of behaviors, speaking.

The range of behavior that is assumed to be specifically human, including our rich and complex language system, is sometimes difficult to grasp. Even harder to believe is that this range ultimately can be reduced to and equated with the mere ebb and flow of minute chemical and electrical changes in tiny but intricate synaptic mechanisms. This contemporary interpretation of neuronal function, reductionist as it appears, highlights the vast and mysterious frontier between mind and brain that faces the neuroscientist. Despite this great gulf between mind and matter, the SLP should remember that this view of neuronal functioning provides the neurophysiologist with a basis for seeing the workings of the brain as a vast abstract complex of neuronal design on the enchanted loom of Sherrington.[7] Despite the sophistication of studying neuronal function, the specifics of the neuronal patterns for understanding and producing language and speech in the brain remain largely a mystery.

DEGENERATION AND REGENERATION OF NEURONS AND THEIR CONNECTIONS

Degeneration

Primary neuronal loss refers to the immediate necrotic degeneration of neurons directly affected by, for instance, anoxia, physical trauma, or vascular insult such as a **cerebrovascular accident (CVA)**. Secondary neuronal loss, on the other hand, refers to the degeneration of neurons that occurs hours, days, or weeks after the primary insult. The secondary neuronal loss is variable and can have an effect on prognosis.

If the axon of the neuron is damaged or severed, degeneration, but not death, of the neuron may occur. In the case of damage to the nerves of the PNS, the damage to the axon may be at a point close to the cell body of origin or to a point far away because they often extend some distance. In the CNS, especially with cortical lesions or lesions in the spinal cord, because the cells are so close in proximity, secondary neuronal loss and degeneration of neurons may occur in the region just adjacent to the primary area of tissue damage. Several variables have an effect on the mechanisms of degeneration. These could include blood flow levels, the integrity of the blood-brain barrier, edema, and inflammation.

Two types of damage may occur in axons. Anterograde degeneration refers to the degradation of axonal structure that spreads away from the cell body. Wallerian degeneration is the most common type of anterograde degeneration and is often considered a synonymous term. Wallerian degeneration is the type of deterioration of axons and the myelin sheath resulting from more proximal axonal or neuronal damage. Deterioration consists of a pulling away of the myelin sheath and swelling of the axon with it eventually breaking into segments. The terminals continue to deteriorate, and the distal segment eventually dies. Glial cells then will go through the area and rid it of the debris.

In the PNS, retrograde degeneration, or spread of deterioration toward the cell body, may occur and the cell body itself may undergo chromatolysis (loss of color) from the loss of the Nissl cells. This may eventually lead to cell death.

Regeneration in the Peripheral Nervous System

Axonal regeneration most likely occurs in the PNS when a peripheral nerve is either compressed or crushed but not severed and permanently damaged. The injured axon degenerates distal to the lesion, and the myelin sheath begins to break up. Monocytes from the blood enter and become macrophages to clean up the debris. The macrophages also signal the Schwann cells to secrete trophic substances to feed and guide the growth of new axonal sprouts. The axonal sprouting begins at the site of injury days to weeks after the injury. If regeneration is to be successful, the sprouting axons must make contact with the Schwann cells of the distal stump. The

---

BOX 4.5   Principles of Divergence and Convergence

Divergence
- Branching of all axons within the human nervous system allows activation of all proximate synapses.
- Creates limitless pathways for potential neuronal activity.
- Allows grouping of neuronal activity: excitation or inhibition.

Convergence
- Individual neurons receive multiple signals simultaneously from many other neurons.
- Signals from multiple neurons can be conflicting (some that excite and some that inhibit).
- Activation or suppression of an individual neuron is based on these incoming signals.

sprouting axons exhibit swellings on their tips. These swellings are called growth cones. The Schwann cells on the distal stump send out processes toward these growth cones. Regeneration usually proceeds at approximately 5 mm/day in the larger nerve trunks, with growth in the finer branches at approximately 2 mm/day.

If the nerve trunk of a peripheral nerve has been completely severed, spontaneous regeneration is not as successful because the axonal sprouts are not as likely to reach the appropriate distal stump targets. If the proximal axon sprouts fail to make contact, a neuroma may form, with whorls of these regenerating axons trapped in scar tissue at the injury site. Surgical repair of a severed nerve trunk is not usually attempted for a few weeks; delay is desired so that connective sheaths can thicken somewhat to be able to hold sutures better.

Regeneration in the Central Nervous System

If injury occurs to white matter in the CNS, degeneration distal to the point of injury occurs as it does in the PNS. However, clearance of the debris by the microglial cells and monocytes proceeds quite slowly, with debris found months later. Rather than the chromatolysis noted in parent cell bodies of peripheral nerves, the neurons in the CNS that are injured tend to **necrose**, or die. Surviving neurons in the area may appear wasted and usually do not make many synaptic contacts. This large-scale death of neurons is caused by the process of **orthograde transneuronal atrophy**. Neurons of the CNS normally have a trophic effect on each other—that is, they sustain each other. When the main input to a group of neurons is damaged

and no longer effective, the whole group is likely to waste away. Sometimes a phenomenon called **retrograde transneuronal degeneration** occurs in neurons upstream to those initially affected by the lesion. Astrocytes may initiate the formation of a glial scar, which replaces the neuronal debris in the case of a small lesion. With a large lesion, cystic cavities containing cerebrospinal fluid and blood may be left.

Animal studies in the laboratory have provided hope that CNS neurons have regenerative capacity because they have shown sprouting of axons and invasion of planted peripheral nerves. In the CNS, deterrents to spontaneous regeneration like that seen in the PNS are the glial scar tissue that develops and the growth inhibition caused by breakdown of oligodendrocyte products. Unfortunately, oligodendrocytes of the CNS do not generate growth signals (like the active signaling for growth by the Schwann cells in the PNS). In general the CNS in mammals seems to lack trophic factors required to initiate the significant sprouting of axons. Injured motor and sensory pathways will regenerate only for a few millimeters, and if synapses develop they are usually on nearby neurons.

At this writing, active areas of research for provision of trophic factors for regeneration in the CNS include control of reactive astrogliosis,[8] injection of the substance secreted by stem cells (secretome),[3] and neural tissue engineering using biofabrication of scaffolds for tissue support and transport.[2,5] Athough medical science has yet to find a proven way to regenerate neurons or hasten connections, there is promising research, including clinical trials, giving hope for the future of rehabilitation.

SYNOPSIS OF CLINICAL INFORMATION OR APPLICATIONS FOR THE SPEECH-LANGUAGE PATHOLOGIST

- A neuron is a nerve cell that is the basic anatomic and functional unit of the nervous system.
- Neurons have a cell body that synthesizes proteins.
- The three types of neuronal cells are classified by shape: multipolar, pseudounipolar, and bipolar.
- Each cell contains a nucleus and 1 to 12 projections of varying length that receive stimuli and conduct neural impulses.
- Dendrites receive neural stimuli; shorter ones receive signals from other neurons.
- Axons are longer single fibers that conduct nerve impulses away from the neuron to other parts of the nervous system, glands, and muscles.
- A synapse is the point of contact between the axon of one neuron and another neuron's cell body.
- This action produces neuronal activity or brain activation, thus producing perceptions, thoughts, and voluntary muscle movements.
- Cellular potential is the relative amount of voltage in an electrical field.
- Neurons have two electrical fields—one inside and one outside the cell body.
- Functions of neuron integration (thinking or cognition) depend on electrical properties and how the ions move.

- Resting potential is the ionic difference across the membrane at a steady state in the cell.
- AP is the neural impulse that travels to another cell body, dendrite, or axon.
- APs are brief electrical transients visible when recorded.
- APs occur throughout the body's tissues and regulate secretions of hormones and signal fertilization of the egg by the sperm. In a nervous system, APs integrate neural messages from cell bodies from sense organs.
- Nerve fibers, or axons, are either myelinated or unmyelinated.
- Myelin is a white, fatty, lipid substance that surrounds the axon for protection and transmission.
- Myelin in the CNS is oligodendrocytes.
- Myelin in the PNS is Schwann cells.
- Myelin is white, as opposed to the nonmyelinated cells, which appear gray.
- Myelin develops as the brain develops from the embryonic state.
- Multiple sclerosis is an autoimmune inflammatory response that damages the myelin sheath; it may cause irreversible damage.
- Dysarthria is a speech disorder found in some neurologic diseases.

SYNOPSIS OF CLINICAL INFORMATION OR APPLICATIONS FOR THE SPEECH-LANGUAGE PATHOLOGIST—cont'd

- The synapse is the point at which an electrical nerve impulse in the form of an AP must be transmitted to another neuron, gland, or muscle.
- The presynaptic terminal is at the axon sending the impulse.
- The postsynaptic terminal is the receiving area of the receiving axon.
- The synapse between the presynaptic and postsynaptic space, called the synaptic cleft, is transmitted by chemical reaction.
- Chemical substances known as neurotransmitters are released by the presynaptic terminal; they diffuse across the synaptic cleft and bind with receptors in the postsynaptic terminal.
- Neurotransmitters provide excitatory action from the presynaptic terminal; to ensure completion of the synapse across the cleft, neurotransmitters also provide an inhibitory action from the postsynaptic terminal.
- Neurotransmitters are the fundamental basis for chemical action in the nervous system.
- Neurotransmitter types are named specifically to describe the neurons and axons that are part of the synapse process.
- The neurotransmitter dopamine has cells called dopaminergic neurons; if the cells contain glutamate, they are called glutamatergic cells.
- GABA and glutamate are the most prevalent neurotransmitters.
- Glutamate is a major excitatory neurotransmitter.
- GABA is a major inhibitory neurotransmitter.
- Disorders of neurotransmitter metabolism include Parkinson disease, which is caused by a decrease in dopamine in the substantia nigra.
- Myasthenia gravis is a condition caused by reduced acetylcholine at the synapse between nerve and muscle.
- Primary neuronal loss is necrotic degeneration of neurons affected by anoxia or CVA.
- Secondary neuronal loss is degeneration of neurons that occurs within hours, days, or weeks after a primary insult; it may include effects on blood flow, integrity of the blood-brain barrier, edema, and inflammation.
- Neurons in the adult brain that are lost to trauma or disease are not replaced.
- In Parkinson and Alzheimer diseases, neurons die in large numbers and leave those areas of the brain nonfunctional for motor function or cognition.
- If axons are simply damaged, then regeneration may be possible.
- Axonal damage is categorized as anterograde or retrograde.
- Anterograde damage is disintegration of the myelin sheath that depends on the Schwann cells or oligodendrocytes.
- Retrograde damage is characterized by swollen cell bodies, an enlarged nucleus, and dissolution of endoplasm.
- Large-scale death of neurons is called orthograde transneuronal atrophy.
- Research on astrogliosis, the secretome, and neural tissue engineering is currently being done to investigate neuronal regeneration in the CNS and PNS.

REFERENCES

1. Desmond, A., & Offit, P. A. (2021). On the shoulders of giants—from Jenner's cowpox to mRNA covid vaccines. *New England Journal of Medicine, 384*(12), 1081–1083.
2. Dolgin, E. (2021). The tangled history of mRNA vaccines. *Nature, 597*(7876), 318–324.
3. Drago, D., Cossetti, C., Iraci, N., Gaude, E., Musco, G., Bachi, A., & Pluchino, S. (2013). The stem cell secretome and its role in brain repair. *Biochimie, 95*(12), 2271–2285. http://www.ncbi.nlm.nih.gov/pmc/articles/PMC4061727.
4. Dwyer, T. M. (2018). Chemical signaling in the nervous system. In D. E. Haines & G. A. Mihailoff (Eds.), *Fundamental neuroscience for basic and clinical applications* (5th ed., pp. 54–71). Elsevier.
5. Papadimitriou, L., Manganas, P., Ranella, A., & Stratakis, E. (2020). Biofabrication for neural tissue engineering applications. *Materials Today Bio, 6*, article 100043.
6. Schubert, D., Herrera, F., Cumming, R., Read, J., Low, W., Maher, P., & Fischer, W. H. (2009). Neural cells secrete a unique repertoire of proteins. *Journal of Neurochemistry, 109*(2), 427–435.
7. Sherrington, C. S. (1926). *The integrative action of the nervous system.* Yale University Press.
8. Sofroniew, M. V., & Vinters, H. V. (2010). Astrocytes: Biology and pathology. *Acta Neuropathologica, 119*(1), 7–35.
9. Squire, L. R., Berg, D., Bloom, F. E., du Lac, S., Ghosh, A., & Spitzer, N. C. (2013). *Fundamental neuroscience* (4th ed.). Academic Press.

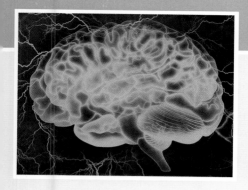

5

Neurosensory Organization

Speech is normally controlled by the ear.

Raymond Carhart, Hearing and Deafness, 1947

KEY TERMS

agnosia
analgesia
anterior spinothalamic tract
astereognosis
atopognosis
audition
auditory agnosia
auditory brainstem responses
   (ABRs)
basilar membrane
cerebellopontine angle
cochlea
cochlear duct
dermatome
dorsal column pathway
endolymph
exteroceptors

fasciculi
helicotrema
hemianopsia
hyperalgesia
hyperesthesia
hypoalgesia
hypoesthesia
interoceptors
lateral spinothalamic tract
mechanicoreceptors
modiolus
nociceptors
optic chiasm
optic disk
organ of Corti
perilymph
peristriate cortex

photoreceptors
proprioceptors
Romberg test
scalae
spinocerebellar pathway
spiral ganglion
splenium
stereocilia
stereognosis
striate cortex
tectal (collicular) pathway
tectorial membrane
temporal visual cortex
tonotopic
visual agnosia

CLASSIFICATION

During the 19th century, neurophysiologists primarily conceived the execution of skilled motor acts as the result of programming in the motor areas of the cerebral cortex, with some additional influences on the descending motor impulses from cerebellar and extrapyramidal mechanisms. This view of the nervous system was modified during the 20th century to include the concept of sensory feedback control in motor acts. Audition, of course, plays a special and primary feedback role in the control of speech. More recently, specific efforts have been directed at determining the nature of other neurosensory controls exercised in speaking. Before discussion of sensory control in speech, an understanding of the general types of sensation mediated by the nervous system is necessary.

Sherrington's Scheme

Charles Sherrington[1,9,11] proposed a classification of sensation that has application for the sensory control of speech. He divided the sensory receptors into three broad classes: exteroceptors, proprioceptors, and interoceptors. **Exteroceptors** mediate sight, sound, smell, and cutaneous sensation. Cutaneous superficial skin sensation includes light touch or pressure, fine touch (also known as two-point or discriminative touch), superficial pain, temperature, itching, and tickling. **Proprioceptors** mediate deep somatic sensation from receptors beneath the skin, in muscles and joints, and in the inner ear. Proprioception includes the senses of movement, vibration, position, and equilibrium. **Interoceptors** mediate sensation from the viscera as well as visceral pain and pressure or distention. Pain receptors, either from cellular or tissue injury, are known as **nociceptors**.

Neurophysiologists have classified the senses as special and general. The term special senses reflects the traditional layperson's concept that certain senses are primary. For the neurophysiologist, hearing, vision, taste, smell, and balance are the special senses. The general senses, in this classification scheme, include the remainder of the senses. Further breakdown into visceral and somatic sensations has also been added to the classification schemes. General visceral afferent interoceptors monitor events within the body, including bladder distention and pH changes in the blood. Special visceral afferent receptors are those of taste and smell (olfaction). Special somatic afferent receptors are concerned with vision, audition, and balance or equilibrium.

Sensory Association Cortices

In Chapter 2 the functional typology of association cortex was discussed, with unimodal and polymodal association cortices found in the sensory processing areas of the brain. Afferent projections of sensory information initially are processed in unimodal cortex found in the primary sensory cortices, including the visual cortex (area 17 along the calcarine fissure), the auditory cortex (areas 41 and 42 in Heschl gyrus), and the somatosensory cortex (areas 1–3 in the postcentral gyrus). Areas around the primary sensory cortices usually are polymodal association cortex. The visual association cortex includes the entire medial surface of the occipital lobe beyond the primary area, the lateral surface of the occipital lobe (areas 18 and 19), the inferior and middle temporal gyri, and the entire inferior surface of the temporal lobe (areas 20, 21, and 37). The auditory association cortices include the areas around Heschl gyrus and area 22, a portion of the superior temporal gyrus. Area 22 in the left temporal lobe, however, is considered more of a supramodal association area than simply a polymodal processor because of the language processing capability.

Recognition and identification or classification of a sensory stimulus is a critical function and can preclude or complicate evaluation of communication skills. Perception of a word requires adequate hearing acuity, but the stimulus must also be recognized to be a word. The features must be visually, audibly, or tactilely perceived before an object can be recognized. Sensory disorders resulting in an inability to interpret a sensory stimulus and recognize it are called agnosias.

The term **agnosia** was introduced to neurology by Sigmund Freud (1856–1939) in 1891. Agnosia is a disorder of recognition caused by cerebral injury. Classic theory places the lesion responsible for the disorder in the sensory association areas of the cerebral cortex, leaving the primary sensory receptor areas intact. To diagnose the classic disorder correctly, certain precautions must be observed. First, the lesion must be determined to be at the level of the cortical association area rather than at the level of the sensory receptor, the sensory pathway, or the primary sensory receptor area in the cortex. Second, unfamiliarity with the test item must be ruled out as a reason for failure to recognize the sensory stimuli. To establish basic knowledge of an item, the patient should match items. If an item can be matched or recognized in other modalities, unfamiliarity can be ruled out as a possible cause for the lack of recognition. For example, prosopagnosia is a type of visual agnosia where faces are no longer recognized following brain injury, in the absence of other visual impairments. In other words, the person can see and recognize all visual stimuli but is unable to identify faces. The affected individual continues to be able to match identical faces to each other in an array, demonstrating intact visual abilities, but demonstrated difficulty identifying familiar people from their faces alone. Many degrees of impairment in prosopagnosia have been described, with the most severe cases being those in which patients do not recognize their own image in a photo or their own reflection in a mirror.[2,4]

The concept of agnosia has been highly criticized in contemporary neurology. Although true agnosias are not common, some patients in clinical practice appear to demonstrate a tactile, visual, or auditory agnosia. Table 5.1 defines the various types of agnosias that may be seen in a clinical practice specializing in neurobehavioral disorders.

THE SENSE OF HEARING

A major aspect of speech and language function depends on audition. **Audition** generally is classified as one of the special senses and as an exteroceptive sense. Knowledge of the neurologic functions of the central auditory pathways is crucial for an understanding of the mechanisms of the communicative nervous system.

Before discussing the specific levels of the central auditory pathway, a review of how sound is transmitted to the inner ear and the auditory nerve, cranial nerve VIII, is warranted. The physical signal known as sound undergoes a series of complex transformations for it to be heard. These transformations begin when a mechanical disturbance causes molecules in the air to alternately expand and compress (vibrate) and sets up a displacement that is passed along among the molecules. The resulting sound waves are channeled by the external ear structures into the external auditory meatus, or ear canal, the resonating canal that ends at a taut membrane called the eardrum, or tympanic membrane (Fig. 5.1). The eardrum is at the entrance to the middle ear, an air-filled cavity containing

the three tiniest bones of the body: malleus, incus, and stapes, collectively known as the ossicles. This ossicular chain has one end attached to the eardrum and the other to a small opening at the inferior part of the cavity called the oval window. Mechanical transmission of vibration through the ossicular chain helps increase the force that reaches the oval window. The force causes the oval window to move and transmit the movement into the fluid-filled cavity of the inner ear. The inner ear contains the coiled **cochlea** (Fig. 5.2). On the membranes of the cochlea are the sensory hair cells that contain neurotransmitters to be released to stimulate the auditory nerve, cranial nerve VIII. This auditory nerve then carries this signal to the cochlear nucleus in the brainstem and on to its final destination, the auditory cortex.

Receptor Level

The cochlea of the inner ear serves as an acoustic transducer, changing fluid vibrations to nerve impulses. The design and function of the cochlea are incredibly complex and intricate. A summary of this fascinating structure for study by the speech-language pathologist (SLP) is, of necessity, brief. More in-depth information can be found in other texts.[3,11]

Fig. 5.2 depicts a cross section of the cochlea. This coiled structure has a central bony, hollow core called the **modiolus**, which is in the axis of the internal auditory meatus. Running through the modiolus is the cochlear division of cranial nerve VIII, the acoustic-vestibular nerve. The cell bodies of its neurons form the **spiral ganglion**, and these are the primary or first-order neurons of the auditory pathway.

Forming a coil of two and a half turns around the modiolus are three separate fluid-filled columns called **scalae** (see Fig. 5.2). The upper compartment is the scala vestibuli, and the lower chamber is the scala tympani. These two chambers communicate at the apex of the modiolus at a site called the **helicotrema**. Between these two compartments is a third chamber called the scala media, also known as the **cochlear duct**.

TABLE 5.1	**Agnosias**
Type of Agnosia	**Characteristics**
Agnosia	A disorder of recognition caused by damage to cortical sensory association areas or pathways
Visual agnosia	Inability to recognize objects, colors, and pictures
Auditory agnosia	Inability to comprehend speech or nonspeech sounds (pure forms: auditory nonverbal agnosia and pure word deafness)
Tactile syndrome	Inability to recognize objects by touch; characterized by bilateral parietal lobe lesions
Gerstmann syndrome	Includes finger agnosia, right-left disorientation, acalculia, and agraphia; usually characterized by left parietal lobe lesions

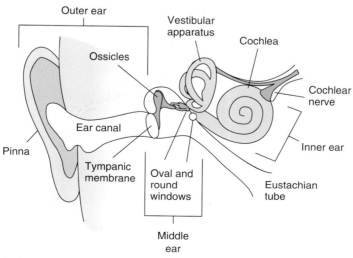

Fig. 5.1 Three divisions of the ear. In the outer ear sound waves are directed to the middle ear, where they are converted to oscillations of the ossicles. In the inner ear the oscillations are converted to pressure waves, which in turn are converted to neuronal activity. (From Castro, A., Neafsey, E. J., Merchut, M. P., & Wurster, R. D. [2002]. *Neuroscience: An outline approach.* Mosby/Elsevier.)

The scala vestibuli and the scala tympani are filled with a fluid called **perilymph**. The cochlear duct is filled with a different fluid, **endolymph**. These two fluids do not mix because of a tight barrier of epithelium lining the cochlear duct. The vestibular membrane, or Reissner membrane, separates the cochlear duct and the scala vestibuli, and the basilar membrane separates the cochlear duct from the scala tympani.

Membranes of fibrous connective tissue also run between the epithelium and the bones of the cochlea. The spiral lamina projects from the modiolus. Attached to the tip of the spiral lamina is the **basilar membrane**.

This membrane reaches across the cavity of the cochlea, forming the floor of the cochlear duct, and attaches to the spiral ligament on the outer wall of the cochlea. Fig. 5.3 shows a cross section of the cochlear duct, looking at the cochlea in an upright position rather than its usual position on its side.

The basilar membrane is an important structure because it contains the **organ of Corti**, the sensory epithelium of hearing. When sound occurs, causing vibration of the tympanic membrane and movement of the ossicles of the middle ear, movement of the oval window leading into the scala vestibule occurs. This creates a pressure wave in the perilymph in the scala vestibuli. The pressure waves are transmitted through the vestibular membrane to the basilar membrane. This movement then sets up a neural chain of events in the organ of Corti.

In the organ of Corti are several types of cells, with the two most important being the inner hair cells and the outer hair cells. These cell types are separated by a central tunnel, with the outer hair cells located on the outer side of the tunnel. The hair cells rest on supporting cells; other ancillary cells also are in the structure. On the top of the hair cells are **stereocilia**, extremely long microvilli extending from the surface. Overlying the hair cells and their stereocilia is a gelatinous structure called the **tectorial membrane**. The stereocilia of the inner hair cells lie just below the tectorial membrane, whereas those of the outer hair cells are embedded in the tectorial membrane (see Fig. 5.3). The outer hair cells outnumber the inner cells by approximately 3:1, but most of the neurons of the spiral ganglion innervate inner hair cells, with up to 20 large afferent neurons synapsing on each inner hair cell. These myelinated neurons innervating the inner hair cells are called type I cells, and each one responds best to a certain frequency.

The organ of Corti also receives efferent innervation coming from the olivocochlear bundle of the superior olivary complex in the brainstem.[8] Thus, some information comes from the brain to the cochlea rather than it all being unidirectional, from cochlea to brain. Some neurons go to the outer hair cells. These well-myelinated efferent neurons (medial olivocochlear bundle) typically cross the midline and exit the

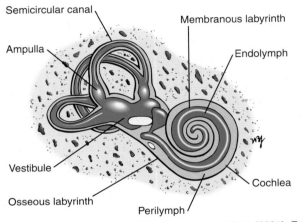

Semicircular canal
Membranous labyrinth
Ampulla
Endolymph
Vestibule
Cochlea
Osseous labyrinth
Perilymph

Fig. 5.2 Cross section of the cochlea. (From Swartz, M. H. [2021]. *Textbook of physical diagnosis: History and examination* [8th ed.]. Elsevier.)

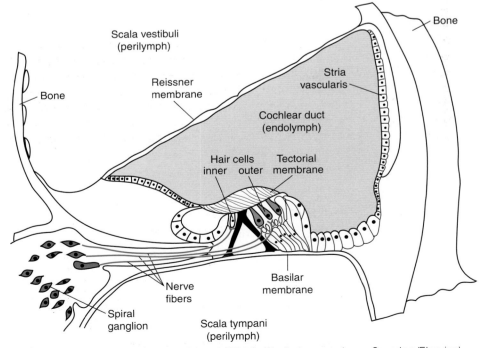

Scala vestibuli (perilymph)
Bone
Reissner membrane
Stria vascularis
Bone
Cochlear duct (endolymph)
Hair cells
inner outer
Tectorial membrane
Nerve fibers
Basilar membrane
Spiral ganglion
Scala tympani (perilymph)

Fig. 5.3 Cross section of the cochlear duct. (From Nadeau, S., et al. [2004]. *Medical neuroscience*. Saunders/Elsevier.)

brain with the vestibular portion of cranial nerve VIII. They eventually join the cochlear division and travel in the spiral ganglion. They then enter the organ of Corti and synapse on the outer hair cells. Although none of the efferent fiber functions of the auditory system is well understood, these cells are believed to inhibit or reduce the movement of the outer hair cells, effectively reducing the sensitivity of the cochlea at that particular region.

Some efferent neurons also go to the inner hair cells (lateral olivocochlear bundle); these are unmyelinated, usually do not decussate, and follow the same pathway to synapse just under the inner hair cells. These fibers appear to influence the type I spiral ganglion cells by making them more difficult to excite. These efferent pathways of innervation to the cochlea are believed to combine to assist the auditory system in selective listening so that certain auditory input can be attuned to in background noise or other input can be ignored.

CRANIAL NERVE LEVEL

The nerve of hearing, cranial nerve VIII, has two divisions: the cochlear branch, associated with hearing, and the vestibular branch, associated with balance. Central processes of the cochlear nerve (the first-order neurons) proceed from the spiral ganglion through the internal auditory canal. The cochlear nerve is accompanied by cranial nerve VII, the facial nerve, in the auditory canal. The two nerves enter the brainstem at the sulcus between the pons and the medulla, an area known as the **cerebellopontine angle**. The cochlear nuclear complex spans the border between the pons and the medulla.

Brainstem Level

The fibers of the cochlear division of cranial nerve VIII end in the dorsal and ventral cochlear nuclei, which are draped around the inferior cerebellar peduncle. The cochlear nuclei contain the second-order neurons of the auditory pathway. From the cochlear nuclei, most fibers of the auditory pathway proceed to the upper medulla and pons and cross the midline. Other fibers ascend in the brainstem ipsilaterally. Fibers course upward in the ascending central auditory pathway of the brainstem called the lateral lemniscus. The fibers take one of several routes, and synapses in the auditory system may occur at one or more of the following structures: the superior olives, the inferior colliculus, and the nucleus of the lateral lemniscus. The superior olivary nuclei play an important role in localizing sound through neural response to the time and intensity differences arriving from both ears. All of the ascending auditory fibers terminate in the medial geniculate body, a thalamic nucleus.

Auditory Radiations and Cortex

The fibers arising from the medial geniculate body, coursing to the temporal cortex, are called auditory radiations. They pass through the internal capsule in their route to the bilateral primary auditory areas of the brain in the superior and transverse temporal gyri. These areas are numbered 41 and 42 and are known as Heschl gyrus.

The nuclei of the auditory pathway—the superior olivary complex, the nucleus of the lateral lemniscus, and the inferior colliculi—serve as relay nuclei as well as reflex centers. The reflex centers make connections with the eyes, head, and trunk, where automatic reflex actions occur in response to sound.

Descending efferent fibers, in addition to the ascending afferent fibers, are present in all parts of the central auditory pathway. They probably serve as feedback loops within the pathways. Fig. 5.4 shows a simplified schema of connections along the auditory pathway.

Auditory Physiology

Sound is transmitted to the central auditory pathways by a traveling wave set up on the basilar membrane of the cochlea. The basilar membrane is narrower at the base of the cochlea than at its apex. The mechanics of the membrane on which the organ of Corti is located vary slightly from base to apex. Traveling pressure waves of a specific frequency cause the basilar membrane to vibrate maximally at a specific point along the length of the membrane. Higher pitched sounds (high-pitched frequency waves) cause the shorter fibers at the basal turn of the cochlea to absorb their energy, whereas lower pitched sounds are absorbed by the longer fibers at the apical

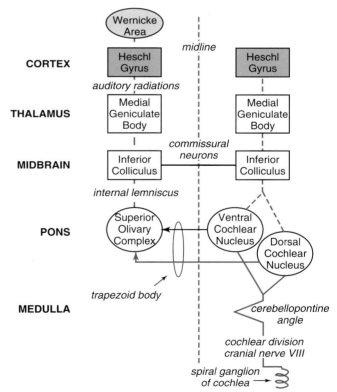

Fig. 5.4 The afferent pathways of the central auditory system and the major auditory waystations. The *bold lines* indicate that the majority of fibers in the auditory pathways decussate, although some do travel ipsilaterally *(dotted lines)*. For most of the population, perceptual sensitivity and comprehension of language occur in Wernicke area of the left hemisphere, and information coming in to the left ear has to cross to Wernicke area on the left after reaching Heschl gyrus in the right hemisphere.

turn of the cochlea. Thus, the basilar membrane is said to be **tonotopic** in its organization of fibers. This tonotopic organization extends to the inner hair cells as well. These hair cells receive afferent input from the peripheral processes of the spiral ganglion cells. When a local response to a certain frequency occurs in the hair cells, the vibration produces shearing forces, causing depolarization. Electrical charges in the dendrites of the spiral ganglion are set up and, in turn, cause the nerve cells to fire, releasing excitatory neurotransmitters.

Auditory nerve impulses ascend in the pathways of the central auditory nervous system. The organ of Corti serves as an analyzer of sound frequencies. Because of its tonotopic organization, the highest frequencies stimulate hair cells in the most basilar portion of the cochlea, where the basilar membrane is narrowest. The lowest frequencies stimulate the portions of the membrane at the apex. Frequency discrimination is therefore dependent on the frequency of the tone and the spatial response of the basilar membrane. Intensity discrimination depends on the length of the basilar membrane set in motion and the amplitude of the vibration. Displacement of a longer area of the membrane activates more nerve fibers, and a greater amplitude of vibration increases the frequency of the neural discharge.

Localizing the source of a sound depends on a comparison between the arrival time and the intensity of the sound at the two ears. Localization of sound occurs at higher levels in the auditory pathways. Central auditory structures, generally above the level of the inferior colliculus, are capable of making appropriate comparisons for sound localization. Thus, in mammals and human beings the temporal auditory cortex is not needed for simple sound recognition, but it is essential for sound localization and recognition of changes in the temporal sequencing of sounds.

Temporal sequencing is a crucial higher auditory function because it is a significant aspect of speech. Sound localization probably requires the inferior colliculus and auditory cortex, whereas temporal sequencing may require the cochlear nuclei, the medial geniculate nuclei, and the auditory cortex. A tonotopic organization is present in all the central auditory nuclei, but the nuclei are used for analysis of several auditory properties of sound other than the recognition of tones or different frequencies.

Lesions of the Auditory System

The integrity of part of the central auditory system, the auditory brainstem, may be assessed by recording **auditory brainstem responses (ABRs)**. Surface electrodes are placed on the mastoid bone and on the top of the head. Repetitive clicks are presented, evoking responses in a large number of central fibers of cranial nerve VIII. These responses stimulate activity at the cochlear nuclear level, the superior olivary complex, the lateral lemniscus tracts, and the inferior colliculi. The combined potential is enough to be picked up by the skin electrodes. This method may be used to assess hearing objectively in infants and persons who cannot cooperate in subjective testing. A normal ABR is a strong indication that the middle ear, cochlea, and auditory brainstem are functioning normally. Abnormal ABRs may be caused by a middle ear

or cochlear problem or may indicate a pathologic condition at sites in the brainstem such as at the level of the geniculate bodies, the medial colliculus, and the lateral lemniscus. If abnormal ABRs are found, further testing is necessary.

If a lesion occurs unilaterally and involves the auditory nerve in its path from the ear and includes the cochlear nuclei, the person will be deaf in one ear. The results of unilateral cortical damage do not produce complete deafness. Lesions in Heschl gyrus bilaterally may produce cortical deafness, nonverbal agnosia, or auditory agnosia.

The term **auditory agnosia** usually refers to the inability to identify auditory nonlinguistic stimuli, although many use the term when referring to the inability to recognize nonlinguistic as well as verbal stimuli. Most appropriate is the label *auditory nonverbal agnosia* for a pure deficit in which identification of nonlinguistic stimuli is impaired and *pure word deafness* if referring to the disorder in which nonverbal stimuli can be identified but speech cannot be understood. All auditory agnosias occur in the face of normal hearing acuity. The site of lesion for auditory nonverbal agnosia is in dispute but is assumed to be in the auditory association areas of both hemispheres.

Pure word deafness is an uncommon syndrome in which the patient cannot comprehend verbal language but usually reads, speaks, and writes functionally. Errors in speech are often noted, and a mild measurable language disorder (aphasia) may be present.[10] Both unilateral and bilateral temporal lobe lesions have been described. Unilateral lesions occur deep in the temporal lobe in the fibers projecting to Heschl gyrus. In the vast majority of cases, these lesions were lateralized to the left hemisphere. In bilateral lesions, auditory input from either hemisphere is unable to reach speech processing centers (i.e., Wernicke area). In either case, because the auditory input is disconnected from speech processing areas, this agnosia is often described as a disconnection syndrome.[10] It is important to remember that auditory stimuli continue to be received in Heschl gyrus, allowing for comprehension of other auditory inputs such as environmental sounds.

Anatomically, the bilateral lesion is thought to occur in the midportion of the superior temporal gyri of both hemispheres but spares Heschl gyrus. The lesions on the left are assumed to cut off connections between the primary auditory receptor cortex and Wernicke area. A lesion on the right would cut off the origin of the callosal fibers from the right auditory cortex. If auditory nonverbal agnosia co-occurs with pure word deafness, the unfortunate patient may present with cortical deafness. In this disorder, the ears receive sound normally, but the person is unable to recognize sounds and becomes functionally deaf. Anatomically, cortical deafness is caused by bilateral lesions to the primary auditory cortex of both temporal lobes.

THE SENSE OF TOUCH

Somatic Sensation

The neuroanatomy of the senses is complex. The general somatic sensory pathways—those dealing with bodily sensation—use the spinal cord and spinal nerves. Sensation to

TABLE 5.2   The Sensory Modalities Represented by the Somatosensory Systems

Modality	Submodality	Sub-Submodality	Somatosensory Pathway (Body)
Pain	Sharp cutting pain Dull burning pain Deep aching pain		Lateral spinothalamic Anterior spinothalamic, tectospinal, and reticulospinal tracts Older multisynaptic diffuse tract through reticular formation and periaqueductal gray sends fibers to hypothalamus and limbic system; mediates visceral, emotional, and autonomic reactions
Temperature	Warm/hot Cool/cold		Anterior spinothalamic, tectospinal, and reticulospinal tracts Lateral spinothalamic
Touch	Itch/tickle and crude touch Discriminative touch	Touch Pressure Flutter Vibration Muscle tension Joint pressure	Anterior spinothalamic, tectospinal, and reticulospinal tracts Medial lemniscal

the head and vocal mechanism—larynx, pharynx, soft palate, and tongue—uses the cranial nerve pathways. When these pathways are assessed for integrity during a routine office examination, the attempt is made to isolate a sensory function, like touch to a particular part of the body. Keep in mind that when you actually touch something and can describe or at least crudely perceive features of it (e.g., weight, temperature, pressure, location of touch on the body), you are using many integrated pathways. In general, most sensory pathways are three-neuron pathways from the periphery to the cerebral cortex, although some variation exists within this three-neuron organization for the sensations of touch, pain, temperature, and proprioception. For most bodily sensations carried to the brain through spinal nerves, the first-order, or prime, neuron is found on the dorsal or posterior spinal root in a mass known as a spinal ganglion. The axons then ascend and synapse on a second-order neuron. A general name for the tract formed by the axon of the second-order neuron is lemniscus. In most systems, fibers of the second-order neuron then cross the midline and ascend to the third-order neuron in the thalamus. Table 5.2 summarizes the touch pathways for the body, excluding the pathways for the oral musculature, which is discussed in Chapter 7.

Lateral Spinothalamic Tract

The crossed ascending sensory pathway in the spinal cord, known as the **lateral spinothalamic tract**, transmits the sensations of pain and temperature and perhaps itch (Fig. 5.5). The fibers enter the cord through the spinal root ganglion, travel up or down a few segments in Lissauer tract, and end in the dorsal root of the gray matter. At this point the first-order neuron synapses with the second-order neuron and promptly crosses to the other side of the spinal cord. There, the fibers enter the lateral white column or the lateral spinothalamic tract and ascend to the ventral posterior lateral nucleus in the thalamus. The axons of the lateral spinothalamic tract synapse

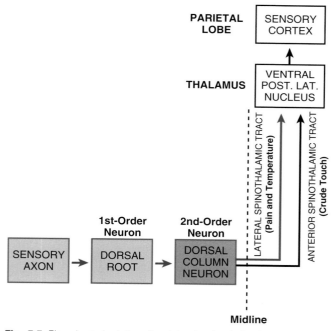

Fig. 5.5 Flowchart depicting the lateral spinothalamic tract, which mediates pain and temperature, and the anterior spinothalamic tract, which mediates light or crude touch. *POST. LAT.,* Posterior lateral.

with a third-order neuron that leaves the thalamus, ascends in the internal capsule, and reaches the postcentral cortical gyri in the parietal lobe (areas 3, 1, and 2).

Anterior Spinothalamic Tract

Approximately 10% of the spinothalamic fibers are sometimes separated in anatomic texts and presented to be fibers of the **anterior spinothalamic tract**. The anterior (or ventral) spinothalamic tract carries sensory information of crude (nondiscriminative) touch, as well as itch and tickle sensations (see Fig. 5.5). These fibers synapse within the dorsal gray horn cells in the spinal cord, cross midline, and ascend in the anterior spinothalamic tract to the brainstem and the posterior ventral nucleus of the thalamus. The fibers associated with crude touch particularly branch extensively. The anterior spinothalamic tract also ends in the postcentral gyrus of the parietal lobe.

As the fibers of the spinothalamic tracts ascend, axon collaterals provide for additional neuronal connections, most notably to the reticular nuclei in the brainstem. The reticular nuclei then send projections to the thalamus, hypothalamus, and hippocampus. Descending fibers from these structures provide for mediation of somatic and visceral responses to pain, such as changes in respiration and heartbeat as well as nausea and fainting.

Effect of damage

Damage to the spinothalamic tracts of pain and temperature usually results in loss to the opposite side of the body. Because of the extensive branching of ascending crude touch fibers, this type of touch is unlikely to be abolished by injury to a specific pathway in the spinal cord.

Proprioception Pathways

Proprioception, two-point discrimination, vibration, and form perception follow different pathways than do those of the spinothalamic tracts. Proprioception is the sense of knowing exactly where body parts are in space and in relation to one another. Two-point discrimination allows two adjacent points on the skin to be distinguished. Two-point sensitivity varies over the brain surface. The lips and fingertips are the most sensitive, and the back the least sensitive. Vibratory sensation allows the recognition of vibration from touch. Form perception allows recognition of objects by touch alone. Table 5.3 summarizes the human proprioceptive pathways.

Spinocerebellar tract. Proprioception is conveyed by fibers from muscle tendons and joints and takes two major routes after entering the spinal cord. One of these major pathways is the **spinocerebellar pathway**, and the other is the **dorsal column pathway**.

The spinocerebellar pathways are of lesser importance in human neurology because of the poor localizing information available about these tracts. The spinocerebellar pathway has two tracts, dorsal and ventral. These tracts arise from the posterior and medial gray matter of the cord. The dorsal tract ascends ipsilaterally, but the ventral tract crosses in the cord. Both tracts terminate in the cerebellum and allow proprioceptive impulses from all parts of the body to be integrated in the cerebellum. The spinocerebellar pathway has been proposed to function in unconscious perception of already-learned motor patterns.

Dorsal columns. Conscious proprioception, two-point discrimination, and form perception have been called the sensory modalities of the dorsal, or posterior, columns of the spinal cord. The first-order neuron of the posterior column pathway can be found in the dorsal root ganglion (Fig. 5.6). The axon of the first-order neuron enters the spinal cord and ascends to the medulla aggregately as the dorsal white columns. However, two fiber bundles, or **fasciculi**, comprise these columns. Axons entering the cord at the sacral and lumbar regions, which mediate proprioception from the leg and lower body, travel in the fasciculus gracilis, which comprises the medial dorsal column. Axons from the thoracic and cervical regions, generally related to the arm and upper body, travel in the fasciculus cuneatus, comprising the lateral dorsal columns. These first-order neuron axons terminate in the nucleus gracilis and nucleus cuneatus in the medulla. The second-order neuron axons then cross over to the other side of the medulla, where they form a bundle called the medial lemniscus. Fibers of the medial lemniscus ascend to the third-order neuron in the ventral posterior nucleus of the thalamus and then proceed to the somatosensory cortex in the parietal lobe.

Proprioceptive Deficits

Damage to the postcentral gyrus of the parietal lobe, the dorsal columns, or the dorsal root ganglion may produce a loss of proprioception, astereognosis, loss of vibratory sense, and loss of two-point discrimination in the trunk or extremities. If damage to these dorsal column fibers occurs below the level of the medulla (i.e., below the decussation of the fibers), the loss in proprioception is ipsilateral (on the same side) of the injury. Damage above the level of decussation in the medulla produces a loss in proprioception on the opposite side of the body (contralateral to the site of injury).

SENSORY EXAMINATION

The neurologist uses several traditional and standard procedures for determining sensory loss. These are incorporated into the standard neurologic examination (see Appendix C).

The senses of light touch, pain, and temperature are mediated by the fibers of the dorsal root of the spinal cord, which come from a circumscribed area of the skin known as a **dermatome**. In peripheral nerve injuries, impairment of touch corresponds to dermatomal zones; however, at the boundary of each segmental dermatome is an overlap area supplied by the adjacent segmental nerves. For instance, if the fifth thoracic nerve (T5) is severed, T3 and T6 will carry many of the pain and temperature sensations supplied by T5. This segmental overlap also is present in the spinal cord. Thus, overlap is greater for pain and temperature than for touch.

TABLE 5.3 Human Proprioceptive Pathways	
Pathway	**Description**
Proprioception	Allows temporal and spatial comprehension among body parts
Two-point discrimination	Cognition of adjacent points on dermis
Vibratory sensation	Sensory pathway to detect vibrations by touch
Form perception	Recognition of objects by touch

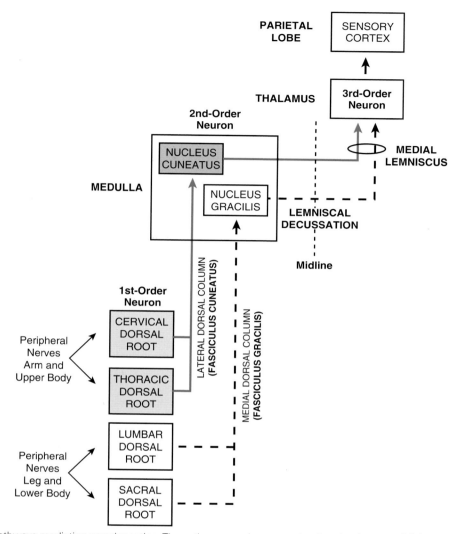

Fig. 5.6 Flowchart of pathways mediating proprioception. The pathways are known as the dorsal column modalities.

Light Touch

The sense of light touch is tested by determining the patient's ability to perceive light stroking of the skin with a wisp of cotton. Disorders of the sensory pathways from skin to cortex show abnormal sensory reactions. Decreased tactile sensation is called **hypoesthesia**, and complete loss of sensation is called anesthesia. Abnormally increased tactile sensation is known as **hyperesthesia**.

Inability to localize touch is called **atopognosis**. Topagnosis is tested by touching the patient's body. With the eyes closed, the patient is asked to point to the spot where touch occurred. The neurologist compares similar areas on both sides of the body. Atopognosia usually is associated with a lesion of the parietal lobe.

Two-Point Discrimination

Two-point discrimination, or the ability to discriminate the shortest distance between two tactile points on the skin, is sometimes tested with points of a caliper. Right and left sides of the body are compared. Loss of discrimination suggests a parietal lobe lesion.

Double stimulation may also be used to determine a cortical sensory disorder. Two simultaneous tactile stimulations are presented to both sides of the body in similar areas or to different areas. Lateralized sensory loss can then be determined. Sensory pathway or cortical sensory losses frequently accompany lesions that produce cerebral language disorders.

Pain and Temperature

Pain and temperature disturbance are more likely to be sensory pathway disorders, and lesions of the ventral and lateral spinothalamic tracts may be present. Pain perception is lost on the side contralateral to the lesion. Pain is tested by the ability to perceive a pinprick or deep pressure. Increased pain, or tenderness, is called **hyperalgesia**. A diminished sense of pain is **hypoalgesia**, and a complete lack of pain sensibility is **analgesia**.

Temperature disturbances are tested by the ability to distinguish between warm and cold. For this test, the neurologist usually asks the patient to identify a test tube of warm water and one of cold water.

Recognition of Limb Position

The patient with proprioceptive deficits may not be able to determine, without looking, whether a joint of an arm, hand, or leg is in flexion or extension and may have difficulty identifying the direction of displacement of limbs or digits during movement.

Stereognosis

Stereognosis is the ability to perceive the weight, form, and other details of a body by touch. **Astereognosis** is the inability to recognize common objects, such as coins, keys, and small blocks, by touch. The examiner has the patient close the eyes and then places various objects in the patient's hand, first one and then another, to be identified.

If this recognition disorder is caused by a cortical sensory lesion rather than a dorsal column proprioceptive lesion, it is called tactile agnosia. A lesion in the right somesthetic association area or in the corpus callosum may produce a true tactile agnosia in the right hand.

Vibratory Sensibility Test

The sensation evoked when a vibrating tuning fork is applied to the base of a bony prominence is lost with dorsal column problems. The patient cannot differentiate a vibrating tuning fork from a silent one on bony surfaces.

Body Sway Test

This test, called the **Romberg test**, requires the patient to stand with feet together. The neurologist notes the amount of sway with the patient's eyes open and compares it with the amount of sway with the eyes closed. An abnormal accentuation of swaying with the eyes closed or actual loss of balance is called a positive Romberg sign. The visual sense can compensate for this loss of proprioception of muscle and joint position if it is caused by a dorsal column disorder, so the patient may correct balance problems by opening the eyes. If the lesion is in the cerebellum rather than the dorsal columns, the cerebellar ataxia of balance will not be corrected by visual compensation, as is the case in the sensory ataxia of the dorsal column.

NEUROANATOMY OF ORAL SENSATION

The neuroanatomy of oral sensation is different from that of the trunk and extremities in that the cranial and oral sensations are mediated by the cranial nerves, as opposed to mediation by the spinal nerves, as in bodily sensations. The sensory innervation of the speech mechanism is summarized in Table 5.4. Of particular importance to oral sensation is the trigeminal nerve (cranial nerve V). This cranial nerve is the primary somatic sensory nerve for the skin of the face, the anterior portion of the scalp, the anterior

TABLE 5.4	**Sensory Innervation of the Speech Mechanism**	
Structure	Cranial Nerve	Function
Face	V	Pain, temperature, touch to face
	VII	Proprioception to face
Tongue	V	Touch to anterior two-thirds
	IX	Touch to posterior third
Palate	IX	Sensory to soft palate
Pharynx	IX	Sensory to lateral and posterior pharyngeal walls
	X	Sensory to lower two-thirds of pharynx (forms pharyngeal plexus with cranial nerve IX)
Larynx	X	Sensory to most of the laryngeal muscles

two-thirds of the tongue, the teeth, and the outer surface of the eardrum. It mediates the sensations of pain, temperature, touch, pressure, and proprioception for the oral and cranial regions.

The glossopharyngeal nerve (cranial nerve IX), which is primarily sensory, also plays a role in mediating general somatic sensation in the cranial and oral regions. It mediates sensation from the posterior third of the tongue, the palatopharyngeal mucosa, and the external ear. Cranial nerve X mediates laryngeal sensation as well as sensation from the lower two-thirds of the pharynx. The cranial nerves, their distribution and anatomy, motor innervation, and sensory mediation function are detailed further in Chapter 7.

ORAL SENSORY RECEPTORS

Sensory receptors in the oral region and respiratory system generally are excited by chemical or mechanical stimulation. Taste, of course, is based on chemical stimulation. **Mechanicoreceptors** respond when stimuli distort them. For instance, the tongue touching the teeth, alveolar ridge, or palate compresses mechanicoreceptors, and the receptors in turn generate electrical impulses to the fibers.

The tongue mucosa and the tongue surface in particular are served by many types of mechanicoreceptors. The endings in these receptors have been divided into diffuse, or free, endings and compact, or organized, endings. Some speech experts believe that free endings provide a general sense of touch in sensory control of speech articulation and that organized endings provide sensitive acuity in speech articulation. Fig. 5.7 illustrates the sensory innervation pattern for the tongue. Further discussion of oral sensation and its role in speech and swallowing are discussed in Chapter 7.

THE SENSE OF VISION

Retina

The visual system processes and decodes a wealth of information, more than any other afferent system in the body. To begin this processing, the eye absorbs the light from an image and passes it through the pupil. The image is then passed into the lens, where it is reversed and inverted. The lens focuses and projects the light onto the retina, which is a light-sensitive 10-layer formation of nerve cells lining the inside of the eyeball. The retina is composed of two types of **photoreceptors** (rods and cones) and four types of neurons (bipolar cells, ganglion cells, horizontal cells, and amacrine cells). Rods play a special role in peripheral vision and in vision under low light. Cones, on the other hand, function under bright light and are responsible for discriminative vision and color detection. The rods and cones synapse with the first-order neurons, the

bipolar cells. These cells in turn synapse with the ganglion cells, which are second-order neurons. The axons of these cells converge to leave the eye within the optic nerve. After leaving the eye, the axons acquire myelin sheaths.

This series of transmissions from first- to third-order sensory neurons is modified by horizontal cells and amacrine cells. They essentially sharpen the response of the ganglion cells to certain formations of light.

Path of the Optic Nerve

The point of exit for the optic nerve is called the **optic disk**, which can be seen through an ophthalmoscope. Because rods and cones do not overlay the optic disk, it is essentially a small blind spot in each eye. The area on the retina for central fixated vision during good light is the macula. A small central pit in the macula called the fovea centralis is composed of closely packed cones, and vision here is sharpest and color vision most acute.

The optic nerve conveys visual impulses. It consists of approximately 1 million nerve fibers, which course through the optic canal of the skull to form the **optic chiasm** (see Fig. 5.4). The fibers from the retina of each eye originate from two different areas on each retina. The retinal fibers can be thought of as exiting either as temporal fibers, which come from the lateral half of the retina nearest the temple, or as nasal fibers, which originate from the lateral half nearest the nose. As Fig. 5.8 shows, at the optic chiasm the nasal fibers from each eye decussate while the temporal fibers continue ipsilaterally. This shift makes stereoscopic three-dimensional vision possible.

Fig. 5.8 shows that the optics of the eye are such that the temporal half of one retina and the nasal half of the other retina receive information from the same half of the visual field. In

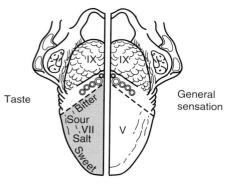

Fig. 5.7 Cranial nerve sensory innervation for mediation of taste and general sensation for the tongue.

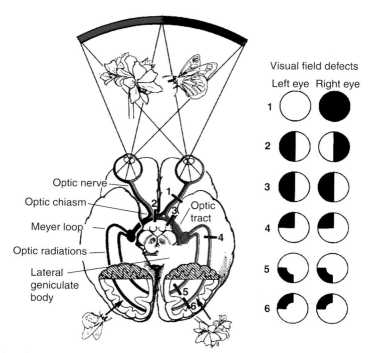

Fig. 5.8 Visual pathways with lesion sites and resulting visual field defects. The occipital lobe has been cut away to show the medial aspect and the calcarine sulci.

other words, the temporal fibers of the left retina and the nasal fibers of the right retina carry information from the right half of the visual field, and the temporal fibers of the right retina and the nasal fibers of the left retina receive information from the left side of the visual field. Because of the decussation of the nasal fibers at the optic chiasm, all the information from the contralateral side of the visual field travels in one pathway down the optic tract to the visual cortex. The visual cortex in the left hemisphere receives information about the contralateral right side of the visual field, whereas the right hemisphere processes information from the left visual field. This information is critical to understanding how a visual field deficit occurs after brain injury.

After passing the point of the optic chiasm, most of the axons forming the optic tract course to the lateral geniculate body, which is a small swelling located under the pulvinar of the thalamus. They then pass through the internal capsule and around the lateral ventricle, curving posteriorly. Some fibers travel far over the temporal horn of the lateral ventricle and form the temporal (Meyer) loop (see Fig. 5.8). These fibers terminate in the visual cortex below the calcarine sulcus. Meyer loop carries fibers representing the upper part of the central visual field. Other optic fibers travel from the lateral geniculate body to the visual cortex above the calcarine sulcus. These fibers represent the lower part of the central visual field.

Some retinal ganglion cells terminate in the superior colliculus of the midbrain. The superior colliculus also receives synapses from the visual cortex. Fibers from the superior colliculus project to the spinal cord through the tectospinal tracts. These tracts control reflex movements of the head, neck, and eyes in response to visual stimuli.

Primary Visual Cortex

The characteristics of neurons in the visual cortex and the responses of individual cells have been studied in a wide variety of experimental animals. Scientists are interested in how patterns are perceived and recognized by the eye. Hubel and Wiesel,[4] among others, have found many different types of receptive fields in the neurons of the visual cortex. These receptive fields are termed simple, complex, hypercomplex, and higher order hypercomplex. Simple receptive field cells respond to a slit of light of particular width, slant, or orientation and place on the retina. Complex receptive fields respond to slit-shaped stimuli over a large area of the retina rather than a specific place. For hypercomplex fields, the line stimulus must be of a certain length. Cells with higher order hypercomplex fields require more elaborate visual stimuli to respond.

The visual cortex is organized in columns of cells with similar properties. Some columns respond only to one eye and are monocular. Others respond to both eyes and are binocular. Because the eyes are located in different positions on the head, a difference of position exists on the retinas for a stimulus, giving binocular disparity to the columnar cells. This provides information about the depth of objects.

In addition to the primary visual pathways, two other major visual pathways can be distinguished: the **tectal**, or **collicular pathway**, and the pretectal nuclei pathway. Thus,

fibers from the optic tracts do not all go to the lateral geniculate body. Some of them project to the subcortical pretectal nuclei and ascend to the thalamus and out from there to various regions of the cortex. This system seems to be important in the control of certain visual reflexes, such as the pupillary reflex, and certain eye movements.

The tectal (collicular) pathway projects to the superior colliculi in the brainstem and to the thalamus and out to many regions of the cortex. The superior colliculi also receive input from somatosensory and auditory systems. The tectal pathway seems to be involved in a major way in the ability to orient toward and follow a visual stimulus.

The visual pathways do not operate independently. They are interconnected at every level from retina to cortex, and each receives descending input from the cerebral cortex, providing for the richness of visual perception.

Visual Association Cortex

The area surrounding the **striate cortex**, the **peristriate cortex** (Brodmann areas 18 and 19), is composed of neurons that have firing properties much like those of the primary visual cortex; however, these neurons also tend to show regional specialization for analyzing more complex aspects of visual stimuli such as motion, color, and form. Anatomists have been able to identify at least five regions of this peristriate area, each with a different processing role.

The second major part of the visual association cortex is the **temporal visual cortex** located within the middle and inferior temporal areas. This association area receives input from the peristriate cortex and has four major cortical output pathways: (1) to the contralateral temporal visual area, (2) to the prefrontal cortical area, (3) to the ipsilateral posterior association cortex of the superior temporal area, and (4) to the paralimbic and limbic areas of the medial temporal lobe. As with other neurons in primary and secondary visual cortex, neurons in the temporal visual association areas are sensitive to properties of the visual stimulus such as wavelength, size, length, and movement. These neurons, however, also seem to trigger in response to specific objects, including faces. Thus, this part of the visual system may extract complex features from visual stimuli so that neurons become responsive to individual patterns rather than to isolated stimulus features. This may provide the mechanism for object discrimination. Box 5.1 outlines the two cortices associated with vision.

Visual Integration

As Mesulam[5] points out, object recognition or identification requires interaction between the visual representation in the association areas and other components of mental operation, including integration with past experience. This process requires relay of information from these temporal visual association areas to paralimbic and limbic areas of the brain.

Damage to the association areas in the peristriate cortex or temporal lobes or to their connections to other parts of the brain may have a number of different effects on visual processing. Mesulam[5] lists the following four consequences as possibilities:

BOX 5.1   Cortical Output Regions and Pathways for Vision Association

Peristriate Cortex
- Consists of five regions, each having a different role in processing visual stimuli
- Includes neurons that function as those of the primary visual cortex *and* show regional specialization for analyzing complex stimuli

Temporal Visual Cortex
Consists of cortical output pathways to the following four areas:
1. Contralateral temporal visual area
2. Prefrontal cortical area
3. Ipsilateral posterior association cortex of the superior temporal area
4. Paralimbic and limbic areas of the medial temporal lobe
   a. Neurons trigger in response to specific objects and individual patterns
   b. May play key role in object discrimination

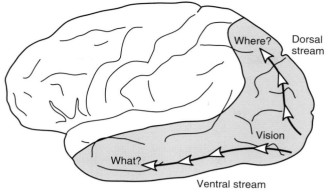

Fig. 5.9 Dorsal and ventral parallel processing streams shown emerging from the primary visual cortex in the occipital lobe. The dorsal stream, directed toward the parietal lobe, processes where the stimulus is, its direction of movement, and its speed of movement. The ventral stream, directed toward the temporal lobe, processes stimulus shape, what the stimulus is, and what it is called. (From Castro, A., Neafsey, E. J., Merchut, M. P., & Wurster, R. D. [2002]. *Neuroscience: An outline approach.* Mosby/Elsevier.)

1. Impaired specialized visual processing and impaired formation of visual templates
2. Loss of visual templates previously formed
3. Disconnection of visual-auditory, visual-motor, visual-somatosensory, and visual-verbal pathways caused by interruption of input from the visual association areas to the frontal and parietal association areas
4. Interruption of pathways providing input to paralimbic and limbic structures from the visual association area

Lesions in the peristriate areas have been noted to cause specific disorders, such as difficulty with color vision or movement perception, yet they cause no disturbance to other visual functions. In 1982 Mishkin and Ungerleider,[6] scientists at the National Institutes of Health, published a study discussing two cortical pathways separating the function of object perception and recognition from location and movement perception. Nadeau et al.,[7] referred to these as the "what" and "where" systems in vision. This differentiation of visual processing capabilities begins at the retina, with rod and cone receptors projecting to both pathways. The "where" system allows visually guided hand and eye movements, permitting individuals to direct the eyes at specific objects and coordinate the touching or capture of a desired object with part of the body. The "where" pathway is described as beginning in the occipital cortex and extending dorsally and medially into the parietal cortex (Fig. 5.9).

The "what" system is critical because it allows perception and recognition of objects located anywhere in the visual field—that is, independent of location, the abstract features of an object can be perceived and recognized. The pathway for this system begins in the occipital cortex and extends ventrally along the inferior temporal cortex, progressing into anterior areas of that cortex (see Fig. 5.9). With anterior progression, neurologic responsiveness of the visual receptive fields increases both in the number of neurons responding and the complexity of the stimulus

features that generate a response. As Mesulam[5] implies, a point exists at which what is seen is paired with what is already known, and the stimulus can be recognized in many orientations and backgrounds. Lesions in this pathway may result in impairment of object recognition or a visual agnosia.

Visual Agnosia

Analyzed in disconnection terms, classical **visual agnosia** is produced when visual associations are lost because of a disconnection of the visual areas from the language area. Also known as associative visual agnosia, the condition results in difficulty in recognizing pictures and objects along with a surprisingly good ability to describe, copy, and match visual stimuli. Patients correctly name the stimulus after tactile or auditory presentation. Bilateral occipital lobe lesions with extension on one side or the other into the medial temporal lobe involving the hippocampus have been found on autopsy. With such lesions both the naming and the memory of objects presented visually are affected.

Visual agnosia may also result from unilateral lesions. With destruction of the left visual cortex in addition to a lesion of the **splenium** of the corpus callosum, or extensive involvement of the white matter of the association cortex of the left occipital and parietal lobes, a unilateral left visual agnosia may result.

In cases of visual agnosia, associated findings are common. These may include **hemianopsia** and prosopagnosia, discussed earlier in this chapter. Other associated disorders include constructional impairment, alexia without agraphia, amnesia, and some degree of anomia. A color-naming deficit may also be present, in which the affected individual is unable to match seen colors to their spoken names. Lesions in the calcarine fissure and splenium are usually present, which are thought to disconnect the right visual cortex from the left language areas.

SYNOPSIS OF CLINICAL INFORMATION AND APPLICATIONS FOR THE SLP

- The SLP should be quite familiar with the auditory pathways and vigilant in identification of possible hearing loss.
- The central auditory pathway is complex, with the primary auditory receptor in the spiral ganglion of the organ of Corti of the cochlea of the inner ear. The auditory nerve (cranial nerve VIII) enters at the pontomedullary juncture, and damage in this area or to the auditory nerve often results in accompanying damage to cranial nerve VII (the facial nerve) because it also runs through the auditory canal.
- Bilateral damage to Heschl gyrus or the temporal lobe auditory processing areas produces a spectrum of deficits, including cortical deafness, nonverbal agnosia, and auditory agnosia. Unilateral cortical damage to Heschl gyrus does not produce total deafness.
- A unilateral lesion along the auditory nerve pathway from the ear and including the cochlear nuclei causes deafness in one ear.
- The lateral and anterior spinothalamic tracts carry sensory impulses of pain and temperature, light touch and pressure, and tactile discrimination from the periphery to the sensory cortex.
- Cerebral lesions marked by language loss may have accompanying sensory loss involving the parietal lobe or subcortical pathways.
- An agnosia is a disorder of recognition of a sensory stimulus. Agnosias result from bilateral damage to the primary cortical receptor areas associated with the particular sensory input affected.
- The oral cavity is rich in sensory receptors and the tactile receptors of the mouth, tongue, pharynx, and teeth; however, the role of sensory feedback in speech production is currently not clear, and no standard clinical method of assessment is widely accepted.
- Interruptions of the visual pathway from the retina to the occipital cortex cause visual field deficits, with the extent and type of deficit depending on the point of interruption in this double-crossed pathway.
- Patients with language disorders caused by posterior lesions are most at risk for visual field deficits that particularly affect reading and writing.

CASE STUDY

A 26-year-old male soldier was on duty in Iraq, driving a supply truck. An improvised explosive device detonated on the road near the left side of the truck, causing some damage to the truck and breaking the left window. The soldier had some cuts to his face and arm from the glass and experienced severe difficulty hearing from both ears after the incident. Fortunately, rupture of the tympanic membranes was ruled out on examination. In approximately 2 weeks, he found that he could hear out of the right ear much better than from the left. He was sent for audiometric testing and consequent radiographs. The radiographs showed a fracture of the left temporal bone.

QUESTIONS FOR CONSIDERATION

1. What type of hearing loss would the audiogram show as resulting from a fracture of the temporal bone?
2. What part of the ear would most likely be affected?
3. What cranial nerve would be involved?

REFERENCES

1. Burke, R. E. (2007). Sir Charles Sherrington's The integrative action of the nervous system: A centenary appreciation. *Brain*, *130*(4), 887–894. https://doi.org/10.1093/brain/awm022.
2. Kumar, A., & Wroten, M. (2022). *Agnosia*. StatPearls Publishing. PMID 29630208.
3. Lundy-Ekman, L. (2018). *Neuroscience: Fundamental for rehabilitation* (5th ed.). Elsevier.
4. Martinaud, O. (2017). Visual agnosia and focal brain injury. *Revue Neurologique*, *173*(7–8), 451–460. https://doi.org/10.1016/j.neurol.2017.07.009.
5. Mesulman, M. M. (2000). *Principles of behavioral neurology*. Oxford University Press.
6. Mishkin, M., & Ungerleider, L. G. (1982). Contribution of striate inputs to the visuospatial functions of the parieto-preoccipital cortex in monkeys. *Behavioural Brain Research*, *6*(1), 57–77.
7. Nadeau, S. E., Ferguson, T. S., Valenstein, E., Vierck, C. J., Petruska, J. C., Streit, W. J., & Ritz, L. A. (2004). *Medical neuroscience*. Elsevier.
8. Seikel, J. A., Drumright, D. G., & King, D. W. (2016). *Anatomy & physiology for speech, language and hearing* (5th ed.). Cengage.
9. Sherrington, C. S. (1926). *The integrative action of the nervous system*. Yale University Press.
10. Slevc, L. R., & Shell, A. R. (2015). Auditory agnosia. *Handbook of Clinical Neurology*, *129*, 573–587. https://doi.org/10.1016/B978-0-444-62630-1.00032-9.
11. Webster, D. B. (1999). *Neuroscience of communication*. Singular.

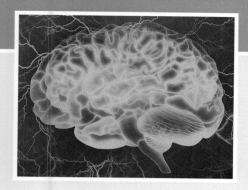

6

Neuromotor Control of Speech

We cannot state exactly the number of muscles that are necessary for speech and that are active during speech. But if we consider that ordinarily the muscles of the thoracic and abdominal walls, the neck and the face, the larynx and pharynx, and the oral cavity are all properly coordinated during the act of speaking, it becomes obvious that over 100 muscles must be controlled centrally.

Eric H. Lenneberg, Biological Foundations of Language, 1967

CHAPTER OUTLINE

KEY TERMS

action tremor
adiadochokinesia
   (dysdiadochokinesia)
akinesia
alpha motor neuron (AMN)
apraxia
areflexia
asynergia
ataxia
ataxic dysarthria
athetosis
atrophy
Babinski sign
bilateral innervation
bilateral symmetry
caudate nucleus (CN)
chorea
clonus
contralateral innervation
contralateral motor control
corona radiata
corpus striatum

corticonuclear fibers
corticopontine tract
corticospinal tract
decussation
denervation
direct activation pathway
dyskinesia
dysmetria
dystonia
extrafusal fibers
extrapyramidal system
feedback
feedforward
flocculi
genu
globus pallidus (GP)
Golgi tendon organs
hemiparalysis
hemiplegia
hyperkinesia
hyperreflexia
hypertonia

hypokinesia
hyporeflexia
hypotonia
indirect activation pathway
intention tremor
intrafusal fibers
lateral corticospinal tract
lower motor neuron (LMN)
motor unit
muscle spindle
muscle tone
myoclonus
neocerebellum
nucleus accumbens
nystagmus
paralysis
paresis
peduncles
phasic tone
postural tone
premotor
putamen

KEY TERMS—CONT'D

pyramidal tract	striatum	tardive dyskinesia
rest tremor	substantia nigra (SN)	tremors
servomechanism control systems	subthalamic nucleus (STN)	upper motor neuron (UMN)
spasticity	synergy	volitional

Speech is one of the most complex behaviors performed by human beings. On average, a person utters approximately 14 recognizable speech sounds per second when asked to produce nonsense syllables as rapidly as possible. This unusually brisk rate is maintained even when speaking conversationally or reading aloud. The number of separate neural events supporting this complex coordination of the articulatory muscles is, of course, quite large, and the degree of neural integration in the motor system for routine, everyday talk is truly amazing. The statement that normal speech production requires the finest motor control in the body is no exaggeration.

SPEECH PRODUCTION VERSUS LIMB AND TRUNK MOVEMENT

The competent speech-language pathologist (SLP) of today must be familiar with how limb, trunk, and speech production muscles work. SLPs work on teams with respiratory, physical, and occupational therapists. It is important that SLPs understand such things as how to reposition a child for the best motor control for feeding or what muscles of the trunk and limbs were affected in a spinal cord injury and how that injury may affect work on speech and language. But, of course, what is most critical to the SLP is an understanding of the muscles of speech production. As we reviewed in Chapters 2 and 3, the most obvious difference in these muscles and limb and trunk muscles is that the muscles of speech production receive sensory and motor innervation through the cranial nerves, whereas limb and trunk muscles rely on the spinal nerve innervation. In his discussion of the uniqueness of the speech muscles, Kent[16] provides information retrieved from a search of the literature on how the speech muscles are different in their genetic, developmental, functional, and phenotypical properties as well as their innervation. It would be useful for the student of speech-language pathology to read this article, but the main points are summarized in Box 6.1. Review this information before moving on to the discussion of the levels and systems of motor control for both spinal and cranial muscles.

The Motor System in Speech Ontogeny

The student of speech-language pathology about to explore the motor system underlying the production of speech should also keep in mind the structure of the basic unit of speech and how speech is thought to have evolved in humans. Although a great deal of time is spent in early academic classes learning all the phonemes of our language and their distinctive

> **BOX 6.1   Some Differences in Biomechanical and Functional Properties between Speech Muscles and Limb Muscles**
>
> - Muscles of speech production are more complex in nature. The >100 muscles involved are composed of several types of muscles that can be grouped into structural and functional classes:
>   - Joint related (e.g., masseter and digastric muscles)
>   - Sphincteric (e.g., orbicularis oris; palatal and pharyngeal constrictors)
>   - Muscular hydrostat (e.g., intrinsic muscles of the tongue)
>   - Specialized for vibration and airway valving (e.g., intrinsic laryngeal muscles)
>   - Respiratory muscles that inflate and deflate the lungs
> - With the exception of the muscles that close the jaw, muscles of speech production are specialized more for speed than for force.
> - Speech muscles are capable of more precise coordination of movement sequences.
> - The kinematics and force features of speech muscle movements are maintained at normal and fast rates but are different at slow rates.
> - Like the skeletal muscles, there is contralateral motor control of the lips, tongue, and jaw with ipsilateral innervation to many of the muscles as well; however, the ipsilateral pathway provides much more assistance in speech muscles, generating bilateral synergistic movements though the contralateral innervation is stronger.

Data from Kent, R. (2004). The uniqueness of speech among motor systems. *Clinical Linguistics & Phonetics, 18*(6–8), 495–505.

features, it is not the phoneme but the syllable that is the basic unit of speech. The basic or modal syllable frame in English is that of a vowel nucleus alternating with a consonant (usually a CV structure).[20]

This text also adopts the frame/context (F/C) theory of the evolution of human speech as a basis for looking at why motor control evolved as it did, resulting in the complicated motor pathways and relationships between structures. In formulating the F/C theory,[19] MacNeilage acknowledged the relatively well-accepted theory that before speech output, the content elements (consonants and vowels) are inserted into a syllabic structure or frame. This is based on the fact that when speech errors are made by adults, whether neurologically intact or brain damaged, the syllable structure does not change; the consonants and vowels never occupy each other's positions in the syllable.[20] For example, a person may switch the consonants in a phrase ("gad birl" for "bad girl") or the vowels ("bag cit" for "big cat"); however, consonants do not change places with vowels. Furthermore, when phonemes are switched, they do so with the phonemes that occupy the same place in the syllable, such as the consonants in the syllable initial positions in the previous example.[20]

MacNeilage has suggested in his F/C theory that in the evolution of human speech the rhythmic and repetitive opening and closing of the mandible necessary for the intake of food (and thus survival) was combined with vocalization to produce syllables. The open mandible for vowels and the more closed posturing for consonants thus were perpetuated through the evolutionary cycles and never biologically had an opportunity to be substituted for one another. MacNeilage[19] theorizes that there may have been an intermediate stage in evolution of speech where the open/close mandible cycle was combined with other structure movements to produce tongue clicks or lip smacking, for instance; these types of oral gestures appear to be used for communication by some primates whose evolution preceded that of humans.[8]

In the study of normal stages of speech development in children, the progression or refinement of the motor movements necessary for increasingly more varied consonant and vowel production can easily be seen. The progress a child makes when going from babbling to reduplicative babbling to variegated babbling to word production to sentence production showcases the advancement of the ability of the motor system to quickly and effortlessly respond to the commands of the language system. This progression in such a short time appears miraculous and is the result of the development and coordination of the nervous system structures we are about to explore.

A HIERARCHICAL SYSTEM

The motor system for all voluntary and reflexive movement is considered a hierarchical system that becomes progressively less sophisticated as it is descended or more sophisticated as it is ascended. The great neurologist Hughlings Jackson asserted that each level of this hierarchy has a certain autonomy, but the autonomy at the lower levels is partially constrained by the higher levels of the motor system. This is also true for sensation, cognition, and emotion. Speech production requires, as does most motor activity, the action of major mechanisms at every significant motor integration level of the nervous system. The Jacksonian principle that higher centers bring more refinement to neuronal processing while also inhibiting the neural activity of certain lower centers is often demonstrated when disease or injury to the motor system occurs. This loss of refinement and/or effect of disinhibition will become clear when signs and symptoms of the different motor speech disorders are discussed in subsequent chapters. An attempt must first be made to understand the functioning of the motor system as a whole. Though we are most interested in speech, we will also look at how movement for extremities occurs since the corticospinal pathway is important to total patient rehabilitation. As we did when discussing the motor system in Chapters

2 and 3, we begin with the higher levels of control and work our way through subcortical systems and out to the muscle.

Neuroanatomically, the frontal lobe is the largest lobe, and it is divided into three major areas defined by their anatomy and function. These areas are the primary motor cortex, supplemental and premotor cortex, and prefrontal cortex. Damage to the primary motor, supplemental motor, and premotor areas leads to weakness and impaired execution of motor tasks of the contralateral side. The prefrontal cortex is a large association area of the frontal lobe and is involved in higher reasoning and executive functioning. The primary function of the motor cortex is to plan and execute voluntary movements. The motor cortex is part of the frontal lobe (Fig. 6.1) and consists of the primary motor cortex, premotor cortex, and supplementary motor area (SMA). Other areas important for speech production include Broca area and the insula.

Motor Execution and Planning Centers
Motor Strip

The precentral gyrus is situated just anterior to the central sulcus (hence its name), Brodmann area 4. It is also known as the motor strip. The strip has been well mapped; different regions of the motor strip serve specific regions of the body. This representation of body regions on the motor strip is known as the homunculus (see Fig. 2.7).

Neurons of the motor cortex synapse directly with motor neurons of the spinal cord. Because these neurons originate in the cortex, they are called the **upper motor neurons (UMNs)**, which is easy to remember as the top neurons in the hierarchy of the motor system.

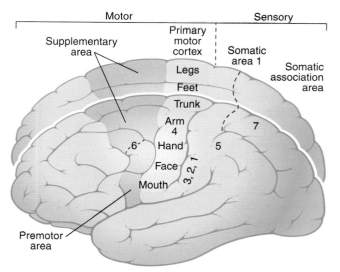

Fig. 6.1 Motor and somatosensory functional areas of the cerebral cortex. The numbers 4, 5, 6, and 7 are Brodmann cortical areas. (From: Hall, J. E, Guyton, M. E. [2021]. Cerebral cortex, intellectual functions of the brain, learning and memory. In: *Guyton and Hall textbook of medical physiology* [pp. 727–740, fig. 58.4]. Elsevier.)

Premotor Area

Immediately anterior to the motor strip is the premotor cortex, which is important for the preparation of movement. The **premotor** area (a part of Brodmann area 6) is usually active bilaterally. It has a major projection to the brainstem nuclei that gives origin primarily to the reticulospinal tracts and has minor projections to the major motor tracts. Its primary function appears to be preparation for movement, especially of proximal muscles.[29] This area receives cognitive input from the prefrontal cortex in terms of motor intention and from the parietal lobe in terms of tactile and visual signals. It gets quite active when motor routines are run in response to visual or somatosensory cues (e.g., reaching for an object).

Supplementary Motor Area

The SMA is involved in the programming of complex sequences of movement and the coordination of bilateral movement. Evidence suggests that the SMA selects movements based on remembered sequences. In one study, subjects in a positron emission tomography (PET) scanner were required to perform certain movements. When the movements were simple, such as moving a finger repeatedly, the motor strip as well as the sensory strip were activated in the contralateral hemisphere. However, when the subjects performed a complex sequence of finger movements, the SMA was activated bilaterally in addition to activation of the contralateral motor and sensory strips. Interestingly, in the final task, the subjects were asked to remain motionless but to mentally rehearse the complex sequence of finger movements. In this condition, the motor and sensory strips were silent, but the SMA was active. The study concluded that the SMA is involved in bilateral movements and in the rehearsal of complex sequences of movement.[17]

The most anterior portion of the SMA is called the pre-SMA region; this region appears to have a different specialization as compared to the SMA proper. The pre-SMA region appears to be associated with new sequence acquisition, while the SMA proper is involved in sequential movement automatization.[28] The different roles of the SMA and pre-SMA regions in word production were investigated using functional magnetic resonance imaging and intricate research design involving word generation versus reading and repetition. Alario et al.,[1] found the SMA proper to be involved in actual execution of the motor movements for articulation. A later study[7] found that the pre-SMA area was sensitive to tasks that require both articulation and cognitive demands, such as decision making and speech production. In contrast, the SMA was sensitive to tasks requiring articulation but which placed little or low cognitive demands.

Broca Area

Located in the inferior frontal gyrus, Broca area is a critical region for speech production. It is typically larger in the left hemisphere, an asymmetry that has been correlated with language dominance. As was previously discussed in Chapter 2, Broca area is found in the motor association cortical area at the foot of the primary motor and the premotor cortices, roughly the third left frontal convolution. Broca area includes the pars opercularis (Brodmann area 44) and the pars triangularis (Brodmann area 45) in the posterior inferior frontal gyrus[9] (see Fig. 2.5 and 2.6). Interestingly, our closest relatives, the chimpanzees, have no asymmetry associated with areas 44 and 45, suggesting that Broca area enlarged in the left hemisphere during evolution, possibly as an adaptation for our dependence on language.[25]

Broca area was named for the French neurologist Pierre Paul Broca, who first described the expressive language disorder we now refer to as Broca aphasia. Patients with expressive aphasia may partially lose the ability to produce spoken and written language. Both their spoken and written language may retain content words, but often these patients will omit articles, prepositions, and other words that only have grammatical significance, leading to the description of their language as "telegraphic." Broca aphasia varies in severity, with some patients only able to speak in single words or not at all, and others able to carry on conversations with minimally noticeable changes. Most patients with expressive aphasia retain good language comprehension.

Price et al.,[21] used PET scanning technology to look at the possible participation of Broca area as a site of internal models or "higher level representations" of already learned words that enable the speaker to unconsciously predict the auditory output of a spoken word and send these predictions to auditory processing areas in the temporal lobe. This would perhaps allow adjustments to be made in articulation after a mismatch occurs, improving the precision of speech. This predictive/comparative/corrective system seems reasonable and important in such situations as early language acquisition, speech output with a hearing loss, or learning a new language. As the authors note, this theory requires connectivity studies to be done to confirm and clarify the functional pathways.

Insula

Apraxia is a disorder that impairs performance of voluntary learned motor acts while similar automatic gestures remain intact. It is caused by a lesion in motor association areas and association pathways. Apraxia of speech (AOS) is a disorder of motor planning for speech production. A person with acquired AOS shows difficulty with accurate and rapid movement of the articulators to produce purposeful speech in the absence of paralysis or weakness of the articulators. Movement of the oral mechanism for motor activities such as eating, blowing out a match, or licking an ice cream cone, for example, are typically unaffected. AOS in adults with brain damage most often co-occurs with a language disorder, and this disorder is often diagnosed as a Broca aphasia (although the apraxic component is not necessary for a diagnosis of Broca aphasia to be warranted). The anatomic etiology of AOS had generally been placed in the traditional Broca area. Recent studies localize the neuroanatomic correlate of AOS to the insula,[4] and in the case of pure AOS with no concomitant aphasia to the premotor cortex and adjacent precentral gyrus.[13]

Trunk and Limb Movement: The Pyramidal Tract

The **pyramidal tract** is the major voluntary pathway for all movement mediated by the spinal cord (trunk and limbs). This tract is named the pyramidal tract because it passes through and actually makes up the bulk of a certain point in the medulla that looks like a small pyramid. This tract controls the skilled movements in the distal muscles of the limbs and digits and is particularly responsible for the precise movements made by the hands and fingers.

The **corticospinal tract** descends from the cerebral cortex to different levels of the spinal cord; it begins in the motor cortex of the two cerebral hemispheres, specifically from the motor strip and the SMA. These UMNs receive afferent input from the primary sensory cortex and the dorsal column sensory nuclei in the spinal cord. The basal ganglia and the cerebellum also serve as "consultants" to the cortical motor system, influencing timing and coordination of movement. The influence of these inputs occurs before neural firing initiated in the motor cortex and through the corticospinal tract.

Descending pyramidal fibers also originate from the postcentral gyrus and the parietal lobe. Those fibers are of sensory area origin and terminate on sensory, rather than motor, relay nuclei in the brainstem and in the dorsal horn of the spinal cord; they modulate sensory transmission.

The pyramidal system is actually composed of two tracts that innervate muscles controlled by peripheral nerves. The two divisions of the pyramidal tract indicate where the UMN fibers synapse. Fibers that synapse with spinal nerves belong in the corticospinal tract (the name describes it well, as these fibers originate in the cortex and terminate in the spine). Fibers that synapse at the brainstem level belong to the corticonuclear tract, or the corticobulbar tract in older terminology. Before a recommended terminology change, the corticonuclear fibers were called the corticobulbar fibers, a term that is still in use by some authors. Because that name erroneously implies that all fibers terminate in the medulla (the old term for the medulla was the bulb because of its rounded shape), corticonuclear replaced corticobulbar in the international terminology of neuroanatomic terms in 1998. The **corticonuclear fibers** of the pyramidal tract innervate the cranial nerves and make up the voluntary pathway for the movements of all speech muscles, except those of respiration. They are the most important motor fibers for the SLP.

Both tracts descend from the motor cortex in each hemisphere to subcortical white matter in a fan-shaped distribution of fibers called the **corona radiata**, or radiating crown. The fibers converge to enter into an L-shaped subcortical structure called the internal capsule, passing through the posterior limb of the internal capsule (in the case of the corticospinal fibers) and the genu or bend of the internal capsule (for the corticonuclear tract).

As the axons pass through the internal capsule, they join axons from other areas, such as those projecting to and from other cortical areas, the thalamus, and the brainstem. Damage in the pathway through the internal capsule can result in devastating motor deficits because of the number of fibers going through this narrow point.

From the internal capsule, they descend below the thalamus and lie on the ventral brainstem surface, forming part of the cerebral peduncles of the midbrain. These white matter tracts are found in the ventral portion of the peduncles, a portion called the crus cerebri. Some of the descending fibers may end in or send collaterals to the red nucleus at this point.

Descending to the level of the pons, some cortical axons may begin to intermix with pontine neurons at the base (basis pontis). Many of these axons will synapse on the pontine neurons and become part of the **corticopontine tract**, which exits through the cerebellar peduncles and out to the cerebellum. This tract allows input from the cortex to be conveyed to the cerebellum. At this point in the pons, some other fibers of the descending cortical axons may synapse in the pontomedullary reticular formation and provide cortical input to the reticulospinal system.

The pyramidal tract neurons that continue to descend collect at the point called the pyramids of the medulla situated at the medullary-cervical juncture. More collaterals are given off by the axons, innervating nuclei of the inferior olivary complex, the posterior column nuclei, and some reticular nuclei of the medulla. At the level of the pyramids, approximately 85% to 90% of the corticospinal fibers cross over (decussate) to the other side of the neuraxis, providing **contralateral motor control** of the extremities. In contrast, only about 50% of the corticonuclear fibers decussate, which has clinical implications that are discussed next.

Decussation

The crossing of the right and left corticospinal tract is known as **decussation**, sometimes called the decussation of the pyramids. The majority of the corticospinal fibers decussate at the level of the pyramids of the medulla. The few fibers that do not cross are collectively known as the anterior corticospinal tract. The primary crossed corticospinal tract is the **lateral corticospinal tract**. The decussation means that a lesion interrupting the fibers above the crossing has an effect on the side of the body opposite the site of the lesion. If the corticospinal tract is interrupted in the cerebrum or at any level above the pyramids of the medulla, voluntary movement of the innervated structure is limited on the contralateral side of the body. By contrast, a lesion below the decussation impairs voluntary movement on the same, or ipsilateral, side.

After the corticospinal fibers enter the spinal cord, they synapse in the anterior horn cells of the spinal cord segment dedicated to control of the particular body part associated with that level of the spinal cord (remember cervical, thoracic, lumbar, sacral, and coccygeal segments from Chapter 3). At the point of synapse, a new axon is sent out to the muscle fiber controlling or adding to control of a particular muscle or muscle group. At this point, the new fibers resulting from this synapse are called the **lower motor neuron (LMN)** fibers.

Brainstem Centers for Tone and Posture

When a cross section of the spinal cord is examined, other descending motor tracts besides the lateral and anterior corticospinal tracts can be seen. These additional descending motor tracts found terminating in the spinal cord are the reticulospinal tracts, vestibulospinal tracts, tectospinal tracts, and rubrospinal tracts. These tracts are the major tracts in what is sometimes called the **extrapyramidal system**, defined as being made up of fibers descending to the spinal cord outside of the corticospinal tracts. Duffy[10] refers to these tracts as the **indirect activation pathway**. These fiber pathways provide primary input to motor neurons for maintenance of normal tone, body posturing, and reflex responses to sensory stimuli.

According to Duffy,[10] the components of the indirect activation pathway consist of many short pathways and interconnections with structures between the origin of the pathway in the cortex and its termination at the LMN. The nuclei and tracts considered to be components of the indirect activation system are listed in Table 6.1.

The reticular formation itself is also thought of as part of the subcortical extrapyramidal system. The extrapyramidal system is concerned with coarse stereotyped movements. It has more influence over proximal (midline) than distal (peripheral) muscles. It maintains proper tone and posture. Even with destruction of the pyramidal tract, it can allow a person to eat and walk.

Because muscle tone and body posture are important to the neurologist's examination of the body, this is a good point to discuss those terms as they relate to the neurologic control. **Muscle tone** is the resistance of the muscle to stretch. The two types of tone are phasic and postural. **Phasic tone** is a rapid contraction in reaction to a high-intensity stretch (or change in muscle length) and is assessed by testing tendon reflexes. **Postural tone** is a prolonged contraction in response to a low-intensity stretch. Gravity provides a low-intensity stretch on antigravity muscles, which respond with prolonged contraction and the normal posturing of the head,

neck, and extremities that persons without neurologic damage usually maintain.

Facial and Oral Movement: The Corticonuclear Tract

Their course is not as direct as that of the corticospinal fibers. Corticonuclear fibers begin with the corticospinal fibers at the cortex, as the two components of the pyramidal tract. Chapter 7 discusses these neuron pathways individually for the cranial nerves. However, the corticonuclear fibers terminate at the motor nuclei of the cranial nerves located at various points in the brainstem. Unlike the corticospinal fibers, the corticonuclear fibers have many ipsilateral (terminating in motor nuclei in the brainstem on the same side of the brain as the primary site from which the axon began) as well as contralateral fibers (terminating in nuclei on the opposite side from which they began). After the axons of the corticonuclear fibers leave the cortical motor areas, they travel the same path that the corticospinal fibers do through the corona radiata and the internal capsule. The corticonuclear fibers, however, transverse the **genu**, or bend, of the internal capsule rather than the posterior limb.

The corticospinal and corticonuclear fibers separate at the upper brainstem level. Each of the different cranial nerve axons terminates at its own designated nuclei at some point along the brainstem. Some decussate and others primarily travel ipsilaterally. If they cross, they do so at various levels of the brainstem. The general location of each of the nuclei for the cranial nerves most important to speech is discussed in Chapter 7.

UPPER AND LOWER MOTOR NEURONS

This point in our discussion of the motor system seems like an appropriate place to briefly discuss a useful concept in clinical neurology: the notion of UMNs and LMNs. This division of designation of the general location in the neural pathway of the axon has been applied in clinical neurologic teaching and practice for a very long time. Knowledge of the different symptoms and signs of damage to each type of neuron pathway will often be useful to SLPs performing motor speech examinations or to the SLP in general trying to understand the basis of the neurologic examination findings in their patients.

Upper Motor Neurons

All the neurons of the anterior and lateral corticospinal tracts, which send axons from the primary motor area in the cerebral cortex down to the anterior horn cells of the spinal cord, are considered UMNs. The neurons of the corticonuclear tracts that send axons from the primary motor area in the cerebral cortex to the nuclei in the brainstem also are UMNs. An important concept in trying to learn the difference between UMNs and LMNs is this: No axons of UMNs leave the neuraxis. In other words, they are contained within the brain, brainstem, and spinal cord. The pyramidal tract,

Components (Nuclei or Tracts)	Functional Role in Motor Control
Reticular formation or reticulospinal tracts	Excitation or inhibition of flexors and extensors; facilitation or inhibition of reflexes and ascending sensory information
Vestibular nuclei or vestibulospinal tract	Facilitation of reflex activity and spinal mechanisms controlling muscle tone
Red nucleus or rubrospinal tract	Facilitation of flexor and inhibition of extensor neurons

TABLE 6.1 Major Components of the Indirect Activation Pathway of the Extrapyramidal System

Modified from Duffy, J. R. (2005). *Motor speech disorders: Substrates, differential diagnosis, and management.* Mosby/Elsevier.

with its UMN activation, can be thought of as the **direct activation pathway**, or direct motor system, because of the direct connection of its UMNs with the LMNs that subsequently send their axons outside the neuraxis.[5] These UMNs in the primary motor area have a major activating influence on their LMN targets.

Lower Motor Neurons

LMNs are all the neurons that send motor axons outside the neuraxis into the peripheral nerves: both cranial and spinal nerves. LMNs are designated second-order neurons. Sherrington[27] called the LMN "the final common pathway." By this he meant that the peripheral nerves, both cranial and spinal, serve as a final route for all the complex motor interactions that occur in the neuraxis above the level of the LMNs. The final muscle contraction is the product of all the interactions that have occurred in the central nervous system (CNS).

The concept of the **motor unit** helps explain the LMN pathway (Fig. 6.2). A motor unit is a structural and functional entity that can be defined as (1) a single anterior horn cell in the spinal cord or cranial nerve neuron in the brainstem, (2) its peripheral axon and its branches, (3) the myoneural juncture, which is the point where the nerve synapses on the muscle fiber, and (4) each muscle fiber innervated by the branches. Lesions may occur at many points within the motor unit and produce LMN signs.

Bilateral Symmetry

Because the movements of limbs and digits would not be efficient or effective if the movement of one side mirrored the other, the corticospinal system allows for control of one side of the body to come from only one source (for at least 90% of the fibers), the opposite hemisphere's cortical motor areas. In comparison, because the oral musculature movements on one side of the body typically are mirrored by the same movements on the other side, the majority of the midline speech muscles work in **bilateral symmetry**, making speech more efficient. This is the result of the **bilateral innervation** to the cranial nerve nuclei that the corticonuclear fibers provide. If a cranial nerve's nuclei are said to receive bilateral innervation, the nuclei on the right side of the brainstem (in

this example) receive axons from the primary motor cortices of both hemispheres. However, if that cranial nerve were to be one of those only receiving contralateral innervation, the axons providing neural input would come only from the left hemisphere's cortical motor areas. The majority of the paired muscles of the face, palate, vocal folds, and diaphragm work together in synchrony most of the time in wrinkling the forehead, smiling, chewing, swallowing, and talking and thus are bilaterally innervated.

This bilateral input to most of the speech muscles has important implications for the effect of damage to the nervous system on the speech musculature in cases of the motor speech disorders we call the dysarthrias (see full discussion in Chapter 8). After damage to the corticonuclear pathway, this bilateral innervation provides a safety feature or compensatory mechanism for speech production. For example, if the left corticonuclear fibers coming from the motor cortex to the nuclei of a cranial nerve are damaged, the motor nuclei of a bilaterally innervated neuron will still receive impulses by way of the intact right corticonuclear tract, and paralysis of the muscle will not be severe. The innervation of the limbs, on the other hand, is primarily contralateral rather than bilateral. Therefore, if the pyramidal tract input from the left side of the brain to the spinal motor nuclei were damaged, there would be little input to those spinal neurons from the opposite side; a severe right limb paralysis would result. Unilateral lesions to corticonuclear fibers typically do not produce a severe weakness because of redundancy provided by the bilateral innervation.

Contralateral and Unilateral Innervation

Even though the cranial nerve nuclei are primarily bilaterally supplied, some of the muscle groups moving the facial and oral musculature have mixed innervation patterns with much variation among the nuclei regarding the amount of unilateral innervation versus contralateral innervation each receives. Areas with a greater ratio of unilateral supply suffer more damage after a unilateral lesion. Because of their primarily **contralateral innervation**, the muscles of the lower face and the trapezius muscles are most affected by unilateral damage (to the contralateral side). An intermediate paralytic effect, meaning significant weakness but not paralysis, is found in the tongue with a unilateral lesion because the mixture contains a greater ratio of bilateral innervation to the different muscles of the tongue. The diaphragm, ocular muscles, upper face, jaw, pharynx, and muscles of the larynx show little paresis with a unilateral lesion because of primarily bilateral innervation of the muscles controlling movement of these structures.

The nuclei for the facial nerve are complex. The facial nucleus is made up of a ventral and a dorsal component and combines bilateral innervation with contralateral innervation. The muscles of the upper half of the face, supplied by the ventral portion, are far more bilaterally innervated than the muscles of the lower half of the face, which are supplied by the dorsal portion of the motor nucleus and receive more contralateral innervation. In practical terms, among

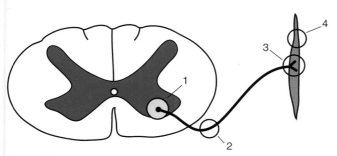

Fig. 6.2 The motor unit and typical lesion sites producing different signs and symptoms of lower motor neuron damage: *1,* Anterior horn cell—motor neuron disease; *2,* nerve axon—denervation, neuropathy; *3,* myoneural juncture—neuromyopathy, myasthenia gravis; *4,* muscle fiber—myopathy or dystrophy.

the healthy population most people can wrinkle the forehead or lift both eyebrows together. Only a few people, with more contralateral fibers, are able to lift their eyebrows one at a time. The muscles of the midface receive a more equal combination of bilateral and contralateral innervation. Most, but not all, people can wink one eye at a time because of the increase of contralateral fibers to eyelid muscles compared with forehead muscles.

In the lower face the innervation is primarily contralateral. Most people are able to retract one corner of the mouth alone when asked to do so because of the limited bilateral innervation of the lower face muscles. Table 6.2 summarizes the innervation for the cranial nerves of speech production. Fig. 6.3 shows the difference in effect on facial movement of an UMN lesion compared with an LMN lesion as a result of this unusual innervation pattern. The principles of bilateral and contralateral innervation are practically applied when a speech cranial nerve examination is performed to determine whether lesions are present affecting the corticonuclear fibers, cranial nerve nuclei, or the cranial nerves themselves.

The concepts of bilateral symmetry and contralateral independence are of crucial clinical utility when analyzing and understanding muscle involvement in dysarthria. This is explained further in Chapter 7 in the discussion of testing the cranial nerves involved in speech.

Indicators of Upper versus Lower Motor Neuron Damage

Once an understanding has been grasped of the anatomy of the pyramidal tract and the final common pathway, the concepts of UMNs and LMNs, and the concept of bilateral versus contralateral innervation, it is important to understand and be able to identify the signs of UMN versus LMN damage.

Lesions of the UMNs and LMNs produce fairly different sets of signs and symptoms. Many of the symptoms are easier to identify in the gross muscles of the limbs, but it is critical to the SLP that these signs/symptoms are recognized and considered whenever an examination is done on the oral musculature. Table 6.3 presents a contrast of the signs

of damage to these two systems. This distinction provides the neurologist with a powerful tool in neurologic examination for deciding where a lesion is located in the nervous system. The most striking sign of a lesion in both UMNs and LMNs is paralysis. The type of paralysis, however, is

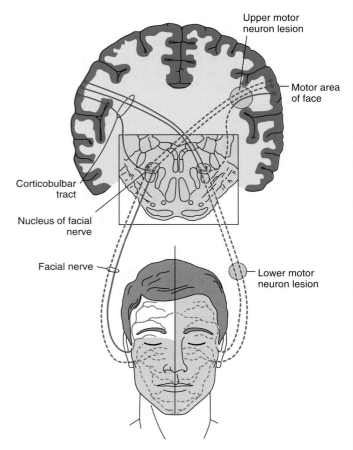

Fig. 6.3 Upper versus lower motor neuron facial paralysis. The *shaded areas* of the face show the distribution of the facial muscles paralyzed after an upper motor neuron lesion and a lower motor neuron lesion. (Modified from Gilman, S., & Winans, S. S. [1987]. *Manter and Gatz's essentials of clinical neuroanatomy and neurophysiology* [7th ed.]. F. A. Davis.)

TABLE 6.2 Corticonuclear Innervation in the Cranial Nerves for Speech

Trigeminal (V)	Bilateral innervation
Facial (VII)	Mixed bilateral and contralateral innervation
Glossopharyngeal (IX)	Bilateral innervation (motor innervation of IX is only to a single muscle)
Vagus (X)	Bilateral innervation
Spinal accessory (XI)	Contralateral innervation
Hypoglossal (XII)	Primarily bilateral innervation with contralateral innervation of one muscle (genioglossus)

TABLE 6.3 Signs of Upper (UMN) and Lower (LMN) Motor Neuron Disorders

UMN Disorders	LMN Disorders
Spastic paralysis	Flaccid paralysis
Hypertonia	Hypotonia
Hyperreflexia	Hyporeflexia
Clonus	No clonus
Babinski sign	No Babinski sign
Little or no atrophy	Marked atrophy
No fasciculations	Fasciculations
Diminished abdominal and cremasteric reflexes	Normal abdominal and cremasteric reflexes

quite different depending on the site of the lesion that produces the paralysis. The neurologist would note paresis or paralysis and proceed by assessing muscle tone, muscle strength, and reflexes. Understanding the differences in the type of paralysis, tone, and other confirmatory signs is a large step toward establishing a correct diagnosis of a neurologic disease involving motor disturbance. The differences in strength, tone, and reflexes are much more difficult to assess in the oral musculature than in the larger limb muscles. However, there are differences that can be identified. It is also important that the SLP help confirm these signs, if possible, in the oral musculature to assist in a correct diagnosis of the underlying etiology. It is also important that the SLP recognize these signs in the larger limb muscles so that identification of new problems can be made early or progression could be questioned.

Paralysis, Paresis, and Plegia

A gross limitation of movement is called **paralysis**, and an incomplete paralysis is known as **paresis**. A complete or near-complete paralysis of one side of the body is **hemiparalysis** or, more commonly, **hemiplegia**. The presence of right-sided hemiplegia or hemiparesis is an extremely important sign for the SLP. Paralysis or paresis on the right side of the body suggests left hemisphere involvement. As previously noted, the left hemisphere is the primary site of brain mechanisms for language, so right hemiplegia is often associated with language disorders. Lesions of the bilateral motor strip or the corticonuclear tract alone may produce the motor speech disorder of dysarthria.

Upper Motor Neuron Signs and Symptoms

Damage to the corticospinal tract anywhere along its course produces spastic paralysis. Spastic muscles display increased tone, or resistance to movement, a condition called **hypertonia**. Spastic hypertonicity can be identified by moving a limb through its full range of motion so that the joint is flexed or bent. The neurologic examiner puts an increased stretch on the muscles during range-of-motion testing and thereby elicits a muscle stretch reflex, an increase in tone or tension that resists the flexion of the joint. The examiner can feel this increased resistance to movement. (The muscle stretch reflex controls the degree of contraction in a normal muscle and provides muscles with tonus, or tone.) When an injury occurs to the corticospinal or corticonuclear tract, such as in a vascular stroke, this spasticity may take several days to weeks to develop and stabilize. Temporary flaccid hemiplegia may initially be present, with a more permanent spastic paralysis developing over time. The increasing spasticity of the muscles after a corticospinal injury may be caused by a buildup of collagen in the muscles as well as biochemical changes.[2]

A "clasp knife" reaction occurs in a spastic muscle when the neurologist feels increased tone or resistance to movement in the muscle after the joint has been briskly flexed and then feels the resistance fade. This reaction, which identifies spastic hypertonicity, is analogous to the resistance felt when a knife blade is first opened, followed by the reduction of resistance when the blade is straightened. This reaction occurs more typically in extension rather than in flexion of the elbow. A short span of no tone is usually present, then a rapid buildup of tone and a sudden release as the joint is moved, just as with opening a clasp knife.

Spasticity is also associated with exaggerated muscle stretch reflexes, resulting in **hyperreflexia**. Reflex action is tested at joints by putting stretch on tendons. This elicits the exaggerated muscle stretch reflex. Spastic paralysis, hypertonia, and hyperreflexia have most often been associated with pyramidal tract damage, particularly lesions of the corticospinal tract. However, the corticonuclear tracts are often also involved when a lesion interrupts the corticospinal tract, and signs of spasticity may be found in the midline speech muscles as well as in the distal limb muscles. Therefore, the clinical signs of **spasticity**, or an UMN lesion, are of equal interest to the SLP and neurologist. Spastic speech muscles may be weak, slow, and limited in range or movement. Hypertonia may decrease muscle flexibility of the articulators and limit the ability to achieve a full range of motion of the speech muscles.

Other confirmatory signs. Several signs, in addition to a clinical demonstration of clasp knife spasticity, hypertonia, and hyperreflexia, are used by the neurologist to help verify the diagnosis of spasticity and localize the lesion to the pyramidal tract.

The **Babinski sign**, or extensor plantar sign, in particular has been identified as an abnormal reflex sign that develops with corticospinal damage. The lesion causes the release of cortical inhibition. The sign has achieved considerable status in the diagnosis of UMN lesions because it is a highly reliable abnormal reflex, is new behavior released by the presence of a lesion, and is clearly associated with a relatively specific lesion site—the cortex or the corticospinal tract. The SLP is not directly interested in it because it does not involve the midline speech muscles, but its presence as a confirmation of a UMN lesion of the spastic type is important to all who manage neurologic patients.

The Babinski sign is observed as a reflex toe sign. It is elicited by stimulating the sole of the foot with a strong scratching maneuver. The normal response to stimulation of the sole, or plantar portion of the foot, is a slight withdrawal of the foot and downward turning or curling under of the toes. With a corticospinal lesion, the great toe extends upward, and the other toes fan as the foot withdraws slightly. Physicians test this response several times to convince themselves that the upturning great toe sign can be repeatedly and automatically elicited. Automatic repetition of a given response such as this defines it as a reflex. The presence of a repeatable abnormal reflex sharply increases the probability of predicting with accuracy the possible site(s) of a neurologic lesion, though it may not be present if the patient with a vascular lesion is tested early after onset of the insult.

The Babinski sign is more reliable in adults than in infants and children. Normal infants are highly variable in display of the sign. The explanation usually given for this variability is that the immature nervous system and the damaged nervous system often show similar symptoms and signs. Damage to the nervous system often releases early reflex behavior that has become inhibited by development of higher centers, so signs of damage at that point in time are signs of immaturity at an earlier time. Clinical neurologists believe that the extensor plantar sign usually reaches stability by age 2 years. Other signs, such as a persisting asymmetric tonic neck reflex and the Moro reflex, can be tested to suggest a UMN lesion in young children (see Chapter 11).

Another confirmatory sign of spasticity is **clonus**. Hyperactive muscle stretch reflexes associated with spasticity may show a sustained series of rhythmic beats or jerks when a neurologic examiner maintains one tendon of a muscle in extension. To test for clonus, the Achilles tendon in the ankle is often put under extension. If a UMN lesion is present, the ankle and the calf show sustained jerks. A few clonic jerks, called abortive clonus, are not clinically significant, but if the clonus is sustained over time, it is considered pathologic and an indicator of hyperreflexia. This sign is part of the clinical syndrome resulting from a UMN lesion.

With bilateral UMN lesions, a characteristic dysarthria may be present. This motor speech disorder, called spastic dysarthria, is discussed in Chapter 8.

Lower Motor Neuron Signs and Symptoms

If a lesion directly damages a cranial or peripheral nerve, or is in the cell bodies of the anterior horn cell in the spinal cord or the nuclei of cranial nerves in the brainstem, neural impulses will not be transmitted to the muscles. This condition is called **denervation**. The result is that the muscles innervated by the cranial or spinal nerve become soft and flabby from a loss of muscle tone. This is an LMN paralysis.

The loss of muscle tone is called **hypotonia**. Hypotonia results in flaccid muscles, thus the term flaccid paralysis. Hypotonia may be an acquired condition, with disease or injury affecting the peripheral nervous system pathway, but it may also be a condition found at birth or developing shortly after birth. Infantile hypotonia may result from conditions such as chromosome disorders (e.g., Prader-Willi syndrome), genetic defects, spinal cord disorders, spinal muscular atrophy, muscular dystrophy, metabolic myopathies, or other problems that affect the peripheral pathways.[12] Fig. 6.4 shows the posture, the frog-leg position, typically assumed by an infant with hypotonia.

LMN paralysis also is sometimes associated with loss of muscle bulk, a condition called **atrophy**. Muscles undergoing atrophy display some degree of degeneration because they have become denervated. Signs of this degeneration can be observed clinically. Atrophic muscles show fibrillations and fasciculations. These signs are caused by electrical disturbances in muscle fibers resulting from denervation. Fibrillations are fine twitches of single muscle fibers. These generally cannot be seen on clinical examination but must be detected by electromyographic examination. Fasciculations, on the other hand, are contractions of groups of muscle fibers that can be identified, with training, in skeletal muscles through the skin.

When muscle bulk is lost through atrophy in motor neuron disease (e.g., amyotrophic lateral sclerosis), fasciculations

are sometimes seen in the muscles of the head and neck as well as other parts of the body. These muscle twitches may be particularly observed in the relatively large muscle mass of the tongue if the bulbar muscles are involved. Fasciculations have no direct effect on speech itself but serve as a sign of LMN disease.

Interruption of a peripheral nerve by an LMN lesion also damages the reflex arc involved with that nerve. The result is that normal reflex responses mediated through the sensory and motor limbs of the arc become diminished. Reduced reflex response is called **hyporeflexia**. Complete lack of reflex is known as **areflexia**. Hyporeflexia and areflexia are also associated with LMN disease.

Referring back to Fig. 6.2 with some explanations of typical disorders can help the reader understand damage caused by more typical types of LMN disorders. The most obvious example of a disorder is a lesion or cut in the spinal nerve (point 2). This damage paralyzes the muscle innervated by

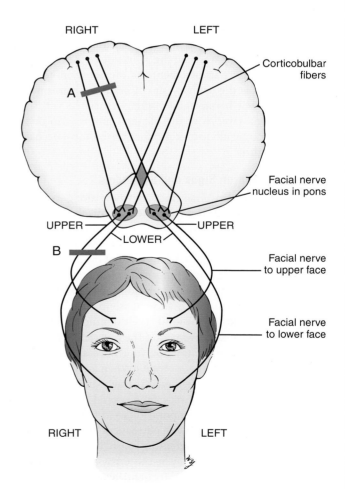

Fig. 6.4 Central contributions to upper and lower face. A. Lesion to the upper motor neurons (from the motor cortex to the brainstem) causes paralysis of the contralateral lower face but spares the contralateral forehead. B. Lesion of the facial nerve nucleus and the lower motor neurons causes total paralysis of both the upper and lower face. (From Swartz M. H. *Textbook of physical diagnosis: History and examination.* 8th ed. Philadelphia: Elsevier; 2021).

the nerve. In addition, the denervated muscle becomes hypotonic, areflexic, and atrophic. Finally, fasciculations appear. If a cranial nerve is denervated, weakness of speech muscles results from hypotonia and loss of muscle bulk.

A lesion may also occur in the cell body itself and produce paralysis and related LMN signs (see point 1 of Fig. 6.2). An example is acute bulbar poliomyelitis, which attacks the high cervical anterior horns as well as the cranial nerve nuclei of the bulbar muscles controlling speech. Speech muscles again may become weak and atrophic.

Lesions of the LMN type may also directly occur in muscles (point 4). An example of this type of disorder is seen in muscular dystrophy. Speech muscles lose strength and show disturbances of muscle bulk. This LMN disease within a muscle is called a myopathy, as opposed to a disease of the peripheral nerves, which is called a neuropathy. Lesions may also occur at the neuromuscular junction (point 3), as seen in myasthenia gravis. Speech muscles show weakness as well as notable fatigue with use in this myoneural disorder.

A pause to review. The study of the levels of control of the motor system and the terms associated with the different levels and different disorders is complicated. Here we will pause and review what has been discussed so far. Basic movement is generated by a neural impulse generated by motor neurons of the primary motor cortex and sent down to either the spinal cord (for movement of the extremities and trunk) or to the cranial nerve nuclei (for movement of eyes, face, mouth structures, and neck) located primarily in brainstem structures. Before the neural firing to muscles of speech production from the motor cortex, there is cortical activity that takes place in the SMA (pre-SMA portion) and insula (rostral portion), with perhaps some participation of part of Broca area. This cortical activity is concerned with motor planning or motor programming of the movements that need to occur to accomplish the task at hand. If the task is to produce speech, current research suggests that the motor planning takes place primarily in the pre-SMA segment, in the insula, and in a small part of Broca area.

The corticospinal (pyramidal) tract and the corticonuclear (corticobulbar) tract follow similar descending pathways for a short while. They both descend in a fan-shaped manner forming the corona radiata. Both then pass through the narrow space called the internal capsule with the corticospinal fibers traversing the posterior limb and the corticonuclear fibers passing through the genu. From this point the corticobulbar fibers will descend to synapse on their various target nuclei, primarily in the structures of the brainstem. Some of these fibers will decussate and others will continue ipsilaterally. Many of the cranial nerve nuclei receive bilateral innervation, meaning that fibers from both sides of the brain will synapse on the motor nuclei in the brainstem.

There is a different path for the corticospinal fibers from the point of the internal capsule. They descend below the thalamus and form part of the cerebral peduncles of the midbrain, a part called the crus cerebri. They will give off some fibers to nuclei in the pons, and these will become part of the corticopontine fiber pathway taking neural signaling out to the cerebellum. Most fibers will continue descending, though some collaterals are given off to the red nucleus, the olivary nuclei, reticular formation nuclei, and posterior column nuclei. Ninety percent of pyramidal tract fibers will decussate at the level of the pyramids of the medulla at the junction of the medulla and the cervical spinal cord. These fibers make up the lateral corticospinal tract. The other 10% will continue into the spinal cord ipsilaterally and make up the anterior corticospinal tract.

There are other descending tracts of fibers that form indirect activation pathways and make up the extrapyramidal tracts. These are the reticulospinal tract, the vestibulospinal tract, and the tectospinal tract. They consist of many short pathways with interconnections between the motor cortex and the spinal cord. They are concerned with coarse, stereotyped movements and with maintaining body tone and posture.

Two important concepts of clinical neurology were also discussed: UMNs and LMNs. The neurons and their axons that make up the pathway from the motor cortex down to the nuclei on which they synapse in either the spinal cord (for the corticospinal tract) or the brainstem (for corticobulbar fibers) are known as UMNs. They provide direct input into those targeted nuclei, carrying motor directives planned and implemented in the cortex. The second-order neurons found in the nuclei of either the anterior horn cells of the spinal column (for the corticospinal tract) or in the nuclei of the cranial nerves (for corticobulbar fibers) are known as LMNs. The axons of the LMNs take the transmitted information or motor directive out to the peripheral nervous system, exiting the brain or the spinal cord and synapsing on the muscle fibers. The motor unit is a helpful concept in understanding LMNs.

Other terms and concepts included as important to understanding the effect of damage to the pyramidal, corticobulbar, and extrapyramidal tracts are unilateral and contralateral innervation, bilateral symmetry, tone (hypertonicity and hypotonicity), Babinski sign, reflexes, paralysis, and muscular weakness. If these terms and concepts are not firm in your mind at this point, then go back and study this section before advancing to the next sections, which will take you to more in-depth information about neural control within muscles and then will introduce other influences on the motor pathways.

Neuromuscular Control

In the final analysis, motor control of speech muscles, or any other musculature, is brought about by muscle contraction. At one time it was believed that the only route for control of voluntary muscle contraction was by way of the several descending motor pathways in the nervous system that end in nerve cells called **alpha motor neurons (AMNs)**. In the spinal cord these motor neurons are called anterior horn cells and are in the largest cells in the spinal cord. Homologous motor neurons are the cranial nerve neurons of the brainstem. Along with gamma motor neurons (GMNs), the AMNs supply skeletal muscles. They discharge impulses through the spinal nerves to contract muscles of the trunk and limbs in the corticospinal system. Most motor commands for a given articulatory act, other oral-motor acts, or facial movement are transmitted by the AMN system through contraction of muscles innervated by cranial nerves.

Alpha Motor Neurons

The AMN innervates the main fibers that cause muscle contraction. These fibers lie within the muscle and are called **extrafusal fibers**. Fig. 6.5 illustrates the structure of a muscle fiber, including the input from the AMN. The axon of each AMN branches to supply the fibers. An axon may supply only a few fibers, as in the case of a small muscle with precisely controlled contraction, or it may control several hundred fibers, as in the case of large muscles with strong, crude movements. This fact is consistent with that shown on the homunculus in Fig. 2.7. The oral musculature involved in speech and

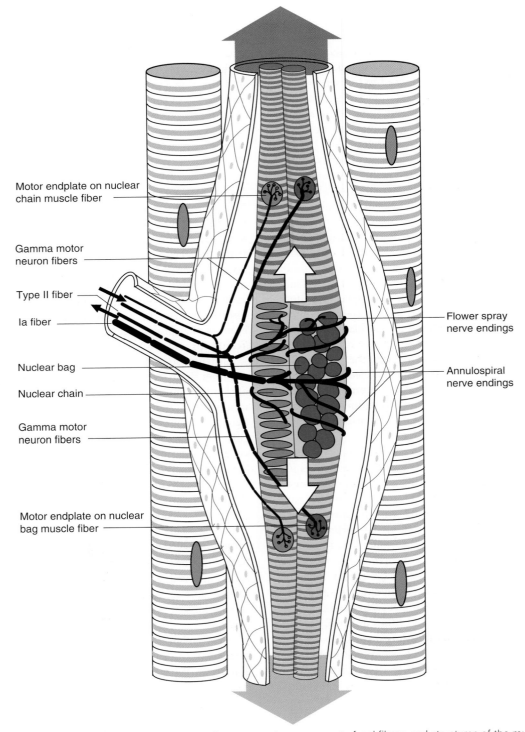

Motor endplate on nuclear chain muscle fiber

Gamma motor neuron fibers

Type II fiber

Ia fiber

Nuclear bag

Nuclear chain

Gamma motor neuron fibers

Motor endplate on nuclear bag muscle fiber

Flower spray nerve endings

Annulospiral nerve endings

Fig. 6.5 A muscle fiber showing the alpha motor neuron and gamma motor neuron, extrafusal fibers, and structures of the muscle spindle.

swallowing requires a much larger area on the motor strip because the innervation and control of these muscles require the involvement of a vastly larger number of neurons to allow fine and precise motor control for these acts.

The AMN supplies the trophic, or nutritional, factors, which direct differentiation of muscle fibers and keep the muscle healthy. These substances are called myotrophic factors. The motor neuron also supplies the acetylcholine that stimulates contraction of muscle.

Three types of extrafusal fibers can be differentiated in skeletal muscle. All muscles contain all three types of fibers, but all muscle fibers in one motor unit are of the same type. The type is determined by the myotrophic influences of the innervating neuron. The first of the three types of fibers are slow twitch (type I) fibers that contract slowly and are resistant to fatigue. These fibers predominate in sustaining postural activities, including standing. Fast twitch fibers (type IIx in humans) contract faster but fatigue more rapidly. They exert a more powerful force and are primarily found in superficial muscles. An intermediate fiber (type IIA) has properties between the other two types in terms of speed of contraction and amount of force; it is considered a fast twitch fiber, however.

Muscle Spindles

Another level of neuromuscular control has been identified at the level of the **muscle spindle** (see Fig. 6.5). Muscle spindles serve as sensory, or afferent, receptors within some striated muscles. They provide sensory information on the status of the normal stretch mechanisms in muscle. In muscles that have muscle spindles, the spindle is the mechanism through which, in passive stretch, the muscle contraction is elicited. The spindles receive efferent innervation through GMNs. Because muscle spindles serve as afferent (sensory) receptors yet they themselves receive efferent (motor) innervation, they are considered more complex sensory receptors than those found in the tendons and joints. Muscle spindles are most commonly found in the slow twitch (type I) fibers and are plentiful in the muscles along the vertebral column, the muscles of the neck, and the intrinsic muscles of the hand. They have been found to be present in large numbers in the muscles that close the jaw as well. The muscle spindle is encapsulated and fusiform (i.e., tapered at both ends). It contains a limited number of short fibers that are parallel to other muscle fibers. The extrafusal muscle fibers are outside of the spindle. Fibers of the muscle spindle itself are called **intrafusal fibers**, and they connect to those extrafusal fibers outside the spindle. Intrafusal fibers provide the nervous system with information about the length and the rate of change in length of the muscle. The number of intrafusal fibers within a spindle varies. To accomplish monitoring and informing the nervous system about length as well as rate of change, there are two types of fibers within the intrafusal fibers: nuclear chain and nuclear bag fibers. There are also two types of sensory endings associated with these fibers: primary (annulospiral) and secondary (flower spray) endings.

Nuclear bag fibers look chubby in the middle due to a clustering of nuclei there in this central region. The nuclear chain fibers have nuclei that are arranged in single file and are thinner appearing. These two types of fibers are the sensory receptors within a muscle and need to be associated with a sensory neuron to get the information to the nervous system about the status of stretch on the muscle. This information is conveyed to the CNS by the primary fibers, the annulospiral endings, and secondary afferent fibers, the flower spray endings. The annulospiral endings are wrapped around the center of both nuclear bag and nuclear chain fibers and are rapidly conducting afferent fibers. The flower spray endings are the more slowly conducting secondary afferents and are found mainly on nuclear chain fibers. These two types of fibers carry information toward the CNS and are thus afferent pathways. Because a majority of the muscle spindles are associated with spinal nerves (as opposed to cranial nerves), most of the body's information regarding muscle stretch enters the spinal cord and goes through the dorsal root ganglion associated with that body part. Muscle spindles associated with cranial nerve innervated muscles will synapse on sensory nuclei associated with that cranial nerve.

When the muscle is stretched, the sensory neurons wrapped around the intrafusal fibers act as length detectors and send information about the stretch into the CNS. The nuclear bag fibers can sense the onset of stretch, and the nuclear chain fibers sense sustained stretch. Both types of fibers will respond immediately, however, to rapid stretch, which is a protective mechanism for the muscle. The rate of firing of these fibers is proportional to the change in length of the muscle. The greater the stretch on the muscle, the more rapid the rate of firing.

Upon the onset of stretch on the muscle, muscle spindles are elongated. Both primary (annulospiral) and secondary (flower spray) afferents are stimulated by the lengthening of the intrafusal fibers within the muscle spindle and the rate of change of their length. This will result in the initiation of action potentials traveling through these afferents to the spinal cord (or the nuclei of the cranial nerve) and synapsing with the AMN, which in turn will fire neural impulses to the extrafusal fibers. It is the efferent signal of the AMN to the extrafusal fibers of the muscle that causes the muscle to contract.

Gamma Motor Neurons

Recall that both the AMNs and the GMNs synapse with the sensory afferents coming into the CNS. As with the AMNs, the GMNs are part of a motor nerve. They are relatively small in size compared with the alpha efferents, but they make up ~30% of the motor neurons leaving the spinal cord. Whereas the AMN signals the extrafusal fibers causing muscle contraction, the GMNs supply efferent innervation to the muscle spindle fibers, the intrafusal fibers.

The central region of an intrafusal fiber does not contract; only the ends have contractile properties. The GMNs innervate the muscle spindle at each end. At the same time as the sensory afferent synapses in the CNS with the AMN, there is also a synapse with GMNs. The firing of the GMN carries an efferent signal back to the ends of the intrafusal fiber causing it to contract. This is an important part of the muscle contraction because when muscle contraction takes place, the muscle spindle's intrafusal fibers tend to go a little slack. Proper functioning of the sensory afferents of the muscle spindle depends heavily on the appropriate amount of tension on the nuclear bag and nuclear chain fibers in the central region of the intrafusal fiber. The coactivation of both the AMN and the GMN allows the contraction of both extrafusal and intrafusal fibers. The GMN activation is at a slightly slower pace than the AMN action. When the ends of the intrafusal fibers contract, the appropriate amount of tension is reset within the muscle spindle so that it can be sensitive to any stretch placed on the muscle. This functional contractile process is known as the gamma loop system. Through this system the GMNs form an important muscle stretch reflex mechanism that acts in conjunction with the AMNs. This sensitivity to stretch provides fine compensations of muscle length and velocity and helps maintain muscle tone.

The speed with which the spindles convey sensory feedback information to the central nervous system would seem to mark them as likely candidates for the neural mechanisms controlling the fine and rapid movements of speech muscles. Evidence from the speech science laboratory indicates that rapid compensatory motor behavior is necessary for intelligible speech. Motor speech acts are rarely performed exactly the same way twice, but in most cases motor speech production meets the broad specifications of the motor commands in such a way that the listener can recognize an individual speech sound, or phon, as a member of a phoneme class. In the case of density of muscle spindles, the jaw-closing muscles have been found to be rich with muscle spindles.[7] Liss[18] used cadaver study with particular staining and light microscopy and identified a significant density of spindles in the levator palatini and palatoglossal muscles of the velum. A cadaver study by Cooper[6] in 1953 found the presence of muscle spindles in the intrinsic muscles of the tongue, particularly the superior longitudinal muscle at a point proximal and posterior to the tip. Studies by Saigusa et al.,[22,23] found muscle spindles present in the transverse lingual muscles at the base of the tongue and in the genioglossus muscle with the primary distribution being toward the base of the tongue. Muscle spindles have also been found in the digastric and mylohyoid muscles, important for mastication.[24]

Golgi Tendon Organs

Beyond the muscle spindle system are joint receptors and special tendon receptors called **Golgi tendon organs**, which are involved in sensorimotor control of some muscles of the body. The Golgi tendon organs are directly attached to the tendons of muscles. They respond when either stretching or contraction places tension on the tendon, or they signal the force of muscle contraction. The Golgi tendon organs temper motor activity and inhibit activity in muscles when high levels of tension are placed on the tendon. Golgi tendon organs dampen oscillation of the limbs, at times producing joint stiffness. If these afferents allow too much freedom (such as in Parkinson disease), the tendency to oscillate is not inhibited and tremor is seen.

A pause to review. In the foregoing section, the neural anatomy concerned with muscle fiber and neural innervation of muscle contraction was discussed. The main fibers within muscles that result in muscle contraction are the extrafusal fibers. These are innervated by the large neuron AMNs. The axon of an AMN will branch out to control more than one muscle fiber depending on the precision of muscle control needed to accomplish that movement. Therefore, a large number of fibers may be controlled by only a few AMNs when the movements are cruder, large movements (e.g., muscles of the quadriceps); muscles requiring fine, precise movements to accomplish the motor task (e.g., muscles of the finger or tongue) will require many AMNs because each axon will branch to control only a small number of fibers. The AMNs supply the trophic factors that determine the type of muscle fibers in a motor unit (type I, IIx, or IIA most frequently in skeletal muscle in humans). AMNs also supply the primary neurotransmitter, acetylcholine.

Another important level of control at the muscle fiber level is the muscle spindle, which is the sensory mechanism or afferent receptor present in some striated muscles. The muscle spindle contains intrafusal fibers. The muscle spindle provides the AMN information on the status of stretch on a muscle and can elicit muscle contraction. The spindle is a complicated structure with both afferent and efferent mechanisms. Most of the muscles under spinal control contain muscle spindles, but research has shown that some of the oral muscles also contain muscle spindles, which is important to the successful use of neuromuscular therapy methodology in treatment of oral-motor deficits.[15]

Other mechanisms or terms in the previous section include nuclear bag and nuclear chain fibers, annulospiral and flower spray endings, GMNs, and Golgi tendon organs. Please review these if needed before advancing to study other influences on the motor system.

THE INFLUENCE OF OTHER SYSTEMS ON MOVEMENT

Even if you have only limited experience with patients with neurologic disorders, you likely realize that there are many patients for whom subconscious planning of the movement pattern or grossly implementing movement does not seem to be the main problem. For many patients it is the finer aspects of motor control, the efficiency and coordination of the movements, that appear to be the locus of the disorder. There may be no problem in the direct corticospinal or corticonuclear tracts but, instead (or, sometimes, in addition) there may be damage to pathways associated with the basal nuclei (or basal ganglia as many texts still use) and/or the cerebellum. These structures and their input and output pathways are quite complex, and this text will not attempt to fully explain them.

However, it is important for the SLP to be somewhat familiar with their composition and their contribution to movement control so that the effects of damage to these structures can be better understood.

The Basal Ganglia (or Basal Nuclei)

Before beginning the discussion of the basal ganglia, review Figs. 2.13 and 2.14. The terminology for these structures as a whole has changed through the years with many contemporary texts using basal nuclei in place of basal ganglia. To acquaint the student with both, the terms are used interchangeably here. These structures include the **caudate nucleus (CN)**, the **putamen**, the **nucleus accumbens**, the **globus pallidus (GP**, both the internal and external segments), the **subthalamic nucleus (STN)**, and the **substantia nigra (SN)**. With the exception of the nucleus accumbens, these deep subcortical nuclei serve to modulate the activity of the motor cortex and brainstem nuclei of the motor system.

The CN lies just medial to the anterior limb of the internal capsule and adjacent to the wall of the lateral ventricle, close to the thalamus. The structure is divided into a head, body, and tail by some neuroanatomists, but others divide the caudate into only a head and a tail. The entire caudate cannot be illustrated in a coronal section because of its C shape. Only a part of it (or none at all) will be seen depending on where the sectioning occurs in the anterior-posterior plane. It follows the body of the lateral ventricle with the tail end at about the level of the temporal lobe; it terminates at the amygdaloid nucleus.

The putamen is located anterior to the genu of the internal capsule. In humans, the caudate and the putamen are separated structurally by the internal capsule. Functionally, together the caudate and the putamen make up the **striatum** or, in some texts, the neostriatum. The putamen and caudate are connected by bridges of cells that span across the internal capsule; these strands give the area its striped or striated appearance, thus earning its name at some point. Converging excitatory input comes into the striatum from almost the entire cortex, but especially the sensorimotor and frontal areas of the cortex. The thalamus also provides input into the striatum.

The nucleus accumbens lies between the caudate and the putamen and is sometimes called the ventral striatum or dorsal striatum. It is part of a mesolimbic circuit involved in dopamine signaling that seems to be involved in establishing associations between rewarding or adversive stimuli and the environment surrounding that experience. It has minimal involvement in control of movement and will not be discussed here further.

The GP is located medial to the putamen and rostral to the hypothalamus. In primates the GP is separated by a fiber tract (the internal medullary lamina) into two segments, an internal segment (GP_i) and an external one (GP_e). The putamen and GP (as a whole) together comprise the lentiform nucleus, a thumb-sized structure wedged against the internal capsule. The lentiform nucleus (i.e., the putamen and the

GP), combined with the CN, comprises the **corpus striatum** (Table 6.4).

The other structures of the basal nuclei, the STN and the SN, are found near the reticular formation of the midbrain. The STN is located at the junction of the diencephalon and the midbrain, ventral to the thalamus. The SN is located in the ventral part of the midbrain between the red nucleus and the crus cerebri; although it is located in the midbrain, it is functionally part of the basal ganglia system. There are two segments comprising the SN: the pars reticulata (SNpr), which is composed of few cells, and the pars compacta (SNpc), which is densely packed with cells. The SNpc provides a critical supply of dopamine to the neostriatum.

Excitatory afferent input to the basal nuclei is primarily through the striatum and comes from the entire cerebral cortex and parts of the thalamus. There are projections from frontal, temporal, parietal, and occipital cortical areas stratified throughout the basal ganglia; the head of the caudate receives the largest number of input fibers, those coming from the frontal lobe. The basal ganglia also contain a motor homunculus similar to the one in the primary motor cortex. The projections from the motor cortex to the basal nuclei maintain this somatotopic organization from the source area to the targeted basal ganglia region and could be traced.

Only two structures of the basal ganglia transmit outside of this circuitry: the GP (internal segment, GP_i) and the SN (pars reticulata segment, SNpr). Output transmissions from the basal nuclei project primarily to the thalamus and are relayed back to parts of the cortex. A limited number of fibers also project to the brainstem, and some of the SNpr fibers project to the superior colliculus for control of eye movement.[3]

The neurotransmitter secreted by these output basal ganglia structures is gamma-aminobutyric acid (GABA), and the transmission is inhibitory. The strength of the final inhibitory transmission will depend on the pathway taken between the striatum and the output neurons of the GP_i or the SNpr. There is more than one pathway, particularly between the striatum and the GP_i; there are some excitatory and many inhibitory connections along the various routes. These intervening connections and the neural signaling involved could

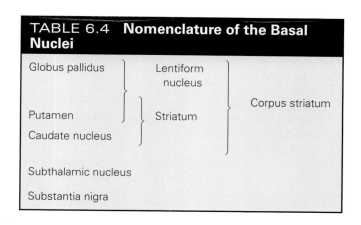

TABLE 6.4 **Nomenclature of the Basal Nuclei**

significantly alter the effectiveness of the final transmission from the output basal ganglia structure (the GP_i or the SNpr) and, subsequently, the thalamus.

There is a somatotopic organization of the output of the basal ganglia such that output associated with leg and arm movement is from the GP_i and from the face and eyes, the SNpr. The GP_i sends ~70% of its output to the thalamus and the brainstem. The thalamic nuclei in turn send projections to different parts of the cortex, including the motor, premotor, supplementary motor, and prefrontal areas. Some project back to the striatum for possible feedback loops. Brainstem connections in the midbrain and pons project to reticulospinal neurons. There are some output neurons of the GP_i whose eventual connections are unknown at this time.

The other structures of the basal nuclei transmit only within the circuitry. Box 6.2 lists the output targets and the type and target of transmission of the structures. Note that within the basal ganglia circuitry, the SNpc is the source of dopamine to the striatum and that dopamine transmission may result in an eventual transmission that is excitatory or inhibitory. It just depends on what type of receptor (D1 = excitatory; D2 = inhibitory) within the striatum receives the neural signal. Please keep in mind that most connections within this circuitry are inhibitory so that the net effect (strength of inhibition or excitation) of the output transmission of the GP_i and the SNpr depends on how many inhibitory versus excitatory connections have been made before the final output. The ramifications of too little or too much inhibition or excitation of the cortical motor areas will be obvious when we review the motor speech disorders associated with damage to the basal ganglia.

The basal ganglia indirectly affect motor function. The input fed into the thalamus and then to the cortex or brainstem can facilitate initiating movement, executing movement or terminating movement. Through this complex circuitry, learned movement patterns can be selectively activated or suppressed so that the intended movement can be accomplished with involvement of appropriate muscle tone, body posturing, and without interference from other unnecessary or disruptive movements.

Damage to the Basal Ganglia

Lesions of the basal ganglia generally produce two major types of movement disorders: poverty of movement (**akinesia**)

BOX 6.2 **Basal Ganglia**

Internal Connections
- Caudate and putamen (striatum) = inhibitory (GABA) → GP_i, GP_e, SNpr, SNpc
- Globus pallidus internal (GP_i) = inhibitory (GABA) → subthalamic nucleus
- Globus pallidus external (GP_e) = inhibitory → subthalamic nucleus
- Subthalamic nucleus = excitatory (glutamate) → GP_i, GP_e, and SNpr
- Substantia nigra (SNpc) = mixed (depends on the receptor) dopamine → striatum

---

and excessive involuntary movement (**dyskinesia**). Akinesia is often accompanied by muscular rigidity, as in Parkinson disease. The basal ganglia particularly influence movements related to posture, automatic movements, and skilled voluntary movements.

The basal ganglia appear to be important in the automatic execution of learned motor plans, based on learning through error. This set of structures appears to filter out competing motor plans and to block unwanted movements.[11] Older models of the function of the basal ganglia have not been altered and include subconscious selection, sequencing, and delivery of the motor programs of a learned or practiced motor strategy, such as playing an instrument or writing by hand. When the basal ganglia are damaged, the individual appears to revert to slower, less automatic, and less accurate cortical mechanisms for motor behavior. Civier et al.,[5] provide a review of studies that support the possibility that the basal ganglia-thalamocortical circuit plays an important role in the pathophysiology of stuttering.

Dyskinesia. Damage to some parts of the basal ganglia produces motor disturbances usually classified as involuntary movement disorders. The most commonly used technical term for them is dyskinesia (*dys*, "disordered"; *kinesia*, "movement"). These disorders encompass a full range of bizarre postures and unusual movement patterns. The dyskinesias have long been described by such terms as tremor, writhing, fidgeting, flailing, restlessness, jerking, and flinging. Often, the unusual movements that dominate the trunk and limbs of the dyskinetic patient are also reflected in the face and speech mechanism. The result is a serious and typical dysarthria classified under hyperkinetic dysarthria (see Chapter 8). In general, the dysarthria reflects the specific symptoms of each specific type of dyskinesia.

Dyskinesia may be used in a broad sense to include any excess of movement (hyperkinesia) or reduction in movement (akinesia). **Hyperkinesia** has been used to indicate dyskinesias that present too much movement. **Hypokinesia** and akinesia, on the other hand, refer to too little movement and reduced movement, respectively. In actual clinical use, the terms may not always be strictly applied to a person with an identified neurologic lesion. For instance, neurologists may apply hyperkinesia to the well-known twitching or fidgeting of Huntington chorea as well as the abnormal hyperactivity of children in whom there may not be evidence of an organic lesion in the nervous system, let alone knowledge of a lesion localized to the CNS.

Hypokinesia also may be used to describe the reduced activity level of a depressive patient with no suspected neurologic lesion. By tradition, neurologists do not apply the term to limitations in movement resulting from lesions of the pyramidal tract or peripheral nerves. In other words, lesions that paralyze voluntary movement are not labeled hypokinetic. Thus, hemiplegia, quadriplegia, and paraplegia are not considered hypokinetic disorders.

Dyskinetic types. The responsibilities of SLPs do not extend to the identification of lesion sites in the complex circuitry of the motor system, but SLPs should attempt to recognize the standard dyskinesias and determine the effect of the symptoms of specific dyskinesias on the accompanying dysarthria. Undiagnosed cases of movement disorders demand referral to a neurologist. Dyskinesia has several distinct patterns, but not all of them are related to the dysarthrias. Described next are only those motor signs that can produce motor speech symptoms.

Tremors. **Tremors** are defined as purposeless movements that are rhythmic, oscillatory, involuntary actions. Normal (or physiologic) and abnormal (or pathologic) tremors are usually distinguished. Tremors are pathologic if they occur in a disease and are characteristic of that disease. Normal tremor is called physiologic tremor. Several classifications of tremor are in use today. The SLP should be familiar with three types of tremor associated with vocal performance in normal and pathologic conditions.

Rest tremor. **Rest tremor** designates a tremor that occurs in Parkinson disease. A tremor of three to seven movements per second occurs in the patient's limbs and hands at rest. The tremor is temporarily suppressed when the limb is moved, and it sometimes can be inhibited by conscious effort. The voice may be affected by the tremor. Tremulous voice has been described in ~14% of a large sample of parkinsonian patients. It is a salient vocal deviation that is easily recognized among the other vocal deviations of the hypokinetic dysarthria of parkinsonism.

Physiologic, or action, tremor. Healthy people demonstrate a fine tremor of the hands when maintaining posture. The rate may vary with age but usually falls within the range of 4 to 12 cycles per second. This normal tremor is distinguished from pathologic tremors associated with known neurologic diseases such as Parkinson and cerebellar disorders. An abnormal **action tremor** may affect the laryngeal muscles and produce a voice disorder known as organic or essential voice tremor.

Intention tremor. **Intention tremor** refers to a tremor that occurs during movement and is intensified at the termination of the movement. Intention tremor has been associated with the ataxic dysarthria seen in cerebellar disease. It is often seen in cerebellar disorders but is not exclusive to cerebellar dysfunction.

Chorea. **Chorea** refers to quick, random, hyperkinetic movements simulating fragments of normal movements. Speech, facial, and respiratory movements, as well as movements of the extremities, are affected by choreic symptoms in this dyskinesia. The movement is close to what is popularly described as fidgets. Chorea is one symptom of a hereditary disorder known as Huntington disease, or Huntington chorea, and is seen in other movement disorders as well.

Athetosis. The hyperkinesia of **athetosis** is a slow, irregular, coarse, writhing, or squirming movement. It usually involves the extremities as well as the face, neck, and trunk. The movements directly interfere with the fine and controlled actions of the larynx, tongue, palate, pharynx, and respiratory mechanism. As with most other involuntary movements, the involuntary movements of athetosis disappear in sleep. In congenital athetosis, the most common type of spastic

paralysis may also be observed. Lesion sites in pure athetosis are often in the putamen and the CN. Hypoxia, or lack of oxygen at birth, is a common cause, producing death of brain cells before or during birth. Choreoathetotic movements have also been described; they appear to be a dyskinesia that lies somewhere between choreic and athetoid movements in terms of rate and rhythm of movement or that includes both types of movement. In fact, many of the involuntary movement disorders appear to blend one or more of the different clinical dyskinesias, as the term choreoathetosis implies.

Dystonia. In **dystonia** the limbs assume distorted static postures resulting from excess tone in selected parts of the body. The dyskinetic postures are slow, bizarre, and often grotesque, involving writhing, twisting, and turning. Dysarthria and obvious motor involvement of the speech mechanism are common. Often, differential motor involvement occurs in the speech muscles, and some dysarthrias have been observed that primarily affect the larynx. Others affect the face, tongue, lips, palate, and jaw. A rare dystonic disorder of childhood is called dystonia musculorum deformans. It may be accompanied by dysarthria in its later stages.

Fragmentary, or focal, dystonias have been described, and some neurologists assert that they contribute to spastic or spasmodic dysphonia, a bizarre voice disorder that mixes aphonia (lack of voice) with a strained, labored whisper. The etiology of spastic dysphonia is unclear. Injections of botulinum are often effective in reducing the dystonia.

Myoclonus. **Myoclonus** has been used to describe differing motor abnormalities, but basically a myoclonic movement is an abrupt, brief, almost lightning-like contraction of muscle. An example of a normal or physiologic myoclonic reaction occurs when a person is drifting off to sleep but suddenly is awakened by a rapid muscle jerk. This muscle jerk is myoclonus.

Pathologic myoclonus is most common in the limbs and trunk but also may involve the facial muscles, jaws, tongue, and pharynx. Repetitive myoclonus in these muscles, of course, may affect speech. Myoclonic movements in the muscles of speech have been described as having a rate of 10 to 50 per minute, but they can be more rapid. The pathology underlying these movements has been debated, but because they have been associated with degenerative brain disease, the cerebral cortex, brainstem, and cerebellum have all been considered as possible lesion sites.

A special myoclonic syndrome involving speech muscles called palatal myoclonus has been described. It involves rapid movements of the soft palate and pharynx and sometimes includes the larynx, diaphragm, and other muscles. The symptoms most often present in later life and are characteristic of several diseases. This myoclonus has a specific pathology in the central tegmental tract of the brainstem, but the etiology can be varied. The most common cause is a stroke, or cerebrovascular accident, in the brainstem.

Orofacial dyskinesia (tardive dyskinesia). In orofacial or **tardive dyskinesia**, bizarre movements are limited to the mouth, face, jaw, and tongue. This movement includes grimacing, pursing of the mouth and lips, and writhing of the tongue. These dyskinetic movements often alter articulation of speech. The motor speech signs of orofacial dyskinesia usually develop after the prolonged use of powerful tranquilizing drugs, the most common class of which are phenothiazines. Drug-induced dyskinesias associated with the phenothiazines and related medications may even produce athetoid movements or dystonic movements of the body. Parkinsonian signs and other symptoms associated with movement disorders are also caused by these drugs. Orofacial dyskinesia also occurs in elderly patients without drug use. A rare disorder that includes dyskinesia of the eyelids, face, tongue, and refractory muscles is Meige syndrome.

Other dyskinesias are included in the spectrum of movement disorders but generally do not include motor involvement of the speech mechanism. These include hemiballismus, which causes forceful, flinging unilateral movements and may involve half of the body. Akathisia refers to motor restlessness or the inability to sit still. Restless leg syndrome is an example of this dyskinesia. Box 6.3 summarizes the dyskinesias.

The Cerebellar System

The third major subcomponent of the motor system that affects speech is the cerebellum. Interacting with the other systems of motor control we have been studying, the cerebellum is known to provide significant coordination for motor speech. As noted, the cerebellum is located dorsal to the medulla and pons. The occipital lobes of the cerebral hemispheres overlap the top of the cerebellum. The anatomy of the cerebellum is complex, and the SLP need only understand it in a gross sense to see the relation of the cerebellum to speech performance.

Anatomy of the Cerebellum

The cerebellum can be divided into three parts. The thin middle portion is called the vermis because of its serpentine, or snakelike, shape. The vermis lies between two large lateral masses of the cerebellum, the cerebellar hemispheres (Fig. 6.6). The vermis connects these two hemispheres. The vermis and hemispheres are divided by fissures and sulci into lobes and into smaller divisions called lobules. The division into lobes and lobules is helpful in clarifying the physiologic function of the cerebellum. Although the lobes and lobules have been classified differently by different investigators, this text uses a classification system that divides the cerebellum into three lobes.

Three cerebellar lobes. The three cerebellar lobes are the anterior lobe, posterior lobe, and flocculonodular lobe. The anterior lobe, which is modest in size, is superior to the primary fissure. This part of the cerebellum roughly corresponds to the paleocerebellum, the second oldest part of the cerebellum in a phylogenetic sense. The anterior lobe receives most of the proprioceptive impulses from the spinal cord and regulates posture.

The posterior lobe, the largest part of the cerebellum, is located between the other two lobes. It comprises the major portion of the cerebellar hemispheres. It is the newest part

BOX 6.3 Common Dyskinetic Types

- *Tremors:* Purposeless movements that are rhythmic, oscillatory, involuntary actions. Designated as either normal (physiologic) or abnormal (pathologic).
  - Rest tremor: Designated tremor caused by Parkinson disease. Presenting signs include tremor when affected limb is at rest and may include tremulous voice. Range of three to seven movements per second.
  - Action (physiologic) tremor: Fine tremor of hands while maintaining posture. Can affect laryngeal muscles, causing voice tremor. Range of 4–12 cycles per second.
  - Intention tremor: Tremor intensified at termination of movement. Associated with ataxic dysarthria and other cerebellar disorders.
- *Chorea:* Quick, random, hyperkinetic movements simulating fragments of normal movement. Movements are close to what is commonly described as fidgets and present as a symptom of Huntington disease.
- *Athetosis:* Slow, irregular, coarse, writhing, or squirming movement. Involves extremities and can directly interfere with fine and controlled actions of the swallowing and respiratory mechanisms.
- *Dystonia:* Limbs assume distorted, static postures resulting in excess tone in selected body parts. Movements include slow, bizarre, and often grotesque writhing, twisting, and turning motions.
- *Myoclonus:* Abrupt, brief, almost lightning-like contraction of muscle. Pathology is still debatable. Has been associated with degenerative brain disease, cerebral cortex, brainstem, and cerebellum. Palatal myoclonus is a special type involving rapid movements of the soft palate and pharynx, commonly caused by stroke or cerebrovascular accident in the brainstem.
- *Orofacial (tardive) dyskinesia:* Bizarre movements limited to mouth, face, jaw, and tongue characterized by grimacing, pursing of mouth and lips, and writhing of the tongue. Shown to develop from prolonged use of tranquilizing drugs, especially phenothiazines. A dyskinesia called Meige syndrome affects the eyelids, face, tongue, and refractory muscles.

Non-Speech-Related Dyskinesias
- Hemiballismus: Forceful, flinging, unilateral movements that may involve the whole body
- Akathisia: Motor restlessness or the inability to sit still (e.g., restless leg syndrome)

of the cerebellum and is therefore also known as the **neocerebellum**. The posterior lobe receives the cerebellar connections from the cerebrum and regulates coordination of muscle movement.

The flocculonodular lobe consists of two small wispy appendages, known as **flocculi**, in the posterior and inferior region of the cerebellum. The flocculi are separated by the nodulus, the inferior part of the vermis. The flocculonodular lobe, the oldest portion of the cerebellum, contains the fastigial nucleus, which is composed of fibers that travel from the

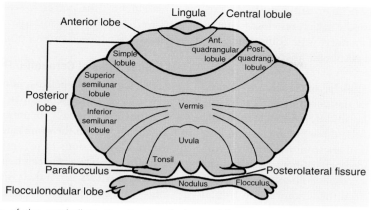

Fig. 6.6 A schematic illustration of the cerebellum showing hemispheres, lobes, and lobules. *Ant.,* Anterior; *Post.,* posterior; *Quadrang.,* quadrangular.

nucleus to the four vestibular nuclei in the upper medulla. The cerebellum mediates equilibrium by way of these fibers.

Longitudinal zones and deep nuclei. The cerebellum is also in some texts divided into longitudinal zones that relate to deep nuclei within the cerebellum. The nuclei receive input from the cerebellar cortex and are named (going from medial to lateral placement deep within the cerebellum): fastigial, interpositus, and dentate nuclei. The longitudinal zones relate to these nuclei and are called the medial, intermediate, and lateral zones. The fastigial nuclei receive input from the medial zone. This zone receives sensory input from sensory systems such as visual, vestibular, and auditory systems. The related fastigial nucleus will output to vestibular, and reticulospinal systems, the thalamus, and the superior colliculus. The interpositus nuclei receive input from the longitudinal division called the intermediate zone. This zone receives information from the spinal cord and receives input from the motor cortex via the corticopontine fibers. The interpositus nuclei send output to the red nucleus and to the contralateral thalamus. The third zone, the lateral zone, gets input from widespread areas of the cortex, through the corticopontine fiber tracts. This zone projects to the dentate nucleus, which primarily communicates with the thalamus and the reticular formation.

Synergy and asynergy. The connections that the cerebellum has with other parts of the CNS are important to its function. Through these connections the cerebellum sends and receives afferent and efferent impulses and executes its primary function: a synergistic coordination of muscles and muscle groups. **Synergy** is defined as the cooperative action of muscles. Ensuring the smooth coordination of muscles is the prime task of the cerebellum. Specifically, the cerebellum, along with other structures of the nervous system, maintains proper posture and balance in walking and in the sequential movements of eating, dressing, and writing. It also guides the production of rapid, alternating, repetitive movements, such as those involved in speaking, and smooth pursuit movements. Voluntary movement, without assistance from the cerebellum, is clumsy, uncoordinated, and disorganized. Motor defect of the cerebellar system has been called asynergia or dyssynergia. **Asynergia** is a lack of coordination in agonistic

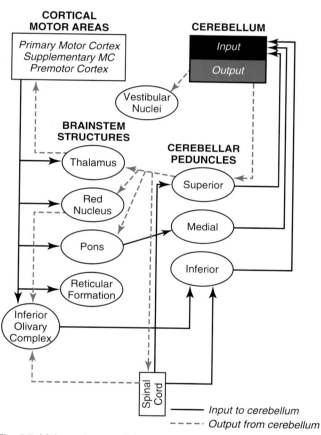

Fig. 6.7 Major pathways of the cerebellum. *MC,* Motor cortex.

and antagonistic muscles and is manifested as deterioration of smooth, complex movements.

Cerebellar peduncles and pathways. The cerebellum is connected to the rest of the nervous system by three pairs of **peduncles**, or feet. The cerebellar peduncles anchor the cerebellum to the brainstem. All afferent and efferent fibers of the cerebellum pass through the three peduncles and the pons to the other levels of the nervous system. The pons, which means bridge, is aptly named; it is literally a bridge from the cerebellum to the rest of the nervous system (Fig. 6.7).

The inferior cerebellar peduncle, or restiform body, carries primary afferent fibers from the structures close to it: the medulla, spinal cord, and cranial nerve VIII. Thus, spinocerebellar, medullocerebellar, and vestibular fibers pass through the inferior peduncle.

The middle cerebellar peduncle, or brachium pontis, connects the cerebellum with the cerebral cortex by the pathways that traverse it. The middle peduncle is easily recognized; it is the largest of the three peduncles and also conveys the largest number of fibers from the cerebral cortex and pons. It carries pontocerebellar fibers as well as the majority of the corticopontocerebellar fibers. These fibers convey afferent information from the temporal and frontal lobes of the cerebrum to the posterior lobe of the contralateral cerebellum.

The superior cerebellar peduncle, or brachium conjunctivum, conveys the bulk of efferent fibers that leave the cerebellum. The primary efferent fibers arise from an important nucleus deep in the cerebellum called the dentate nucleus. The rubrospinal and dentatothalamic pathways, along with several other tracts, leave by way of the superior peduncle and terminate in the contralateral red nucleus and ventrolateral nucleus of the thalamus. From here impulses are relayed to the cerebral cortex.

Cerebellar Role in Speech

The major pathways and structures of the cerebellum have been outlined to suggest a rough schematic of the feedback nature of the afferent and efferent connections of the structure. Basic as the presentation is, it still highlights the fact that the cerebellar motor subsystem significantly influences the function of the other motor systems in the production of motor speech. The fact that the cerebellum plays an important part in the synergy of rapid alternating movements and the fine coordination of muscles suggests that it interacts in a crucial way with the corticonuclear fibers to provide the specialized rapid and precise motor control needed for ongoing connected speech.

Auditory, tactile, and visual areas also exist in the cerebellum. These centers in the cerebellum, both cortical and subcortical, project back to corresponding cerebellar areas. The cerebellum therefore is neither completely vestibular, proprioceptive, nor motor in function. Rather, it serves to reinforce or diminish sensory and motor impulses, acting as a critical modulator of neuronal function. There is an abundance of sensory and cortical information conveyed to and from the cerebellum, resulting in indirect influence on motor nuclei. There are also many connections with nonmotor areas, leading to the conclusion that the cerebellar role is to evaluate sensory and motor information during a movement. In swallowing, recent research[26] suggests the cerebellar role is to compare movements prior to initiation to the ideal movement. As the cerebellum compares the intended movement with the actual movement, it sends corrective information back to the cortex and brainstem to modify the movement without major disruption to the

movement. This correction takes place for large muscles as well as for the respiratory, articulatory, and phonatory muscles for speech production.

Clinical Signs of Cerebellar Dysfunction

Cerebellar or cerebellar pathway lesions manifest themselves by affecting coordination of **volitional** movements and often volitionally maintained postures. Clinical signs usually appear on the same side of the body as the cerebellar lesion. UMN lesions of pyramidal pathways yield contralateral effects, whereas the cerebellum and its pathways manifest ipsilateral effects. Several classic signs of cerebellar disorders follow and are summarized in Table 6.5, along with tests used to determine the abnormality.

Ataxia. **Ataxia** is the prime sign of a cerebellar lesion (*taxis,* "ordering in rank and file"). The term is often used in several senses. It may refer to the general incoordination of motor acts seen with cerebellar system lesions. In this sense it often describes a staggering or reeling gait and abnormal posture seen with cerebellar lesions. The patient compensates for the ataxic gait by standing and walking with feet wide apart in what is called a broad-based gait.

Decomposition of movement. Decomposition of movement is also related to ataxia. The patient breaks a complex motor act into its components and executes the act movement by movement so that the act seems as if it were being performed by a robot. Decomposition of movement is considered an ataxic movement.

Dysmetria. **Dysmetria** is the inability to gauge the distance, speed, and power of movement. A patient may stop before the movement is performed or may overshoot the motor goal.

TABLE 6.5	Cerebellar Dysfunction Signs and Tests
Abnormality	**Signs and Tests**
Gait ataxia	Broad-based gait seen on tandem walking test
Arm ataxia	Finger to nose test, hand pronation to supination test results in overshooting of nose and slowed pronation and supination
Overshooting	Rebound noted on arm-pulling test
Hypotonia	Flaccid muscle tone noted on passive movement testing; pendular reflexes elicited on reflex testing; "rag-doll" postures observed
Nystagmus	Pupil oscillation seen when patient attempts to follow finger through field of gaze
Dysarthria	Ataxic dysarthria with disturbance in speech rate and prosody; often associated with left cerebellar hemisphere lesion

Adiadochokinesia or dysdiadochokinesia. **Adiadochokinesia**, or **dysdiadochokinesia**, is the inability to perform rapid alternating muscle movements. Often, the rate of alternating movement may be recorded in a neurologic examination. This measure is called an alternate motion rate. Diadochokinetic rate measures of the muscles of the oral mechanism during speech and nonspeech activities have long been used as an assessment task by the clinical SLP. These rates, however, are used as measures of the integrity of the oral muscles in speech pathology and have not specifically been related to cerebellar function.

The neurologist may test alternating movements in many muscle groups in persons suspected of cerebellar disorders. Successive pronation or supination of the hands, rapid tapping of the fingers, and rapid opening and closing of the fists are all diadochokinetic diagnostic tests. During the testing of diadochokinesis or alternate motion rates, awkwardness or clumsiness of alternate movements may be seen.

Rebound. The rebound phenomenon is the inability to check the contraction of the flexors and rapidly contract the extensor. It may account for the lack of smooth diadochokinetic movements.

Hypotonia. Hypotonia (or muscle flaccidity) with a decrease in resistance to passive movement is seen in cerebellar dysfunction. The muscles of the body are flabby and lack normal tone.

Tremor. Tremor is seen as part of cerebellar disease. It is usually an intention or kinetic tremor not present at rest.

Nystagmus. **Nystagmus** involves oscillatory abnormalities of the pupil of the eye often seen in cerebellar disorders. The rhythmic oscillations may be vertical, horizontal, or rotary.

Muscle stretch reflexes. Muscle stretch reflexes are normal or diminished. Pendular reflexes often may be seen in cerebellar disease. When the knee-jerk reflex is elicited, a series of smooth to-and-fro movements of the limb often occur before it comes to rest, as seen with a pendulum. This pendular reflex differs from a normal knee-jerk response.

Dysarthria. Dysarthria associated with damage to the cerebellum is called **ataxic dysarthria**. Its characteristics are discussed in Chapter 8.

A pause to review. In the last section we concentrated on the basal nuclei and the cerebellum and their influence on the coordination, efficiency, and effectiveness of movement initiated at the cortex. The basal nuclei (aka, basal ganglia) structures are the CN, the putamen, the GP, the STN, and the SN. The nucleus accumbens is also part of the basal ganglia but is not involved in movement control. As is typical in neuroanatomy, some structures have been combined and the combination given a different name: the caudate and the putamen together are called the striatum (or neostriatum); the putamen and the GP together are called the lenticular nucleus; the three structures together make up the corpus striatum. As is also typical in neuroanatomy, some structures have been found to be segmented into different functional parts. The GP can be segmented into an internal part (GP_i)

and an external part (GP_e) with the internal part sending transmission outside the basal nuclei. The SN can be separated into the pars reticulata (SNpr) and the pars compacta (SNpc) with the SNpr sending transmission outside of the basal ganglia and the SNpc supplying dopamine to the structures of the basal nuclei. The neurotransmitter of the output of the basal ganglia is GABA, and the transmission is inhibitory. The strength of the final transmission depends on the complicated dopamine transmissions within the circuitry, some being excitatory and some inhibitory to the circuit structures. The output transmission of the basal ganglia is primarily to the thalamus, which then relays the transmission to the cortex. There is some transmission to brainstem structures, particularly the superior colliculus, contributing to control of eye movement. Some of the terms and concepts to be learned and associated with basal ganglia function are akinesia, dyskinesia, hyperkinesia, hypokinesia, tremor, chorea, dystonia, athetosis, and myoclonus.

The cerebellum contributes significantly to coordination of movement for speech and other motor activities. It is located at the base of the brain and is connected to the brainstem by cerebellar peduncles through which corticopontine fibers traverse. It has three parts: two hemispheres and a middle portion called the vermis. There are also three lobes of the cerebellum, each concerned with a different function, including proprioception, motor coordination, and equilibrium. The cerebellum is also made up of different zones and nuclei, which are deep inside the cerebellum. These zones and their nuclei receive input from the cortex, spinal cord, and sensory systems such as the auditory, vestibular, and visual systems. They then will project output to the thalamus, the reticular formation, or various sensory systems. The cerebellar system has been found to be critical to synergistic motor control to enable movements to be smooth, well timed, and coordinated. The cerebellum has been supported in research as functioning to compare the actual movement with intended movement. It appears to send corrective information back to the cortex and brainstem about mismatch between the two, enabling "online" nondisruptive modification of the motor program. It is believed that the cerebellum participates in this manner in the coordination of respiration, articulation, and voice for speech production.

SERVOMECHANISM THEORY AND SPEECH MOTOR CONTROL

Feedback

Several fruitful engineering concepts have been applied to neuronal transmission problems in the nervous system. These concepts have been particularly useful in explaining the possible control of neural impulses in the speech mechanism. The basic concept, known as the theory of **servomechanism control systems**, implies the concept of **feedback**. Feedback describes the functioning principle in self-regulating systems, either mechanical or biologic. Feedback assumes that the output of any self-regulating system, such as a thermostat, is fed back into the system at some point to control or regulate the output of the system. This concept of self-monitoring is most appropriate for understanding the biologic system known as the speech motor control system. For instance, the questions of how a speaker monitors speech and what neuronal feedback mechanisms are available to control speech movements seem likely ones for explanation by servomechanism theory.

Open and Closed Control Systems

Two types of bioengineering control systems have been described as applicable to neuronal transmission in speech production: closed-loop and open-loop control systems. A closed-loop system uses positive feedback in which output is returned as input to control further output. For example, when copying a complex and delicate drawing, the sensory input to the visual system guides the motor output of the hand. Similarly, hearing one's own speech while talking may at times control the motor speech output as one continues to talk more. In these two examples, motor output by hand or speech is assumed to be guided by the sensory input of vision or audition. Furthermore, if the sensory feedback were blocked, the drawing or speech would be assumed to go awry.

In an open-loop system, the output is generally preprogrammed, and the performance of the system is not matched with the system. For instance, if a person has memorized a short poem and has practiced it repeatedly, that person may be able to say the phonemes of the words in the poem without error even when the ears are stuffed with cotton. In an open-loop system the notion of **feedforward**, rather than feedback, is important. Once a phrase of a well-learned poem has been uttered, it cues the next preprogrammed phrase of speech without the need to hear what was said through auditory feedback. An open-loop system thus typically generates another input by its output system. The term *negative feedback* is also used in control systems of the servomechanism type. That term implies that when errors are fed back into the system, the error information acts to keep a given output activity within certain limits. Correcting an articulation error on hearing it is an example of the use of negative feedback in speech activity.

Much speech research has viewed speech motor control as the product of a closed-loop feedback system with sensory monitoring from hearing, touch, and deep muscle sense guiding the movements of the speech muscles. Circumstantial evidence for this position has come from studies of sensory dysfunction in some speech disorders. Yet evidence exists that much of speech motor control is preprogrammed by the brain and that feedforward control is also critical to speech output. Guenther et al.,[14] developed a model of feedforward control that works in concert with auditory and somatosensory feedback called DIVA (Directions into Velocities of Articulators) (Fig. 6.8) that can be implemented in computer simulations producing

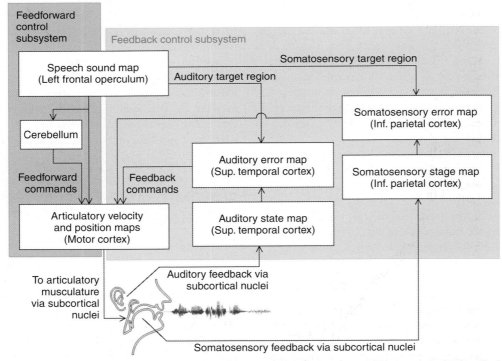

Fig. 6.8 Schematic of the DIVA (Directions into Velocities of Articulators) model of speech acquisition and production. Projections to and from the cerebellum are simplified for clarity. (From Guenther, F. H. [2006]. Cortical interactions underlying the production of speech sounds. *Journal of Communication Disorders, 39*(5), 350–365.)

articulation and acoustic signals. This model theorizes the probable feedback and feedforward mechanisms that may be in play in neural processing for speech production. Neurologic control of speech may well involve combinations of both open and closed loops in a multiple-pathway, hierarchic system that provides the necessary flexibility, speed, and precision to program and execute the everyday movements of speech with such complexity and ease.

SYNOPSIS OF CLINICAL INFORMATION AND APPLICATIONS FOR THE SLP

- The motor system has a hierarchy. It becomes progressively more sophisticated as the paths ascend and progressively less sophisticated as the paths descend.
- The lower levels of the motor system are partially constrained by the upper levels, but all have a certain autonomy.
- The levels of the motor system can be enumerated as Broca area and the motor association cortex areas, the corticospinal and corticonuclear tracts, the spinal cord and the brainstem nuclei (LMN), the basal nuclei, the cerebellum, and the extrapyramidal or indirect activation pathway tracts.
- Motor speech commands are organized in the premotor and SMA (motor association areas) and Broca area as well as the insula. AOS is the disorder associated with damage to the motor speech programming areas.
- The pyramidal system includes the corticospinal tract for motor control of limbs and the corticonuclear tract, which provides motor control for muscles of the face, tongue, pharynx, and larynx.
- The corticospinal tract is a primarily contralateral innervation system, with 90% of the fibers decussating at the level of the pyramids of the medulla and terminating in the opposite side of the spinal cord.
- The corticonuclear tract provides primarily bilateral innervation for the majority of the musculature innervated, with the decussation occurring at various levels of the brainstem. Although most of the nuclei receive both unilateral and contralateral fibers, the amount of unilateral versus contralateral innervation varies.
- UMNs are the first-order neurons in the corticospinal and corticonuclear tracts. The UMNs send axons to the nuclei of the spinal cord or the cranial nerves in the brainstem. They comprise the first fiber pathway of the direct activation pathway that is the pyramidal tract.
- LMNs are the second-order neurons in the direct activation pathway. They send axons out of the spinal cord or brainstem and become the peripheral nerves. Sherrington[28] called the LMN the final common pathway because it is the final route for all the complex motor activity occurring above the level of the LMNs.
- The motor unit is a useful concept when studying the LMNs. The motor unit consists of the cell body, axon (the nerve itself), junction of the nerve and muscle fiber (neuromuscular juncture), and muscle fiber.
- The facial nerve (cranial nerve VII) is unusual in that it has a dorsal and ventral component to its nucleus. The ventral portion, supplying the upper face, is far more bilaterally innervated than the dorsal part, which supplies the lower part of the face. The clinical implication of this is that a unilateral UMN lesion affecting this nerve results in paresis or paralysis of the opposite side of the lower face, whereas the upper half of the face is relatively unaffected because of its bilateral innervation.
- Lesions of the UMN tract produce different clinical symptoms than lesions of the LMN tract. The SLP must be able to recognize these signs. Damage to either of the two pathways produces different types of dysarthria as well.
- AMNs are the nerve cells that comprise the LMN. They are found in the anterior horn cells in the spinal cord and in the nuclei of the cranial nerves in the brainstem. They supply skeletal muscles through innervation of the extrafusal fibers of the muscles.
- The muscle spindle is present in many skeletal muscles and provides the sensory feedback to the muscle regarding length. This feedback results in the muscle stretch reflex. With the exception of the jaw-closing muscles, muscle spindles are few and scattered in the muscles concerned with speech and swallowing.
- The extrapyramidal system is composed of the descending indirect activation pathways (vestibulospinal, reticulospinal, rubrospinal, and tectospinal tracts). The reticular formation can also be included.
- The primary structures of the basal ganglia are the CN, GP, and putamen. The SN and STN are also included. Four different functional circuits seem to operate in the basal ganglia system: motor loop, limbic loop, cognitive loop, and oculomotor loop.
- Basal ganglia disease can cause movement disorders and associated dysarthrias. The dysarthria of Parkinson disease is an example of a hypokinetic dysarthria, and the motor speech disorder associated with Huntington chorea is an example of hyperkinetic dysarthria. Both result from damage to parts of the basal ganglia.
- The small hemispheres at the base of the brain are the lobes of the cerebellum. The cerebellum, like the basal ganglia, is a consultant to the motor system and provides coordination needed for smooth, synergistic movement. Signs of cerebellar damage include ataxia, nystagmus, dysmetria, dysdiadochokinesis, and sometimes an ataxic dysarthria.
- Speech motor control seems to be a product of both an open-loop and a closed-loop feedback system according to servomechanism theory. The open-loop system contains feedforward control, with the brain partially preprogramming movements that will be made to accomplish certain productions. The concept of speech motor control as a product of a closed-loop system has been generally accepted as the prime system controlling speech output, meaning that sensory monitoring from hearing, touch, and deep muscle sense guides production. Sufficient evidence exists that feedforward occurs, and both types of systems are probably in operation.

CASE STUDY

A 63-year-old man awoke in the early morning with disorientation, inability to speak, and inability to move his right side. He was admitted through the emergency department with a preliminary diagnosis of acute left hemisphere cerebrovascular accident (also known as a stroke). A computed tomography scan was done early to rule out hemorrhage but did not show a lesion site. He was put on blood-thinning medication and began to show some movement of the right lower extremity and some ability to speak, although speech was very hesitant, nonfluent, and difficult to understand. He was able to answer yes/no questions accurately and could read fairly well. Further testing during the next few days revealed difficulty following body movement commands involving facial and oral movements and found him "awkward and slow" in following commands involving movements of the left hand. He was diagnosed with a mild nonfluent aphasia with accompanying apraxia of speech, right hemiparesis, mild right facial weakness affecting the movement of the right side of the lips, and "clumsy hand syndrome" (sympathetic apraxia) on the left side. He was discharged to an acute rehabilitation center, where he participated in occupational therapy, physical therapy, and speech therapy. He did well in treatment. At discharge 3 weeks later, he was walking with a cane, and movement and use of the right arm had improved, providing some gross functional use. Speech was still effortful with simple sentence structure and was distorted though intelligible.

Questions for Consideration

1. Considering the right hemiparesis, mild nonfluent aphasia, apraxia of speech, and sympathetic apraxia, what are the likely structures damaged by this stroke?
2. What is meant by a "sympathetic apraxia"? (You will have to research this outside of this text.) How might this complicate the SLP's treatment plan for this patient?

REFERENCES

1. Alario, F.-X., Chainay, H., Lehericy, S., & Cohen, L. (2006). The role of the supplementary motor area (SMA) in word production. *Brain Research, 1076*(1), 129–143.
2. Booth, C. M., Cortina-Borja, M. J., & Theologis, T. N. (2001). Collagen accumulation in muscles of children with cerebral palsy and correlation with severity of spasticity. *Developmental Med Child Neurol, 43*(5), 314–320.
3. Bostan, A. C., Dum, R. P., & Strick, P. L. (2018). Functional anatomy of basal ganglia circuits with the cerebral cortex and the cerebellum. *Prog Neurological Surg, 33*, 50–61. https://doi.org/10.1159/000480748.
4. Chenausky, K., Paquette, S., Norton, A., & Schlaug, G. (2020). Apraxia of speech involves lesions of dorsal arcuate fasciculus and insula in patients with aphasia. *Neurol Clin Practice, 10*(2), 162–169. https://doi.org/10.1212/CPJ.0000000000000699.
5. Civier, O., Bullock, D., Max, L., & Guenther, F. H. (2013). Computational modeling of stuttering caused by impairments in a basal ganglia thalamo-cortical circuit involved in syllable selection and initiation. *Brain and Language, 126*(3), 263–278.
6. Cooper, S. (1953). Muscle spindles in the intrinsic muscles of the human tongue. *J Physiol, 122*, 193–202.
7. Cummine, J., Cribben, I., Luu, C., Kim, E., Bakhtiari, R., Georgiou, G., & Boliek, C. A. (2016). Understanding the role of speech production in reading: Evidence for a print-to-speech neural network using graphical analysis. *Neuropsychology, 30*(4), 385–397. https://doi.org/10.1037/neu0000236.
8. Davis, B. L., & MacNeilage, P. F. (2004). The frame/content theory of speech evolution: From lip smacks to syllables. *Primatologie, 6*, 305–328. https://www.researchgate.net/publication/251275645_The_framecontent_theory_of_speech_evolution_From_lip_smacks_to_syllables.
9. Dronkers, N. F., Plaisant, O., Iba-Zizen, M. T., & Cabanis, E. A. (2007). Paul Broca's historic cases: High resolution MR imaging of the brains of Leborgne and Lelong. *Brain, 130*(5), 1432–1441.
10. Duffy, J. R. (2005). *Motor speech disorders: Substrates, differential diagnosis, and management* (2nd ed.). Mosby: Elsevier.
11. Fazi, A., & Fleisher, J. (2018). Anatomy, physiology, and clinical syndromes of the basal ganglia: A brief review. *SemPediatric Neurol, 25*, 2–9. https://doi.org/10.1016/j.spen.2017.12.005.
12. Fenichel, G. M. (1993). *Clinical pediatric neurology: A signs and symptoms approach*. W. B. Saunders.
13. Graff-Radford, J., Jones, D. T., Strand, E. A., Rabinstein, A. A., Duffy, J. R., & Josephs, K. A. (2014). The neuroanatomy of pure apraxia of speech in stroke. *Brain Lang, 129*, 43–46. https://doi.org/10.1016/j.bandl.2014.01.004.
14. Guenther, F. H. (2006). Cortical interactions underlying the production of speech sounds. *J Commun Disord, 39*(5), 350–365.
15. Inoue, T. (2015). Neural mechanisms of mastication. *Brain and Nerve, 67*(2), 141–156. https://doi.org/10.11477/mf.1416200107.
16. Kent, R. (2004). The uniqueness of speech among motor systems. *Clin Linguist Phonetics, 18*(6–8), 495–505.
17. Knierim, J. (2020). Motor cortex. *Neuroscience Online*. https://nba.uth.tmc.edu/neuroscience/m/s3/chapter03.html#:~:text=The%20supplementary%20motor%20area%20.
18. Liss, J. M. (1990). Muscle spindles in the human levator veli palatini and palatoglossus muscles. *J Speech Hearing Res, 33*(4), 736–746.
19. MacNeilage, P. F. (1998). The frame/content theory of evolution of speech production. *Behav Brain Sci, 21*(4), 499–511.
20. MacNeilage, P. F., & Davis, B. L. (2001). Motor mechanisms in speech ontogeny: Phylogenetic, neurobiological and linguistic implications. *Current Opinion in Neurobiology, 11*(6), 696–700.
21. Price, C. J., Crinion, J. T., & MacSweeney, M. (2011). A generative model of speech production in Broca's and Wernicke's areas. *Front Psychol, 2*, 1–9.
22. Saigusa, H., Niimi, S., Yamashita, K., Gotoh, T., & Kumada, M. (2001). Morphological and histochemical studies of the genioglossus muscle. *Ann Otology, Rhinology Laryngology, 110*(8), 779–784.
23. Saigusa, H., Yamashita, K., Tanuma, K., Saigusa, M., & Niimi, S. (2004). Morphological studies for retrusive movement of the human adult tongue. *Clin Anat, 17*(2), 93–98.
24. Sasegbon, A., & Hamdy, S. (2021). The role of the cerebellum in swallowing. *Dysphagia* https://doi.org/10.1007/s00455-021-10271-x.

25. Saverino, D., De Santanna, A., Simone, R., Cervioni, S., Cattrysse, E., & Testa, M. (2014). Observational study on the occurrence of muscle spindles in human digastric and mylohyoideus muscles. *Biomed Res Int*, 294263. https://doi.org/10.1155/2014/294263.

26. Schenker, N. M., Hopkins, W. D., Spocter, M. A., Garrison, A. R., Stimpson, C. D., Erwin, J. M., Hof, P. R., & Sherwood, C. C. (2010). Broca's area homologue in chimpanzees (*Pan troglodytes*): Probabilistic mapping, asymmetry, and comparison to humans. *Cereb Cortex, 20*(3), 730–742. https://doi.org/10.1093/cercor/bhp138.

27. Sherrington, C. S. (1926). *The integrative action of the nervous system*. Yale University Press.

28. Shimizu, T., Hanajima, R., Shirota, Y., Tsutsumi, R., Tanaka, N., Terao, Y., Hamada, M., & Ugawa, Y. (2020). Plasticity induction in the pre-supplementary motor area (pre-SMA) and SMA-proper differentially affects visuomotor sequence learning. *Brain Stimulation, 13*(1), 229–238. https://doi.org/10.1016/j.brs.2019.08.001.

29. Yip, D.W., & Lui, F. (2022). *Physiology, motor cortical*. StatPearls Publishing. PMID 31194345.

7

The Cranial Nerves

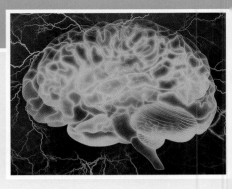

To those I address, it is unnecessary to go further than to indicate that the nerves treated in these papers are the instruments of expression from the smile of the infant's cheek to the last agony of life.
Charles Bell, 1824

CHAPTER OUTLINE

KEY TERMS

abducens	flaccid	primary olfactory cortex
abduction	genioglossus	ptosis
branchial	glottal coup	secretomotor
central pattern generator	hyoglossus	solely special sensory
chorda tympani	internuncial	styloglossus
cranial nerves	lacrimal	tinnitus
diplopia	palpate	

This chapter is intended to help the speech-language pathologist (SLP) understand one of the most important components of the nervous system in regard to the acts of hearing, speaking, and swallowing. The **cranial nerves** comprise a part of the peripheral nervous system that provides crucial sensory and motor information for the oral, pharyngeal, and laryngeal musculature and the auditory and vestibular systems. The SLP should be familiar with the names, structure, innervation, testing procedures, and signs of abnormal function of the cranial nerves. This information is especially critical when working with an adult or child with dysarthria and/or dysphagia.

ORIGIN OF THE CRANIAL NERVES

Names and Numbers

Twelve pairs of cranial nerves leave the brain and pass through the foramina of the skull. They are referred to by their numbers, which by convention are written in Roman numerals, as well as by their names. The names sometimes give a clue to the function of the nerves, but the number, name, and concise descriptions of the various functions should all be learned (Table 7.1). Many students use a suggested mnemonic device to help them remember the cranial nerves (e.g., "**O**n **O**ld **O**lympus' **T**owering **T**op **A** **F**inn

TABLE 7.1   The Cranial Nerves

Number	Name	Summary of Function
I	Olfactory	Smell
II	Optic	Vision
III	Oculomotor	Innervation of muscles to move eyeball, pupil, and upper lid
IV	Trochlear	Innervation of superior oblique muscle of eye
V	Trigeminal	Chewing and sensation to face, teeth, anterior tongue
VI	Abducens	Abduction of eye
VII	Facial	Movement of facial muscles, taste, salivary glands
VIII	(Vestibular) acoustic	Equilibrium and hearing
IX	Glossopharyngeal	Taste, swallowing, elevation of pharynx and larynx, parotid salivary gland, sensation to posterior tongue, upper pharynx
X	Vagus	Taste, swallowing, elevation of palate, phonation, parasympathetic outflow to visceral organs
XI	Accessory	Turning of head and shrugging of shoulders
XII	Hypoglossal	Movement of tongue

And German Vend At Hops") or create their own, maybe more interesting, mnemonic to aid their memory. In addition to a mnemonic for the name of the cranial nerves, it is helpful to have a separate aid to remember the function of each nerve. In the following example, **S** stands for "sensory," **M** for "motor," and **B** for "both sensory and motor": Some Say Money Matters But My Brother Says Big Brains Matter More. This example of a memory aid then helps remind us that the first two cranial nerves are sensory, the second two are motor, and so on.

Embryologic Origin

As you will learn in Chapter 11, the body develops in the embryo from transverse segments as well as from longitudinal tubes. The viscera, including the neuraxis, are developed from the elaboration, or diverticulation, of the hollow longitudinal tubes. The transverse segments are of two types: somites and arches. Somites eventually give rise to muscle, bone, and connective tissue of the body wall. The arches are the branchial or pharyngeal arches, and these give rise to structures of the face and neck.

The nuclei of the cranial nerves are of three different types. The motor nuclei are distinguished by the embryologic origin of the muscles they innervate. In the development of the embryo, the branchial (gill) arches are responsible for the structure, muscles, and nerves of the face and neck. Cranial nerves V, VII, IX, X, and XI are thus known as the **branchial** set. Cranial nerves III, IV, VI, and XII are derived from this somatic segmentation and thus are called the somatomotor, or somitic, set. The elaboration of the longitudinal tubes gives rise to three cranial nerves (I, II, and VIII) known as the **solely special sensory** set.

Some branchial and somitic cranial nerves have a visceral component: III, VII, IX, and X. Cranial nerves V, VII, IX, and X also have a general sensory component (i.e., they participate in sensation of pain, pressure touch, vibration, and proprioception).

The Corticonuclear Tract and the Cranial Nerves

The cranial nerves themselves are part of the peripheral nervous system and consist of efferent motor fibers that arise from nuclei in the brainstem and afferent sensory fibers that originate in the peripheral ganglia. The motor nuclei of the cranial nerves receive impulses from the cerebral cortex through the corticonuclear tracts. The tracts begin in the upper motor neurons found as pyramidal cells in the inferior part of the **precentral** gyrus and in the adjacent part of the postcentral gyrus. The tracts then follow the path illustrated in Fig. 6.2. They descend through the corona radiata and the genu of the internal capsule and then pass through the midbrain in the cerebral peduncles. They then synapse either with the lower motor neuron directly or indirectly through **internuncial** neurons, a chain of neurons situated between the primary efferent neuron and the final motor neuron.

The majority of the corticonuclear fibers to the motor cranial nerve nuclei cross the midline, or decussate, before reaching the nuclei. All the cranial nerve motor nuclei have bilateral innervation except for portions of the trigeminal, facial, and hypoglossal fibers, which are discussed later.

The motor fibers of the cranial nerves are formed by axons of nerve cells within the brain, but the sensory, or afferent, fibers of the cranial nerves are formed from processes of nerve cells found outside the brain. These sensory nerve cells are usually found in clumps of nerve cells called peripheral ganglia. They are situated on the nerve trunks or in the sensory organ itself (e.g., the nose, ear, or eye). The central processes of these cells enter the brain and terminate by synapsing with cells grouped together to form the nuclei of termination. These cells have axons that cross the midline and ascend and synapse on other sensory nuclei, such as in the thalamus. The axons of the resulting cells then terminate in the cerebral cortex.

CRANIAL NERVES FOR SMELL AND VISION

Cranial nerve I, the olfactory nerve, is a plexus of thin fibers that unite in ~20 small bundles called fila olfactoria. The olfactory receptors are situated in the mucous membrane of the nasal cavity. The nerve fibers synapse with other cells in the olfactory bulb and finally end in the olfactory areas of the cerebral cortex, the periamygdaloid and prepiriform areas. Together these are known as the **primary olfactory cortex**. They also send fibers to many other centers within the brain to establish connections for automatic and emotional responses to olfactory stimulation.

Cranial nerves II, III, IV, and VI are concerned with vision. The optic nerve (II) is the primary nerve of sight. Its nerve fibers are axons that come from the retina, converge on the optic disk, and exit from the eye on both sides. The right nerve joins the left to form the optic chiasma. In the optic chiasma, fibers from the nasal half of the eye cross the midline, and fibers from the temporal half continue to run ipsilaterally. Most of the fibers synapse with nerve cells in the lateral geniculate body of the thalamus and then leave it, forming optic radiations. The optic radiations formed by these fibers terminate in the visual cortex and the visual association cortex.

Cranial nerve III is the oculomotor nerve, the nucleus of which is located at the level of the superior colliculus. Cranial nerve III has a somatomotor component that innervates the extraocular muscles to move the eyeball and a visceral component responsible for pupil constriction. Dysfunction of the third cranial nerve causes **ptosis** (drooping) of the eyelid. The eye may also be in **abduction** and turned down. If the visceral component is impaired, the pupillary reflex is lost and the pupil is dilated. Fig. 7.1A illustrates a complete paralysis of the left oculomotor nerve.

Cranial nerve IV is the trochlear nerve, the nucleus of which is at the level of the inferior colliculus. This nerve innervates the superior oblique muscle, which is primarily responsible for intorsion of the eyeball, helping to maintain its position toward the midline of the face. Confirmed lesions cause **diplopia** (double vision).

Cranial nerve VI, the **abducens**, has its nucleus on the floor of the fourth ventricle. Dysfunction prevents lateral movements of the eyeball. Fig. 7.1B shows a complete paralysis of the left cranial nerve VI.

The remaining seven cranial nerves are vital for the production of normal speech and thus are given more attention, focusing on the pathway, structures innervated, functional purpose, signs of dysfunction, and testing procedure for each nerve. Learn them one by one. Test yourself on them until you are firmly acquainted with each nerve. Review Fig. 3.2 for attachment sites of the cranial nerves to the brainstem.

CRANIAL NERVES FOR SPEECH AND HEARING

Cranial Nerve V: Trigeminal
Anatomy

Both the motor and sensory roots of the trigeminal nerve are attached to the lateral edges of the pons. The motor nuclei are restricted to the pons, but the sensory nuclei extend from the mesencephalon to the spinal cord.

Innervation

The motor part of the trigeminal nerve innervates the following muscles: masseter, temporalis, lateral and medial pterygoids, tensor tympani, tensor veli palatini, mylohyoid, and the anterior belly of the digastric muscle. The sensory fibers have three main branches:

1. The ophthalmic nerve, which is sensory to the forehead, eyes, and nose
2. The maxillary nerve, which is sensory to the upper lip mucosa, maxilla, upper teeth, cheeks, palate, and maxillary sinus
3. The mandibular nerve, which is sensory to the anterior two-thirds of the tongue, mandible, lower teeth, lower lip, part of the cheek, and part of the external ear

Fig. 7.2 shows a sensory map of the trigeminal nerve supply to the areas of the face and oral structures.

Function

Cranial nerve V is primarily responsible for mastication and for sensation to the face, teeth, gums, and anterior two-thirds of the tongue for general sensation (e.g., temperature and texture). Innervating the tensor velar palatini, cranial nerve V is partially responsible for flattening and tensing the soft palate and for opening the eustachian tube. Innervating an extrinsic laryngeal muscle (the anterior belly of the digastric), it also assists in the upward and anterior movement of the larynx. Innervating the mylohyoid and part of the digastric, this nerve contributes to retraction of the tongue. Also innervated by CN V, the tensor tympani in the middle ear works with the stapedius muscle to dampen oscillation of the eardrum in the presence of loud noise.

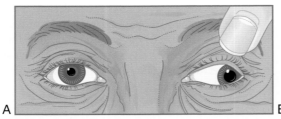
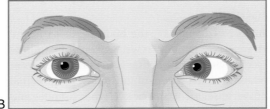

Fig. 7.1 (A) Complete left III (oculomotor) nerve paralysis with a fully abducted eye, which is also depressed. The pupil of the eye is nonreactive and fully dilated. The ptosis of the left eye requires the examiner to lift the lid to examine movement. (B) Complete left VI (abducens) nerve paralysis showing a fully adducted eye resulting from the unopposed pull of the medial rectus. (Reprinted from FitzGerald, M. J. T., & Folan-Curran, J. [2002]. *Clinical neuroanatomy and related neuroscience* [4th ed.]. Saunders/Elsevier.)

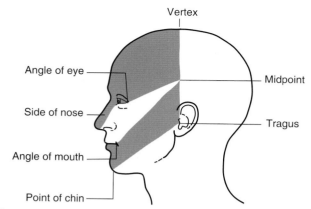

Fig. 7.2 Trigeminal nerve sensory map. (Reprinted from FitzGerald, M. J. T., & Folan-Curran, J. [2002]. *Clinical neuroanatomy and related neuroscience* [4th ed.]. Saunders/Elsevier.)

Testing

The jaw-closing and grinding lateral movements of chewing are the result of the function of the masseter and temporal, medial pterygoid, and lateral pterygoid muscles. The first three contribute to closure of the jaw, but only the masseter can be directly tested. To evaluate the masseter, **palpate** the area of the muscle (2 cm above and in front of the angle of the mandible) as you bite down firmly and then relax. During the bite, the bulk of the muscle can be felt. Try this to become familiar with the masseter. The muscle body should feel firm and bulky. The temporal muscle cannot be well palpated; however, if it is atrophied (shrunken) from a lower motor neuron lesion, the temple of the face will be sunken.

The strength of jaw closure should also be evaluated. To do so, place your hand on the tip of the patient's mandible as the jaw is held open. Place the other hand on the forehead to prevent neck extension. Ask the patient to bite down hard against the resistance of your hand. The patient should be able to close the jaw against a moderate resistance.

The lateral pterygoids enable the jaw to lateralize in chewing. To evaluate these muscles, ask the patient to open the jaw against resistance of your hand and note how the tip of the mandible lines up with the space between the upper medial incisors. Ask the patient to move the jaw from side to side and observe the facility of movement.

Finally, ask the patient to lateralize the jaw against resistance. Have the patient move the jaw to one side and hold it while you gently try to push it toward the center. Place your other hand against the opposite cheekbone so the patient cannot use the neck muscles to help.

The patient with a unilateral paralysis of cranial nerve V may show a deviation of the jaw to the side of the lesion and an inability to force the jaw to the side opposite the lesion. Atrophy may also be noted after a period. These problems result from lower motor neuron lesions. Upper motor neuron lesions that are unilateral do not affect cranial nerves as much because the nuclei receive so many axons from the other hemisphere. Therefore, the paresis is usually transitory or mild unless bilateral upper motor neuron lesions are present.

Bilateral upper motor neuron lesions result in an observable limitation of jaw movements. Opening and closing movements of the jaw, though possible, are restricted. Gross chewing movements are seen, but chewing and biting may lack vigor and are performed slowly.

To evaluate the sensory component of the trigeminal nerve, sensation to the face may be tested. The patient is asked to close the eyes, and a cotton swab is used to stroke the face in the three different distribution areas of the nerve. The examiner should stay in the central part of the face because, as shown in Fig. 7.2, considerable overlap exists on the periphery. The ophthalmic division may therefore be tested by stroking above the eyebrows; the maxillary division tested by stroking the upper lip in an upward movement toward the cheekbone; and the mandibular division tested by stroking between the lower lip and the chin in an upward movement toward the cheekbone. Left and right sides should be done separately and compared. Stroking should be done with firm pressure and kept consistent across all trials.

Sensation to the anterior two-thirds of the tongue may also be tested during the examination, especially if chewing and swallowing are of concern. The two sides of the tongue may be compared for sensitivity to the touch of a cotton-tip swab on the anterior as well as medial portion of the tongue.

Cranial Nerve VII: Facial

Anatomy

The facial nerve is a complex nerve carrying two motor and two sensory components. It involves several different nuclei, all within the pons near the reticular formation.

The special sensory component of the facial nerve involves the taste fibers (known as gustatory sensation) for the tongue and palate. These fibers have their primary sensory neurons in the geniculate ganglion. They enter the brainstem in the sensory root of the facial nerve, called the nervus intermedius. They run in a bundle, or fasciculus, called the tractus solitarius and are joined in that bundle by the taste fibers from cranial nerves IX and X.

The gustatory fibers split off from the facial nerve in the middle ear as the **chorda tympani**. This joins the lingual branch of cranial nerve V. These fibers then terminate in the nucleus of the tractus solitarius and are then distributed to the taste buds of the anterior two-thirds of the tongue. Some fibers also terminate in the taste buds in the hard and soft palates. Ascending fibers from the nucleus solitarius run to the ventroposterior thalamus and then project to the cortical area for taste located at the lower end of the postcentral gyrus in the parietal lobe.

The general sensory component of VII is a small cutaneous component whose nerve cells are found in the geniculate ganglion in the temporal bone. Impulses travel in the nervus intermedius, descending in the spinal tract of the trigeminal nerve and synapsing in the spinal nucleus of the trigeminal nerve located in the upper medulla. This sensory component may supplement the mandibular portion of cranial nerve V, providing sensation from the wall of the acoustic meatus and the surface of the tympanic membrane.

The visceral motor component of cranial nerve VII is composed of cell bodies that are preganglionic autonomic motor neurons. These cell bodies are collectively called the superior salivatory nucleus and the lacrimal nucleus. The fibers from the nucleus travel in the nervus intermedius and divide in the facial canal, becoming the greater petrosal nerve and the chorda tympani. The petrosal nerve fibers follow a complicated path and join fibers of the trigeminal to reach the lacrimal and mucosal glands of the nasal and oral cavities, where they stimulate secretion.

The branchial motor component of the facial nerve is of critical importance to the SLP. The fibers of the motor nucleus extend to the floor of the ventricle, curve around the nucleus of the abducens (cranial nerve VI), and exit the brainstem near the inferior margin of the pons. These fibers then join those from the nucleus of the tractus solitarius and the autonomic or parasympathetic nuclei and enter the internal auditory meatus as they extend through the facial canal of the petrosal bone. They leave the skull through the stylomastoid foramen. While coursing through the facial canal, the facial nerve travels through the tympanic cavity, innervating the stapedius muscle. The facial nerve can therefore be involved in pathologic conditions related to the ear as well as the oral musculature. Surgeons removing acoustic tumors must be mindful of the location of the facial nerve.

The dorsal motor nucleus of cranial nerve VII innervates the lower part of the face and receives most of its corticonuclear fibers from the opposite hemisphere; thus innervation to these structures is primarily contralateral. The ventral motor nucleus that supplies the upper part of the face receives fibers from both cerebral hemispheres (i.e., receives crossed and uncrossed fibers), and innervation is bilateral.

Innervation

The parasympathetic nuclei are also known as the superior salivatory and the lacrimal nuclei. The superior salivatory nucleus receives afferent information from the hypothalamus and olfactory system as well as taste information from the mouth cavity. It supplies the sublingual salivary glands and the nasal and palatine glands.

The lacrimal nucleus solitarius receives information from afferent fibers from the trigeminal sensory nuclei for reflex response to corneal irritation. The sensory nucleus receives information concerning taste from fibers from the anterior two-thirds of the tongue, the floor of the mouth, and the soft and hard palates.

The motor nucleus gives the face expression by innervation of the various facial muscles (i.e., the orbicularis oculi, zygomatic, buccinator, orbicularis oris, and labial muscles). Other muscles innervated are the platysma, stylohyoid, and stapedius and the posterior belly of the digastric.

Function

Most important to the SLP is that the facial nerve is responsible for all movements of facial expression. All facial apertures are guarded by muscles innervated by the facial nerve: the eyes, nose, mouth, and external auditory canal. Cranial nerve VII enables the actions of wrinkling the forehead, closing the eyes tightly, closing the lips tightly, pulling back the corners of the lips, pulling down the corners of the lips, and tensing the anterior neck muscles.

Beyond these important movements in speech and swallowing, the facial nerve also helps pull the larynx up and back (through the belly of the digastric muscle). It provides motor innervation to the sublingual and submaxillary salivary glands, and it guards the middle ear by innervating the stapedius muscle, which, with the tensor tympani muscle, dampens excessive movement of the ossicles in the presence of a loud noise. Finally, the facial nerve is partially responsible for taste.

Testing

Tests of facial expression are the primary tests in the oral-motor examination for cranial nerve VII. Before any motor testing, however, the patient's face at rest should be visually inspected, especially noting the symmetry. Then begin movement testing at the upper part of the face, focusing first on the forehead, then the eyes, and finally the mouth. Box 7.1 outlines what to observe and note before commencing with speech testing.

The patient with a lower motor neuron lesion of cranial nerve VII has involvement of the entire side of the face on the side of the lesion (ipsilateral). Fig. 7.3 is an example of unilateral facial paralysis. Although speech may be distorted,

---

BOX 7.1   Facial Assessment

Forehead
Ask the patient to wrinkle the forehead and look up at the ceiling. Note the symmetry of the wrinkling on both sides. Keep in mind that this ability or inability is diagnostic for localization. Because the upper part of the face is innervated bilaterally, only a lower motor neuron lesion would cause complete paralysis of this function. An upper motor neuron lesion causes some weakness on the opposite side, but it will not be nearly as perceptible because of the ipsilateral fiber innervation.

Eyes
Ask the patient to close the eyes as tightly as possible. Note the contraction of the orbicularis oculi and the consequent wrinkling around the eyes. Bilateral innervation is also present in this part of the face, although not to the degree that the forehead displays. The lower motor neuron-upper motor neuron difference holds true for dysfunction of this part of the face.

Mouth
Take a close look at mouth movements. First ask the patient to smile or pull back the corners of the lips. It helps to tell the patient to show the teeth when doing this, exaggerating the smile somewhat. Again, observe the symmetry of the two sides. Then ask the patient to pucker the lips; observe the symmetry of constriction. Finally, ask the patient to pull down the corners of the lips (as in pouting) or try to wrinkle the skin of the neck. Inspect for symmetry. Also test for the strength of movement against resistance and compare the two sides of the mouth.

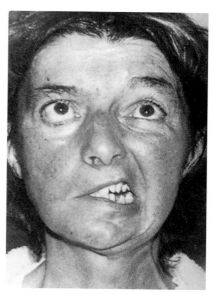

Fig. 7.3 Patient with complete facial nerve paralysis on the right side. The patient was asked to show her teeth and look up at the ceiling. Note the inability to raise the eyebrow, drooping of the lower eyelid, inability to retract the mouth, and lack of webbing on the neck (effect on the platysma muscle). This patient also was unable to abduct the eye because of involvement of the abducens. The patient was found to have demyelination affecting the facial nerve and abducens nerve, resulting from multiple sclerosis. (From Parsons, M. [1986]. *Diagnostic picture test in clinical neurology.* Wolfe Medical.)

it is usually not significantly hindered by peripheral involvement of cranial nerve VII. The patient with an upper motor neuron lesion shows complete involvement of the contralateral lip and neck muscles, some degree of involvement of the area around the eyes, and little difficulty with the forehead or frontalis muscle. It should be noted that the paralysis occurs on voluntary movement. The patient may have almost normal movement for emotionally initiated movements, such as a true smile, but be unable to lateralize the lips on the affected side when asked to do so voluntarily.

Because the facial nerve innervates the stapedius muscle, it may be paralyzed by a lesion. If this occurs, the patient may report that ordinary sounds seem uncomfortably loud.

The sensory component of the facial nerve may be assessed by testing the patient's sense of taste on the anterior two-thirds of the tongue. Sensitivity of the two sides of the tongue should be compared. The patient should be able to identify the four primary tastes (salty, sour, bitter, and sweet) if the sensory pathways are intact.

Cranial Nerve VIII: Acoustic-Vestibular or Vestibulocochlear

The following explanation assumes the reader has studied the anatomy of the ear and is well versed in the structure and function of the cochlea and semicircular canals. A good working knowledge of the anatomy of the ear is imperative; review of the information provided in Chapter 5 on the auditory system is suggested.

Anatomy

As can be ascertained from its name, the acoustic-vestibular, or vestibulocochlear, nerve consists of two distinct parts: the vestibular nerve and the cochlear, or acoustic, nerve. Both take afferent information from the internal ear to the nervous system, but as their names imply, they carry different types of information.

The vestibular nerve consists of nerve cells and their fibers, which are located in Scarpa ganglion located in the internal acoustic meatus. The fibers enter the brainstem in a groove between the lower border of the pons and the upper medulla oblongata in a sulcus called the cerebellopontine angle. This location is the site of one of the most common brain tumors, a vestibular schwannoma, also known as an acoustic neuroma. A few of the axons terminate in the flocculonodular lobe of the cerebellum. Most axons enter the vestibular nuclear complex, which consists of a group of nuclei located in the floor of the fourth ventricle.

The cochlear nerve consists of nerve cells and fibers located in the spiral ganglion around the modiolus of the cochlea. Nerve fibers wrap around each other in the modiolus, with a layering effect. Fibers from the apex, carrying low-frequency information, are found on the innermost part of the core, whereas fibers from the basal part of the cochlea, carrying high-frequency information, are found on the outermost layers. The nerve fibers from these cell bodies enter the brainstem at the lower border of the pons on the lateral side of the facial nerve. They are separated from the facial nerve fibers by the vestibular nerve. Fig. 7.4 illustrates the relation of cranial nerve VIII to the inner ear.

When the cochlear fibers enter the pons, they divide into two branches. One branch enters the dorsal cochlear nucleus (high frequencies), and the other enters the ventral cochlear nucleus (low frequencies). Both nuclei are situated adjacent to the inferior cerebral peduncle.

From this point the axons take varied and complex paths. The system is largely contralateral. Most fibers decussate after the cochlear nuclei, although there are a few ipsilaterally projected fibers. The fibers form a tract called the lateral lemniscus as they ascend through the posterior portion of the pons and midbrain. All ascending fibers terminate in the medial geniculate body and from there project to the auditory cortex by way of the auditory radiations. Between the cochlear nuclei and the medial geniculate body, the fibers take one of several pathways, including synapses at one or more of the following structures: the superior olives, the trapezoid body, the inferior colliculus, and the nucleus of the lateral lemniscus.

Innervation

Both portions of the vestibulocochlear nerve are primarily sensory in nature. The vestibular nerve receives afferent information from the utricle, saccule, and semicircular canal of the inner ear and from the cerebellum. The vestibular nerve also sends out efferent fibers that pass to the cerebellum through the inferior cerebellar peduncles and to the spinal cord, forming the vestibulospinal tract. Efferent fibers are also sent to the

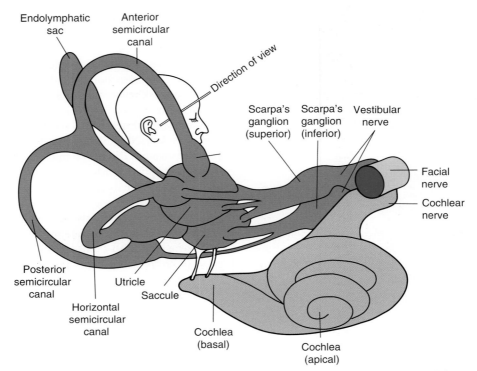

Fig. 7.4 Relation of the vestibular, cochlear, and facial nerve to the inner ear. (Reprinted from Nadeau, S. E., Ferguson, T. S., Valenstein, E., Vierck, C. J., Petruska, J. C., Streit, W. J., & Ritz, L. A. [2004]. *Medical neuroscience.* Saunders/Elsevier.)

nuclei of cranial nerves III (oculomotor), IV (trochlear), and VI (abducens) through the medial longitudinal fasciculus. As previously outlined, the cochlear nerve carries afferent fibers from the cochlea to the auditory cortex.

Function

Cranial nerve VIII takes afferent information from the internal ear to the nervous system. It is responsible for sound sensitivity and innervates the utricle and the saccule of the inner ear, which are sensitive to static changes in equilibrium. In addition, innervation of the semicircular canals takes place through this nerve, controlling sensitivity to dynamic changes in equilibrium.

Testing

Although the SLP may perform hearing threshold screening or testing that may provide information about the cochlear nerve, the audiologist usually is responsible for thorough assessment of hearing and cochlear function. Neurologists often perform simple tuning fork tests for acuity and sound lateralization, and some prefer to use whispered words.

Testing the vestibular function is also not in the purview of the SLP. Vestibular function usually is investigated with caloric tests that involve raising or lowering the temperature of the internal auditory meatus, thereby inducing current in the semicircular canals and stimulating the vestibular nerve for testing. Neurologists also use maneuvers of changing head position. Dynamic platform posturography is a technique developed in recent years to perform a functional assessment of how senses are used for balance.

The patient reporting reduced hearing acuity, **tinnitus** (ringing in the ears), or dizziness should always be seen by an otologist and receive an audiologic evaluation. The dizzy patient may be referred to a neurologist or a neurotologist, who typically will also refer for extensive audiologic and vestibular testing.

Cranial Nerve IX: Glossopharyngeal
Anatomy

The glossopharyngeal nerve carries two motor components and three sensory components. It can be found emerging from the medulla between the olive and the inferior cerebellar peduncle. The main trunk of the nerve exits the skull through the jugular foramen. Three nuclei in the brainstem are concerned with the functions of the glossopharyngeal nerve: the nucleus ambiguus, the inferior salivatory nucleus, and the nucleus solitarius.

Innervation

The nucleus ambiguus receives corticonuclear fibers of cranial nerve IX from both hemispheres and supplies the efferent innervation to the stylopharyngeus muscle, which contributes to the elevation of the pharynx and larynx. The inferior salivatory nucleus receives afferent information concerning taste from the hypothalamus, olfactory system, and mouth cavity. Efferent fibers supply the otic ganglion of the ear and the parotid salivary gland. The nucleus solitarius receives fibers arising from the inferior ganglia. Peripherally, these visceral afferent fibers of cranial nerve IX mediate general sensation to the pharynx, soft palate, posterior third of the tongue, fauces, tonsils, ear canal, and tympanic cavity. The fibers decussate and travel upward to the opposite thalamic and some hypothalamic nuclei. From here the axons pass through the internal capsule and carry this sensory information to termination points in the lower postcentral gyrus.

Function

Cranial nerve IX is efferent to one muscle only—the stylopharyngeus. This muscle dilates the pharynx laterally and contributes to the elevation of the pharynx and larynx. It thereby serves to help clear the pharynx and larynx for swallowing. **Secretomotor** fibers are efferent fibers provided for the parotid gland's production of saliva. Sensory fibers carry taste information from the posterior third of the tongue. The glossopharyngeal nerve mediates the sensory portion of the palatal and pharyngeal gag. Cranial nerve IX also carries sensory information to the faucial pillars and posterior section of the tongue. This sensory input is responsible for triggering the swallow response.

Testing

Most functions of cranial nerve IX cannot be tested separately from those of cranial nerve X because the vagus has predominant control over laryngeal and pharyngeal sensory and motor function. However, testing the sensory portion of the pharyngeal gag provides information about the integrity of cranial nerve IX. Testing the pharyngeal gag is not easily done in most people because getting so far back in the oral cavity without touching any other structure is difficult. To do the testing, the examiner should use a cotton-tipped applicator with a long wooden end (as used in medical clinics). The examiner carefully puts the cotton tip back against one side of the posterior pharyngeal wall, avoiding any contact with the base of the tongue or the velum. With a gentle poking of the wall, a gag should be elicited. Both sides of the pharynx should be tested.

If stimulation procedure (poking in correct spots) appears to be adequate but pharyngeal gag cannot be elicited, the examiner should ask whether the patient feels the pressure of the touch. If the stimulus is felt and no gag occurs, only the motor portion of the gag (mediated by the vagus) may be impaired. This situation is rare. Because sensation precedes motor activity, the absence of sensation and the gag implicates cranial nerve IX and gives the clinician information about the integrity of sensation to the upper pharynx, which can be important information in swallowing assessment.

Cranial Nerve X: Vagus
Anatomy

Like the glossopharyngeal nerve, the vagus nerve also has three associated nuclei: the nucleus ambiguus, the dorsal nucleus, and the nucleus solitarius, also located in the medulla. Axons from vagal cell bodies in the nucleus ambiguus have two major branches: a pharyngeal branch and a laryngeal branch. The laryngeal branch will branch again into the recurrent laryngeal nerve and the superior laryngeal nerve. The superior laryngeal nerve further splits into two branches, the internal laryngeal and the external laryngeal.

The recurrent laryngeal nerve does not divide again. It arises considerably below the larynx and ascends to terminate at the larynx. The right recurrent nerve runs in a loop behind the common carotid and subclavian arteries. The left recurrent nerve is longer, leaving the main laryngeal branch of the vagus at a lower level than does the right. The left recurrent loops under and behind the aortic arch. It then ascends to the larynx in a groove between the trachea and esophagus and enters through the cricothyroid membrane. Damage to the recurrent laryngeal nerve sometimes occurs during surgery, especially heart and thyroid surgery. Following the path of the branching, one can see how this nerve would be vulnerable because of the location within the neck and in the chest cavity.

Innervation

The nucleus ambiguus receives an approximately equal number of corticonuclear fibers of cranial nerve X from both hemispheres; these fibers are efferent to the constrictor muscles of the pharynx and the intrinsic muscles of the larynx. The efferent fibers of the dorsal or parasympathetic nucleus are associated with autonomic functions and innervate the involuntary muscles of the bronchi, esophagus, heart, stomach, small intestine, and a portion of the large intestine. The afferent fibers from the nucleus of the tractus solitarius follow much the same path as those of the glossopharyngeal nerve and terminate in the postcentral gyrus.

Function

Vagus means "wanderer," an apt name considering the many functions of the vagus nerve. It is motor to the viscera (heart, respiratory system, and most of the digestive system). It supplies primary efferent innervation to the palatal muscles (except for innervation of the tensor palatini by the trigeminal nerve). The vagus is also the primary efferent for the pharyngeal constrictors. On its own, the vagus innervates all of the intrinsic muscles of the larynx, primarily through the recurrent laryngeal branch. The cricothyroid, however, is innervated by the external laryngeal branch of the superior laryngeal nerve. This can be an important difference to remember during clinical examinations for speech or swallowing.

The vagus has both a visceral and a general sensory component in its afferent pathways. The visceral component carries visceral sensation that is not appreciated at a conscious level. Sensory information from the mucous membranes of the epiglottis, base of the tongue, aryepiglottic folds, and the majority of the larynx is carried in the internal laryngeal branch of the superior laryngeal nerve. Visceral sensation from below the larynx is carried in the recurrent laryngeal nerve.

General sensation (pain, temperature, and touch) from the larynx, pharynx, skin of the external ear, and the external auditory canal is carried in the vagus as well. From the vocal folds and below the larynx, general sensation is carried in the recurrent laryngeal nerve. From above the vocal folds, sensation travels in the internal laryngeal division of the superior laryngeal nerve. Damage to one or both of these sensory components of these nerves could result in silent aspiration (aspiration with no reflexive cough) because of the decreased sensory input. The sensory information would normally cause the cough reflex to trigger or cause a tickle in the throat or airway, indicating that something foreign is on the membranes and needs to be coughed out.

Testing

Remember that evaluation of palatal function involves testing both cranial nerves IX and X. Palatal function is controlled primarily by cranial nerve X, with the tensor veli palatini innervated by V. Intrinsic laryngeal muscle function is covered solely by cranial nerve X.

Palatal function is tested by first observing the palate at rest as the patient opens the mouth to allow viewing. Look at the palatal arches and observe their symmetry. Note if one arch hangs lower than the other. Next ask the patient to phonate "ah" and observe. The soft palate should elevate and move posteriorly and symmetrically. If the palate does not elevate, the palatal gag reflex, primarily innervated by cranial nerve IX, should be tested by touching the tongue blade against the palatal arches or against the base of the tongue. The gag is a reflex activity, and it is preserved in an upper motor neuron lesion because the reflex arc is still intact. As in all reflexes, it may be lost acutely after an upper motor neuron lesion; then it may become hyperactive. If both volitional and reflex activities of the palate are diminished, a lower motor neuron lesion is evidenced. Bear in mind that palatal elevation is also reduced by a cleft palate, congenital oral malformations, and soft tissue palatal lesions. Do not overlook these vital facts in vigorously searching for an upper or lower motor neuron lesion.

Laryngeal function evaluation is adequately completed only by direct or indirect laryngoscopy in which the vocal cords can be seen. A finer analysis of vocal cord movement patterns can be done by using laryngeal stroboscopy. Damage to the vagus nerve may cause paralysis or paresis of the vocal cord. Innervation is bilateral to the larynx, with the crossed and uncrossed fibers being approximately equal. Therefore, complete paralysis of a vocal cord from an upper motor neuron lesion is rare.

Preliminary assessment of laryngeal function is performed by traditional clinical voice evaluation procedures. The patient is asked to phonate and prolong a vowel such as /a/. Maximum phonation time varies for normal adults. If the patient can phonate for a 7- to 8-second duration, laryngeal and respiratory control is presumed acceptable. Perceptual analysis of the voice is done by the clinician during this phonation and during conversation. The patient may be asked to demonstrate laryngeal function and control by raising and lowering the pitch of a prolonged vowel or singing up and down the scale. Remember that the ability to change pitch depends on proper function of the cricothyroid muscle, which is innervated by the superior laryngeal nerve rather than the recurrent nerve. Estimate of the strength of laryngeal closure can be made perceptually by asking the patient to perform the **glottal coup**, which is essentially to make a short, sharp grunting sound. A voluntary (as opposed to reflexive) cough should also be requested. The clinician listens for the sound made at the larynx in these two maneuvers to be strong and sharp. Stress testing of the vocal mechanism is done by asking the patient to count to 300 or to keep talking for a prescribed length of time. More sophisticated analyses of the voice may be performed with instrumentation for acoustic analysis.

In cases of spastic dysarthria from an upper motor neuron lesion, a rough, harsh quality is heard on phonation. In bilateral upper motor neuron lesions (pseudobulbar palsy), a characteristic voice quality is heard, characterized by what Darley et al.,[3] describe as "strain-strangle." This voice is harsh, with a strained, tense quality as if the person is fighting to push the air flow through the larynx and supralaryngeal areas.

A lower motor neuron lesion causes complete paralysis of the ipsilateral vocal cord, resulting in a hoarse, breathy voice. In some lower motor neuron diseases, the voice will initially be strong; however, after the patient talks for a while, the voice becomes progressively weaker and more breathy. Hoarseness sometimes results from direct damage to the recurrent laryngeal nerve during carotid artery or thyroid surgery. The hoarseness is transient unless the nerve was severed.

Cranial Nerve XI: Spinal Accessory

Anatomy

The spinal accessory nerve consists of a cranial and a spinal root. The nucleus of the cranial root is found in the nucleus ambiguus of the medulla. It receives corticonuclear fibers from both cerebral hemispheres. These fibers then join the glossopharyngeal, vagus, and spinal accessory nerves.

The spinal root's nucleus is located in the spinal nucleus of the anterior gray column of the spinal cord. The fibers pass through the lateral white column and eventually form a nerve trunk, which joins the cranial root to pass through the foramen magnum. The spinal root then separates from the cranial root, however, to find its way to the sternocleidomastoid and trapezius muscles.

Innervation

The cranial root joins the vagus to innervate the uvula and the levator palatini. As previously mentioned, the spinal root innervates the sternocleidomastoid and trapezius muscles.

Function

The spinal accessory nerve's primary function is as a motor to the muscles (including the sternocleidomastoid) that help turn, tilt, and thrust the head forward or raise the sternum and clavicle if the head is in a fixed position. It provides innervation also to the trapezius muscle, which is responsible for shrugging the shoulders.

Testing

When testing cranial nerve XI, the spinal part is evaluated. The accessory part is accessory to the vagus and cannot be tested alone.

Initially, look at the size and symmetry of the sternocleidomastoid muscles and palpate them. (Do this on yourself and others to become familiar with normal muscle size and firmness.) Ask the patient to turn the head to one side and hold it there while you try to push it back to the middle. Put one hand on the patient's cheek and the other on the shoulder to brace the patient. Gently push against the cheek and observe and palpate the sternocleidomastoid on the opposite side of the neck.

Next have the patient try to thrust the head forward while you gently resist the movement with your hand against the forehead. Again, observe and palpate the sternocleidomastoid muscle.

Finally, ask the patient to shrug the shoulders while you press down on them. You should feel the shoulders elevate against your gentle resistance.

Cranial Nerve XII: Hypoglossal

Anatomy

The hypoglossal nerve runs under the tongue and controls tongue movements. The nucleus, called the hypoglossal nucleus, is located in the medulla beneath the lower part of the fourth ventricle. It receives fibers from both cerebral hemispheres, with one exception. The cells serving the genioglossus muscle receive only contralateral fibers. The nerve fibers pass through the medulla and emerge in the groove between the pyramid and the olive. Other apparent branches of the hypoglossal are not connected with the hypoglossal nuclei but rather are derived from the ansa cervicalis of cervical vertebrae C1, C2, and C3. Ansa means "loop," and some branches of these spinal nerves form a loop and join the hypoglossal nerve to help innervate the sternothyroid, sternohyoid, and omohyoid muscles.

Innervation

The hypoglossal nerve innervates the intrinsic muscles of the tongue. It also innervates four extrinsic tongue muscles: the genioglossus, hyoglossus, chondroglossus, and styloglossus.

With the branches from the ansa cervicalis, cranial nerve XII contributes to the innervation of the sternothyroid, sternohyoid, and omohyoid muscles, thus contributing to the elevation and depression of the larynx.

Function

The hypoglossal nerve innervates the muscles responsible for tongue movement. The four intrinsic muscles of the tongue control tongue shortening, concaving (turning the tip and lateral margins upward), narrowing, elongating, and flattening. The extrinsic muscles innervated account for tongue protrusion (**genioglossus**), drawing the tongue upward and backward (**styloglossus**), and retraction and depression of the tongue (**hyoglossus**). The hyoglossus also acts with the chondroglossus to elevate the hyoid bone, thus participating in phonation.

Testing

Ask the patient to open the mouth and let you look at the tongue at rest. Inspect it for signs of atrophy. With a unilateral lower motor neuron lesion, one side of the tongue may look shrunken or atrophied. This atrophy occurs on the same side as the lower motor neuron lesion. A lower motor neuron lesion may cause fasciculations, seen as tiny ripples under the surface of the tongue. Normal tongues may also show some ripples when they are not completely relaxed. Therefore, if fasciculations seem present, ask the patient to move the tongue around and then relax it; again observe the surface for fasciculations. Even in a normal tongue, however, ripples may still be present. Therefore, the clinician does better to rely on atrophy and weakness as signs of lower motor neuron damage. The tongue should also be observed for tremor or random movements at rest.

Next ask the patient to protrude the tongue; evaluate the symmetry of this posture. The tongue tip should be at midline. If the patient has weak lip musculature on one side, that side may be lower, causing the tongue to look as if it deviates to that side. Therefore, try to align the tip of the tongue with the midline of the jaw visually. That side of the lip can be pulled back so that it is symmetric with the other side of the lip; then ask the patient to protrude the tongue. If the cranial nerve is dysfunctional, the genioglossus will not be able to push its side out; the stronger side will overcome the weaker, and the tongue will deviate to the weaker side (Fig. 7.5).

In lower motor neuron damage the weakness is on the same side as the lesion. In upper motor neuron damage, because of the contralateral control, the tongue deviates to the side opposite the lesion. For example, in many stroke patients with left hemisphere damage to the area of the motor strip, the tongue shows a characteristic deviation to the right on protrusion. This is usually less marked than in lower motor neuron tongue weakness.

The patient who has bilateral XII nerve damage has weakness on both sides and is unable to protrude the tongue beyond the lips. Strength of tongue protrusion may be tested by asking the patient to push against a tongue blade held directly in front of the lips.

Other movements of the tongue must be evaluated to document precisely the range, rate, and strength of the tongue for follow-up in treatment and for diagnostic purposes. Ask the patient to lateralize the tongue (i.e., move it from one corner of the mouth to the other). The tongue should move the full range from corner to corner. Evaluate the strength of lateral movement by asking the patient to push the tongue against the inside of the cheek (i.e., make a "ball" in the cheek) against your fingers placed for resistance on the outside of the cheek. A tongue blade can also be placed along the side of the tongue, with the patient pushing against a light resistance.

The ability to elevate the tongue can be evaluated by having the patient open the mouth to a moderate degree while you hold down the mandible with your finger on it. Ask the

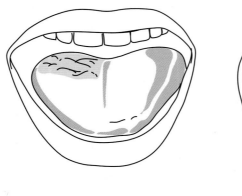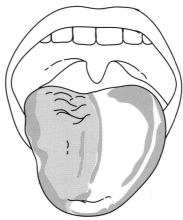

Fig. 7.5 Unilateral paresis of the tongue. *(Left)* The resting tongue shows a smaller weak side (atrophy) with a corrugated surface suggesting fasciculations and the effects of atrophy. These tongue signs suggest denervation. *(Right)* The protruded tongue deviates to the weak side. In a lower motor neuron lesion, the deviated tongue points to the side of the lesion. (Modified from Darley, F., Aronson, A., & Brown, J. [1975]. *Motor speech disorders*. W. B. Saunders.)

patient to try to touch the top lip and the alveolar ridge with the tongue. This should be done with full range of movement and little effort.

Strength of elevation of the tip, blade, or back of the tongue is difficult to assess with tongue blade resistance. A quick perceptual analysis may be a better informal assessment of strength of elevation. The tip of the tongue should be able to make firm contact to produce /t/, /d/, /t ʃ/ (as in "chum"), and /dz/ (as in "judge") and to elevate fully for /l/ and /n/. The blade of the tongue should elevate well to produce a distinct /i/ (*e* as in "eat") and /j/ (*y* as in "young"). Elevation of the back of the tongue is necessary for production of the velar consonants /k/ and /g/. Careful examination of the production of these consonants and vowels as well as others, in isolation and in context, may provide the most information regarding tongue elevation and strength.

INSTRUMENTAL MEASUREMENT OF STRENGTH

If your clinic or practice is fortunate enough, you may have access to instrumentation that could provide you with objective measures of lip and tongue strength. The Iowa Oral Pressure Indicator (IOPI) was introduced to our field through research on dysphagia in 1995. The IOPI is a small handheld medical device designed to objectively measure lip and tongue strength as well as provide quantitative measurement of tongue fatigability. Since its introduction it has been made available not only to researchers but to practicing clinicians who utilize it for therapy. It has been widely used in research providing validation and normative data for these measures. A systematic review of the available literature found that there is sufficient evidence for the use of the IOPI in measuring tongue strength and endurance, as well as in intervention.[1]

Table 7.2 summarizes the five cranial nerves (V, VII, IX, X, and XII) involved in the oral musculature.

CRANIAL NERVE COOPERATION: THE ACT OF SWALLOWING

The act of swallowing is highly complex and must be studied independently in regard to its cranial nerve innervation. Normal deglutition consists of four phases: oral preparatory, oral, pharyngeal, and esophageal.[6]

Oral Preparatory Phase

In the oral preparatory phase, the food or liquid stimulates sensory receptors (taste, touch, temperature, and pressure). These receptors are activated by saliva. Mastication mixes the food with saliva and forms it into a cohesive bolus. Food and liquid are held by the tongue against the hard palate prior to swallow initiation, though some will also collect in the valleculae and be held there at the base of the tongue. The oral preparatory stage is variable in duration depending on ease of mastication, oral motor efficiency, and individual preference in savoring flavor.

Taste is also enhanced by the presence of saliva, which dissolves flavors in foods and distributes them around the oral cavity to taste buds. Saliva also allows flavors to travel into the nasopharynx, allowing for the interaction of smell and taste. The sense of smell contributes greatly to the appreciation of taste, with smell carried directly into the nares or indirectly through the salivary action. Smell receptors that enhance taste have been found in the brain, airway, digestive tract, and testis, in addition to the nose.[4]

The oral preparatory stage actively involves cranial nerves I, V, VII, IX, and XII for smell, taste, salivation, general sensation regarding where food is in the mouth, lip closure, chewing, and movement of the tongue.

Oral Phase

The oral stage begins when the lips form a seal, and the back of the tongue begins moving the bolus posteriorly. The tip and sides of the tongue contract against the hard palate, gradually

TABLE 7.2   Summary of Cranial Nerve Function for the Oral Musculature

Cranial Nerve	Muscles Innervated	Movements and Sensation Innervated	Test Procedure	Signs of Lower Motor Neuron Damage	Signs of Upper Motor Neuron Damage
V: trigeminal	Masseter, tensor tympani, tensor veli palatini, mylo-hyoid, digastric (anterior belly)	Jaw closing, lateral jaw movement, contribution to laryngeal eleva-tion, sensation to face and anterior tongue	Palpation of mas-seter, closing and lateralization against resistance, sensation on face and tongue	Weakness, jaw deviation to lesion side, atrophy	Mild, transitory weakness
VII: facial	Orbicularis oculi and oris, zygomatic, buccinator, pla-tysma, stylohyoid, stapedius, portion of digastric (poste-rior belly)	Forehead wrinkling, closing eyes, clos-ing mouth, smil-ing, pulling down corner of mouth, tensing anterior neck muscles, moving stape-dius to dampen ossicles; taste from anterior two-thirds of tongue and hard and soft palates	Observation of facial symmetry at rest; have patient wrinkle forehead, close eyes tightly, smile, pucker, and pull down lip cor-ners; identification of tastes	Involvement of entire side of face, weakness, limited range of move-ment, decreased taste sensation	Complete involve-ment of lips and neck muscles, less involvement of eye area muscles, little difficulty with forehead mus-cles; weakness, limited range of movement of affected muscles; decreased taste sensation
IX: glosso-pharyngeal	Stylopharyngeus, otic ganglion, parotid salivary gland, part of the middle pharyngeal constrictor	Elevation of pharynx and larynx, pharyngeal dilation, saliva-tion; taste from posterior third of tongue; sensation from posterior tongue and upper pharynx	Tested with cranial nerve X for motor; sensory test for pharyngeal gag	—	—
X: vagus	Inferior, middle, and superior pharyngeal con-strictors; salpin-gopharyngeus, glossopalatine, pharyngopala-tine, levator veli palatini, uvular, cricothyroid, thy-roarytenoid, pos-terior and lateral cricoarytenoid, interarytenoid, and transverse and oblique interary-tenoid muscles; various muscles of the viscera, esophagus, and trachea	Palatal elevation and depression, laryngeal movement, pharyngeal constriction, cricopharyngeal function; visceral and general sensation from base of tongue, epiglottis, larynx, and pharynx	Observation of palatal movement, palatal gag reflex; laryngoscopic evaluation of vocal musculature; abil-ity to change pitch; phonation time; assessment of swallowing	Absence of gag reflex, poor move-ment of palate or pharyngeal wall, absent or delayed swallow response, aspiration, breathy hoarse voice (may be improved by pushing effort)	Poor palatal or pharyngeal wall movement, harsh-ness or strained-strangled voice quality, delayed or absent swallow reflex, aspiration

continued

TABLE 7.2   Summary of Cranial Nerve Function for the Oral Musculature—cont'd

Cranial Nerve	Muscles Innervated	Movements and Sensation Innervated	Test Procedure	Signs of Lower Motor Neuron Damage	Signs of Upper Motor Neuron Damage
XII: hypoglossal	Superior longitudinal, inferior longitudinal, transverse vertical, genioglossus, hyoglossus, and styloglossus	All tongue movements as well as some elevation of the hyoid bone	Observation for atrophy or fasciculations as well as symmetry on protrusion; assessment for lateralization, protrusion, elevation, retraction (to observe range of movement); assessment of movement against resistance for strength testing on lateral, protrusion, and elevation movement; articulation testing	Atrophy, fasciculations, weakness, reduced range of movement, deviation of tongue to side of lesion, decreased tone, consonant imprecision	Weakness, reduced range of movement, deviation of tongue to contralateral side, increased tone, consonant imprecision

squeezing the bolus backwards. Simultaneously, the posterior portion of the tongue forms a central groove that acts as a ramp or chute for the food, allowing for a quick transition into the pharyngeal phase. At some point during the oral stage, the swallow reflex will be initiated (triggered). The swallow reflex occurs through stimulation of sensory receptors on the faucial pillars, tonsils, soft palate, base of the tongue, the posterior pharyngeal wall, and/or the epiglottis. These sensory receptors respond to the presence of liquid, pressure, and possibly even temperature of the bolus. Input from these receptors is carried mainly by cranial nerves VII, IX, and X and is processed in the nucleus tractus solitarius (NTS) in the medulla.[8]

Motor movements during this stage include large cyclical tongue movements that are coordinated with jaw movements. The tongue moves front to back, vertically, and with rotation, while jaw movements are vertical. These movements reduce the size of food, and saliva softens foods. Movements also pump air into the nasal cavity, helping to deliver the aroma of food into nasal receptors. The movements continue until the bolus is ready to be swallowed, at which point the tongue propels the bolus to the oropharynx.[7]

The oral stage motor activity involves cranial nerves V, VII, and XII for salivation, mastication, lip closure, and tongue movement.

Pharyngeal Phase

The pharyngeal phase is a period of rapid muscular activity that is completed in 1 second. This phase accomplishes two crucial biologic functions: the transport of food to the esophagus and airway protection. For food transport, the soft palate (velum) elevates and contacts the lateral and posterior walls of the pharynx; velar elevation seals the nasal cavity from the oral cavity, preventing regurgitation into the former. The pharyngeal constrictor muscles contract sequentially from top to bottom, squeezing the bolus downward, while the upper esophageal sphincter opens to accommodate the bolus.

Airway protection is critical, and several protective mechanisms ensure the prevention of aspiration to the trachea before or during the swallow. The vocal folds seal the glottis and the epiglottis moves backwards to direct food away from the airway. The hyoid bone is pulled upwards, moving the larynx forward and upward, which tucks the larynx under the base of the tongue.

While the oral phases are voluntary, the pharyngeal and esophageal phases are involuntary. Cranial nerves involved in the swallowing reflex include IX, X, and XI, considered the pharyngeal plexus. Additional cranial nerve involvement is provided by V, VII, and XII.

Esophageal Phase

The final phase in normal swallowing, the esophageal phase, occurs as the bolus enters the esophagus through the cricopharyngeus. A wave of contractions (peristalsis), innervated by cranial nerve X, is initiated in the esophagus, and the bolus is passed through into the stomach through the lower esophageal sphincter. This sphincter is tensioned at rest to prevent regurgitation from the stomach. Normal esophageal transit time is 8 to 20 seconds.[7]

Box 7.2 outlines the four phases of deglutition, and Fig. 7.6 illustrates the final three stages.

Coordination of Physiologic Functions

There are several physiologic responses that occur during the swallow: a safe swallow hinges on the coordination of swallowing and breathing. In a normal swallow, breathing ceases briefly because of the closure of the airway as well as the neural suppression of respiration in the brainstem. The respiratory pause ranges from 0.5 to 1.5 seconds, and respiration resumes with exhalation. Exhalation is thought to help maintain safety since an inhalation may drag any food left in the pharynx into the airway. Studies have noted that the respiratory cycle is altered even during mastication, with the cycle decreasing in duration.[7]

Neurally, the afferent transmission to the NTS appears to be required to be in a specifically organized pattern to lead to initiation of swallowing. This stimulus pattern is conveyed to the reticular formation to make connections with efferent nuclei of cranial nerves V, VII, IX, X, and XII in the nucleus ambiguus of the medulla. The efferent response that we call the swallow response or the pharyngeal swallow is an orderly configuration of several physiologic actions occurring in the oropharynx simultaneously: velopharyngeal closure, laryngeal elevation, inversion of the epiglottis, closure of all sphincters (aryepiglottic folds, false vocal folds, and true vocal folds), initiation of pharyngeal peristalsis (squeezing), and relaxation of the cricopharyngeal sphincter (or cricopharyngeus) to allow material to pass from pharynx to esophagus. If the swallow is not neurally triggered, whether this be voluntarily or involuntarily, this physiologic pattern of activity does not occur spontaneously. The bolus may be pushed into the pharynx and come to rest in the valleculae or pyriform sinuses and eventually will spill over into an unprotected airway (i.e., aspirated) unless it is expectorated before this happens.

While the pharyngeal phase is primarily involuntary, there are some maneuvers that can be learned to compensate for a slow or impaired swallowing response. These maneuvers mimic intact swallowing actions. Foremost is airway protection, by temporary cessation of breathing and closure of the vocal cords if possible. Other voluntary movements include elevating the larynx, inverting the epiglottis, and opening the cricopharyngeus, but these movements are difficult to pattern and maintain without the neural swallow initiation.[5]

BOX 7.2   Four Phases of Deglutition

1. **Oral preparatory phase:** Tongue forms the liquid or solid into a cohesive bolus after the solid has been chewed and mixed with saliva. Some of the solid bolus may fall into the valleculae during mastication; the rest of the bolus is held as a cohesive unit against the hard palate.
2. **Oral phase:** Lips seal and tongue moves food to the back of the mouth.
3. **Pharyngeal phase:** Swallow response is triggered, causing several physiologic activities to occur simultaneously and pushing food from the pharynx into the esophagus.
4. **Esophageal phase:** Food passes, by peristaltic action, through the esophagus to the stomach.

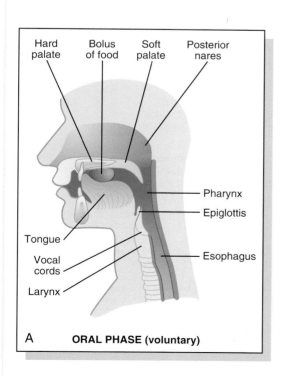

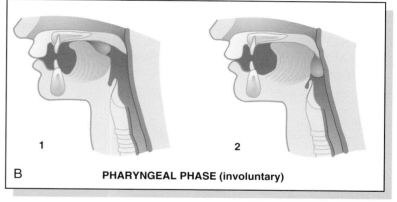

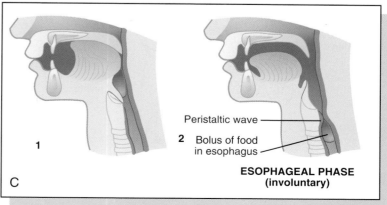

Fig. 7.6 The initial phase of swallowing, the oral preparatory phase (A), involves mastication and mixture of the food with saliva. It is then followed by oral (B1), pharyngeal (B2 and C1), and esophageal (C2) phases. (Modified from Mahan, K. L., & Escott-Stump, S. [2008]. *Krause's food & nutrition therapy* [12th ed.]. Saunders.)

Efficient swallowing demands cooperation and coordination of the cranial nerves that are also involved in speech production. Fig. 7.7 is a simplified summary of the actions that occur in swallowing and the cranial nerves that are responsible. The trigeminal nerve (V) plays an important part because of the efferent control of the muscles of mastication and the afferent control for general sensation to the anterior two-thirds of the tongue. Cranial nerve VII, the facial nerve, controls taste for the anterior two-thirds of the tongue and controls the lip sphincter and the buccal muscles, allowing food to be held inside the mouth.

The hypoglossal nerve (XII) controls the movement of the tongue. This action of the tongue has been compared with that of a plunger and is called the tongue driving force.

The vagus nerve (X) mediates the action of the cricopharyngeus, which relaxes to allow the bolus to pass from the hypopharynx to the esophagus. The movement of the intrinsic muscles of the larynx to close the entrance to the airway is also innervated by the vagus. The elevation and anterior movement of the larynx are significant mechanical forces contributing to the opening of the cricopharyngeus. Therefore, cranial nerves V, VII, IX, X, and XII, all with efferent innervation to one or more extrinsic muscles of the tongue and larynx, are important to this aspect of swallowing. The opening of the cricopharyngeus creates a negative pressure and thus a suction pump effect, which significantly increases the rate of bolus flow and contributes to the elimination of the bolus before the larynx reopens.

The hypoglossal, glossopharyngeal, and vagus nerves are major contributors to clearing the bolus through the pharynx. The tongue driving force and the pharyngeal clearing force, combined with the hypopharyngeal suction pump, produce a rapid transit through the pharynx once the swallow response has been triggered.[2]

The glossopharyngeal nerve is thought to be the primary afferent of the swallow response, and the vagus is thought to be the secondary afferent. As stated previously, the brainstem center of neural control for swallowing is located in the medulla in the nucleus solitarius and in the nucleus ambiguus. Afferent fibers converge on the nucleus solitarius in the medulla. They communicate with neurons in the nucleus ambiguus by way of interneurons, thereby stimulating the motor response. The medullary swallowing center has been referred to as the **central pattern generator**[9] rather than a reflex center for swallowing due to the observation of the timing and sequence of the muscle contractions that follow the onset of the pharyngeal swallow. This physiologic response to a sensory event is obviously more complex than a mere reflex. Regulation of swallowing by the nervous system is likely carried out not only by the innervation of cranial nerves and patterns of muscle response but also by involvement of different levels of the central nervous system, including the cerebellum, limbic and other subcortical structures, and areas of the neocortex. We can and do swallow differently for different textures and in different settings or situations. We can talk while eating; we can put swallowing under much greater (although not total) voluntary control in situations such as swallowing a pill; we can eat faster or slower; although rare (and very dangerous), some of us can even control the opening of the esophageal sphincters to "swallow" a sword! These variations in swallowing control support the input of supranuclear structures to swallowing.

If swallowing is inefficient and aspiration occurs, a reflexive cough should occur as one of the respiratory system's defenses against foreign matter. The cough reflex is induced by irritation of the afferent fibers of the pharyngeal distribution of the glossopharyngeal nerve along with the sensory endings of the vagus nerve in the larynx, trachea, and larger bronchi.

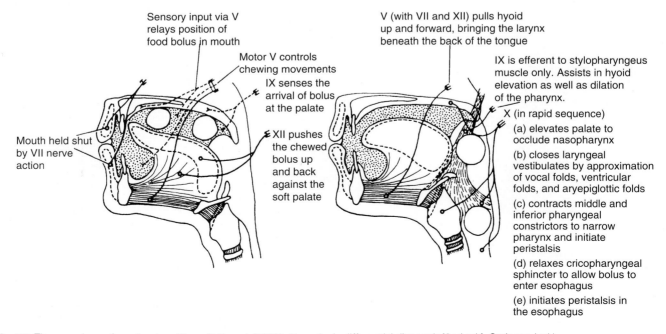

Fig. 7.7 The neurology of swallowing. (From Patten, J. [1998]. *Neurologic differential diagnosis* [2nd ed.]. Springer, Ltd.)

Assessment of Swallowing

The cranial nerve examination is critical to the assessment of swallowing. Careful evaluation of the sensory component of the cranial nerves is probably more important in the swallowing evaluation than when the examination is for a speech disorder alone.

Taste, carried by cranial nerves VII and IX, is not a typical part of the assessment of the sensorimotor control for speech or for swallowing. However, if the etiology and characteristics of a swallowing disorder are particularly difficult to figure out or if treatment is not going as well as planned, taste should be tested with some of the primary tastes (salt, sweet, bitter, and sour). The testing must be done on both sides of the anterior two-thirds of the tongue and on both sides of the posterior third of the tongue to include cranial nerves VII and IX. In these cases, smell should probably also be evaluated, as the sense of smell is critical to normal taste perception. Smell is carried by cranial nerve I. It can be assessed by having the patient identify certain smells that are typically readily identifiable in the patient's culture (e.g., the smell of sulfur [rotten eggs], roses, vanilla, peppermint [for Americans]). This of course would not be relevant for a patient who reports a poor premorbid sense of smell, a laryngectomy or tracheostomy patient, or a patient with cognitive deficits.

General sensation to the tongue, carried by cranial nerves V and IX (posterior third), should be tested with the two sides compared regarding sensitivity to touch. As previously mentioned, testing of the pharyngeal gag can be attempted.

The motor examination for swallowing should consist of the same maneuvers as for the speech examination with additional time for dedicated swallowing assessment. In most settings, if the patient is not so compromised as to be unable to cooperate or to be too at risk for injury, a cursory screening examination of swallowing is performed (often called a bedside swallowing evaluation). For this screening, the clinician first does the oral-motor and cognitive testing and then observes the patient's attempt at swallowing a variety of textures and bolus sizes. Typically, water, ice chips, a puree, and a soft and a hard chewable are introduced. This swallowing should only be done if the clinician judges it safe to try in the clinic setting. If patient safety is a concern or if the cranial nerve examination has pointed to a likely swallowing disorder, a modified barium swallow (MBS, aka a videofluoroscopic swallow study [VFSS]) or perhaps a flexible endoscopic evaluation of swallowing (FEES) should be requested. These examinations should be performed only by an SLP or other professional with appropriate training and experience in their administration and interpretation. The purpose of any instrumental examination should be to document problems and evaluate therapeutic alternatives that may improve oral intake.

A VFSS is obviously a radiographic study that exposes the patient (and clinician) to a small amount of radiation; it does require that barium be mixed with the food consistencies or that a barium solution duplicating normal consistencies be used. The MBS is the gold standard for instrumental evaluation because of the complete view of all stages of the swallow. Fig. 7.8 presents a lateral view used during the study and labels the structures.

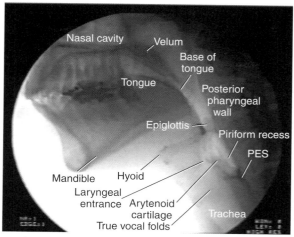

Fig. 7.8 Lateral radiographic view of normal swallowing mechanism in an adult. *PES*, Pharyngoesophageal segment. (From Groher, M. E., & Crary, M. A. [2016]. *Dysphagia: Clinical management in adults and children* [2nd ed.]. Mosby.)

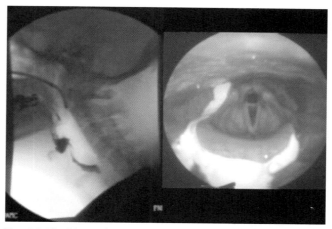

Fig. 7.9 Flexible endoscopic evaluation of swallowing image of tracheal aspiration. (Modified from Leder, S. B., & Murray, J. T. [2008]. Fiberoptic endoscopic evaluation of swallowing. *Physical Medical & Rehabilitation Clinics of North America, 19*(4), 787–801.)

FEES is another instrumental procedure that may be helpful when a pharyngeal stage disorder is suspected. For this study, a flexible endoscope is passed nasally to allow a view superior to the pyriform sinuses and the vocal folds. Once the scope is placed, the patient can be asked to swallow liquids, soft solids, or solids with the only addition being perhaps some food coloring.

The major drawback for the use of the FEES study is that the image is blocked at the peak of the swallow when the material being swallowed covers the tip of the scope, and this is followed by a brief period of whiteout as the vocal folds close and the larynx rises, blocking any image. It is at this point that aspiration may be missed. Fig. 7.9 presents the view during a FEES examination after the whiteout but showing residual aspirated material at the entrance to the airway. This residue at the entrance to the vocal folds does not always occur, and the possibility of missing aspiration, especially silent aspiration, is a concern; however, if residue is not coated with barium, the MBS study may miss potential aspiration as well.

SYNOPSIS OF CLINICAL INFORMATION AND APPLICATIONS FOR THE SLP

- The SLP must be knowledgeable regarding the function and assessment of the cranial nerves, which are vital for speech production and swallowing.
- Twelve pairs of cranial nerves can be found exiting the brainstem; seven are concerned with communication and/or swallowing.
- Cranial nerves I (olfactory), II (optic), III (oculomotor), IV (trochlear), and VI (abducens) are concerned with smell and vision as well as movement of the eyes.
- Cranial nerve VIII (vestibuloacoustic) is the auditory nerve carrying the sensation of sound to Heschl gyrus. The vestibular portion of the nerve controls the sense of equilibrium.
- Cranial nerve XI (spinal accessory) contributes to movement of the uvula and the levator palatini through its cranial root.

- Testing of the spinal part of the nerve is the only possible test of the nerve's viability.
- The five remaining cranial nerves (V, trigeminal; VII, facial; IX, glossopharyngeal; X, vagus; XII, hypoglossal) are main motor and sensory nerves for oral-motor and sensory function, enabling speech production, oral feeding, and swallowing.
- Table 7.2 summarizes pertinent clinical information for these five cranial nerves on anatomy, innervation, signs of damage, and testing procedures that can be done during an extended oral-motor examination.
- Beyond a limited bedside swallow examination, FEES and/or MBS would be necessary to adequately evaluate cranial nerve function during swallowing.

CASE STUDY

A 34-year-old female welder sought help from her physician for persistent ringing (medically known as tinnitus) and "wave crashing" sounds in her right ear. These symptoms were initially attributed to occupational noise exposure. However, a year later she continued to experience the same sounds but with additional symptoms that brought new concern. She now demonstrated a clumsy gait, had pain in her right ear, and reported dizziness. She also thought that her hearing in her right ear had decreased. Her symptoms worsened, and she went to the emergency department. She reported in the emergency department that she had suddenly begun having difficulty seeing clearly out of her right eye, was having some difficulty with swallowing, and had some slurring of speech.

Examination showed moderate facial weakness and right-sided weakness of her mouth and tongue. Voice and speech production were notably weak. The physician diagnosed classic signs of a **flaccid** dysarthria.

Questions for Consideration

1. What, if any, cranial nerves are involved here?
2. Could this patient's symptoms be explained as noise-induced hearing loss with cranial nerve damage?
3. The final diagnosis for this patient was a vestibular schwannoma (or acoustic neuroma). What are some of the characteristics of this tumor? (The answer to this question will involve some research.)

REFERENCES

1. Adams, V., Mathisen, B., Baines, S., Lazarus, C., & Callister, R. (2013). A systematic review and meta-analysis of measurements of tongue and hand strength and endurance using the Iowa Oral Performance Instrument (IOPI). *Dysphagia, 28*(3), 350–369. https://doi.org/10.1007/s00455-013-9451-3.

2. Costa, M. (2018). Neural control of swallowing. *Gastroenterology, 55*(S1), 61–75. https://doi.org/10.1590/S0004-2803.201800000-45.

3. Darley, F., Aronson, A., & Brown, J. (1975). *Motor speech disorders*. W. B. Saunders.

4. Dawes, C., Pedersen, A. M., Villa, A., Ekström, J., Proctor, G. B., Vissink, A., Aframian, D., McGowan, R., Aliko, A., Narayana, N., Sia, Y. W., Joshi, R. K., Jensen, S. B., Kerr, A. R., & Wolff, A. (2015). The functions of human saliva: A review sponsored by the World Workshop on Oral Medicine VI. *Archives of Oral Biology, 60*(6), 863–874. https://doi.org/10.1016/j.archoralbio.2015.03.004.

5. Ertekin, C., & Aydogdu, I. (2003). Neurophysiology of swallowing. *Clinical Neurophysiology, 114*(12), 2226–2244. https://doi.org/10.1016/s1388-2457(03)00237-2.

6. Lancaster, J. (2015). Dysphagia: Its nature, assessment and management. *British Journal of Community Nursing, 20*(Sup6a), 28–32. https://doi.org/10.12968/bjcn.2015.20.Sup6a.S28.

7. Matsuo, K., & Palmer, J. B. (2008). Anatomy and physiology of feeding and swallowing: Normal and abnormal. *Physical Medicine and Rehabilitation Clinics of North America, 19*(4), 691–707, vii. https://doi.org/10.1016/j.pmr.2008.06.001.

8. Steele, C. M., & Miller, A. J. (2010). Sensory input pathways and mechanisms in swallowing: A review. *Dysphagia, 25*, 323–333. https://doi.org/10.1007/s00455-010-9301-5.

9. Steuer, I., & Guertin, P. A. (2019). Central pattern generators in the brainstem and spinal cord: An overview of basic principles, similarities and differences. *Reviews in the Neurosciences, 30*(2), 107–164. https://doi.org/10.1515/revneuro-2017-0102.

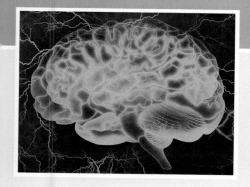

8

Clinical Speech Syndromes of the Motor Systems

Speech is deranged in a variety of ways by disease of the brain. The process of articulation is immediately affected by a mechanism of nerve nuclei situated in the pons and medulla, but these are excited to action by centers in the cerebral cortex. Thus, there are higher and lower mechanisms; the former is cerebral, the latter is bulbar.

William R. Gowers, A Manual of Disease of the Nervous System, 1888

CHAPTER OUTLINE

KEY TERMS

amyotrophic lateral sclerosis (ALS; Lou Gehrig disease)
apraxia of speech
ataxic dysarthria
athetosis
cerebrovascular accident (CVA)
childhood apraxia of speech
cogwheel rigidity
diplegia
dystonia
essential tremor
excess and equal stress
explosive speech

fasciculations
flaccid
flaccid dysarthria
Huntington chorea
hypernasality
hypokinetic dysarthria
L-dopa
monoloudness
monopitch
myasthenia gravis
oral apraxia
palilalia
parkinsonism

pathologic tremor
pseudobulbar (supranuclear bulbar) palsy
scanning speech
Shy Drager syndrome
spasmodic dysphonia
spastic dysarthria
Sydenham chorea
tardive dyskinesia
unilateral upper motor neuron dysarthria

Speech-language pathologists (SLPs) must have an understanding of the function of the cranial nerves and the rest of the motor and sensory system for the treatment of motor speech disorders. Data kept at the Mayo Clinic between 2009 and 2016 showed that of the 9430 people whose primary diagnosis was an acquired neurologic communication disorder, roughly half were diagnosed with a motor speech disorder, with the main complaint being dysarthria (47.3%).[12] These data indicate that SLPs whose practice is primarily with adult clients must be well versed in the anatomy and physiology of the motor speech system and familiar with the clinical signs and symptoms of diseases and conditions producing them. This knowledge will be important to the treatment of children with motor speech disorders as well, which is discussed in Chapter 12.

DYSARTHRIAS

Dysarthria is a motor speech disorder that can be classified according to the underlying neuropathology and is associated with disturbances of respiration, phonation, articulation, resonance, and prosody. People with dysarthria exhibit difficulties in the quality of their speech and in reduced intelligibility. Dysarthria is a frequent symptom of many neurologic conditions and is particularly common in progressive neurologic diseases. The presence of dysarthria often has a profound effect on both patient and family, as impaired communication impacts personal and social relationships.[17] More recently, a study of the impact of dysarthria on social relationships found a correlation between reduced intelligibility and a risk of being judged negatively on physical and mental capability.[7]

In the classic Mayo Clinic study, Darely et al.,[7] defined dysarthria as the speech disorder resulting from paralysis, weakness, or incoordination of the speech musculature that is of neurologic origin. Their definition encompasses any symptoms of motor disturbance of respiration, phonation, resonance, articulation, and prosody. Remarkably, these definitions have changed very little in the ensuing decades.

There are six major types of dysarthria, classified by the underlying neuropathology, as well as by auditory-perceptual judgments of speech. These are spastic (upper motor neuron [UMN]), flaccid (lower motor neuron [LMN]), ataxic (cerebellar), hypokinetic (basal ganglia), hyperkinetic (basal ganglia), and mixed. Figure 8.1 shows the distribution of dysarthria types in a study by Duffy.[12] SLPs should be familiar with the motor system as well as the features of the various dysarthrias as familiarity can assist with diagnosis of disease etiology as well as with treatment.

Damage to the motor system responsible for speech production may occur at any point along the pathway from the cerebrum to the muscle itself. The following discussion does not include an exhaustive listing of neurologic diseases that can produce dysarthria; any disease or trauma affecting movement, coordination, and timing of the oral musculature may produce a dysarthria.[32]

Like speech difficulties, swallowing disorders are symptoms of underlying lesions. The same neurologic and muscular symptoms that produce speech difficulties will likely also result in dysphagia. In a screening of all stroke patients admitted to the Ghent University hospital in an 18-month period, researchers found a 23% incidence of dysphagia and a 44% incidence of dysarthria in patients with a novel stroke,[10] although other researchers have found a higher incidence of dysphagia.[21] For example, in a study of 100 stroke patients in 2019, Stipancich et al.,[42] found an incidence of

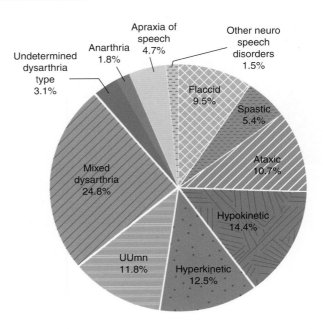

Fig. 8.1 Distribution of neurologic communication disorders, speech pathology, Department of Neurology, Mayo Clinic, 1987–1990 and 1993–2001. (Reprinted from Duffy J. [2005]. *Motor speech disorders: Substrates, differential diagnosis, and management* [2nd ed.]. Mosby.)

dysphagia in 32% and dysarthria in 26% of patient with first stroke. In a review article investigating the prevalence of dysphagia in neurogenic disorders, Wang et al.,[47] analyzed 24 research articles and found that dysarthria and dysphagia were prevalent in neurogenic disorders and particularly in neuromuscular diseases. The authors concluded that the presence of dysarthria is a strong clinical indicator of dysphagia. Because of this high incidence of co-occurrence of dysphagia and dysarthria in neurogenic disorders, typical swallowing characteristics are included in each of the six major dysarthria types.

Spastic Dysarthria

UMN damage may result in a spastic paralysis. Speech may sound strained and harsh, and it is often accompanied by hypernasality and hyperactive reflexes. The lesion that causes spastic dysarthria is most frequently bilateral in the direct and indirect activation systems.

A unilateral UMN dysarthria has been described in the literature and will be summarized in this section. The dysarthria associated with unilateral UMN lesions is called unilateral UMN dysarthria. The dysarthria associated with bilateral UMN lesions is known as spastic dysarthria. An overview of UMN lesions is found in Box 8.1.

Etiology

Bilateral UMN damage may result from stroke, head trauma, tumor, infection, degenerative disease, and inflammatory or toxic-metabolic diseases. In most instances of **spastic dysarthria**, bilateral damage occurs to both the

---

BOX 8.1   Upper Motor Neuron Lesions

Unilateral Upper Motor Neuron Dysarthria
- Primarily caused by stroke but can also result from trauma or tumors
- Imprecise articulation; slow rate and irregular articulatory breakdown may also occur
- Harshness, reduced loudness, and hypernasality common
- Difficulty with oral stage transit

1 Spastic Dysarthria
- May be caused by stroke, head trauma, tumor, infection, degenerative disease, or inflammatory or toxic-metabolic disease
- Loss of skilled movement, hyporeflexia, positive Babinski sign, muscle weakness, loss of muscle tone
- Usually severe impairment in the range and rate of movement of oral musculature
- Harsh voice with strained-strangled quality, low pitch, and monoloudness; often accompanied by hypernasality and imprecise consonant production
- Aspiration common, often with moderate to severe dysphagia

---

direct activation pathway (pyramidal system) and the indirect activation pathway (extrapyramidal system). Bilateral damage can occur because the two pathways are in close proximity from cortex to the internal capsule to termination at the cranial nerve or spinal nerve. The resulting oral-motor disorder from bilateral UMN damage to both systems is sometimes called **pseudobulbar** (or **supranuclear bulbar) palsy**. This name indicates the impact of damage on cranial nerves, with symptoms including facial paresis or paralysis, dysarthria, dysphagia, and dysphonia. This syndrome is commonly associated with emotional lability and a hyperactive jaw reflex.[15,17]

Associated Neurologic Characteristics

Direct activation pathway damage results in the characteristic loss of skilled movement, hyperreflexia, a positive Babinski sign, and muscle weakness and loss of tone. Damage to the indirect activation pathway causes increased muscle tone (spasticity) and hyperactive stretch reflexes. The gag reflex may be absent in the acute stages, but it later returns and may be hyperactive. This hypertonicity and hyperreflexia dominate if both systems are damaged, which is usually the case. Although tone is increased, the muscles are weak, range of movement is limited, and rate of movement is slow because of the direct activation motor system damage.

Oralfacial Motor Movements

In spastic dysarthria, the oral musculature usually shows severe impairment of range and rate of movement. The tongue may extend only to the lips on protrusion. The lips move slowly, and excursion is limited. Palatal movement is severely reduced and sluggish on phonation. Due to the limited range of motion of the orofacial structures, chewing and swallowing

are both frequently affected. Drooling is frequently present due to poor saliva management.

Auditory-Perceptual Speech Characteristics

The typical presentation of spastic speech includes hypernasality, slowed rate, and poor control of the volume of speech and poor intonation patterns.[9]

Phonation. The voice of the patient with spastic dysarthria is described as harsh, and many have a characteristic strained-strangled quality. An effortful grunt is often heard at the end of vocalizations. Excessively low pitch is frequently found, with pitch breaks in some cases.

Articulation. As in most dysarthrias, imprecision of consonant production is a noticeable part of the speech disorder in spastic dysarthria. Vowel distortion has been noted in some cases. Impaired acceleration of the moving articulators accounted for part of the distortion and the increase in production time often noted in these speakers.

Resonance. Hypernasality is a frequent component of spastic dysarthria. Nasal emission is uncommon, however.

Prosody. Little variation in loudness (**monoloudness**) and reduced stress (**monopitch**) are also noted. Occasionally heard in spastic dysarthria is excess and equal stress (i.e., inappropriate stress on monosyllabic words and the usually unstressed syllables of polysyllabic words).

Swallowing

The following symptoms associated with dysphagia are often observed in patients with bilateral UMN damage: reduced labial, lingual, and mandibular strength and sensation; delayed swallow response; reduced pharyngeal peristalsis; incomplete laryngeal elevation and closure; and cricopharyngeal dysfunction. The dysphagia may be severe, and drooling may be noted. With mild dysphagia, the patient may unconsciously alter the eating pattern to eat more slowly and carefully, denying any difficulty.[21]

Unilateral Upper Motor Neuron Dysarthria

As discussed by Duffy,[13] the dysarthria associated with unilateral UMN damage has been given scant attention in the literature probably because the symptoms are usually mild and sometimes transitory. This section on UMN lesions is primarily devoted to a discussion of spastic dysarthria for the same reasons. However, a brief review of unilateral UMN dysarthria, as termed by Duffy, is warranted because it is as frequently encountered as the other types discussed in this chapter.

Etiology

The primary etiology of **unilateral upper motor neuron dysarthria** is stroke. Many other etiologies of UMN damage cause more diffuse brain injury and result more often in bilateral damage to the pyramidal pathways. Trauma and tumors can result in injury confined to a single hemisphere and can produce a unilateral UMN dysarthria. Unilateral UMN dysarthria can result from damage to either hemisphere.

Auditory-Perceptual Speech Characteristics

Only a small number of studies have looked at the speech characteristics of unilateral UMN dysarthria.[15,24] The collective findings of these studies indicate that the most prominent deviant characteristic of speech is imprecise articulation. Slowed rate and irregular articulatory breakdown were also noted in a number of cases. Other characteristics present in some cases were harshness, reduced loudness, and hypernasality. Most characteristics were described as mild to moderate in severity, although some patients had more severe dysarthria. Many patients demonstrated significant recovery during the spontaneous recovery period, but in some cases the dysarthria symptoms persisted and required speech therapy to address the reduced intelligibility.

Swallowing

Swallowing difficulty is generally less severe in unilateral UMN dysarthria, likely due to the bilateral representation of motor functions. If the dominant hemisphere is impaired, an initial difficulty may be present, which tends to resolve due to cortical plasticity. In some patients, mild swallowing difficulty persists, which may require intervention.[21]

Flaccid Dysarthria

Damage to the LMN system affects the final common pathway for muscle contraction. The muscles become hypotonic or flaccid. Thus, every type of movement is involved (voluntary, automatic, and reflexive movement are all impaired), and flaccid dysarthria may be seen.

Etiology

Any disease that affects part of the motor unit—the cell body, its axon, the myoneural junction, or the muscle fibers themselves—may yield LMN symptoms. Viral infections, tumors, trauma to the nerve itself, or a brainstem stroke with involvement of the nerve fibers may be the cause of flaccid dysarthria. Myasthenia gravis results from impairment of transmission across the myoneural junction or the synapse between the nerve and muscle. Bulbar palsy results from damage to the motor units of the cranial nerves. Möbius syndrome (congenital facial diplegia) involves bilateral sixth (abducens) and seventh (facial) nerve palsies of congenital origin rather than generalized bulbar palsy. Most patients with these palsies exhibit only mild dysarthria predominantly characterized by articulatory imprecision. Direct muscle involvement is found in diseases such as muscular dystrophy, myotonia, and myositis.

Associated Neurologic Characteristics

Damage to the LMN system causes flaccid paralysis. Reflexes are reduced (i.e., hyporeflexia is present). The affected muscles become atrophied over time and fasciculations (tiny spontaneous muscle contractions, typically only involving a few muscle fibers at a time) can be observed. The fasciculations appear as spontaneous dimpling of the tongue, which may look as though tiny worms are moving just beneath its surface.

Orofacial Movements

Because the cranial nerve nuclei are dispersed throughout the brainstem rather than being clustered together, the oral structures may be selectively impaired and should be carefully evaluated.

Muscle tone in LMN damage is flaccid or hypotonic. Muscles are weak. The affected side of the lips sag, and in some cases drooling may be present. In bilateral weakness the whole mouth may sag, and the lower lip may be so weak that habitual open-mouth posture results. As a result of the weakened orofacial musculature, the patient may have difficulty puckering the lips or pulling up the corners of the lips to smile.

Weakness of the mandibular muscles may not be readily evident in unilateral involvement. Careful observation reveals that the jaw deviates to the side of weakness upon opening the mouth and lowering the jaw. With bilateral damage the jaw obviously sags at rest.

With damage to any component of the motor unit supplying the tongue, the muscles become atrophied over time, and the tongue is atonic. This tends to affect tongue protrusion, lateralization, and elevation, particularly of the posterior portion of the tongue.

Palatal weakness or immobility may also be present, and the gag reflex is reduced or absent. Pharyngeal involvement may occur, causing swallowing difficulty and possibly nasal regurgitation of fluids.

Auditory-Perceptual Speech Characteristics

SLPs are most likely to be consulted concerning patients with flaccid dysarthria resulting from vascular disease, head trauma, or disease processes. These patients may exhibit a flaccid dysarthria and show some of the following characteristics during dysarthria testing.

Phonation. Unilateral vocal fold paralysis is relatively unusual in disease processes affecting the brainstem nuclei. If unilateral damage is present, the quality of phonation depends on the position of the vocal fold. If it is paralyzed in an adducted position, the voice is harsh, and loudness is reduced. If it is in the abducted position, more breathiness is heard with reduced loudness. More likely is bilateral vocal cord involvement resulting in breathy voice, inspiratory stridor (or audible inhalation), and abnormally short phrases.

Articulation. Imprecise consonant production may be present ranging from mild to severe (unintelligible speech) degree. The consonants requiring firm contact with the palate from tongue tip elevation are particularly vulnerable. Plosives such as /p/, /t/, and /k/ and fricatives such as /f/ and /s/ are frequently distorted because of the lack of intraoral pressure that results from palatal dysfunction or insufficient tongue-palate, bilabial, or labiodental constriction.

Resonance. Hypernasality is noted as a prominent characteristic of the patients with flaccid dysarthria whose disease or injury affected velopharyngeal function. Nasal emission of air is also found in a high percentage of such patients.

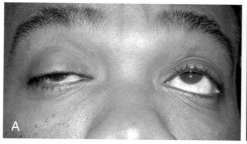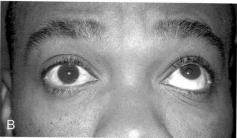

Fig. 8.2 (A) Ptosis of the left eyelid. (B) Left eyelid elevates during the tensilon test.

Prosody. Flaccid dysarthria is often accompanied by monotony of pitch and loudness.

Swallowing

A brainstem **cerebrovascular accident (CVA)** can cause flaccid dysarthria with lesions affecting the motor nuclei. A study of over 500 stroke patients admitted to a rehabilitation unit found that 15% were admitted with brainstem strokes,[22,47] with many patients exhibiting flaccid dysarthria. Of these patients, roughly half (47%) are estimated to also exhibit dysphagia.[22] Aspiration in this population occurs more often because of reduced airway protection or large amounts of stasis (insufficient clearing of food) in the pharyngeal recesses, particularly in the piriform sinuses. Incomplete as well as delayed relaxation of the cricopharyngeal sphincter was also noted in some of these patients.

Myasthenia Gravis

Myasthenia gravis is a neuromuscular disease that often produces flaccid dysarthria. This is a chronic autoimmune disease resulting from a reduction in available acetylcholine receptors at the neuromuscular junction due to the disease process that produces acetylcholine antibodies. It may be associated with other autoimmune diseases, such as rheumatoid arthritis. A tumor of the thymus gland in the chest can occur in some patients. Symptoms of myasthenia gravis may include changes in the eyes such as drooping of the eyelid, known as ptosis (Fig. 8.2). Double vision may also occur. In myasthenia gravis, oral muscles may be weak, with jaw sagging accompanied by weak chewing. Swallowing difficulty is not uncommon.[1]

Some patients present with dysphonia as their primary and only initial symptom, with no other sign of dysarthria. The flaccid dysphonia of myasthenia should be suspected when, despite normal laryngoscopic findings, the voice nevertheless becomes progressively breathier and more reduced in intensity as the client speaks. Respiratory weakness, in addition to extremity weakness, may be present, and myasthenia can occur with no oral motor involvement. Administration of an anticholinesterase agent, known as the tensilon test, is a diagnostic procedure used to confirm a diagnosis of myasthenia. Fig. 8.2 shows improvement in eyelid elevation during the tensilon test. For speech, the client would be asked to continue to speak until the dysarthric symptoms are noted in articulation, resonance, or voice. The tensilon would then be injected a

---

BOX 8.2 Lower Motor Neuron Lesions

2 Flaccid Dysarthria
- May be caused by any disease that affects part of the motor unit (viral infections, tumors, nerve trauma, brainstem stroke)
- Selective impairment of a muscle or muscle group can occur, resulting in a flaccid paralysis, brainstem cerebrovascular accident, or bulbar palsy
- Damage resulting in flaccid paralysis, hyporeflexia, and shrunken or atrophied muscle
- Hypernasality and nasal emission common; selective consonants, plosives, and fricatives often affected
- Frequent aspiration
- Myasthenia gravis, a chronic autoimmune disease caused by reduced acetylcholine receptors at neuromuscular junctions, results in a unique symptomatology
  - Ptosis, double vision, muscle weakness, and dysphagia common
  - Flaccid dysphonia, progressive breathiness, and reduced voice intensity common

---

little at a time, and if myasthenia is the correct diagnosis, dramatic improvement in speech would result in a short period of time as the client continues to speak. Treatment for myasthenia gravis includes drugs such as cholinesterase inhibitors, corticosteroids and immunosuppressants, plasma exchange, immunoglobulin infusion (IVIg), and thymectomy to remove the source of abnormal antibody production. Box 8.2 summarizes the lower motor lesions.

MIXED UPPER AND LOWER MOTOR NEURON LESIONS

Amyotrophic Lateral Sclerosis

A common finding in clinical practice is a lesion or disease process that has not confined itself to one motor system but instead has affected both UMN and LMN systems. The most frequently encountered example of this damage is **amyotrophic lateral sclerosis (ALS,** also known as **Lou Gehrig disease).**

Etiology

ALS causes progressive degeneration of the neurons of the UMN and LMN systems and is of unknown etiology. Onset is typically in the fifth decade, although it may be earlier or later, and early symptoms depend on which motor neurons initially are affected. About 25% of ALS patients experience a bulbar (UMN) onset with the remaining experiencing spinal or limb onset (LMN).[44] In both cases the disease progression ultimately affects both the UMN and the LMN systems. As the disease progresses, verbal communication and oral feedings become progressively difficult. The patient with this type of ALS has a variable life expectancy but typically may survive only 1 to 3 years after onset. Pneumonia is frequently the cause of death. ALS has no known effective treatment or cure, although many palliative treatments are available, including physical therapy, drugs for reduction of muscle pain, and speech therapy, which focuses on improving communication and managing swallowing. The primary involvement of the SLP is to help prepare the patient for worsening speech and swallowing functions and to establish compensatory strategies, including augmentative and alternative communication (AAC) systems.

Associated Neurologic Characteristics

Signs may be present from damage to both UMN and LMN systems. Muscles are weak, but reflexes are hyperactive. Spasticity is usually present unless the LMN damage is well advanced.

Orofacial Movements

The motor neuron disease impairs tongue functions in all ALS groups. As a consequence, tongue movements are more impaired during speech than jaw and lip movements. With disease progression, tongue speed becomes slower while jaw speed increases. It is currently unclear if the increase in jaw movements and speed is a compensatory mechanism or part of the disease.[11,29]

Auditory-Perceptual Speech Characteristics

Speech characteristics in ALS are typically mixed spastic-flaccid dysarthria progressing to total anarthria. In bulbar onset ALS, speech tends to have more spastic qualities, while speech in patients with a spinal onset tends to be more flaccid. With involvement of both UMN and LMN systems, a mixed pattern of dysarthria is exhibited, including slow rate, strain-strangled and/or harsh vocal quality, low pitch, breathy weak voice, hypernasality, nasal emissions, audible inspiration, and short breath groups.[9]

Swallowing

The degree of dysphagia in patients with ALS varies greatly depending on the extent of involvement of the oral musculature and the type of motor system involvement predominating. Evidence of poor lingual control is frequently found, with lingual stasis and aspiration before the swallow. A delayed swallow response may also be present, causing aspiration before the swallow. Poor tongue propulsion, weak pharyngeal contractions, and/or cricopharyngeal dysfunction may also result in pharyngeal stasis and aspiration after the swallow. Airway protection may be significantly better in patients with predominantly spastic (UMN) symptoms than in those with primarily LMN symptoms. The amount of aspiration may thus be reduced in these patients despite a severe dysarthria.

Dysphagia can either parallel or follow the loss of speech. Managing secretions and maintaining appropriate amounts of fluid intake are often huge challenges for patients with ALS.

Box 8.3 presents an overview of ALS, the most common example of mixed upper and motor neuron lesions.

Ataxic Dysarthria

The cerebellum serves as an important center for the integration or coordination of sensory and motor activities. It receives fibers from the motor and sensory cortex either directly or through intervening nuclei. Damage to the cerebellum and/or its pathways causes a disorder called ataxia, and the motor speech symptoms yield an **ataxic dysarthria**. Box 8.5 summarizes ataxic dysarthria.

Etiology

Ataxic dysarthria is often thought to be caused by cerebellar lesions. However, ataxia may be caused by damage at any point in the cerebellar control circuit. Damage may be localized to the cerebellum alone or may be part of more generalized damage affecting several systems. For example, abnormal sensory inputs into the cerebellum, such as diseases involving the proprioceptive system (dorsal column), can result in ataxia. Hence, ataxia may have both motor and sensory components, and not all patients with ataxia have disease pathology in the cerebellum.[27] Some degenerative diseases can also produce ataxia, such as Friedreich ataxia, olivopontocerebellar atrophy, and multiple sclerosis. Other etiologies include stroke, trauma, tumors, alcohol toxicity, drug-induced neurotoxicity (from such drugs as phenytoin [Dilantin], carbamazepine [Tegretol], lithium, or diazepam [Valium]), encephalitis, lung cancer, and severe hypothyroidism.

Associated Neurologic Characteristics

Ataxia is a disruption in the smooth coordination of movement with failure to coordinate sensory data with motor performance. A gait imbalance is often the first symptom of ataxia. Patients may have difficulty going up and down stairs and may need to hold on to railings. In more severe manifestations, ataxic patients may experience frequent falls. Visual difficulties may also be experienced, including double vision (diplopia). A gait test includes observation of walking.

BOX 8.3 Amyotrophic Lateral Sclerosis

- Most common example of mixed upper and lower motor neuron lesions; also known as Lou Gehrig disease
- Causes progressive motor neuron degeneration; usually appears in fifth decade; etiology unknown
- Weak muscles, hyperactive reflexes, and spasticity common
- Weakness in lips, tongue, and palate with reduced range of movement and/or atrophy
- Mixed upper and lower motor neuron symptoms, frequent hypernasality, and imprecise consonant production
- Degree of dysphagia variable; usually follows or parallels degree of dysarthria

Presence of ataxia is signaled by an unsteady, staggering gait, which may be wide based in more severe cases. If a patient is required to close the eyes, a balance disturbance may be observed because of proprioceptive difficulties.

A typical neurologic examination includes finger-nose-finger test, finger-chase test, and a diadochokinetic evaluation. In the first test, patients are required to touch the examiner's finger followed by their own nose, then the finger again. Patients with ataxia may exhibit tremor, particularly when reaching for their nose. In the finger-chase test, the patient is instructed to follow the examiner's moving finger as precisely as possible. A patient with ataxia may over- or undershoot the target, called dysmetria. The diadochokinetic test checks for rapid, alternating movements, such as alternately moving the hand on the thigh in pronation-supination sequences or sliding the heel from knee to shin on the opposite leg repeatedly. A patient with ataxia may demonstrate irregular movements (under- and overshoot) that results in an unsteady rhythm on this task.

Because alcohol affects cerebellar function, law enforcement officers will often use tests of some of these skills in sobriety tests (e.g., walking on a narrow line, alternating hands touching finger to nose). With ataxia, movement is slow to be initiated and slow through the range. Repetitive movements may be irregular and poorly timed, a condition called dysdiadochokinesia. Muscle tone is hypotonic. Intention or kinetic tremor (tremor during purposeful movement) is also present.[27]

Orofacial Movements

The oral mechanism examination is often normal in terms of size, strength, and symmetry of orofacial structures. Drooling is uncommon. However, alternating and sequential motor movements may show irregularity of movement, with overshoot and undershoot on occasion.

Auditory-Perceptual Speech Characteristics

Ataxic dysarthria is often described as **scanning speech**, a pattern of breaking up syllables that impacts prosody.[27] The term was introduced by Charcot[6] to describe the speech of a patient with multiple sclerosis. Charcot described the speech as being very slow, with a pause after each syllable as if the words were being measured or scanned.

Scanning speech is more typically described as "equal and excess stress" prosodic pattern in our field. Other characteristics of ataxic dysarthria include articulatory and phonatory difficulties, described next.

Phonation. Phonation is often perceived as harsh, with monopitch and monoloudness tendencies. In more severe cases, excessive loudness variations and a voice tremor may also be noted.

Articulation. Imprecise consonant production, vowel distortion, and irregular articulatory breakdown mark the speech of ataxic dysarthria. Duffy[12] postulates that in some patients the irregular articulatory breakdown may predominate over prosodic differences, giving the speech an intoxicated, irregular character that overrides the measured aspect of excess and equal stress patterns. Speech diadochokinetic tasks often reveal these irregular breakdowns as well as a variable articulatory rate.

Resonance. Velopharyngeal functioning is usually intact, with normal resonance characteristics, although some patients may demonstrate hypernasal resonance. Nasal emission is less frequently demonstrated.

Prosody rate. Prosody rate is usually slow and often variable. Prosodic changes are usually readily observable in ataxic dysarthria. The prosody characteristic termed **excess and equal stress** by Darley et al.,[7] is a predominant feature, although it is not found in all speakers with ataxic dysarthria. This description refers to the tendency to put excessive vocal emphasis on typically unstressed syllables and words. Some phonemes and intervals between phonemes may be prolonged. Rate is usually slow and often variable. Excessive loudness variability has been noted in a third of the patients; the term **explosive speech** is used to describe these loudness variations. Although they do not occur often, they are striking when present.[14]

Swallowing. Swallowing difficulty is often not recognized in ataxic disorders, although potential dysphagia should become more recognized in this population. A recent study in Germany screened 119 patients with progressive (vs. static) ataxia over a 30-month period. The study excluded patients with dementia or progressive cognitive decline. The researchers found that 17% of this population experienced unrecognized dysphagic symptoms, but only 1% reported dysphagia as a disabling symptom. The study also found an association between dysphagia and reduced health-related quality of life, with aspiration pneumonia a major factor.[40] Ataxic dysarthria is summarized in Box 8.5.

DYSKINETIC DYSARTHRIAS

Hypokinetic Dysarthria

Hypokinetic and hyperkinetic dysarthrias are types of dyskinesias and are due to basal ganglia lesions. The basal ganglia control circuit contributes to complex movements by integrating and controlling the component parts of the movements and by inhibiting unplanned movement. Lesions to the basal ganglia produce dyskinetic movements. If movements are reduced, the dyskinesia is termed hypokinetic. If movements and/or tone are increased, the dyskinesia is termed hyperkinetic, as summarized in Box 8.4.

Parkinsonism

The most common disease associated with **hypokinetic dysarthria** is Parkinson disease. This disorder is characterized by degenerative changes in the substantia nigra, which cause a deficiency in the chemical neurotransmitter dopamine in the caudate nucleus and putamen.

Etiology

Parkinson disease is usually idiopathic (i.e., spontaneous, not caused by another disease). It is a progressive disease that affects movement; the first sign is often a tremor in the hands. Symptoms progress slowly but gradually, with significant variability in disease progress. There are other illnesses that share features with Parkinson disease and which are

BOX 8.4   Basal Ganglia Lesions

3 Hypokinetic Dysarthria: Parkinsonism

- Parkinson disease: most common disease associated with hypokinetic dysarthria; usually idiopathic
- Three cardinal features: tremor, rigidity, and bradykinesia
- Slow rate of movement of tongue, lips, and palate
- Speech varies considerably with pathology, but hypophonia and accelerated speech rate are key features in most patients
- Dysphagic symptoms in all four stages of swallow

4 Hyperkinetic Dysarthria
4.1 Essential Tremor
- Encountered as organic voice tremor when larynx involved; may be pure with no other tremor present
- Involuntary alternations of noted in mild cases; in severe cases, voice stoppage

4.2 Chorea
- Two major types: Sydenham's chorea (childhood complication following infection, typically resolving spontaneously) and Huntington's chorea (progressive and fatal genetic disease)
- Huntington disease characterized by dementia and involuntary movements
- Variable presence of hypotonia and involuntary movement
- Harsh, strained-strangled voice quality common, along with transient breathiness, excessive loudness, and problems with pitch; often imprecise consonants and distorted vowels
- Dysphagia common in Huntington disease; oral swallowing stages significantly affected

4.3 Dystonia and Athetosis
- Classified as the slow hyperkinesias; no well-established etiologies
- Dystonic (excessive tone) trunk, neck, and proximal limb parts; athetotic (writhing) movements of arms, face, and trunk
- Dysarthric features of dystonia and dysarthric features of athetosis: harsh, strained-strangled voice, imprecise consonants, vowel distortion, hypernasality, and velar control
- Dysarthric features of dystonia and dysarthric features of athetosis: excessively loud or breathy; problems with jaw, tongue, and lip movement
- Limited information on dysphagia

4.4 Tardive Dyskinesia
- Caused by long-term use of phenothiazines and similar classes of drugs
- Choreiform, myoclonic, peculiar rhythmic movements and abnormal oral movement
- Usually mild speech disorders
- Possible poor coordination in any stage of swallow

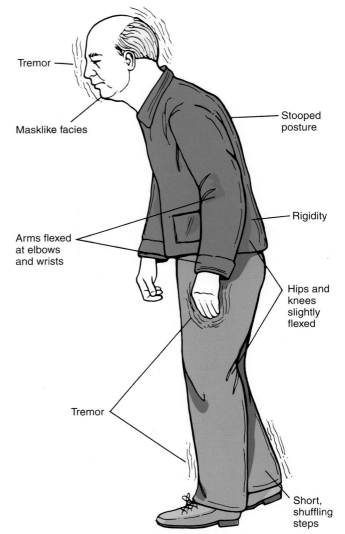

Fig. 8.3 Parkinson's disease. (From Monahan, F. D., Drake, T., & Neighbors, M. [1994]. *Nursing care of adults.* WB Saunders.)

Associated Neurologic Characteristics

The three cardinal features of parkinsonism are tremor, rigidity, and bradykinesia.[27] A tremor may be present at rest that tends to subside on movement and is absent during sleep. It is often called a pill-rolling tremor because of the pattern of movement of the fingers, as if rolling a small pill between the thumb and the fingers. Rigidity is a common characteristic and is elicited by passive movement of the limb, which induces involuntary contractions in the muscle being stretched. The rigidity may be smooth or intermittent (referred to as **cogwheel rigidity**). Bradykinesia is defined as slowness of movement of a muscle through its range. Hypokinesia, or reduced amplitude of movement, is a prime characteristic as well. Fig. 8.3 depicts characteristic posturing and tremor of Parkinson disease.

Cognitive changes occur at any stage in Parkinson disease, particularly as the disease progresses or the patient ages. Dementia prevalence is found in about 30% of more advanced cases,[23] with predominant deficits in executive functions, visuospatial perception, attention, and memory. Language is also impacted in parkinsonian dementia, with impaired

collectively called **parkinsonism** (or Parkinson-like symptoms). Etiology of parkinsonian illnesses can be caused by carbon monoxide poisoning, arteriosclerosis, manganese poisoning, and some tranquilizing drugs (e.g., prochlorperazine [Compazine], trifluoperazine [Stelazine], and haloperidol [Haldol]).

receptive vocabulary, difficulty comprehending the meanings of ambiguous sentences, difficulty with verbal description, and impaired ability to identify a speaker's intention. Analysis of discourse in patients with Parkinson disease found a higher percentage of incomplete and erroneous cohesive ties than in normal control subjects, which supports the conclusion that the basal ganglia play a role in cognitive-communicative functioning.[16]

There are additional features of parkinsonism. One is micrographia, the tendency for the height of the handwritten letters to get smaller as the person writes. Micrographia may occur before other motor symptoms and may assist with early diagnosis of Parkinson disease. Micrographia may also occur with other disorders of the basal ganglia.[26]

Other features show the effect of reduced movement (hypokinesia). Reduced facial expression, often termed a masked face or masked facies, is observed with disease progress. Posture in Parkinson disease is characteristic: stooped and leaning slightly forward. Gait is also characteristic and is described as a festinating gait, with short, slow, shuffling steps. Other features include impaired salivation and a dysphonia (see later).

Treatment for parkinsonism usually involves both pharmacologic and nonpharmacologic approaches. In terms of medications, patients are often treated with a dopamine agonist drug, such as levodopa (L-**dopa**), or a combination of carbidopa/levodopa, such as Sinemet or bromocriptine (Parlodel). Nonpharmacologic approaches include exercise and rehabilitative therapies (physical, occupational, and speech).[2] With medication-resistant tremor or worsening motor symptoms, a surgical procedure called deep brain stimulation (DBS) has demonstrated clinical usefulness in the treatment of tremor, rigidity, slowness, difficulty walking, and dystonia.[19] In DBS a surgically implanted battery-operated medical device called an implantable pulse generator is placed in the brain. In Parkinson disease the target area is most often the subthalamic nucleus, although implantation in the GP_i (globus pallidus) is not uncommon. The mechanism through which stimulation affects neurotransmission in different brain regions has not been determined, although it does not appear to be limited to inhibition or excitation of the basal ganglia. The effects of DBS vary over time. For example, the effects on tremor are immediate, while the effects on dystonia appear over several weeks after implantation.[3] DBS does not cure the disease and does not slow neurodegeneration, but it can provide substantial relief for some symptoms.

Orofacial Movement

Typical findings from the standard oral examination include slow rate of movement of the lips and tongue as the major finding, with some reduced range of movement. Palatal movement may be sluggish. Diadochokinetic rate testing often yields more interesting information. During syllable repetition, reduced range of movement becomes more evident. The patient also tends to show an accelerated or rapid rate of speaking. As repetition continues, oral movements become less distinct and syllables may seem to run together. Some patients may use so little movement that, combined with a rapid rate, no differentiation can be made between syllables and more of a humming or whirring sound.

Auditory-Perceptual Speech Characteristics

Speech difficulties in parkinsonism are common, with an estimated 89% of the population exhibiting impaired speech production. Despite this staggering number, fewer than 5% of patients receive a referral to speech therapy. Speech impairments may be early indicators of Parkinson disease, with hypophonia a particular complaint. Impairments in phonation and articulation are the most frequently observed characteristic of parkinsonian speech.[8]

Phonation. Impairments in the respiratory system is common in Parkinson disease. Some patients were found to have smaller rib cage volume,[43] resulting in hypophonia, or an abnormally weak voice. Hypophonia is common in Parkinson disease and may be an early indicator of its presence. In addition to the reduced speech volume, breathiness, pitch fluctuations leading to a harsh vocal quality, and vocal tremor are strong characteristics of Parkinson disease and are collectively known as parkinsonian dysarthria or hypokinetic dysarthria.[8]

Duffy[12] notes that, even when not pervasive, a strained, whispered aphonia is occasionally noted in the midst of a breathy, harsh vocal quality, occurring toward the end of a vowel-prolongation task and persisting for several seconds. Like gait festinations, oral festinations are sometimes noted in parkinsonian speech, an involuntary acceleration of the rate of speech along with reduced pitch variations, resulting in rapid, unintelligible bursts of speech.[8]

Improving hypophonia is frequently targeted in speech therapy. One methodology is called the Lee Silverman Voice Treatment (LSVT). Studies have demonstrated strong evidence for immediate posttherapy voice improvement and some evidence of long-term maintenance.[8,17]

Articulation. Articulation disorders occur in a significant proportion of patients with Parkinson disease. Most descriptions of the articulatory differences in Parkinson disease report imprecise consonants, irregular articulatory breakdowns, prolonged phonemes, and distorted vowels. The imprecision of consonants may be the most salient articulatory change, most likely due to impaired movement of the articulators. The consonants that require the greatest degree of constriction in the vocal tract tend to be the most distorted in Parkinson disease, specifically high vowels, plosives, fricatives, and affricates.[43]

Resonance. Perceptual analysis of the speech of patients with Parkinson disease showed mild to moderate resonance differences, with increased and intermittent hypernasality in 65% of patients. Nevertheless, hypernasality does not appear to be a cardinal feature of hypokinetic dysarthria when compared to articulation and phonation traits.[37]

Prosody. Prosodic changes are prominent in Parkinson disease. Reduced pitch and loudness leads to the impression of monotonous speech, worsening with disease progress. Speaking rate is variable, with some syllables prolonged and others shortened, and pause duration is variable. In some patients, short rushes of speech and inappropriate silences have been noted.

The presence of **palilalia** has also been described in Parkinson disease. Palilalia is characterized by repetitions that usually involve words, phrases, or sentences and is usually associated with bilateral subcortical damage. This compulsive repetition of phonemes and syllables, noted as dysfluency, has been frequently observed in patients with Parkinson disease as well as in other neurologic and psychiatric disorders. A recent case study reports on the presence of palilalia in a patient who contracted Covid-19 and encephalitis.[30]

Swallowing

More than 80% of parkinsonian patients develop dysphagia during the course of the disease, until the advanced stages of the disease when all patients will present with some form of dysphagia.[46] Swallowing difficulty reduces quality of life, complicates medication intake, and may lead to malnutrition and aspiration pneumonia, a major cause of death in Parkinson disease, with estimates of 30% of deaths resulting from aspiration pneumonia. Despite the high prevalence, only 20% to 40% of parkinsonian patients report awareness of swallowing difficulty.[45] This reduced awareness of swallowing difficulties is particularly problematic in the early stages, when symptoms are more subtle.[46]

Dysphagic symptoms have been identified in all four stages of swallowing. The muscle rigidity and bradykinesia that are iconic in parkinsonian patients contribute to swallowing difficulty. In the oral preparatory phase, reduced sense of smell and taste, reduced proprioceptive feedback from oral structures, weakness and rigidity of oral structures, and disturbed motion of tongue and jaw are prominent factors in dysphagia. In the oral phase, festination of the tongue and soft palate have been reported, in addition to reduced oral bolus control. In the pharyngeal phase, reduced and disturbed motion of the velum and pharyngeal structures along with insufficient laryngeal vestibule closure and dysfunction of the epiglottis and intrinsic phonatory muscles contribute to dysphagia. In the esophageal phase, muscular discoordination and slowness impact esophageal sphincter action.[46]

Impaired salivation has also been reported in Parkinson disease. Some studies report xerostomia (reduced salivation), while other researchers found excessive salivation.[45] In either case, this impaired salivation can have an impact on the swallowing function.

The clinical assessment of dysphagia in parkinsonian patients is challenging and often delivers unreliable results. A modified water test assessing maximum swallowing volume can be used to evaluate oropharyngeal dysphagia. Other evaluation methods include flexible endoscopic evaluation of swallowing and videofluoroscopic swallowing studies, considered the gold standard for this disorder. In addition, parkinsonian-specific questionnaires and high-resolution manometry can further the evaluation.[46]

Treatment of dysphagia includes optimizing dopaminergic medications, particularly in the earlier phases when fluctuations in motor control occur. A promising novel method is an intensive training of expiratory muscle strength. While deep brain stimulation can help reduce the impact of tremors, it has no clinical relevance to swallowing dysfunction.[46]

Hyperkinetic Dysarthrias

While hypokinesia is related to reduction of movement, hyperkinesia is due to an increase in involuntary movement, although both dyskinesias stem from extrapyramidal system damage. Hyperkinetic disorders are varied and heterogeneous. The types most pertinent to our field will be discussed in this section, including tremor, chorea, athetosis, and dystonia.

Essential Tremor

Tremor can be classified as either normal or abnormal/pathologic depending on whether it is associated with a disease state. Both normal and **pathologic tremor** may occur at rest, in static postures, or with movement.

Essential tremor, also called isolated voice tremor, primary voice tremor, or organic voice tremor, is the tremor most often encountered by SLPs. In this condition the extrinsic and intrinsic muscles of the larynx may show tremor either independently or along with tremor of other parts of the body, such as the hands, jaw, or head. The age at onset of this tremor is over 60 years, and the vast majority of cases affect women (75–93%).[28]

Auditory-Perceptual Speech Characteristics

In essential tremor, affected structures include larynx, velum, pharynx, and base of the tongue. The perceptual equivalent of this distribution is disordered phonation in the setting of relatively intact articulatory and resonance characteristics. During a vowel prolongation task, the mildly affected patient's voice has a regular tremor of altering pitch and loudness. With more severe disease the voice may simply stop, resembling the disorder known as spastic dysphonia. However, significant differences have been found between the two disorders in terms of regularity of voice arrest and accompanying characteristics. Patients with essential tremor also demonstrate excessively low pitch and monopitch, intermittent or constant strained-strangled harshness, and pitch breaks.

Chorea

Chorea describes the presence of movements that are irregular and involuntary, affecting the limbs and trunk, and involving the respiratory and orofacial musculature. Chorea is associated with basal ganglia dysfunction; however, the underlying neural mechanism is not well understood. Any process that damages the basal ganglia or related brain structures can cause hyperkinesias; these processes include degenerative, vascular, traumatic, inflammatory, toxic, and metabolic disorders. The two major diseases in this group are **Sydenham chorea** and **Huntington chorea**. Several medical conditions are associated with chorea although chorea is mainly associated with Huntington's Disease. Sydenham's chorea is also well described in the pediatric literature.

Huntington disease is an inherited, neurodegenerative disease characterized by progressive motor, cognitive, and behavioral decline. It follows an autosomal dominant inheritance, and the child of an affected individual has a 50% chance of developing the disease. Onset of this disease is typically between ages 35 and 50, although there is a juvenile variant and a late onset variant, above age 60. The cause of this disease is unknown, but it is progressive and fatal with the majority of patients dying from complications of aspiration pneumonia.[25] Brain changes documented usually include loss of neurons from the basal ganglia, including the caudate nucleus and pallidum, as well as loss of neurons from the cerebral cortex.

Sydenham chorea (called St. Vitus's dance in ancient terminology) is a noninherited infection/immune-related childhood disease that may follow such conditions as strep throat, rheumatic fever, or scarlet fever. The symptoms usually clear within 6 months.

Associated Neurologic Characteristics

Chorea is characterized by rapid, involuntary, usually purposeless movements. They occur unpredictably and may involve any group of muscles but are more likely to involve distal rather than proximal muscles. Voluntary and automatic movements may be interrupted so that coordinated breathing and speech may be quite difficult. The limbs are hypotonic and postures cannot be maintained. Cognitive changes accompany the progression of the disease, eventually resulting in an associated dementia, and some psychiatric symptoms are also associated, with depression being the most common.

Orofacial Motor Characteristics

The presence of hypotonia and involuntary movement of the orofacial musculature is variable in chorea. A common characteristic of Huntington disease is the inability to keep the tongue protruded for more than a few seconds. Sydenham chorea often involves involuntary movements of the mouth and larynx. Even if little involuntary movement of oral musculature is present, speech will probably be affected by the movements of other parts of the body.

Auditory-Perceptual Speech Characteristics

In the Mayo Clinic study of 30 adults with chorea, the following problems were noted.[14]

Phonation. A harsh voice quality and/or a strained-strangled sound were found in many patients. Intermittent breathiness also occurred. Excess loudness variations were prominent because of poor movement control. Lower-than-average pitch levels, voice stoppages, and pitch breaks were also noted. Sudden forced inspiration or expiration was observed in some patients.

According to Duffy,[12] hyperkinetic dysarthria is the only dysarthria in which abnormal noises can interrupt speech; because these abnormal noises are involuntary, they can occur at any point and not only during speech.

Articulation. The involuntary muscle movements impact articulatory precision. In some patients, vowel distortion is also noted. The articulatory difficulty is typically intermittent and is referred as irregular articulatory breakdown.

Resonance. Intermittent hypernasality is a feature of chorea presumably because of choreatic movements of the velopharyngeal mechanism.[37] The interference with resonance also contributed to articulatory problems, including imprecise consonants and short phrases.

Prosody. Chorea also impacts prosody. Hyperkinetic dysarthria features include reduced stress, short phrasing, prolonged intervals, and variable rates. These features contribute to the perception of prosodic deviations and highly bizarre speech patterns.

Swallowing

Dysphagia is common, and aspiration pneumonia is a leading cause of death in Huntington disease.[39] The severity of dysphagia varies from patient to patient primarily because of the constantly changing postures and interpatient variability inherent in the clinical population. All stages of swallowing are affected by choreatic movements. The oral stages of the swallow are significantly affected by the irregular and uncoordinated tongue movements and changes in facial tone. Aspiration before the swallow may occur because these random movements prematurely push the bolus over the base of the tongue. Irregular and uncoordinated movements of the vocal folds and the respiratory musculature as well as neck hyperextension may compromise airway protection. Pharyngeal peristalsis may be weak, and esophageal dysmotility has been reported.[36]

Management recommendations include assessment of dysphagia, starting at the early stages of the disease, and should continue during the course of the disease, based on the recommendations of treating clinicians. Instrumental assessment of swallowing by videofluoroscopy or videoendoscopy is feasible and recommended. Clinical assessment tools and the use of patient-reported outcomes should supplement but not replace instrumental assessments.[39]

Dystonia and Athetosis

Dystonia and **athetosis** are movement disorders classified as the slow hyperkinesias. Movements are characteristically unstable and sustained, suggesting possible conflicts between flexion and extension of the muscles.

Etiology

Most of these disorders do not have well-established etiologies or focal lesion sites. Encephalitis, vascular lesions, birth trauma, and degenerative neuronal disease are often precipitating diseases. Most hyperkinesias show localized damage to the confines of the basal ganglia and are sometimes caused by the effects of drugs such as phenothiazines and related compounds, especially the more powerful tranquilizers.

Athetosis is a rare disorder usually seen as a form of congenital cerebral palsy. It is also seen as a rare progressive disease of adolescence, the cause of which is unknown, and as an accompanying residual deficit with hemiplegia after cerebral infarction. Localization of the lesion is difficult, but the putamen seems to be almost always involved.

Associated Neurologic Characteristics

Dystonia implies excess tone in selected parts of the body. Dystonia mainly affects the trunk, neck, and proximal parts of the limbs. The slow movements are usually sustained for a prolonged period. The movements usually build up to a peak, are sustained, and then recede, although they occasionally begin with a jerk.

Athetotic movements are slow and writhing and predominantly affect the arms, face, and tongue. The movements tend to be exaggerated by attempts at voluntary activity, which make voluntary movements clumsy and inaccurate.

Auditory-Perceptual Speech Characteristics

The dystonic patient usually has a harsh or strained-strangled voice quality. A small subset of patients may demonstrate intermittent breathiness and audible inspiration. Monopitch and monoloudness are also seen in these patients. Because of the involuntary movements, dystonic patients often have voice stoppages and periods of inappropriate silence. Excess loudness variations accompany the excessive movement. Voice tremor is also found among dystonic patients.

Phonation in athetosis is often significantly affected. The patient often has poor respiratory reserve and respiratory patterns. Both dilator and constrictor spasms have been noted in laryngeal functioning. Voicing is often excessively loud or excessively breathy, and it is unpredictable and frequently poorly coordinated with articulation.

Spasmodic Dysphonia

Spasmodic dysphonia is a chronic, task-specific focal dystonia of unknown etiology.[34] This disorder was once known in the literature as spastic dysphonia but has come to be more accurately referred to by its current name. There are three forms of this disorder: adductor, abductor, and mixed. Adductor is the most common by far, but the other two forms are certainly seen, and differential diagnosis is important to treatment.

Adductor spasmodic dysphonia is characterized by a strained voice quality with voice arrests caused by laryngeal adductor spasm. It is frequently associated with pain in the laryngeal area. The interruptions to phonatory airflow are assumed to be caused by hyperadduction of the vocal folds, but indirect laryngoscopy usually reveals normal vocal fold movements. Abductor spasmodic dysphonia is caused by laryngospasms during abduction of the vocal cords resulting in intermittent breathiness or aphonia. Both intermittent strained quality and breathy quality are perceived when there is a mixture of adductor and abductor spasms; the mixed form occurs in a smaller percentage of patients.[31]

Focal dystonias were believed to be caused by dysfunction of the basal ganglia; more recently, this view was expanded to include the cerebellum and sensorimotor cortical regions. Although the pathophysiology of spasmodic dysphonia remains unknown, structural alterations in brain organization were found in patients, including focal reduction of axonal density and myelin in the pyramidal tract. Functional magnetic resonance imaging (fMRI) studies have shown greater activation in cortical motor regions during tasks in spasmodic dysphonia, with greater activation of subcortical structures during symptomatic speech but not asymptomatic

speech. These changes were noted in both adductor and abductor types, suggesting cortical involvement in addition to basal ganglia and thalamic involvement.[33]

The role of the central nervous system (CNS) in spasmodic dysphonia can be seen in the treatments that have been attempted. Initially, treatment focused on restoring voice by altering the innervation of the larynx, including transection of the recurrent laryngeal nerve. Initial reports of this treatment were promising, with a reported 85% to 90% success rate. However, follow-up studies showed that a majority of patients (64%) experienced a recurrence of spasmodic dysphonia. Other procedures included selective laryngeal adduction denervation and reinnervation to alter the impaired laryngeal innervation; long-term results again demonstrated a return to voice breaks in 26% and breathiness in 30% of patients.[33]

Other less drastic treatments include the injection of the neurotoxin botulinum into the affected muscle(s) of the vocal cord. This injection mimics the effect of denervation and reduces laryngeal muscle activity, but it is effective only temporarily and does not treat the underlying CNS disorder.[33]

Auditory-Perceptual Speech Characteristics

Phonation. Spasmodic dysphonia is often described as a strained vocal quality with intermittent and involuntary voice arrests, particularly common in the adductor type. In the abductor type, a breathy vocal quality is often noted. Patients may demonstrate normal voice production during laughing, crying, yawning, singing, whispering, or shouting.[4]

Articulation. As might be predicted, the articulation of patients with these involuntary movement disorders is highly variable, with a range of severity from slight distortion to unintelligible. Distortions include vowels as well as consonants. In the adductor type, vowel distortions are common; in abductor spasmodic dysphonia, voiceless consonants are often distorted.

Resonance. Hypernasality is a prominent feature due to the disturbance in velopharyngeal closure.

Prosody. The prosody in spasmodic dysphonia is impaired, with aberrant rate of speech, short phrases, and prolonged intervals. Prolongation of phonemes has also been observed. Reduction of stress is a relatively prominent characteristic of speech production in spasmodic dysphonia.

Swallowing

Dysphagia in spasmodic dysphonia has rarely been reported except as secondary to botulinum injections. When neurotoxins are introduced to laryngeal muscles, temporary weakness of laryngeal closure and reduced airway protection may occur. In such cases, patients have reported choking on liquids. Within 2 to 6 weeks after injection, the neurotoxin weakens and swallowing difficulties resolve, although phonatory problems may reemerge. The speech pathologist can be instrumental in preparing patients prior to the injection by training to take small sips of liquid and utilizing the chin tuck technique for improved airway protection. In a review article, only one case of dysphagia in spasmodic dysphonia was found that was unrelated to botulinum injection.[4]

Tardive Dyskinesia

Another movement disorder resulting from extrapyramidal damage is **tardive dyskinesia**, which is a movement disorder resulting from chronic use of dopamine receptor blocking medications. Tardive refers to the delayed onset of this disorder because symptoms appear some time after the medication is started. There appears to be a genetic cause for susceptibility to tardive dyskinesia because women and people from African and European ethnicity appear to be more at risk for developing this disorder. Tardive dyskinesia is a potentially permanent condition; stopping the medication does not always relieve the condition.[20]

Symptoms develop insidiously and movements are rhythmic, repetitive, and stereotypical, involving the face, mouth, and tongue, and often involving the trunk and extremities. In terms of oral movements, constant random movements of the lips and tongue may be seen, with a frequent fly-catcher's movement of the tongue in which the tongue involuntarily moves in and out of the mouth. Velar movement may also be involved. Intelligibility is variably affected, with some patients becoming unintelligible because of the random movements. Most patients, however, present with a mild dysarthria only.

The random movements may result in poor coordination in any of the four stages of swallowing. Pocketing of food, pharyngeal stasis, and aspiration before, during, and after the swallow may occur. Reflux of food may be a result of esophageal discoordination. Decreased sensation may also result in lack of reflexive cough or silent aspiration.

MIXED DYSARTHRIAS WITH DIVERSE LESIONS

Multiple Sclerosis

Multiple sclerosis is an acquired, disabling, inflammatory autoimmune disease of the CNS affecting young adults. It is considered the most common nontraumatic disabling disease of young adults, with the first attack between ages 20 and 40. It has an estimated prevalence of 2.3 million people worldwide, with the highest prevalence in North America followed by Europe, and the lowest prevalence in sub-Saharan Africa and East Asia.[13]

The neuroinflammatory nature of multiple sclerosis causes demyelination and a heterogenous array of signs and symptoms, including the involvement of motor, sensory, visual, and autonomic systems. Often, the first symptom of multiple sclerosis is impaired vision, including blurred or double vision and color distortion. In the majority of cases, multiple sclerosis manifests an exacerbating (worsening) and remitting (decreasing) nature. In the remaining one-third of cases, the course of the illness is progressive without remission. On MRI, areas of scar tissue (sclerosis) of varying size are seen in the white matter of brains of persons diagnosed with multiple sclerosis. Microscopic changes reveal more changes in deep and cortical grey matter.[12]

Etiology

There does not appear to be a single cause of multiple sclerosis, although some risk factors have been identified. For example, exposure to the Epstein-Barr virus, sunshine, and smoking along with a genetic susceptibility appear to increase the risks of developing this illness.[12]

Associated Neurologic Characteristics

In the initial stages, signs are typically mild and may go unnoticed. They may include transient paresthesias (altered sensation) of the extremities, transient diplopia or blurring of vision, mild weakness or clumsiness, and mild vertigo. At that stage, axons are relatively preserved. As the disease progresses, symptoms increase in severity and include a marked difficulty with gait, dysarthria, significant weakness, visual disturbances, nystagmus, bladder disturbance, and personality change caused by frontal lobe involvement. Cognitive difficulties are noted in about half this population, with impairments in attention, concentration, memory, and poor judgment, particularly in the later stages.[38] Imaging at these stages shows distinct CNS changes.

There are four identified subtypes of multiple sclerosis. Some patients demonstrate the exacerbating-remitting type in which they have attacks from which they recover completely in the early stages of the disease. In the later stages these patients may accumulate disabilities with each new attack. Other patients may have the primary progressive form that follows a chronic progressive course, which usually involves progressive spinal cord dysfunction. This form may evolve from the relapsing form or be present from the onset of the disease.[12,13]

Fig. 8.4 shows an MRI of a patient with multiple sclerosis, where the lesions involve the entire CNS; the peripheral nervous system is seldom involved.

Auditory-Perceptual Speech Characteristics

Dysarthria is a common occurrence in multiple sclerosis (~47%). Symptoms may be mild initially, progressing as the disease progresses. In later stages, dysarthria may be severe enough to warrant AAC.[35]

Because of CNS involvement, dysarthria manifests in various ways depending on the sites of demyelination. Duffy[12] described a mixed spastic-ataxic dysarthria, which may be the most common type of dysarthria associated with multiple sclerosis but should not be considered the only type found. Other forms or combinations of dysarthria may be present.

Phonation. The most frequently encountered deviation is impairment of loudness control. Harsh voice quality and breathiness are also common. Pitch control and inappropriate pitch levels were also found.

Articulation. Articulatory difficulty due to muscular weakness or incoordination is common and impacts consonant production primarily.

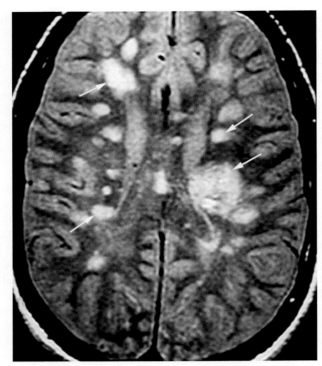

Fig. 8.4 Multiple demyelinated plaques *(arrows)* are seen in this magnetic resonance image of a patient with multiple sclerosis. (Reprinted from Nadeau, S. E., Ferguson, T. S., Valenstein, E., Vierck, C. J., Petruska, J. C., Streit, W. J., & Ritz, L. A. [2004]. *Medical neuroscience.* Saunders.)

Resonance. Multiple sclerosis patients often display some degree of hypernasality due to velopharyngeal weakness.

Prosody. A commonly noted feature is equal and excess stress (scanning speech), typical of ataxic dysarthria. This prosodic feature impacts rate, phrasing, emphasis, and stress.

Swallowing

In a study of 215 consecutive patients with multiple sclerosis, the majority (60%) demonstrated swallowing difficulty on fiber-optic endoscopy regardless of self-report or awareness. In about one-fourth (26.5%) the dysphagia was significant enough to recommend dietary alterations. These subjects tended to have a more severe form of multiple sclerosis.[41]

Multiple System Atrophy (Shy Drager Syndrome)

Shy Drager syndrome was originally classified in 1960 as a neurologic disorder causing atrophy but has since been renamed multiple system atrophy (MSA). MSA is a sporadic, adult-onset, fatal neurodegenerative disease characterized by progressive autonomic failure, parkinsonian features, and a combination of cerebellar and pyramidal features. There are two variants in MSA, depending on whether parkinsonian (MSA-P) or cerebellar (MSA-C) features predominate. The main feature of this disease is atrophy, which affects the cerebellum, pons, and putamen.

Etiology

The exact cause of MSA is unknown; however, research has implicated mitochondrial dysfunction and inflammation,

with a probable genetic susceptibility. MSA affects more men than women, by a ratio of 3:2, and appears most often in the sixth decade of life. MSA-C is largely concentrated in Japan, whereas MSA-P tends to dominate new cases of MSA in Western countries. Prognosis is usually poor, although disease progression is slow.[18]

Associated Neurologic Characteristics

The characteristics associated with MSA include motor dysfunction, sleep disturbances, and autonomic system disorder. In the MSA-P variant, parkinsonian features are prominent, including postural instability, tremor, rigidity, and bradykinesia.[18]

Auditory-Perceptual Speech Characteristics

Consistent with its diagnostic role in other disorders, speech in MSA has been shown to be a sensitive indicator of the presence, and of the type, of MSA. Typical speech patterns include a mixed dysarthria with various combinations of hypokinetic, spastic, and ataxic components. In a study of the speech of 40 consecutive patients with probable MSA, Rusz et al.,[38] found dysarthria to be a prominent clinical feature in all patients, but not in age- and gender-matched controls. Furthermore, the dysarthria characteristics identified the type of MSA. In MSA-P, excess pitch and loudness variations, slow rate, imprecise consonant production, prolonged phonemes, vocal tremor, and strain-strangled voice were prominent features. In MSA-C, prolonged phonemes, audible inspirations, and voice stoppages were dominant features. In both, inappropriate silences, irregular rates, and overall slowness of speech were present.[42]

Phonation. In MSA-P, phonation is marked by excess pitch and loudness variations, vocal tremor, and strain-strangled vocal quality. In MSA-C, phonation is marked by audible inspirations and voice stoppages.

Articulation. Imprecise consonants are a predominant feature of MSA-P.

Resonance. Hypernasality may occur if the involvement of the pyramidal system produces elements of a spastic dysarthria.

Prosody. Prosodic irregularity includes inappropriate silences, irregular rates, and overall slowness of speech.

The dysarthrias associated with multiple sclerosis and multiple system atrophy are summarized in Box 8.6.

BOX 8.5   Ataxic Dysarthria

- Caused by damage to the cerebellum and/or its pathways (e.g., degenerative diseases, stroke, trauma, tumors, alcohol toxicity, drug toxicity, encephalitis, lung cancer, hypothyroidism)
- Failure to coordinate sensory data with motor performance, hypotonic muscle, and kinetic tremor
- Irregular articulatory breakdown, slow rate, and readily observable prosodic changes; harshness, excessive loudness, and voice tremor possible

BOX 8.6 Other Mixed Dysarthrias with Diverse Lesions

5 Multiple Sclerosis
- Unknown etiology, although studies suggest a viral agent may be responsible
- Early signs mild; severe signs include gait difficulty, dysarthria, visual disturbances, nystagmus, bladder disturbances, and personality changes
- Mixed spastic-ataxic dysarthria most common; frequent problems with volume and pitch control
- Possible dysphagia with corticobulbar or lower brainstem involvement

6 Multiple System Atrophy (Shy Drager Syndrome)
- Degenerative disease of the autonomic nervous system
- Early signs: bowel and bladder incontinence, impotence, reduction of perspiration, difficulty maintaining blood pressure while standing
- Later signs: gait disturbance, weakness, limb tremor, dysphagia, dysarthria
- Strained-strangled voice quality, wet hoarseness, hypernasality, imprecise consonants, and a poor ability to change pitch all possible

TABLE 8.1 Apraxias

Type	Description
Apraxia	A disorder in performing voluntary learned motor acts caused by a lesion in motor association areas and association pathways, in which similar automatic gestures are intact
Ideomotor apraxia	A disorder in which motor plans are intact, but individual motor gestures are disturbed
Ideational apraxia	A disorder in performing the steps of complex motor plans
Apraxia of speech	A disorder of motor programming of speech
Oral apraxia (buccofacial apraxia)	A disorder of nonspeech movements of the oral muscles
Childhood apraxia of speech	A disorder in which motor speech programming is disturbed in childhood

BOX 8.7 Apraxias

7 Oral Apraxia
- Inability to perform nonspeech movements with muscles of the larynx, pharynx, tongue, and cheeks
- Paralysis, significant weakness, or incoordination of oral musculature not noted on examination
- Affects voluntary and sometimes imitative movements; reflexive preserved

8 Apraxia of Speech
- Impaired ability to execute speech movements voluntarily in the absence of paralysis, weakness, or incoordination of speech musculature
- May appear independent or in conjunction with oral apraxia
- Most often associated with Broca aphasia
- Speech impaired by inconsistent initiation, selection, and sequencing of articulatory movements; no consistent disturbances of phonation, respiration, and resonance; no related neurologic impairments of oral musculature

APRAXIAS

Praxis is a Greek term (*prassein*, "to do"), hence it means performance of an action. Performing an action that is not reflexive or automatic requires planning, timing, and sequencing. Recall that the motor association cortex of the brain has areas devoted to performing the action of muscle movement to produce speech, called motor planning or motor programming areas.

Apraxia is a disorder of learned movement in which the difficulty with movement is not caused by paralysis, weakness, or incoordination of the muscles and cannot be accounted for by sensory loss, comprehension deficits, or inattention to commands. It has also been defined as a disorder of motor planning. Apraxia is a high-level motor disturbance of the integration of the motor components necessary to carry out a complex motor act. Review the section on motor planning in Chapter 6 while studying the description of the disorders of motor programming described here.

Apraxias are important to the SLP because certain types of apraxia may directly affect the motor programs of the speech muscles. Other forms of apraxia often accompany some aphasia types and other cerebral language deficits associated with the cortical motor association areas and the association pathways of the brain. The types of apraxia important to our field are defined in Table 8.1.

Hugo Liepmann (1863-1925) is credited with elucidating the concept of apraxia around 1900, although John Hughlings Jackson described an apraxic disturbance of the tongue as early as 1866. Liepmann used early disconnection theory to explain apraxia and demonstrated lesion sites to support the variety of apraxias described.[28] Because this text is concerned with clinical speech and language

syndromes, the apraxias that affect movements of other parts of the body are not discussed. Remember, however, that a limb or an ideomotor apraxia may also be present in patients with apraxia of speech. Features associated with oral apraxia and apraxia of speech are summarized in Box 8.7.

Oral Apraxia

SLPs recognize a nonspeech disorder of the oral muscles called **oral apraxia**, the inability to perform nonspeech movements with the muscles of the larynx, pharynx, tongue, and cheeks, although automatic and sometimes imitative movements of the same muscles may be preserved. This disorder is not the result of paralysis, weakness, or incoordination of the oral musculature, and it may be isolated or coexist with an apraxia of speech. Oral apraxia is usually called buccofacial apraxia by neurologists.

Oral praxic disturbance must be differentiated from disorders of the motor pathways involved in UMN and LMN systems. A careful cranial nerve examination usually indicates whether the disturbance is on the higher level of motor planning of praxis as opposed to being a lower-level motor deficit associated with either supranuclear lesions or cranial nerve lesions. In lower-level motor deficits of the central and peripheral nervous systems, motor involvement generally affects both voluntary and reflexive oral acts. Voluntary oral motor acts are limited by paralysis, weakness, and incoordination, and the more reflexive acts of mastication and deglutition are affected as well. Supranuclear lesions are associated with typical tongue deviation, hypertonic oral muscles, palatal paresis, hyperactive gag reflex, and lower facial paresis. LMN lesions are associated with tongue deviation and atrophy, hypotonic oral muscles, palatal paresis, and a hyporeflexive gag reflex. Facial paresis is hypotonic. Extrapyramidal lesions produce involuntary movements of oral muscles, and ataxic movements of oral muscles are found in cerebellar disorders. Disorders of praxis will present different signs on oral and speech examination than these.

Oral apraxia testing is completed on a spontaneous level to verbal command and on an imitative level. Commands requiring oral-facial movements such as "lick your lips" or "clear your throat" may be used. Failure to perform appropriately on a number of similar commands suggests a diagnosis of oral apraxia in brain-injured adults. Love and Webb[29] used a 20-item informal test for assessing oral apraxia. Published tests of apraxia of speech usually include tasks for assessing nonverbal oral apraxia.

Apraxia of Speech

Apraxia of speech is an impaired ability to execute voluntarily the appropriate movements for articulation of speech in the absence of paralysis, weakness, or incoordination of the speech musculature. In 1900 Liepmann[28] discussed a form of apraxia that could be localized to the speech muscles; some 40 years earlier, Broca described elements of this disorder as part of aphemia. Aphemia, the defect in speech and language that Broca believed resulted from damage to the third left frontal convolution of the brain, has become known as Broca aphasia.

Apraxia of speech is characterized by articulatory imprecision, reduced speech rate, visible/audible groping for articulatory postures, and dysprosody, which cannot be explained by a peripheral deficit in muscle paralysis or paresis (i.e., dysarthria), or a linguistic impairment (i.e., aphasia).[5] A developmental form of verbal apraxia is known as **childhood apraxia of speech** (see Chapter 12). The current discussion concerns acquired apraxia of speech in adults.

Oral apraxia and apraxia of speech may appear independently or coexist. Oral apraxia may be the basis of a speech apraxia. Speech apraxia may appear in a pure form but is most often accompanied by a language disorder, as seen in classic Broca aphasia. After an acute stroke, patients may present with a transient mutism in the early stages. As symptoms resolve, an apraxia of speech may become apparent. Basilakos[5] advocates for the use of acoustic speech analysis and neuroimaging techniques to improve differential diagnosis and to provide more objective means to compare participants across studies.

Apraxia of speech must be differentiated from dysarthria. In speech apraxia, articulation is impaired by inconsistent initiation, selection, and sequencing of articulatory movements. In dysarthria, articulatory impairments are more consistent. Speech apraxias worsen with linguistic complexity of the utterance so that multisyllabic words are more difficult than monosyllabic words, whereas such complexity effects are not typically seen in dysarthria. In dysarthria, speech production deficits arise from paralysis, weakness, involuntary movement, and/or ataxia of the articulators. Persons affected by apraxia of speech do not have these neurologic impairments of the orofacial musculature; or if they are present, the apraxia is not the cause of these deficits.

SYNOPSIS OF CLINICAL INFORMATION AND APPLICATIONS FOR THE SLP

- Of the acquired neurogenic communication disorders seen in large speech-language pathology practices, the majority are likely to be motor speech disorders.
- Dysarthria and apraxia of speech are the two primary classifications of motor speech disorders.
- The evaluation of a patient with suspected motor speech disorder should include assessment of hearing and language (to rule out other causes of the communication problem or to define accompanying problems), an oral-motor examination, speech-production tasks, and a screening or full assessment of feeding and swallowing.
- Dysarthria implies true organically based paralysis, weakness, or incoordination of the orofacial musculature that results in distortion of speech.
- The Mayo Clinic classification system categorized the dysarthrias into six major classes: spastic, flaccid, hypokinetic, hyperkinetic, ataxic, and mixed. Unilateral UMN dysarthria has been added more recently as a separate type. Each of these dysarthrias is associated with disorders or diseases affecting certain parts of the motor system. Each has associated unique clusters of auditory-perceptual speech features that the student should learn.
- Other diseases and disorders produce dysarthria but were not included in the discussion of the more common disorders. These can be found in Table 8.2.
- Apraxia of speech is a sensorimotor disorder of motor programming of the speech musculature for the production of speech. The primary symptoms are not the result of weakness, paralysis, or incoordination of the oral musculature.
- Apraxia of speech also is associated with damage to the motor speech planning areas of the motor cortex and has certain perceptual features that should be learned.

TABLE 8.2   Other Neurologic Diseases Associated with Dysarthria

Name	Etiology	Speech Symptoms
Bell palsy	Inflammation or lesion of cranial nerve VII	Slurring caused by unilateral weakness of labial muscles
Polyneuritis	Follows infections or may be caused by diabetes or alcohol abuse	Flaccid dysarthria
Hemiballismus	Lesions of subthalamic nucleus	Hyperkinetic dysarthria
Palatopharyngolaryngeal myoclonus	Brainstem lesions producing rhythmic myoclonic movements of the palate, pharynx, and/or larynx	Hyperkinetic dysarthria, which is sometimes only noted on vowel prolongation
Gilles de la Tourette syndrome	No known etiology	Hyperkinetic dysarthria with spontaneous, uncontrolled vocalizations such as barking, grunting, throat clearing, snorting; echolalia and coprolalia (obscene language without provocation) may be present
Olivopontocerebellar atrophy	Degeneration of olivary, pontine, and cerebellar nuclei	Mixed dysarthria of hypokinetic, spastic, and ataxic types
Progressive supranuclear palsy	Neuronal atrophy in brainstem and cerebellar structures	Mixed dysarthria, which may include hypokinetic, spastic, and ataxic types

CASE STUDY

A 48-year-old accountant reported excess stress in his life. He often made presentations to various companies looking to hire his accounting firm. For the past several months, he reported to his physician that he had been having difficulty speaking and swallowing. He described his speech as "sounding like I am speaking through my nose." He also admitted to noticing mild tremors of his eyebrows and mouth. An oral peripheral mechanism examination revealed bilateral facial weakness, reduced tongue strength, and a hyperactive gag reflex, which was a new finding for him. After an extensive diagnostic workup, the physician diagnosed this patient with ALS.

Questions for Consideration

1. What type of dysarthria is usually present for patients with ALS?
2. What parts of the motor system are impaired with this type of dysarthria?

REFERENCES

1. Abdelmeguid, A., Rojansky, R., Berry, G. J., & Dewan, K. (2021). Dysphagia and dysphonia, a pairing of symptoms caused by an unusual pair of diseases: Castleman's disease and myasthenia gravis. *Annals of Otology, Rhinology & Laryngology*, *130*(3), 319–324. https://doi.org/10.1177/0003489420949581.
2. Armstrong, M. J., & Okun, M. S. (2020). Diagnosis and treatment of Parkinson disease: A review. *JAMA*, *323*(6), 548–560. https://doi.org/10.1001/jama.2019.22360.
3. Ashkan, K., Rogers, P., Bergman, H., & Ughratdar, I. (2017). Insights into the mechanisms of deep brain stimulation. *Nature Reviews Neurology*, *13*(9), 548–554. https://doi.org/10.1038/nrneurol.2017.105.
4. Barkmeier-Kraemer, J. M. (2020). Isolated voice tremor: A clinical variant of essential tremor or a distinct clinical phenotype? *Tremor and Other Hyperkinetic Movements*, *10*. https://doi.org/10.7916/tohm.v0.738.
5. Basilakos, A. (2018). Contemporary approaches to the management of post-stroke apraxia of speech. *Seminars in Speech and Language*, *39*(1), 25–36. https://doi.org/10.1055/s-0037-1608853.
6. Charcot, J. M. (1877). *Lectures on the diseases of the nervous system* (vol. 1). The New Sydenham Society.
7. Darley, F., Aronson, A., & Brown, J. (1969). Clusters of deviant speech dimensions in the dysarthrias. *Journal of Speech and Hearing Research*, *12*(3), 462–496.
8. Dashtipour, K., Tafreshi, A., Lee, J., & Crawley, B. (2018). Speech disorders in Parkinson's disease: Pathophysiology, medical management and surgical approaches. *Neurodegenerative Disease Management*, *8*(5), 337–348. https://doi.org/10.2217/nmt-2018-0021.
9. De Cock, E., Batens, K., Hemelsoet, D., Boon, P., Oostra, K., & De Herdt, V. (2020). Dysphagia, dysarthria and aphasia following a first acute ischaemic stroke: Incidence and associated factors. *European Journal of Neurology*, *27*(10), 2014–2021. https://doi.org/10.1111/ene.14385.
10. Dobson, R., & Giovannoni, G. (2019). Multiple sclerosis—a review. *European Journal of Neurology*, *26*(1), 27–40. https://doi.org/10.1111/ene.13819.
11. Doshi, A., & Chataway, J. (2016). Multiple sclerosis, a treatable disease. *Clinical Medicine*, *16*(Suppl 6), S53–S59. https://doi.org/10.7861/clinmedicine.16-6-s53.
12. Duffy, J. R. (2020). *Motor speech disorders: Substrates, differential diagnosis, and management* (4th ed.). Mosby.
13. Duffy, J. R., & Folger, W. N. (1986). *Dysarthria in unilateral nervous system lesions*. Detroit, MI: Presented at the annual convention of the American Speech-Language-Hearing Association.
14. Ellis, C., Crosson, B., Gonzalez Rothi, L. J., Okun, M. S., & Rosenbek, J. C. (2015). Narrative discourse cohesion in early stage Parkinson's disease. *Journal of Parkinson's Disease*, *5*(2), 403–411. https://doi.org/10.3233/JPD-140476.
15. Enderby, P. (2013). Disorders of communication: Dysarthria. *Handbook of Clinical Neurology*, *110*, 273–281. https://doi.org/10.1016/B978-0-444-52901-5.00022-8.
16. Fecek, C., & Nagalli, S. (2022). *Shy Drager syndrome*. StatPearls Publishing. PMID 32809337.

17. Fox SH, Katzenschlager R, Lim SY, Barton B, de Bie RMA, Seppi K, Coelho M, Sampaio C; Movement Disorder Society Evidence-Based Medicine Committee. International Parkinson and movement disorder society evidence-based medicine review: Update on treatments for the motor symptoms of Parkinson's disease. Mov Disord. 2018 Aug;33(8):1248-1266. doi: 10.1002/mds.27372. Epub 2018 Mar 23. Erratum in: Mov Disord. 2018 Dec;33(12):1992. PMID: 29570866.

18. Frei, K. (2019). Tardive dyskinesia: Who gets it and why. *Parkinsonism Related Disorders, 59*, 151–154. https://doi.org/10.1016/j.parkreldis.2018.11.017.

19. Groher, M. E., & Crary, M. A. (2016). *Dysphagia: Clinical management in adults and children* (2nd ed.). Elsevier.

20. Gupta, H., & Banerjee, A. (2014). Recovery of dysphagia in lateral medullary stroke. *Case Reports in Neurological Medicine*, ID 404871. https://doi.org/10.1155/2014/404871.

21. Hanagasi, H. A., Tufekcioglu, Z., & Emre, M. (2017). Dementia in Parkinson's disease. *Journal of the Neurological Sciences, 374*, 26–31. https://doi.org/10.1016/j.jns.2017.01.012

22. Hartman, D. E., & Abbs, J. H. (1992). Dysarthria associated with focal unilateral upper motor neuron lesions. *European Journal of Disorders of Communication, 27*(3), 187–196.

23. Heemskerk, A.-W., & Roos, R. A. (2012). Aspiration pneumonia and death in Huntington's disease. *PLoS Currents, 4*, RRN1293. https://www.ncbi.nlm.nih.gov/pmc/articles/PMC3269785/.

24. Inzelberg, R., Plotnik, M., Harpaz, N. K., & Flash, T. (2016). Micrographia, much beyond the writer's hand. *Parkinsonism & Related Disorders, 26*, 1–9. https://doi.org/10.1016/j.parkreldis.2016.03.003.

25. Kirshner, H. S. (2002). *Behavioral neurology: Practical science of mind and brain* (2nd ed.). Butterworth-Heinemann.

26. Kuo, S.-H. (2019). Ataxia. *CONTINUUM: Lifelong Learning in Neurology, 25*(4), 1036–1054. https://doi.org/10.1212/CON.0000000000000753.

27. Kwa, L., Larson, D., Yeh, C., & Bega, D. (2020). Influence of age of onset on Huntington's disease phenotype. *Tremor and Other Hyperkinetic Movements, 10*, 21. https://doi.org/10.5334/tohm.536.

28. Liepmann, Dr. phil. et med. H: Das Krankheitsbild der Apraxie ("motorischen Asymbolie") auf Grund eines Falles von einseitiger Apraxie pp. 30–44. Eur Neurol 1900;8:30-44. https://doi.org/10.1159/000221489.

29. Love, R. J., & Webb, W. G. (1977). The efficacy of cueing techniques in Broca's aphasia. *Journal of Speech and Hearing Disorders, 42*(2), 170–178.

30. McHattie, A. W., Coebergh, J., Khan, F., & Morgante, F. (2021). Palilalia as a prominent feature of anti-NMDA receptor encephalitis in a woman with COVID-19. *Journal of Neurology, 268*, 3995–3997. https://doi.org/10.1007/s00415-021-10542-5.

31. Mor, N., Simonyan, K., & Blitzer, A. (2018). Central voice production and pathophysiology of spasmodic dysphonia. *The Laryngoscope, 128*(1), 177–183. https://doi.org/10.1002/lary.26655.

32. Murdoch, B. E. (2015). *Communication disorders*. Louise Cummings (Ed.). Cambridge University Press. https://www.cambridge.org/core/books/cambridge-handbook-of-communication-disorders/acquired-dysarthria/F9926752B0C5134AFF76787AA9A49FF8.

33. Murray, T. (2014). Spasmodic dysphonia: Let's look at that again. *Journal of Voice, 28*(6), 694–699.

34. National Institute of Neurologic Disorders and Stroke. (n.d.). Multiple sclerosis. https://www.ninds.nih.gov/Disorders/All-Disorders/Multiple-Sclerosis-Information-Page.

35. Novotný, M., Rusz, J., Čmejla, R., Růžičková, H., Klempíř, J., & Růžička, E. (2016). Hypernasality associated with basal ganglia dysfunction: Evidence from Parkinson's disease and Huntington's disease. *Peer Journal, 29*(4), e2530. https://doi.org/10.7717/peerj.2530.

36. Pizzorni, N., Pirola, F., Ciammola, A., & Schindler, A. (2020). Management of dysphagia in Huntington's disease: A descriptive review. *Neurological Sciences, 41*, 1405–1417. https://doi.org/10.1007/s10072-020-04265-0.

37. Rönnefarth, M., Hanisch, N., Brandt, A. U., Mähler, A., Endres, M., Paul, F., & Doss, S. (2020). Dysphagia affecting quality of life in cerebellar ataxia—a large survey. *Cerebellum, 19*(3), 437–445. https://doi.org/10.1007/s12311-020-01122-w.

38. Rusz, J., Tykalová, T., Salerno, G., Bancone, S., Scarpelli, J., & Pellecchia, M. T. (2019). Distinctive speech signature in cerebellar and parkinsonian subtypes of multiple system atrophy. *Journal of Neurology, 266*, 1394–1404. https://doi.org/10.1007/s00415-019-09271-7.

39. Schulz, G., Halpern, A., Spielman, J., Ramig, L., Panzer, I., Sharpley, A., & Freeman, K. (2021). Single word intelligibility of individuals with Parkinson's disease in noise: Pre-specified secondary outcome variables from a randomized control trial (RCT) comparing two intensive speech treatments (LSVT LOUD vs. LSVT ARTIC). *Brain Sciences, 11*(7), 857. https://doi.org/10.3390/brainsci11070857.

40. Simons, J. A. (2017). Swallowing dysfunctions in Parkinson's disease. *International Review of Neurobiology, 134*, 1207–1238. https://doi.org/10.1016/bs.irn.2017.05.026.

41. Solaro, C., Cuccaro, A., Gamberini, G., Patti, F., D'Amico, E., Bergamaschi, R., Berra, E., Giusti, A., Rezzani, C., Messmer Uccelli, M., & Grasso, M. G. (2020). Prevalence of dysphagia in a consecutive cohort of subjects with MS using fibre-optic endoscopy. *Neurological Sciences, 41*(5), 1075–1079. https://doi.org/10.1007/s10072-019-04198-3.

42. Stipancic, K. L., Borders, J. C., Brates, D., & Thibeault, S. L. (2019). Prospective investigation of incidence and co-occurrence of dysphagia, dysarthria, and aphasia following ischemic stroke. *American Journal of Speech-Language Pathology, 28*(1), 188–194. https://doi.org/10.1044/2018_AJSLP-18-0136.

43. Suttrup, I., & Warnecke, T. (2016). Dysphagia in Parkinson's disease. *Dysphagia, 31*(1), 24–32. https://doi.org/10.1007/s00455-015-9671-9.

44. Teasell, R., Foley, N., Doherty, T., & Finestone, H. (2002). Clinical characteristics of patients with brainstem strokes admitted to a rehabilitation unit. *Archives of Physical Medicine and Rehabilitation, 83*(7), 1013–1016.

45. Umemoto, G., & Furuya, H. (2020). Management of dysphagia in patients with Parkinson's disease and related disorders. *Internal Medicine, 59*(1), 7–14. https://doi.org/10.2169/internalmedicine.2373-18.

46. Verhoeff, M. C., Koutris, M., de Vries, R., Berendse, H. W., van Dijk, K. D., & Lobbezoo, F. (2022). Salivation in Parkinson's disease: A scoping review. *Gerodontology*. https://doi.org/10.1111/ger.12628. Epub ahead of print.

47. Wang, B. J., Carter, F. L., & Altman, K. W. (2020). Relationship between dysarthria and oral-oropharyngeal dysphagia: The present evidence. *Ear Nose & Throat Journal*. Online ahead of print. https://doi.org/10.1177/0145561320951647.

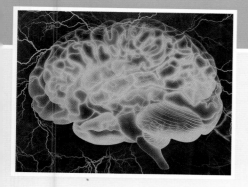

9

Central Language Mechanisms and Learning

Nothing defines the function of a neuron better than its connections.
Marcel Mesulam, 2006

CHAPTER OUTLINE

KEY TERMS

central-executive network
cingulate cortex
cognition
constraint-induced therapy (CIT)
declarative memory
default mode network
episodic memory
executive functions
graceful degradation
hippocampus
input fibers
intrinsic neurons (interneurons)
left fusiform area

long-term memory
metacognition
motor association areas
neocortex (archicortex)
neurogenesis
neuroplasticity
perisylvian cortex
phoneme
prefrontal cortex
presynaptic inhibition
procedural memory
projection neurons
reasoning

reticular formation
salience network
sensory memory
short-term memory
spatial summation
summation
temporal summation
thalamic reticular nucleus
thalamocortical circuit
thalamus
working memory

In the preceding chapters, a foundation has been laid for you to be able to identify where a brain structure is and its primary and associated function(s). Neuronal function as well as the primary motor and sensory systems have been introduced and discussed. Our journey into the clinical world of speech-language pathology began with the motor system and speech and swallowing disorders in adults. The same clinical topics will be discussed for the pediatric population at the end of the text. We now take a simplified, but expanded look at the cortical mechanisms underlying the extraordinary capacity of human beings to use and understand language and to learn and create new ideas. These abilities begin to form a foundation from birth and, barring injury or disease, continue throughout life. This chapter is concerned with the functioning of our brain and includes current research into neuronal circuitry. Also highlighted are the anatomic structures involved in language processing, as well as some of the historically popular models of language underlying explanations of language disorders acquired from brain damage. The more common acquired adult language disorders and cognitive-linguistic disorders are discussed in Chapter 10. Language and learning disorders of children are covered in Chapter 13.

NEOCORTEX

The highest level of cortex in terms of cytoarchitecture is **neocortex** (or **archicortex**), covering ~90% of the brain. The neocortex is a set of layered tissues of the cortex responsible for higher order functions. This vast brain structure was believed to give humans their unique cognitive abilities, including language. The total area of cortex is ~2500 cm², with a range of 2 to 4 mm in thickness; sensory cortex is thinner than motor and association areas. The thickness is determined by the aggregation of neuronal cell bodies. In addition to neuronal cells, brain tissue contains microglial cells. These microglia function as sensors: they respond to injury, the presence of pathogens, and cellular debris. They also play a role in neural plasticity, regulating synaptic formation, maturation, and metabolic-waste elimination.[12]

Until recently the commonly accepted estimated count of neurons was around 100 billion with an 8- to 10-fold greater number of microglial (neuroglial) cells in the cortex. However, recent research using a new counting method called an isotropic fractionator has challenged this notion. The recently validated count, in addition to histologic evidence, has revealed an almost identical glia to neuron number.[4,48]

Additional research into the structure of the human brain has shown that our brain is not the largest or the one with the most folds (sulci and gyri) in the animal kingdom; however, it is seven times larger than expected for our body mass. The cellular composition, including the foldings, relative size of the prefrontal cortex, and cerebellar development, is consistent across primate species and does not account for our unique development. Our larger brain may have contributed to our development in another way: A cortex with more neurons takes longer to develop, which increases the maternal investment period (pre- and postnatally) and increases the age until sexual maturity. A longer period of development provides a greater period to learn from peers and parents, and to form a social group. It also increases opportunities to accumulate knowledge and pass it on to the group and to descendants. These opportunities have fostered human social interactions and increased cultural and technological evolution.[23]

Neural Networks

Early neuroanatomists were acutely aware of and frustrated by the limitations of their knowledge of the brain, being unable to provide much detail about this exceedingly complex and fragile organ. Early advances were made using staining techniques that eventually allowed tracing of some fibers and the identification of association pathways. Clinicopathologic studies added to our knowledge by the study of brains of patients with disorders, and by looking for relationships between the lesioned structures and pathways and the corresponding behavioral changes. All investigation and theorizing in these very early days of neuroscience was constrained by the lack of knowledge about how neurons worked and how neural signals transmitted any information between them. Whole brain integration could not be understood without this knowledge, though most neuroanatomists knew that there existed circuitry and neural networks that communicated in some fashion. Not until 1986 was any complete mapping of a cellular connection network done, this one on the nematode *Caenorhabditis elegans*. Still, there was a lack of ability to record much about physiologic properties of the cells and their synapses. The cellular mapping breakthrough with *C. elegans* did not contribute much to the ongoing early efforts to map mammalian networks.

In the 1980s researchers began to create computational models based on knowledge of anatomy and physiology in an attempt to explain and potentially predict neural interactions. In the late 1980s and early 1990s, anatomic and physiologic studies of the visual cortex of the monkey produced early connectional matrices and promoted the idea that cortical areas were unique in terms of specific input and output fiber connections and could be distinguished by these patterns.

Although the previously accepted thinking was that cognitive functions are attributable to isolated operations of single brain areas, current research has demonstrated that cognitive functions result from the interaction of various brain areas operating in networks. The network approach is not only useful in understanding **cognition**, it also helps explain functional differences in psychiatric and neurologic disorders. The core networks are the **default mode network**, the **salience network**, and **central-executive network**; all three are important to our field.

Large-Scale Brain Networks

The default mode network plays an important role in internally oriented cognitive processes such as daydreaming, reminiscing, and future planning. This network is typically not active during stimulus-driven cognitive tasks, showing decreased activity during tasks such as taking exams or playing games; however, this network shows increased activity during naturalistic situations such as listening to stories or watching movies. The likely role of the default mode network is in integrating extrinsic information with previously acquired knowledge, helping to form rich, context-dependent models of specific situations. This integration of intrinsic and extrinsic information over time provides a shared code for communication in communities and social situations. Anatomically, the default mode netowrk includes the posterior medial cortex, medial prefrontal cortex, and temporoparietal junction.[31,52]

The salience network includes the insula, **cingulate cortex**, and three subcortical structures (ventral striatum, substantia nigra, and tegmental region). The salience network plays a role in the attentional capture of biologically and cognitively relevant events. It communicates with the frontoparietal system for **working memory** and higher order cognitive processing, and is involved in detecting, integrating, and filtering relevant interoceptive, autonomic, and emotional information.[31] In other words, the salience network helps direct behavior to the most pertinent actions.

The central-executive network includes the frontal and parietal cortical regions. This network is important for actively maintaining and manipulating information in working memory. In addition, it is important for rule-based problem solving and decision making and shows strong coactivation during a wide range of cognitively demanding tasks. This network is considered to be crucial to verbal learning and executive functioning.

These three networks are also implicated in cognitive disorders of interest to our field. For example, network dysfunction has been implicated in attention-deficit hyperactivity disorder,[31] depression,[1] and autism spectrum disorders,[14] among others. This finding has significant implications for our field as it demonstrates that cognitive difficulties can result from both focal lesions (such as a stroke) and disruption to the network from a disease process or diffuse damage.

Even our resting brain, which was originally thought to be calm and peaceful, has now been shown to be restless and continuously active, as demonstrated by functional magnetic resonance imaging (fMRI). Intrinsic connectivity networks, the collection of networks that includes the default mode network, central-executive network, and salience network, remain active even during rest.[34]

Small World Networks

In 1998, the concept of small world networks was introduced in a letter in the journal *Nature*.[50] The authors suggested a mathematical method in which a brain area is connected to others that may not be a direct neighbor; however, each node can connect to any others by a small number of steps. This network is similar in human societies where two strangers can be connected to each other by a short chain of acquaintances (much like the six degrees of separation concept).

More recent research has not supported this theory based on cellular level investigation. The proposed small world networks include those pathways that are involved in large-scale brain networks, which have been well evidenced with fMRI and other imaging studies.[24]

Connectomes

A breakthrough in mapping large cortical networks came with the development of new techniques of diffusion imaging and resting state fMRI. A connectome is a comprehensive map of neural connections in the brain, a wiring diagram of sorts. In 2010 the US National Institutes of Health began the Human Connectome Project to map this network as accurately as possible. The website gallery (at http://www.humanconnectomeproject.org/) makes available to the public breathtaking images of brain pathways.

These different connectome representations offer complimentary insights into the inherent functional organization of the brain, but challenges for functional connectome research remain. Interpretability will be improved by future research toward gaining insights into the neural mechanisms underlying connectome observations obtained from fMRI.[8]

Although these studies have generated much excitement, and our knowledge is increasing almost daily, the study of connectivity is not without its limitations and challenges.[8] New imaging methods are being constantly refined and new computational models are being used extensively by researchers in several fields (e.g., neuroanatomy, physiology, psychology, neurology, speech-language pathology). These efforts may help elucidate connectivity in normal brain function and in understanding what happens when there is abnormal development or injury to the brain that changes behavior.

Brain Connectivity

Cortical neurons, like all neurons, transmit and process neural information through synapses and fiber pathways. Synaptic organization is concerned with the way neurons form connections, circuits, and units in the nervous system that mediate the function of different regions of the brain. What abilities do the neurons have in connection building? Obviously they are transmitters, sending millions of signals throughout the brain, but they have many other functions. They are also transducers, for example, converting sound waves into neuronal impulses. Neurons are switches, turning on and off, or causing another neuron to switch on or off in response to a neurotransmitter release. They have the capability to encode information; they then express that code providing information about such things as spatial location, timing, or even higher-level information such as color. Neurons are thought to be minute storage vessels as well; connections at strong synapses are thought to temporarily store memory traces. Finally, another important property of neurons is oscillation. As a neural spike travels down the axon, neurons move back and forth, creating complex waveforms. This signaling can spread from one cellular array to another, resulting in areas or regions of the cortex that are busy sending and resending signals. These oscillations are the signals identified on electrophysiologic studies of the brain.

Connections between neurons are made locally as well as outside their particular region, perhaps a relatively long distance away. Essentially three types of neural elements make the connections possible. **Input fibers** synapse onto the cell body and/or dendrites or dendritic spines found on the dendrites. **Projection neurons** (also called principal or relay neurons) send out a long axon fiber that carries information signals to other regions. The third type is composed of cells concerned only with local processing within a certain region, the **intrinsic neurons**, or **interneurons**. Sometimes a projection neuron takes action locally and behaves as an interneuron; the distinction between the two is not rigid. Inhibitory interneurons have been shown to synchronize the firing of excitatory neurons, enhancing the probability of activation of the target neuron downstream. The relations among these three elements of synaptic organization vary in the different regions of the brain and determine the function of that region.[37]

Spatial Organization

Given the density of neural tissue in the cortex, an astonishing 1000 trillion synapses are estimated to exist in the human brain.[53] These connections form circuits, although they are not of a simple input and output nature. The nervous system is organized in a complex manner from the molecular level to complex behavioral systems. This organization can be viewed in terms of levels of scale. At the microscale level, microcircuits are formed from small bunches of synapses between individual neurons. At the mesoscale level, networks or local circuits are formed in arrangements of columns or mini columns that connect those neuronal populations. Interregional fiber pathways that connect brain regions make up the macroscale level and result in systems of behavior. Fig. 9.1 breaks this organization down further. Microcircuits form dendritic connections and subunits within the connections between dendrites of individual neurons. These neurons with their connections interact, forming local circuits and performing the operations of a particular region of the brain. These regions are organized with interregional pathways, columns, and laminae. Neural impulses traveling by the interregional connections between these multiple local circuits provide for integration of this varying neural information resulting in behaviors.

Laminar Organization

Not only is there columnar organization of the cortex, but also a horizontal laminar organization. You may remember from Chapter 2 that the fully developed neocortex is composed of six layers, with the sixth layer being the innermost. How the laminae develop is discussed in Chapter 11. These cortical laminae are often broken into subareas within the layer for the more finite study of their composition and physiology, but for our purposes we look only at their broad composition. Table 9.1 summarizes the name and some information about the composition of each layer.

Patterns of Synaptic Connection

There is both specificity and variability of the anatomic connections at all levels. You find specificity in the connections between distinct neuronal types, in the branching pattern of the axon collaterals, and in the connections made over long distances between certain cell nuclei and particular brain regions. On the other hand, much variability exists in the shape of neurons and their processes, as well as in size, place, and connection pattern of different brain structures. Across species there is variability in the same brain structure. Across time in the same individual, variability will be found due to development, plasticity, and, perhaps, repair.

In 2016, Sweatt[42] summarized knowledge accrued over the past 60 years of research into neuronal connectivity and its impact on behavior and behavioral change. The review includes the premise that all behavior is the result of underlying activity in the nervous system. In other words, our behavior is a manifestation of the activity of our neural circuits. When we learn a concept that changes our behavior, which occurs with learning of new information, this must be accompanied by an underlying change in neuronal connectivity. Furthermore, because most of the communication between neurons occurs at synapses, new learning implies alterations in the strength or nature of synaptic contacts. This capacity for alterations in synaptic connections is the basis for synaptic plasticity, particularly in relationship to learning and memory. At a neuronal level, our memories are encoded as alterations in the strength of synaptic connections. In addition to synaptic plasticity, plasticity also exists in the neurons themselves.[42]

One of the underlying neuroscience principles of **neuroplasticity** is long-term potentiation (LTP). LTP refers to patterns of synaptic activity that produce long-lasting increases in signaling between two neurons, thus strengthening that particular connection. The effects of LTP are long lasting and input specific, which is reflected behaviorally in new learning. In fact, LTP has been empirically implicated in mediating different types of associative learning, spatial learning, and broad adaptive behavioral change in the central nervous

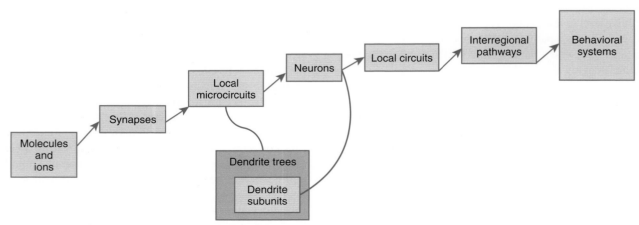

Fig. 9.1 Levels of hierarchical organization in the nervous system. *Arrows* should be read as "organize into." *Curved line connection* indicates that local microcircuits are grouped to form dendritic subunits within the dendritic trees, which are part of the individual neurons.

TABLE 9.1 Summary Description of the Laminar Organization of the Neocortex

Layer Number	Layer Name	Description	Special Features
I	Molecular	Contains mostly horizontal axons and a few neuronal bodies	
II	Outer granular	Contains a mixture of small neurons (granule cells) and slightly larger neurons (pyramidal cells); apical dendrites extend up to layer I and axons descend into and through deeper layers	
III	Outer pyramidal	Contains primarily medium and large pyramidal cells; apical dendrites extend up to layer I and axons descend into and through deeper layers	
IV	Inner granule	Contains stellate (starlike) neurons, smooth and spiny; no pyramidal cells	Primary target layer for ascending sensory information from the thalamus
V	Inner pyramidal	Contains medium and large pyramidal cells; apical dendrites of medium size extend up one or two layers; large cells project to layer I	Large pyramidal = major source of cortical efferent fibers that send axons to corpus striatum, brainstem, and spinal cord; some corticocortical connections
VI	Multiform	Contains an assortment of neuron types	Axons project to subcortical structures such as thalamus; also make corticocortical connections

system (CNS) of mammals, with particular effects on the amygdala, cerebral cortex, and hippocampus.

The opposite of LTP is called long-term depression (LTD), which produces a long-lasting decrease in synaptic strength. LTD also plays a role in plasticity because it weakens connections that are no longer stimulated. Both LTP and LTD vary by brain regions. LTP in the cerebral cortex likely mediates aspects of activity-dependent development in the visual, auditory, and motor systems. In the amygdala, LTP is strongly tied to auditory-cued fear conditioning.

Types of Synaptic Connections

The neural microcircuits are the most localized synaptic patterns that can be studied. Chapter 4 presented two basic patterns of connectivity—divergence and convergence. These are important to remember when thinking about how information processing occurs within these circuits. Microcircuits are built of three types of elements: divergence, convergence, and a variation of convergence called presynaptic control.

Synaptic divergence means that an action potential can trigger multiple excitatory postsynaptic potentials simultaneously, affecting many dendritic terminals at once. This amplifies the activity of a single axon. This kind of divergent synaptic action is found, for example, in the cerebellum, which demonstrates great divergence, and in the sensory afferents of the thalamus. Another method of achieving divergence is also found in the nervous system. Axons branch into collaterals and give rise to multiple terminals, thus resulting in numerous synaptic contacts. This kind of divergence is common in cortical cells.

Synaptic convergence, on the other hand, occurs when multiple synapses occur on one postsynaptic dendrite. When this occurs, two kinds of **summation**, or additive effects, may take place. **Temporal summation** may occur in which the effect of the neurotransmitters may be enhanced (e.g., if all synapses are excitatory). The convergence may also summate with the excitatory and inhibitory potentials canceling each other out, resulting in the resting potential being maintained. The integration of the excitatory and inhibitory synapses usually functions, however, to modulate the action; thus there is a change in potential, but it is not as strong as it would have been without the convergence. Another kind of summation is **spatial summation**, in which the varied sites of synapse along the dendritic surface of the neuron cause responses to rise in the different parts of the neuron. This may increase the possibility of more local mechanisms during activation from the site on one dendritic tree to another.

A third type of action that is similar to convergence is **presynaptic inhibition**, in which two sequential axonic synapses occur. One axon terminates on another with inhibitory action. When the second axon is then presynaptic to a third axon, there is an inhibitory effect on the synapse that will occur on the postsynaptic membrane of the third axon. Box 9.1 summarizes the three kinds of connectivity patterns.

Dendrites and Neurons

The complexity of neuronal processing is exemplified by the extensive variety of patterns of dendritic branching unique to different types of neurons. The different branching patterns are said to impose geometric constraints on activity. These patterns, combined with the different sites of input and the passive and active electronic properties of the membrane of the dendrites, account for the complex nature of the activity of dendrites and consequently the neurons. This text does not go in depth into this complex organization of the dendritic input to the neuron. However, the fact that the dendritic

BOX 9.1   Synaptic Connectivity Patterns

Synaptic Divergence
- Occurs when action potential triggers multiple excitatory postsynaptic potentials, affecting many dendrites; can also occur when axons branch into collaterals, creating multiple terminals and synaptic contacts
- Acts to increase amplification of a single axon
- Commonly found in the cerebellum, the sensory afferents of the thalamus, and in cortical cells

Synaptic Convergence
- Occurs when multiple synapses fire on one postsynaptic dendrite, adding activity from multiple axons to one dendrite
- Two kinds of summation can occur at a synaptic convergence:
  - Temporal summation: effect of neurotransmitter may be enhanced if all synapses are excited or if resulting excitatory and inhibitory potentials create a resting potential
  - Spatial summation: various sites along synapse cause responses in different parts of neuron

Presynaptic Inhibition
- Occurs when two axonic synapses are in sequence and an inhibitory effect occurs on the postsynaptic membrane of the third of three axons

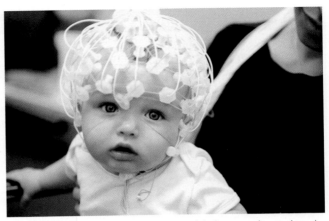

Fig. 9.2 The use of event-related potentials is a popular noninvasive technique to track brain activity in subjects of all ages. (From Haith, M. M., & Benson, J. B. [2008]. *Encyclopedia of infant and early childhood development.* Elsevier, Ltd.)

tree is responsible for the variety of actions the neuron may undertake is important to understand.

Of note is that the smallest functional unit within the dendritic tree is the dendritic spine, which is, as it sounds, a thornlike protuberance on the dendrite. Being quite numerous in the nervous system, they account for most postsynaptic sites in the brain, especially within the cerebellum, basal ganglia, and cortex.

Dendritic spines contain neurotransmitter receptors, organelles, and signaling systems essential for synaptic function and plasticity. They receive most of the excitatory synaptic impulses in the mammalian brain and are considered of critical importance for memory and learning.[9] Numerous brain disorders are associated with abnormal dendritic spines, and changes in size, shape, and density of these spines is observed in a variety of neurodegenerative, neurodevelopmental, and psychiatric disorders.[36]

Within the cortex most excitatory synapses are made onto spines, and an estimated one-third of the inhibitory synapses occur there. Approximately 15% of all dendritic spines carry potential for both kinds. Aside from the obvious function of increasing the surface area available for connective integration, spines are theorized to have significance for rapid signal processing. The foundational study of neuronal functioning in Chapter 4 discussed the basics of impulse initiation and synaptic connection, with the impulse being generated at the axon hillock and traveling down the axon to synapse with another neuron. Also discussed was the graded potential set up in the cell itself. To take this further, evidence exists that to various degrees, electronic backspread of this propagated

current occurs back into the soma and the dendrites. This may be sufficient to activate dendrite-to-dendrite (dendrodendritic) synapses, further facilitating or inhibiting action within that neuron's local circuit.

BASIC CIRCUITS

The basic cortical neuron (usually a pyramidal cell type) is structured well for the integrative actions it serves. The typical cortical neuron has dendritic trees that are divided into apical and basal parts, with dendritic spines on both parts and different excitatory and inhibitory synapses occurring at different levels of the parts of the dendritic tree. It also, of course, has an axon that in most instances gives off collateral axons that synapse within the local circuit as well as at sites some distance from that region.

Brain Waves

We have discussed mapping brain activity through fMRI, but there is another way of trying to observe brain activity, which is to map the oscillatory activity through an electroencephalograph (EEG). Advanced computers have made it possible to separate and analyze the complex waveforms that make up the neural signals. The frequency bands are somewhat arbitrary but have come into common use and are now believed to represent distinct processes coordinated by the brain.

Raw data from an EEG reflect activity of billions of neurons and are difficult to interpret when reading from the scalp even though waveforms can be identified. However, if the EEG signals are averaged over many trials and locked to a specific point in time, the waveforms become more regularized and can yield much more information. This study is called event-related potentials. Because it is noninvasive and the equipment is more accessible now, this technique is becoming more and more common in research in speech-language pathology (Fig. 9.2).

Learning

As you use your brain to study your brain, there are a tremendous number of neural events occurring, with new connections being formed and old connections either enhanced or weakened. What is learning in terms of neural functioning? Learning is simply (well, it's really not simple at all!) the brain increasing the efficiency of synaptic connections. Increasing the efficiency means enabling faster flow of neural signals from one neuron to another. Two of the ways our brains may accomplish this are by growing more synapses between the neurons or by enhancing the neurochemical supply of glutamate, the excitatory neurotransmitter, in the neural circuit to increase the speed of transmission.

When neurons begin to form connections in microcircuits and then in local areas and the connections are strengthened by repeated stimulation and neural firing, these connections and the pattern formed between them in a circuit become stronger. By stronger, we mean that they are more likely to fire when appropriate stimulation is present, and they are more likely to fire together. In turn, when neurons fire together in synchrony, the connections between them are even further strengthened. What has come to be known as the Hebbian learning principle proposed by Donald Hebb[22] in 1949 puts forth that assemblies of spiking cells learn an input pattern by strengthening the connections between cells that fire at the same time. This resulted in the old saying, "Neurons that fire together, wire together." The Hebbian learning principle relies on the theory that synaptic connections are the physical foundation for learning and memory. There is now much evidence gathered from modern techniques of neuroscience that this principle is solid.

The synchronous firing in a neural circuit may result in a representation that we experience as a percept such as a word, a recognizable sound, a familiar shape or visual object, or a combination of facial features that we recognize as a certain person, for example. If the pattern of firing results in a representation that is familiar or meaningful to you, it means that the particular neural input has been transformed across its input into an output pattern that the brain recognizes. A simple example is the transformation of auditory phonologic representations into articulatory phonologic representations. This involves several systems (sensory, cortical association, motor) with repeated neural signaling across those systems strengthening the connection weights (or likelihood of firing together) in a particular pattern. All of the primary and association cortices in the brain are thought to be essentially collections of pattern associator networks, quite often working in parallel. This is where the term *parallel distributed processing* (PDP) came from that is used in explaining computing. It is a simple construct for describing the operation of the brain because the brain is thought to be much more advanced a system than any computer yet built. PDP has been seen as useful, however, in trying to explain some of the aspects of neural networks.

What Parts of the Brain Participate Most Actively in Learning?

There are, as you know, different kinds of learning. Some learning appears to be undemanding and accomplished simply by making ourselves conscious of it—paying attention. We can learn how to do things such as develop motor skills by repetitive practice of the proper movements with the proper timing and force until a motor memory is established. However, our brains are best at tasks we interact with, problems we solve, and, basically, survive. The type of learning that students have to do, however, requiring recall of facts and consolidation of those facts into concepts and principles is different, and our brains have to work even harder! The parts of the brain that are involved may be the same, but they are taxed by the mental effort required to build the more diffuse synaptic circuits that will support consolidation and long-term retention of information.

Take the task you are attempting to do now: learning about the brain areas active in learning. First of all, to commit anything to memory (learning is a process of acquiring lasting brain representations that we call memories), we must attend to the task, obviously requiring that we be conscious and awake. The deep core of the brainstem, the **reticular formation**, must be actively channeling sensory information through the **thalamocortical circuit**, resulting in a state of awakeness. In learning, we are concerned with voluntary attention, not automatic attention, which is the difference between attending to a task and to an environmental sound.

The successful use of voluntary attention allows us to selectively process relevant information. Except for the neurons out in the sensory periphery, selective attention involves activity of neural circuitry at all levels of the sensory system involved. Learning often involves visual, auditory, and tactile senses, and it is usually considered optimal to involve more than one sensory system. Once the sensory information is relayed through the **thalamus** and on to the targeted primary sensory area, executive control systems in subcortical and cortical areas, particularly the cingulate cortex, the parietal cortex, and the **prefrontal cortex**, enable the brain to selectively attend to the stimulus.

In terms of visual-spatial attention, two types of attention have been identified. Endogenous attention refers to our ability to voluntarily monitor information in a location for sustained periods of time. This is the type of attention used when focusing on a set of instructions, for example. Endogenous attention is necessarily sustained to enable successful completion of a task, with an estimated 300 ms required to deploy this ability. In contrast, exogenous attention is transient, peaking at about 100 to 120 ms and decaying quickly thereafter. This type of attention refers to our involuntary noting of a location where sudden stimulation has occurred (e.g., noticing a bird flying because of its motion while engaged in another task). In short, exogenous attention is automatic and inflexible, while endogenous attention is more flexible and under voluntary control.[38]

Once attentional control has been established, the features of the targeted information must be analyzed, and a percept must be established with which a memory can be associated. When learning through reading, an accomplished reader already has the established input-output circuitry in the neocortex to make sense of the shapes the visual cortex encoded. The brain of a skillful reader has automatized the steps necessary to read with understanding: recognition of the letters, the letter combinations into words, the associations between the words and their meaning, and the association of meaning with the particular combination of words in each sentence. In neural terms, strong neural circuits have been established that will easily carry out the reading task without that reader having to switch to controlled processing unless the reader happens upon an unfamiliar word.

For example, before this class, unless you had another class in which it was introduced, you likely had no association for the word *dysarthria*. You may try to sound out the word using phonologic representations stored in the temporal lobe and transformed into articulatory movements in the **motor association areas** of the frontal cortex. Even if you pronounce it correctly (and if you have no experience with the word, you are not sure), you find that there are no memory traces stored for that word. In that case, you may choose to read on, hoping there will be a definition provided in the context or you may go to the glossary or a dictionary. Those strategies are due to cognitive processes we call executive functions—ruled by your prefrontal cortex. Your brain has learned over time what options are available to you to solve this problem, and you employ metacognition, an executive function, to discern what usually works best for you as a learner.

Once you find how to pronounce this word and what it means, your brain can begin the learning process—that is, establish a memory trace associated with both the visual form of the word, the phonologic representation of the word, and the meaning(s) associated with it. Recent research on new word learning indicates that the brain may store written words as pictures in an orthographic lexicon in the **left fusiform area**, which the researchers referred to as the visual word form area.[19] This research indicates that the neural firing associated with recognition of the written word is to the word form as a whole and not to the individual phonemes and letters.

The associations that you learn for a word and commit in the brain as memory traces form what speech-language pathologists (SLPs) call a semantic field around it. For the word *dysarthria* maybe such things as motor system, movement, speech disorder, a particular disease, a particular patient, or a particular teacher are associated. Episodic memories associated with the meaning, for example, in whose class you first heard the term, are likely consolidated in the **hippocampus** in the medial temporal lobe. The semantic associations, the word and the meaning itself, are likely consolidated in the temporal lobe and the neocortex.

Many things that we learn have both episodic and semantic memories associated with them. Over time as you have more experience with the word and concept of dysarthria, associated memories will be stored over a wide area of different brain regions as part of cortical network circuits. The larger the number and type of associations, the more likely you are to remember the meaning.

This system of memory storage in the brain in which the associated information is distributed across many cortical connections helps explain why a breakdown in processing rarely results in a total loss of a percept or concept. The loss of one component of this distributed processing network results in a reduced level of performance but not a complete inability to process. For example, in word retrieval failures, patients often know something about the word; they have not completely lost all information about it. This reduction in performance of the system is called **graceful degradation** in engineering terms and has been a useful concept in neural processing. SLPs often use it to great advantage in treatment.

As you read and process the information, you are establishing concepts you wish to commit to memory. The sentences have been encoded in the temporal lobe and neocortex. In memory consolidation, meaning begins to be established through association with previous learning, previous experience, and recent learning. This may involve sensory memories as well as episodic and semantic memories. The medial temporal lobe and the temporal lobe will begin to resonate with the neocortex to begin establishing the memory. This involves synaptic changes. You may read the text again, you may take notes, you may read aloud to yourself; again, your metacognitive skills are put to work figuring out what typically works best for you. Your professor may go over the same material in class. All this activity helps consolidate the meaning of what you have read because the synaptic changes that take place in the medial temporal lobe, temporal lobe, and neocortex will be strengthened by the repetitive firing in that circuit. The connections also may be adapted and enhanced by new connections to the circuit as you learn more about it or as it makes more sense to you. Repetition and an increased number of associations may eventually result in learning—establishing the concept in **long-term memory**.

Establishing the concept in long-term memory requires protein synthesis. For more permanent memories or representations of knowledge to be established there must be changes at the synapses such as growth of dendritic spikes and increased excitatory (and perhaps inhibitory) connections that need to become efficient and more permanent.

The consolidation of memories and learning takes place most efficiently while we are sleeping. During non-rapid eye movement (NREM) sleep stages, also called slow-wave sleep or delta sleep, consolidation of explicit or declarative memories occurs. During REM sleep, stabilization of memories occurs.[40]

The Power of Connection

The brain is the ultimate information processor. No computer built to date can process information, learn new information, and create from imagination with the efficiency and productivity of the human brain. Because of (1) the properties of the neurons and their links across association cortices; (2) the input from sensory mechanisms, limbic structures, basal ganglia, cerebellum, and so forth; and (3) output back to some of these areas, processing in this supreme network is a two-way function. Processing is from both the bottom up and the top down. From peripheral sensory input comes a forward press of converging neural information, traveling through the intermediate subcortical pathways to early sensory association cortical processing areas (unimodal and polymodal association cortex) to even higher cortical association areas (supramodal or heteromodal cortex). At each local circuit station are also backprojections occurring at the synapses onto the neuron, with this output from the circuits occurring in a mostly divergent rather than convergent manner.

This convergent/divergent action within neuronal circuits enhances or changes the strength of connections within the circuit and thus output to other regions. This allows changes in behavior. These neuronal operations allow translation of what is thought into what is said, written, or signed—in other words, to communicate thoughts.

Language

The contribution of Broca's study of the brain of two patients with language loss was acknowledged earlier in this text. We credit Broca and Wernicke with the first descriptions of the acquired language disorder aphasia. The discovery of specific speech-language areas in the left hemisphere of the brain had dramatic consequences for neurology. It prompted European neurologists to formulate numerous hypothetical models of the central language mechanism. Several of these models were highly speculative and based on limited evidence of the correlation between behavioral deficits and brain lesions. Even today the central mechanism for language is not completely understood, and it remains risky to attempt to formulate a model for normal and abnormal communication. The model formulated by Wernicke is generally thought to be a powerful model, which continues to have clinical relevance. The model was later revived by Geschwind,[18] who, along with his colleagues in Boston, did numerous research studies on patients with acquired language disorders and found this model helpful in explaining some clinical findings. This model became known as a connectionist model, with emphasis on the inferior parietal lobule as important for the association of word sounds and sensory properties of objects. Fig. 9.3 highlights the important perisylvian areas for language function from Broca's, Wernicke's, and Geschwind's research.

Since then, connectionist models have been called parallel distributed processing (PDP) models, and they are often used to model aspects of human perception, cognition, and behavior. These models explain the learning processes and retrieval of information from memory because of their emphasis of the neural processes that underpin cognition.[30]

The connectionist or PDP conception of the higher mental functions of speech and language gives importance to the classic language and speech centers and highlights the significance of the interconnection of the association fibers between major centers. The model has been of significant use to clinical neurologists because it allows a high degree of predictability of symptoms associated with specific lesion sites. In general terms, the model has been confirmed by clinical studies, although our understanding has broadened. The classic language centers postulated by Wernicke and Broca continue to be confirmed as critical to language and comprehension through computerized tomography and other current objective neurodiagnostic procedures.

Geschwind,[18] however, pointed out that some conditions exist under which the model has not always fulfilled its promise. First, the model does not readily explain certain features

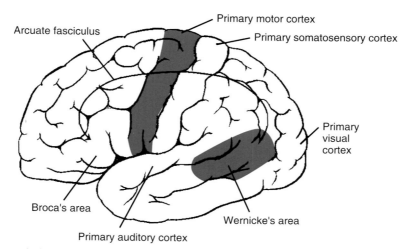

Fig. 9.3 Important perisylvian cortical regions of the central language mechanism. (From Brookshire, R. [2007]. *Introduction to neurogenic communication disorders* [7th ed.]. Mosby.)

of aphasic syndromes. Second, aphasic cases occasionally occur whose existence is not predicted by the model, such as in subcortical aphasia cases. Third, in a few cases, the expected symptoms do not appear when an established lesion site exists. As we will see, research has continued the work of Geschwind with advanced tools that have begun to help clarify the language processing areas of the brain.

Research in acquired communication disorders began to feel the influence of the field of cognitive neuropsychology as experimental psychologists developed information-processing models of cognition and language in individuals with brain damage. Information processing models were highly researched. These information-processing models required that a task be fractionated into its different components, which resulted in inaccurate or inefficient performance. The models usually represented the brain as a specialized computer that has domain-specific modules

associated with defined neural structures, with input and output routes mapped as the model becomes more specific to function. The modules were usually represented as boxes with the input and output routes as arrows. These models appealed to clinicians because techniques for assessment and treatment can be adapted from them. As the use of advanced imaging techniques and electrophysiologic studies have begun to proliferate in literature relevant to speech-language pathology, these models also appealed because of potential relevance to neural circuitry and connectivity.

As imaging and electrophysiologic studies become more common and innovative, we are closer to combining the information gained from them and computational modeling for information processing (e.g., Fig. 9.4 is from a 2002 study on auditory sentence processing). The following sections detail specific language areas and their impact on language and cognition.

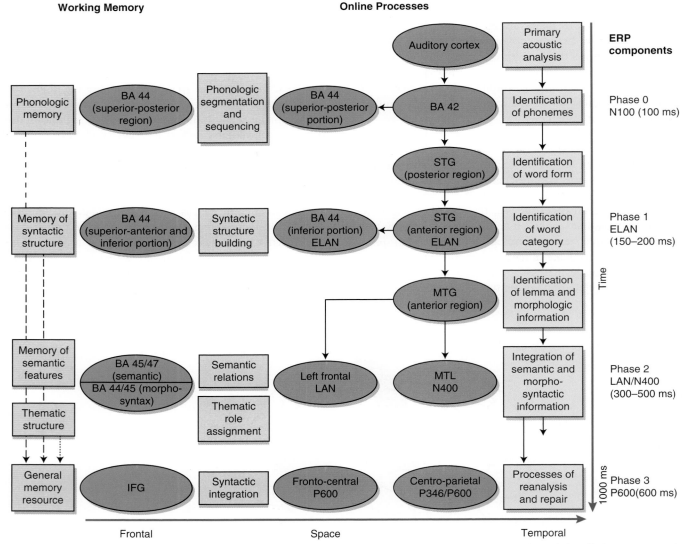

Fig. 9.4 Neurocognitive model of auditory sentence processing. The boxes represent the functional processes, and the ellipses represent the underlying neural correlate identified by functional magnetic resonance imaging (fMRI), positron emission tomography (PET), or event-related potentials (ERP). The neuroanatomic specification (indicated by text in parentheses) is based on either fMRI or PET data. *BA,* Brodmann area; *IFG,* inferior frontal gyrus; *LAN,* language; *STG,* superior temporal gyrus; *MTG,* middle temporal gyrus; *ELAN,* early left anterior negativity; *MTL,* medial temporal lobe. (From Friederici, A. D. [2002]. Towards a neural basis of auditory sentence processing. *Trends in Cognitive Sciences, 6*(2), 78–84.)

NEUROLOGIC SUBSTRATES OF LANGUAGE PROCESSING AND PRODUCTION

Perisylvian Zone

The major neurologic components of language are situated in the dominant hemisphere called the **perisylvian cortex**. Table 9.2 summarizes the components of the language model as hypothesized by Geschwind et al.,[18] from the initial work of Wernicke. This zone contains Broca area, Wernicke area, supramarginal gyrus, and angular gyrus, as well as the major long association tracts that connect the many language centers. These areas are composed of primarily supramodal association cortex. We begin by briefly discussing the areas considered classic in any model of language. We then look at recent research that is expanding the notion of what brain structures may be involved in language and how they are involved.

Before describing these classic areas, describing the basics of language processing within them may be helpful. As mentioned, the smallest unit of language is the **phoneme**, which a SLP can write in phonetic symbols. It is thought that the cortex of the perisylvian area contains a distributed representation of phonemes and that this representation is encoded in all the various forms in which they are used. There are motor, auditory, visual, and tactile representations. Depending on the communication system (e.g., verbal vs. signing), the representation of one type may be stronger than others because of the strengthening of the connections through use. These representations are supported by their links or connections with appropriate cortical processing areas within the perisylvian cortex. These links allow abstract representations of phonemes to be translated into reality. The translation allows a sound to be spoken, a letter representation to be written or signed, and a spoken representation of that phoneme to be correctly understood as that particular phoneme as opposed to other ones. Another functional aspect of the perisylvian cortex is to sequence these individual phonemes into combinations found in a particular language—the phoneme blends, syllables, and words that make up a language. This is the first step, but without a consequent linking to a particular neural pattern that corresponds to meaning, these combinations would have no value.

Recent research using fMRI established a predictive map of the cortical representations of semantic categories. In scanners, subjects listened to natural story stimuli. Semantic categories were found to be represented by distributed and overlapping cortical regions. Both hemispheres supported semantic representations, although the left was more selective to concrete concepts and the right hemisphere more selective for abstract concepts. Moreover, semantic relations that reflected conceptual progressions from concrete to abstract were represented by activation in the default mode network. The authors of this study concluded that the human brain uses distributed networks to encode both concepts and relationship between concepts, and that the default mode network plays a role in semantic processing for abstraction of concepts.[54]

Broca and Wernicke Areas

The location and limits of Broca area in the frontal lobe are well defined by research from several sources (see Chapter 2). However, Broca area is composed of distinct regions, each specializing in a specific function. Experiments have demonstrated that the anterior (pars triangularis) and ventral (pars orbitalis) parts are more involved in semantic processing, and the posterior portion (pars opercularis) is engaged with syntactic and phonologic processing as well as motor control of speech. In addition, the pars triangularis asymmetry between right and left hemispheres was highly correlated with language dominance, which suggests that this cortical site is predictive of language dominance.

Wernicke area, found in the temporal lobe, has long been considered a major component in the model of neurologic language functioning. However, there has never been a consistent anatomic definition for this area. Adding to the confusion is that patients with posterior lesions are often referred to as having Wernicke aphasia even though their presentations were heterogeneous.

Both Broca and Wernicke areas are now considered to be lacking specificity. The large-scale brain networks and connectome maps have demonstrated that these regions have different and discrete functions. Because these areas lack consistent definition of Broca and Wernicke areas, researchers recommend that terms should no longer be used and that they are replaced by more specific terminology, indicating exact anatomic sites.[16,46]

Arcuate Fasciculus

Wernicke[51] must be given credit for developing a language model that highlights the connective association pathways between the frontal and temporal speech-language areas. The arcuate fasciculus (AF) is a large, dense tract of white matter fibers connecting numerous frontal and temporal lobe language centers within each hemisphere. The AF passes dorsally below the parietal lobe. The original model proposed

TABLE 9.2	Major Components of the Central Language Mechanism Model
Structure	Function
Broca area	Motor programming for articulation
Motor strip	Activation of muscles for articulation
Arcuate fasciculus	Transmission of linguistic information to anterior areas from posterior areas
Wernicke area	Comprehension of oral language
Angular gyrus	Integrates visual, auditory, and tactile information and carries out symbolic integration for reading
Supramarginal gyrus	Symbolic integration for writing
Corpus callosum	Transmission of information between hemispheres

by Wernicke was thought to support repetition of verbal information. Later models attributed the importance of the dorsal stream, with the AF a critical component of it, as an interface between acoustic reception and the motor act of articulation. However, recently, studies using brain imaging of patients with aphasia along with more traditional language testing supported the broader role of the AF in language processing. In addition, research demonstrated that different sections of the AF support different language functions in the left hemisphere. In particular, the long segment of this tract contributed to naming abilities. The anterior section was important to fluency and naming. The posterior section of the AF played a role in language comprehension. These results emphasize the importance of this tract to language functioning on the left, with no role of the AF in language on the right in right-handed individuals. The AF does much more than enable repetition: It plays a significant role in comprehension and naming and appears to support residual language abilities.[26]

Inferior Parietal Lobule (Angular Gyrus and Supramarginal Gyrus)

Two gyri are collectively called the inferior parietal lobule: angular gyrus and supramarginal gyrus. The angular gyrus in the left parietal lobe has long been recognized for its role in language. Joseph J. Dejerine (1849–1917) suggested that this area was one of two sites associated with the reading disorder alexia. This gyrus is a distinct region of the cortex, and its functions include integrating and connecting information from surrounding regions. We now recognize various roles of the angular gyrus, including in spatial cognition, attention, memory, and executive functioning, as well as the complex language functions that enable reading and writing.[25]

Anterior to the angular gyrus is the supramarginal gyrus, curving around the posterior end of the sylvian fissure. Sensory information is analyzed and integrated in this area, which is thought to play an important role in perception. Lesions of the supramarginal gyrus in the dominant hemisphere have been associated with agraphia (writing disorders).

New Understanding of the Structures Involved with Language

A review of the evidence from studies of language in aging and after brain damage proposed that the neural basis for language can best be understood by neural multifunctionality. The authors of this review article analyzed research from lesion studies, neuroimaging, and longitudinal language development, and concluded that there are neural networks specialized for cognitive, affective, and praxic skills. In this model, linguistic information is processed through a neural system of component processes in which multiple cognitive tasks contribute simultaneously. The basis of this neural system is a population of neurons that carry out specific functions; these neurons form neural circuits as they connect to one another and eventually form the large-scale brain networks discussed earlier in this chapter.

This model also explains recovery from aphasia as a dynamic development of new neural circuits that interact with nonlinguistic circuits to produce new functional networks.[1,10] Such a model would also help us understand how complex brain functions are possible from a finite set of anatomic structures. Functional networks are constrained by structural connections; however, during a cognitive task, for example, many circuits are recruited to work together, which enables complex task execution and performance.[34]

We know from fMRI studies that mature brains are organized into functional networks that work together to support cognitive and linguistic functions. The developing brain in children is also organized into this kind of network but primarily by anatomic proximity. As the brain matures, the proximal networks become less segregated and become more integrated into regional connections. That is, we develop from more locally organized neural networks to the more distributed networks discussed earlier.

Language learning is subject to large individual differences, yet the vast majority of people learn language despite geographic, socioeconomic, and other factors. Two circuits that appear to be specialized for language learning are the dorsal and ventral pathways. Both arise from the posterior superior temporal gyrus. Fig. 9.5 shows the regions for distributed networks supporting language.

Dorsal Pathways

The dorsal stream projects toward the inferior parietal and posterior frontal lobe through the arcuate fasciculus. These pathways play a role in translating acoustic speech signals into motor/articulatory representations.

Ventral Pathways

The ventral pathways link the superior and middle temporal gyri, inferior parietal lobe, and occipital lobe with the inferior frontal gyrus. This stream is involved in the mapping of auditory speech signals into conceptual and semantic representations for language comprehension.

fMRI data reviewed by Friederici and Gierhan[15] show at least two ventral fiber connection pathways between the frontal cortex and the temporal cortex. These two pathways are the uncinated fasciculus (UF) and the inferior-frontal-occipital fasciculus (IFOF). The IFOF is sometimes referred to as the extreme capsule fiber system (ECFS). The UF connects the anterior frontal cortex with the anterior temporal cortex. The IFOF provides the connection between the frontal cortex and the three posterior cortical areas: temporal, parietal, and occipital cortices. With these pathways, areas in the anterior frontal cortex that are activated during semantic and syntactic processes such as semantic judgment, categorization, lexical-semantic access, and sentence plausibility are linked with the posterior areas in the temporal, parietal, and occipital cortices involved with lexical or sentence semantic processing. In addition to participating in semantic processing, the UF connections between the frontal operculum and the temporal cortex have been found to support syntactic processing for local phrase structure and for sentences that are syntactically simple.

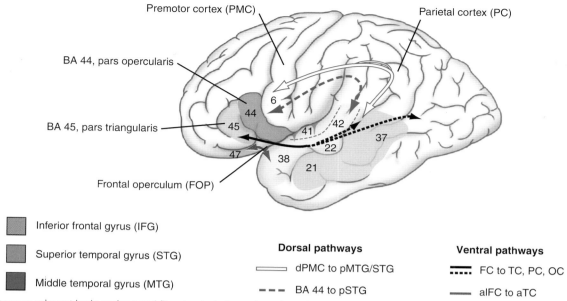

Fig. 9.5 Language-relevant brain regions and fiber tracts (schematic and condensed view of the left hemisphere). The dorsal pathway connecting dorsal premotor (dPMC) with posterior temporal cortex (pMTG/STG) involves the SLF III and/or the SLF II and the SLF-tp (discussed in detail later); the dorsal pathway connecting Brodmann area (BA) 44 with the posterior STG involves the AF. The ventral pathway connecting the frontal cortex (FC; i.e., BA 45 and others) with the temporal (TC), the parietal (PC), and the occipital (OC) cortices involves the inferior-frontal-occipital fasciculus (also called the extreme capsule fiber system); the ventral pathway connecting the anterior inferior FC (aIFC; i.e., BA 47 and others) and the FO, with the anterior TC (aTC) involves the UF. (Modified from Friederici, A. D., & Gierhan, S. M. E. [2013]. The language network. *Current Opinion in Neurobiology, 23*(2), 250–254.)

Subcortical Language Mechanisms

The strictly cortical model of language mechanisms has been questioned numerous times because patients with only subcortical lesions can also have language problems. Wilder G. Penfield and Lamar Roberts were among the first investigators to present evidence for possible subcortical mechanisms for language and speech.[35] They suggested that the pulvinar and ventrolateral nuclei of the thalamus serve as relay stations between Broca and Wernicke areas. They demonstrated massive fiber tracts to and from the thalamus and the major cortical speech and language areas. In addition, direct electrical stimulation of the left pulvinar and ventrolateral nuclei has produced naming problems.

Although subcortical aphasias have been reported since the 19th century, their existence has remained controversial. The language disturbance observed after thalamic infarct or damage to other subcortical mechanisms (caudate, globus pallidus, internal capsule) was originally believed to be a direct result of damage to a cortical structure for language; however, recent imaging has shown this theory to be incorrect. New explanations describe the complicated nature of subcortical-to-cortical connections and their influence on language processing and production when those connections are interrupted by damage.

Thalamic Lesions

The thalamus is a large subcortical structure often described as a relay station because almost all information received cortically is first processed in the thalamus. The thalamus is subdivided into various nuclei, each of which is specialized in processing a specific type of information. As many as 50

distinct nuclei have been identified in the thalamus, some of which have consistently produced language impairments when lesioned. The specific nuclei are the pulvinar/lateral posterior thalamus, anterior thalamic nuclei, and ventral anterior nucleus.

The resultant aphasia from a thalamic lesion is typically described as fluent with paraphasic errors, sometimes degenerating into jargon. Word finding is typically significantly impaired and may contribute to a severe impairment in spontaneous speech. The aphasia presentation may differ depending on the thalamic nucleus.

Pulvinar lesions are well studied; the resulting aphasia is described as fluent with semantic paraphasias and naming deficits. One author stated that the pulvinar's role in language is "most unsurprising," seeing that it projects to temporoparietal cortices as well as Broca area.[39] Anterior thalamic nuceli and ventral nuclei lesions may produce deficits in spontaneous language and verbal fluency as well as anomia. Collectively, these findings demonstrate a clear role for the thalamus in language processing and output. The authors of this review study conclude that because language is organized on a multisynaptic network involving various structural sites, an isolated lesion may impact the "whole functional system, although with different intensity and patterns," irrespective of the lesion location.[39]

In terms of the thalamus, its anatomy and connectivity indicate its role in language processing. Thalamic anatomy and relay fibers were discussed in Chapters 2 and 5, including the vast number of sensory relays that synapse in the thalamus, going from peripheral sensory nerve organs to the cortex, and then from the thalamus to the cortex for higher processing. In fact, the only type of sensory information that bypasses the thalamus is olfactory, as fibers from the nose synapse directly onto cortical tissues. Thalamic axons return into the thalamus and synapse on either relay neurons or on inhibitory interneurons within the thalamus. Connections between thalamic nuclei and cortical tissues are mostly two way, with numerous projections back to the thalamus from the cortex. This connectivity makes the thalamus function similarly to an airport. In this analogy, sensory information is like passengers arriving in a new country. They must be processed by immigration (the thalamus) and either allowed to stay in the country or transit to another place, like the cortex.

For language functions, the two most interesting thalamocortical loops relay from the dorsomedial nucleus and the pulvinar-lateral posterior nucleus of the thalamus to the cortex. The dorsomedial nucleus relays information originating from prefrontal cortical areas involved in executive functioning as well as from some subcortical areas. For the pulvinar-lateral posterior nucleus, projections are from the frontal, temporal, and parietal cortices and back.

Most of the thalamus is covered with a layer of cells that forms the **thalamic reticular nucleus**, a component of the reticular activating system discussed later. The cells of this layer receive inputs from the cortex as well as other sites within the thalamus. The reticular neurons themselves employ gamma-aminobutyric acid and are inhibitory, indicating that their function is to facilitate transmission to the cortex (through inhibition of the inhibitory action of the interneurons) or to block transmission to the cortex (by inhibiting the relay neurons). These reticular neurons are regulated by different brain systems, with two important ones being the reticular formation of the midbrain and projections from the cerebral cortex.

Reticular Activating System

The reticular activating system (RAS) is a complex set of relays connecting the brainstem, cerebellum, cortex, and subcortical structures. The "activating" term in its name refers to its major role in alerting: It guides our attention to stimuli by arousing specific cortical areas to the presence of this stimulus, and it does so by increasing blood flow to the targeted cortical areas. The RAS also suppresses repeated stimuli, such as a beeping car horn or traffic sounds, to prevent sensory overload. In addition to its major functions in arousal, the RAS is important in regulating the sleep-wake cycle and modulation of muscle tone, attention, and autonomic responses, among other functions.[3]

The two main components of the RAS are ascending and descending systems; the ascending system is sensory, delivering sensory information from peripheral cells to the brain. The response, if needed, is delivered via the descending tract, including motor functions and autonomic responses. For example, in a dangerous situation, say, the presence of a rattlesnake, visual and auditory information ascend to the thalamus and then the cortical sites. The motor response to this stimulus is sent to muscles for evasive action and to the autonomic system to increase blood pressure and respiration rates in preparation for flight.

RAS function. The RAS fibers project to the thalamus and to the cortex. The impact of the RAS on thalamic transmission is described as global and nonselective. During high levels of arousal, a strong excitation of the thalamic cells occurs, which inhibits the interneurons and consequently allows ready transmission through the thalamus in an unregulated fashion. During low arousal (with sleep and coma being the most common examples), little can overcome the inhibitory action of the interneurons, and most transmission through the thalamus is blocked, which allows more restful sleep.

In contrast to its impact on thalamic transmission, the impact of the RAS onto the cortical-thalamic-cortical projections is local and selective. Thalamic nuclei are thought to monitor the activity levels in cortical zones, connecting these zones to specific thalamic nuclei. During language activity, the perisylvian zones connect to the basal ganglia as well as to the thalamus, with feedback sent back to the essential cortical areas. This connectivity results in an integrated, feed-forward processing, similar to sensory processing.[33] This cortical-thalamic connection supports **declarative memory** (knowledge of facts and events) and the language function most dependent on declarative memory, which is naming. Naming deficits are seen in the majority of thalamic aphasia, supporting this link.

Nonthalamic Subcortical Lesions

Other subcortical structures besides the thalamus impact language. Lesions in the internal capsule, components of the basal ganglia, and the cerebellum have been documented to produce language disturbances, which will be discussed in more depth in Chapter 10.

In 2017, an evaluation of 38 consecutive patients with aphasia secondary to subcortical stroke divided patients into three groups based on lesion site: basal ganglia, specifically striato-capsular, thalamic, and white matter lesions. Comprehensive language testing found anomic aphasia as the most common aphasia type in all three groups, although aphasic difficulties were not restricted to naming difficulties. The aphasia in these patients was judged as milder than cortical aphasias. Additionally, subcortical aphasias did not show any correlation between lesion location and type and severity of aphasia, indicating that the same subcortical structure could yield different types of aphasia. These results imply that subcortical structures have an indirect and multifaceted effect on language, producing variable language impairments—in direct contrast to cortical aphasias, which have a more predictable correlation.[28]

Right Hemisphere

The contribution to language function from the right hemisphere continues to be a controversial topic, and models to explain can be divided into two main types. The older model attributed a minor language role to this hemisphere centered mainly around the use and comprehension of concrete words. More recent research has resulted in a different view and recognizes the roles of the right hemisphere in higher language functions, such as metaphoric and abstract language, prosody, visual word recognition, and other functions crucial to the competent use of language. This newer appreciation for the contributions of the right hemisphere to language was found from split brain research and lesion studies.

Split brain surgery is a drastic therapy to control intractable seizures, performed by severing the connection between the two hemispheres. Commissurotomy was developed in the 1960s and was successful in controlling seizures in some patients. It also enabled significant research on the function of each hemisphere with the use of split-brain research (see Chapter 2) and heralded a new interest in right brain function.

Lesion studies also helped elucidate the role of the right hemisphere in language. Some researchers estimate that about half the patients with right hemisphere damage present with verbal communication difficulty. Very young children who underwent a left hemispherectomy (removal) were able to learn language sufficiently. In contrast, a greater number of language deficits in this population followed a right hemispherectomy. Researchers speculate that this difference is due to prosodic processing, which may be helpful in language acquisition. However, with either right or left hemispherectomy, speech development and language comprehension were typically normal, indicating that only one hemisphere may be able to promote language.[17]

The current concept of right hemisphere functions shows it to be superior for the following:

- Visuospatial processing and visual perception
- Integration of different types of incoming stimuli
- Comprehending and producing emotion in the face and voice
- Maintaining a normal state of arousal and alertness
- Attending to the left side of space
- Attention in general, selecting what to attend to, and maintaining attention or shifting attention

At approximately the same time that this interest in right hemisphere processes was burgeoning, the concept of communication began to change and expand beyond the traditional informational processing input-output model. Communication style, nonverbal aspects of communication, as well as language use or the pragmatic aspects of language, were now of interest to clinicians and researchers. SLPs, linguists, and neuropsychologists began to look at discourse versus just words, phrases, and sentences and to put much more emphasis on meaning (both literal and implied). As in research with patients with left hemisphere damage, the communication abilities of patients with right hemisphere damage were studied and analyzed. Researchers and clinicians noted that many patients with right hemisphere damage have trouble communicating normally but that these difficulties were not language based in the traditional sense. Communication problems of the patient with right hemisphere damage are discussed in Chapter 10.

Role of Cognition in Communication

The *Oxford English Dictionary* defines cognition as "the mental action or process of acquiring knowledge and understanding through thought, experience, and the senses." However, the definition of cognition varies greatly across the speech-language literature as well as that of other professions. Examining cognition at work is examining functional mental events that take place during behavior, including such activities as perception, recognition, reasoning, judgment, concept formation, and problem solving. The domains of cognition may best be understood by categories. In neuropsychology, these categorizes are sensation and perception, motor skills and construction, attention and concentration, memory, executive functioning, processing speed, and language.[21] In speech pathology, our field requires particular understanding of the domains of attention, memory, executive functioning, processing speech, and language skills; however, it is important to be aware of all the cognitive domains, which will be briefly discussed later. Box 9.2 summarizes the four key concepts that speech pathology clinicians should consider when performing a cognitive assessment.

Sensation and Perception

Sensation refers to the detection of a sensory stimulus, such as the flavor of an apple or the smell of a rose. Perception indicates processing and integrating sensations. Deficits in this domain include loss of a sensory modality, such as blindness, or the inability to identify visual information in the setting of intact sensory inputs, such as visual agnosia.

Motor Skills and Construction

This domain includes fine motor skills, manual dexterity, balance, and other motor functions. These tasks have minimal cognitive and linguistic demands and are helpful in identifying basic motor problems.[21]

Attention and Concentration

Attention and concentration is a multifaceted category, generally divided into selective, alternating, and sustained attention. Selective attention refers to the ability to attend to important stimuli and ignore distracting ones (e.g., attending to a conversation on the phone while ignoring the TV show playing in the same room). Alternating attention is sometimes considered a component of selective attention, particularly in the field of neuropsychology where it is called dual-task processing. This skill enables a person to attend to two stimuli at the same time, such as listening to a podcast while cooking. Sustained attention is also called vigilance in the field of neuropsychology. This is the ability to attend to a task over time, such as listening to a lecture or taking an exam.

Memory

Memory is the retention of experiences over time. Memory functioning is the most complex and most multifaceted of the cognitive domains. The recognized subdomains of memory include sensory, working (short term), and long term. These domains have different names, depending on the particular discipline using them.

Sensory memory. Sensory memory is often considered to be the first step in information processing. We are

BOX 9.2 Cognitive Factors in Communication

Attention and Information Processing

- Attention requires a certain level of arousal (alertness) as well as perception of sensory input.
- Attentional capacity refers to the amount of information one can hold; it is directed by attentional control mechanisms.
- Thought to reside in dorsolateral prefrontal cortex, which also is involved in planning and other executive functions, the orienting response, and additional executive functioning.

Memory

- Retention and recall of internal representations of experience-dependent changes over time.
- Visual and auditory sensory storage can be broken into two types of information processing:
  - Short-term memory: temporary storage that begins to decay in 30 sec to a few minutes
  - Long-term memory: permanent storage of unlimited capacity
- Two kinds of information stored in memory:
  - Procedural (implicit) memory: recalled from performance of repetitive, learned motor behaviors over time
  - Declarative (explicit) memory: recalled through verbal or visual sensory recognition and recall cues

Reasoning and Problem Solving

- Two types of reasoning:
  - Deductive reasoning: evaluation based on a number of facts to create a conclusion about one thing (person, fact, event, etc.)
  - Inductive reasoning: evaluation based on generalization of one fact to create a broad interpretation and conclusion
- Problem solving involves evaluation based on reasoning and application to produce a conclusion
- Lesions to the prefrontal and subcortical areas have been shown to impair both reasoning and problem-solving processes

Metacognition and Executive Functioning

- Metacognition refers to the ability to recognize how and when to use reasoning and problem-solving skills to solve specific problems with the most effective cognitive strategies.
- Executive functions include anticipation, goal direction, planning, monitoring of internal and external events, and feedback interpretation.
- Frontal lobes carry out metacognitive and executive functioning processes.

continuously receiving sensory signals, which are then taken up by sensory receptors and processed in the nervous system. Sensory memory is fleeting, stored for as long as that particular sense is receiving stimulation. For example, as you are walking, you may get a whiff of a sweet fragrance. If you register that smell and recognize it, you have successfully transferred this memory into more cortical control, **short-term memory**. If, however, you keep walking obliviously, that sensory memory fades when your olfactory receptors are no longer stimulated, and you will only be marginally aware of a general pleasantness. In other words, sensory memory does not require attentional effort, but transferring it does.

Working (short-term) memory. Working memory is the skill that allows us to hold information consciously and either maintain it or manipulate it. For example, if a friend tells you their phone number, you may repeat the digits to yourself as you take down the information—called maintenance. If you notice a similarity between those digits and your own phone number, this helps you retain the sequence, and you have now manipulated the information. New information in working memory is temporary, although not as fleeting as sensory memory. If information is rehearsed or manipulated, it may be stored into long-term memory; however, most information in working memory is lost. We have all experienced being given directions to a new place and then promptly forgetting some of the steps; the reason for this lapse is that the directions remained in working memory and were not actively processed—in other words, encoded in long-term storage.

Long-term memory. Long-term memory refers to the unlimited capacity we have to store information and retain it for long periods of time, or even over our entire lifespan. Long-term memory can be explicit or implicit. Explicit memory is further subdivided into episodic and semantic.

Declarative/episodic memory. Declarative or **episodic memory** allows us to encode, maintain, and retrieve information in and out of long-term storage. Information can include sensory, verbal, and nonverbal inputs. The episodic memory system interacts with working memory to transfer information from the brief time it is held in working memory into longer storage. Our ability to recall events of yesterday, for example, is episodic. That we can talk about events that have happened indicates why this type of memory is also called declarative (depending on the discipline). Encoding is part of this type of memory, allowing us to manipulate presented information and analyze it. For example, when required to memorize a list of unrelated words, a student may find relationships between some items, grouping the list into broad categories (e.g., animals, clothing). This categorization allows the items to be encoded and easier to retrieve. The items are now stored and available to the student days or weeks later.

Semantic memory. Our ability to represent information in language enables us to share knowledge and manipulate, associate, and combine concepts. All of science, literature, systems of government, and religion, to name a few, depend on semantic memory. Activities such as reasoning, planning for the future or reminiscing about the past depend on the concepts stored in semantic memory.[11]

Retrieval. Retrieval is also a component of this memory system. In the retrieval stage, a memory can be recalled freely. In the previous example, the student may be able to state the items from the list of words without help. A memory can also be cued, and the cues may be semantic or forced choice. In semantic cueing, the student may be prompted to recall the animals from the list. In forced choice cues, the student may be asked which of two animals was on the list.

Prospective memory. A component of memory that places executive functioning demands, prospective memory enables us to remember an action planned for the future. It is defined as the memory for intentions. Remembering to take your medications as prescribed or pilots checking all systems prior to a flight are examples of this memory. A survey reported that we broadly assign an estimated 30% of memory time to prospective tasks, 55% to present ones, and 13% to recall of previous events.[2]

Considering the amount of processing required in explicit memory, it is not surprising that there are many neural mechanisms activated. Although no consensus exists to date about the number and exact loci involved, the following are some of the cortical centers thought to play a significant role: the inferior parietal lobule, the ventral and lateral temporal lobe, the sensory-motor cortices, and the frontal lobes.[11]

Implicit memory. Implicit memory belongs under long-term memory because implicit information is available for long stretches of time or even the lifetime of a person. Implicit memory encompasses all unconscious memories and skills. There are four recognized subtypes of implicit memory: procedural, associative, nonassociative, and priming.

Procedural memory. Often called muscle memory, this is the type of memory for motor actions or skills acquired through extensive practice and with trial and error. Consider how you learned to ride a bicycle, with numerous wobbles and perhaps even falls. However, once an activity is learned, it is available for life. **Procedural memory** supports daily life by helping with efficient processing of automatic responses.

Procedural memory is neurally encoded differently from episodic memory, which is why a patient with total amnesia can still recall how to ride a bicycle or type. While other types of memory are encoded cortically, the neural basis for procedural memory is subcortical, including the basal ganglia and cerebellum. Patients with degenerative diseases of these structures (e.g., Parkinson and Huntington diseases) have shown more deterioration in procedural memory as compared to declarative recall. The frontal and parietal regions are also thought to be involved in procedural memory, which was demonstrated on patients with isolated lesions in those cortical areas. Other cortical areas, such as the fusiform gyrus, may also play a role.[11]

Associative memory. Associative memory refers to the storage and retrieval of information through association with already acquired information. Associative memory is the basis of operant and classical conditioning, where a new behavior is associated with another stimulus. Pavlov's dog is a classic example.

Nonassociative memory. In nonassociative memory new behaviors are learned through repeated exposure. Habituation is a subtype, where the repetition of a stimulus decreases the response to it, such as when traffic sounds no longer bother someone who resides near a highway. The neural model of habituation is that as acetylcholine is progressively released, its effectiveness decreases. In sensitization, the opposite effect is achieved, where repetition increases the response. For example, schoolchildren can usually tune out ambient school sounds, but they will respond immediately to the bell that signals breaks or the end of the school day. The neural model of sensitization is the presence of serotonin in response to a sensory stimulus that causes an increase in acetylcholine.

Priming. Exposure to a stimulus that later increases the likelihood of a response is called priming. For example, showing a yellow card often evokes a faster response to the word *banana* than to other words. Researchers have demonstrated priming in experimental conditions where they had subjects read words such as *cautious* and *leisurely*. The subjects then walked more slowly than before.[11]

Executive Functioning: Reasoning and Problem Solving

Executive Functions. **Executive functions** are a set of skills that allows us to plan, attend, recall, prioritize, organize, and juggle multiple tasks successfully. The fact that most nonroutine processes are carried out in a deliberate, coordinated manner and that human beings are typically self-regulating and able to inhibit inappropriate behaviors are testament to the executive system of the frontal lobes. These abilities are sometimes called reasoning and problem-solving skills. Executive functioning was sometimes called frontal lobe skills; however, much of the cortex is involved during executive tasks. Interestingly, executive functioning is less affected by aging than other cognitive skills. Older people often demonstrate increased reasoning and problem-solving prowess, as well as improved semantic memory, although processing speech and working memory span decrease. This observation indicates that executive functioning improves over time while the component skills may worsen.[21]

Reasoning and Problem Solving. **Reasoning** is the process of evaluating information and generating conclusions. Two types of reasoning are discussed and evaluated clinically. In deductive reasoning, a number of premises, facts, and opinions are considered, and a conclusion is drawn. In inductive reasoning generalization from one fact or instance is turned into a broad interpretation. In most cases problem solving and reasoning are simultaneous mental activities performed while trying to reach a conclusion needed to solve a problem. Guilford and Hoepfner[20] think of problem solving as having five steps: preparation, analysis, production, verification, and reapplication. These steps obviously point to problem solving (and reasoning) as being a multifaceted process. Impairments in problem solving and reasoning are often associated with lesions in prefrontal regions of the brain, although subcortical damage also can cause difficulties.[45] The prefrontal cortex has been shown to cause difficulty with these skills. For example, researchers in a study of a large group of persons with focal brain damage suggested that social problem solving, psychometric intelligence, and emotional intelligence are supported by a shared network of frontal, temporal, and parietal regions with white matter tracts that connected and bound them into this shared network.[6]

Metacognition and Executive Functions

Metacognition is awareness and understanding of one's own thought processes. Metacognition, then, refers to the seemingly subconscious ability to know how and when to attend, remember, and organize information and recognize and solve certain problems with certain strategies.

Processing Speed

Processing speed refers to the time required for task performance. Prototypical processing speed tasks include coding tasks or connecting sequences while timed. Processing speed is a sensitive measure for several neuropsychiatric conditions, such as schizophrenia, and it is the strongest predictor of overall cognitive performance.[21]

CHANGING THE BRAIN

Any neurology text that is written is behind in its acknowledgment and explanations of new discoveries and research the day it is surrendered for publication. In the past 3 decades the research findings and the technology enabling this science to proceed has exploded. Although still slow, the transmission of these findings to others is much more rapid than was once possible. Many more journals are being published, some online, and many more conferences and other interactions are taking place. This engages other scientists and advances even more discovery.

A text such as this, with the task of teaching students the names, locations, and primary purpose and physiologic mechanisms of parts of the brain most important to a certain function (in this case, communication), is of necessity simplistic in nature. It tends to present the brain as developing over time into an essentially hardwired structure. This is not the impression that students should take away. The mature brain is actually a somewhat flexible organ, capable of more change and development than previously accepted by scientists and medical practitioners.

Neuroplasticity and Neurogenesis

Neuroplasticity

Neuroplasticity refers to the ability of the brain to modify, change, and adapt structure and function in response to experience. Neuroplasticity is variable across individuals and through the lifetime. This variability is attributable to many factors, including age, gender, and psychological traits.

Age is an important variable. Brain changes occur predominantly in early life and are collectively known as critical periods. These periods have been demonstrated in all major sensory systems and in animals. For our field, hearing restoration, visual adaptation, and language acquisition are particularly important. The critical period for language acquisition is well documented and explained in Chapter 13.

In hearing restoration, children with cochlear implantation before age 4 show hearing restoration. However, restoration of hearing has also been found in aging humans who were provided appropriate therapies. Studies of congenitally blind persons have shown CNS changes that lead to improvements in other senses, with expansion of auditory, olfactory, or sensory cortex into the occipital lobe. This neuroplasticity provides affected individuals a greater functionality and compensation for their other senses.[41]

Sex differences have been shown to impact cognition in both animal models and in humans. Estrogen enhances dopamine release, facilitating memory functions.

Psychological traits covary with neuromodulator levels. There is a strong relationship between dopamine receptors and individual differences in risk-taking behaviors.[49]

Just how much neuroplasticity the brain is capable of demonstrating is surprising. Plasticity has even been induced in the human nervous system. Various stimulation methods have been used in the treatment of disease and have produced a corresponding change in brain function. For example, vagal nerve stimulation involves a stimulator implanted surgically in epilepsy patients and people with depression, which is used to impact the functioning of the vagus nerve. This stimulation causes widespread release of neurotransmitters, including acetylcholine, noradrenaline, and dopamine. These brief bursts of stimulation have shown a change in brainstem structures that induces release of acetylcholine and other neuromodulator agents. These studies indicate that brain plasticity may be harnessed for learning and recovery following brain injury or disease.

Neurogenesis

Through studies duplicating earlier findings in animals, scientists now accept that there is **neurogenesis** (birth of new neurons) in some parts of the adult brain.[7] In most mammals there is well-documented neurogenesis for neurons in the olfactory bulb. However, humans are unique in this aspect because there is little if any olfactory neurogenesis in the postnatal period. The evolutionary decrease in dependence on smell and increased dependence on cognitive and social brain areas for human survival is likely related to the finding of no neurogenesis in the olfactory bulb of human brains.

Neurogenesis has been documented for two areas of the adult human brain: the hippocampus[5] and the striatum.[13] The neurons are able to generate because the brain has a reserve of neural stem cells that can differentiate themselves into neurons or other cells of the nervous system. In humans these stem cells or neuroblasts are born in the hippocampus for neurogenesis there. For striatal neurons, they appear to be derived from the subventricular zone (see Chapter 11) and migrate to the striatum. These new neurons can make new connections and establish themselves into functional circuits that already exist, enhancing the structure as well as the function. Thus, even the adult brain is now believed to demonstrate neuroplasticity, although certainly not to as great an extent as that of a young child.

Neurogenesis in the hippocampus appears to be a continuous process[7] with the newborn neurons having specialized electrophysiologic properties for about 1 month. After this period of time, they cannot be distinguished from older neurons.[32] Bergmann and Frisén[7] discuss that these new neurons participate in a process called pattern separation. The neural process of pattern separation allows the brain to discriminate similar experiences and organize them for storage as distinct memories. They use the example of humans being able not only to remember parking a car in a parking lot but remembering where it was parked this time. This process, as you can see from that example, is critical for human adaptation to our increasingly complex environment.

To date, the functional purpose of neurogenesis in the striatum of the mature brain has not been established.[13] The striatum plays an important role in planning and modulating movement, in cognitive flexibility, and in reward/motivation cycles. The adult neurogenesis may help account for individual functionality in these areas with neural integration of these cells. The rate of neurogenesis in the striatum is low under homeostatic conditions for the body and brain. However, the rate increases in response to pathologic conditions, adding small numbers of neurons to the striatum over a long period of time. Investigation of how these new striatal neurons could be used to promote renewal of function in diseases that attack striatal neurons such as Huntington chorea or in disorders such as schizophrenia or addiction, which alter striatal response to reward, could be important to finding treatment modalities for these illnesses.

Recovery in the Damaged Brain

Although not discussed in this chapter, there is evidence for generation of new cells in the mature brain outside of neurons: new neuroglial cells. Oligodendrocytes account for most of the new glial cells produced in the adult brain. The normal function of many nerve fibers depends on myelination of those fibers, as you will remember. As new connections and new fibers appear in the brain, new oligodendrocytes are necessary for new production of myelin to wrap around these fibers enhancing signal transmission. Myelin can be regenerated by these cells to restore some neurologic function. Disease processes may cause incomplete regeneration, resulting in the death of these fibers that have lost myelin. You see this process in action in such diseases as advanced multiple sclerosis.

Astrocytes are another type of glial cell for which there is evidence for limited new generation in the mature nervous system.[7] However, after local injury there is commonly a large increase of astrocytes generated by neural stem cells or by duplication of existing astrocytes. This generation of astrocytes in the damaged brain may not be a positive factor, however. The cells will combine with connective tissue cells and form scar tissue. This scar tissue may then prevent the regrowth of axons, for example, after stroke.

SLPs must believe that the brain can change and reorganize. If they did not, no one would show up to work every day to treat clients attempting to improve their communication skills. Research in neuroscience supports the belief that a permanent change in behavior does involve a change in brain organization. This does not mean change only in the strength of connections in the neural networks involved in the behavior, as takes place when memories are formed. It also may mean a change in the brain where these connections are made or in the pathways used—a type of rezoning or reassignment of the duties of cells in a certain part of the brain. With better technology and more elegant research design, perhaps we will one day be able to know exactly what changes are taking place in the brain during successful (or, in some cases, unsuccessful) treatment for a communication disorder.

One new treatment method that has resulted from the curiosity of a neuroscientist about brain reorganization and its usefulness in rehabilitation is **constraint-induced therapy (CIT)**, introduced by Taub et al.,[44] for improving the use of the paralyzed arm after a stroke. In CIT the functional arm is restrained in a sling, with the hand covered to prevent use. In the initial study, the patients who were 1 year or more poststroke received intensive treatment for 10 days and performed all tasks for most of their waking hours with the paralyzed limb as best they could. At the end of the 10-day period, clients had regained considerable functional use of the formerly paralyzed limb, whereas control subjects who did not receive treatment showed no change. Taub hypothesized a "use-dependent cortical reorganization." Investigation using transcranial magnetic stimulation (TMS) to map the cortical activity before and after CIT proved Taub's hypothesis.[29] Treatment resulted in improved motor functioning and caused the area of the motor cortex controlling the hand to enlarge with recruitment of more neurons in the motor cortex, particularly those adjacent to the area that originally controlled the arm. With more extensive damage to the motor cortex, neurons in the premotor cortex or even in the opposite hemisphere are hypothesized to participate in the network supporting the improved function.

The strong evidence for success with CIT for paralyzed limbs of stroke patients led to interest in CIT for improvement of communication in persons with aphasia. Several studies were initially performed in Europe, showing that constraint-induced aphasia therapy involving the principles of prevention of compensatory communication and massed practice produced significant and stable improvement. Changes in performance on standardized testing as well as in communication as measured by patient and family report and communicative effectiveness ratings were all significantly greater than for patients who participated in the same amount of therapy with more traditional treatment methods allowing compensatory communication use. Since that time several studies have been published with varying methodology and outcomes. A recent review of research articles in this field concluded that CIT may be useful in improving chronic poststroke aphasia; however, there is insufficient evidence about its superiority compared to other aphasia therapies.[43,55]

This chapter ends on a positive note for the clinician because of the work of neuroscientists to prove that the brain can be changed by chemical and surgical intervention as well as by behavioral treatments that replace or supplement other treatments. Chapter 10 describes some of the acquired disorders of communication that adults may experience when damage occurs to language processing areas of the brain. It is hoped that clinicians will not only learn from the literature of neuroscience but will continue to contribute findings that support enhancement of brain function even after the brain has been damaged.

SYNOPSIS OF CLINICAL INFORMATION AND APPLICATIONS FOR THE SLP

- Six layers comprise the neocortex, consisting primarily of pyramidal cells with axons and dendrites ascending and descending from one layer to another.
- Studies using isotropic fractionating have suggested that the ratio of neurons to nonneurons in the brain may be more equal in number than originally thought.
- Synaptic organization is concerned with the way input neurons, projection neurons, and interneurons organize themselves and connect through synapses, becoming neural circuits.
- Dendritic connections and subunits within microcircuits form local circuits in regions of the brain. The connections between these regions and their circuits account for behaviors.
- These connections form small world communities at the microlevel. At the macrolevel, the neuronal processes expand out for long-range connections.
- The brain's vast circuitry is made possible by convergence and divergence of synapses in the nervous system.
- Most postsynaptic sites in the cerebellum, basal ganglia, and cortex are on dendritic spines, increasing the surface area and probably enabling rapid signal processing and LTP.
- A pattern-associator network allows the input patterns to be transformed into output patterns (e.g., sequences of letters transformed into spoken words read aloud).
- All the primary association areas are thought to be collections of pattern-associator networks in which neural representations (percepts, concepts, etc.) are formed.
- The first mapping of cellular connection was done on a nematode in 1986.
- Human brain connectivity is being traced through advanced diffusion tensor imaging methods through a US government-funded multicenter study called the Human Connectome.[47]
- The pattern of neural connections strengthened into a representation is difficult to lose completely. Rather, some components of the representation may be activated, although others are not, degrading the representation. This is called graceful degradation. This often allows people to deal successfully with ambiguous or partial information.
- Learning is the brain increasing the efficiency of synaptic connections.
- Synaptic connections within networks are strengthened by synchronous firing.
- Synaptic connections in neural networks are the physical foundation of learning and memory and account for Hebbian learning.
- Learning requires active participation by multiple brain areas, including the reticular network, sensory and/or motor association areas, thalamocortical circuitry, fusiform area, hippocampus and other medial temporal lobe structures, lateral and superior temporal lobe, cerebellar and striatum circuitry, and diffuse areas of the neocortex.
- Geschwind's model of language, based in large part on the work of Wernicke, is a traditional localization or connectionism model, but has held up over time and is not negated by neural network theory or by evidence from neuroimaging.
- Geschwind's model emphasizes Broca area, Wernicke area, the arcuate fasciculus, and parietal areas of the angular and supramarginal gyrus. These areas comprise the perisylvian language zone. Recent research has identified other connections laid out in a ventral and dorsal stream within the perisylvian zone.
- Language disorders may appear to result from damage to subcortical structures, especially the thalamus and parts of the basal ganglia.[27] However, research into the etiology of the language difficulty has demonstrated that the language disorders result from the indirect effects on cortical language areas.
- Hypoperfusion of the cortex follows basal ganglia and capsular damage because of reduced flow through the lenticulostriate arteries. The language symptoms depend on what area of the perisylvian zone is affected.
- The right hemisphere is dominant for visuospatial processing, integration of different kinds of stimuli, attention, intention, and holistic processing. Right hemisphere damage affects communication in a broader sense with discourse and communication style as well as processing of more intangible input (e.g., humor, sarcasm).
- Cognition is the process of knowing, perceiving, or remembering. It is the examination of mental events, such as perception, reasoning, problem solving, and concept formation.
- Four key aspects of cognition important to the treatment of patients with cognitive-linguistic disorders are (1) attention and information processing, (2) memory, (3) reasoning and problem solving, and (4) metacognition and executive functioning. The study of these cognitive functions involves the dorsolateral cortex, the hippocampus and amygdala, orbitofrontal cortex, and the greater association area in the frontal lobes.
- New neuroimaging techniques and interest in neurogenesis (the birth of new neurons) and neuroplasticity of the brain have spawned exciting research into enhanced learning and recovery after brain damage.

CASE STUDY

A 64-year-old former van driver experienced sudden onset of confusion, slurred speech, and left-sided paralysis of the arm and leg. He was admitted to the hospital stroke unit and started on blood thinners after computed tomography ruled out hemorrhage. He was admitted to the acute rehabilitation unit in 2 days. Testing showed mild unilateral upper motor neuron dysarthria with fair intelligibility, poor pragmatics (poor eye contact, inattention to speaker if on his left, poor topic maintenance, apathy during communication), mild to moderate neglect of left side of space, mild anomia on confrontation naming and questioning, and constructional deficits in drawing and copying. After a

3-week stay, he was ambulatory with a leg brace, had little functional use of his left upper extremity, had improved intelligibility, and was learning to compensate for his left side neglect.

Questions for Consideration

1. What part(s) of the brain was (were) affected by this stroke?
2. Why is neglect more prominent with this location of damage to the brain?
3. What could be the cause of the perception of apathy in the patient's communication interactions?

REFERENCES

1. Albert, K. M., Potter, G. G., Boyd, B. D., Kang, H., & Taylor, W. D. (2019). Brain network functional connectivity and cognitive performance in major depressive disorder. *Journal of Psychiatric Research*, 110, 51–56. https://doi.org/10.1016/j.jpsychires.2018.11.020.

2. Anderson, F. (n.d.). Memory and complex learning lab. Washington University. https://sites.wustl.edu/memoryand complexlearning/prospective-memory/.

3. Arguinchona, J. H., & Tadi, P. (2021). *Neuroanatomy, reticular activating system*. StatPearls Publishing. PMID 31751025.

4. Azevedo, F. A., Carvalho, L. R., Grinberg, L. T., Farfel, J. M., Ferretti, R. E., Leite, R. E., Filho, J., Lent, R., & Herculano-Houzel, S. (2009). Equal numbers of neuronal and non-neuronal cells make the human brain an isometrically scaled-up primate brain. *Journal of Comparative Neurology*, 513(5), 532–541.

5. Baptista, P., & Andrade, J. P. (2018). Adult hippocampal neurogenesis: Regulation and possible functional and clinical correlates. *Frontiers in Neuroanatomy*, 12. https://doi.org/10.3389/fnana.2018.00044.

6. Barbey, A. K., Colom, R., Paul, E. J., Chau, A., Solomon, J., & Grafman, J. H. (2014). Lesion mapping of social problem solving. *Brain*, 137(10), 2823–2833.

7. Bergmann, O., & Frisén, J. (2013). Why adults need new brain cells. *Science*, 340(6133), 695–696.

8. Bijsterbosch, J. D., Valk, S. L., Wang, D., & Glasser, M. F. (2021). Recent developments in representations of the connectome. *NeuroImage*, 243, 118533. https://doi.org/10.1016/j.neuro image.2021.118533.

9. Bliss, T. V., & Cooke, S. F. (2011). Long-term potentiation and long-term depression: A clinical perspective. *Clinics (Sao Paulo, Brazil)*, 66(Supplement 1), 3–17. https://doi.org/10.1590/s1807-59322011001300002.

10. Cahana-Amitay, D., & Albert, M. L. (2014). Brain and language: Evidence for neural multifunctionality. *Behavioural Neurology*, 2014, 260381. https://doi.org/10.1155/2014/260381.

11. Camina, E., & Güell, F. (2017). The neuroanatomical, neuro-physiological and psychological basis of memory: Current models and their origins. *Frontiers in Pharmacology*, 8, 438. https://doi.org/10.3389/fphar.2017.00438.

12. Dos Santos, S., Medeiros, M., Porfirio, J., Tavares, W., Pessôa, L., Grinberg, L., Leite, R. E. P., Ferretti-Rebustini, R. E. L., Suemoto, C. K., Filho, W. J., Noctor, S. C., Sherwood, C. C., Kaas, J. H., Manger, P. R., & Herculano-Houzel, S. (2020). Similar microglial cell densities across brain structures and mammalian species: Implications for brain tissue function. *Journal of Neuroscience*, 40(24), 4622–4643.

13. Ernst, A., Alkass, K., Bernard, S., Salehpour, M., Perl, S., Tisdale, J., Possnert, G., Druid, H., & Frisén, J. (2014). Neurogenesis in the striatum of the adult human brain. *Cell*, 156(5), 1072–1083. https://doi.org/10.1016/j.cell.2014.01.044.

14. Fedorenko, E., & Blank, I. A. (2020). Broca's area is not a natural kind. *Trends in Cognitive Sciences*, 24(4), 270–284. https://doi.org/10.1016/j.tics.2020.01.001.

15. Fernández, M., Mollinedo-Gajate, I., & Peñagarikano, O. (2018). Neural circuits for social cognition: Implications for autism. *Neuroscience*, 370, 148–162. https://doi.org/10.1016/j.neuroscience.2017.07.013.

16. Friederici, A. D., & Gierhan, S. E. (2013). The language network. *Current Opinion in Neurobiology*, 23(2), 250–254.

17. Gainotti G. Lower- and higher-level models of right hemisphere language. A selective survey. Funct Neurol. 2016 Apr-Jun;31(2):67-73. doi: 10.11138/fneur/2016.31.2.067. PMID: 27358218; PMCID: PMC4936799

18. Geschwind, N. (1969). Problems in the anatomical understanding of aphasia. In A. L. Benton (Ed.), *Contributions to clinical neuro-psychology*. Aldine.

19. Glezer, L. S., Kim, J., Rule, J. S., Jiang, X., & Riesenhuber, M. (2015). Adding words to the brain's visual dictionary: Novel word learning selectively sharpens orthographic representations in the VWFA. *Journal of Neuroscience*, 35(12), 4965–4972.

20. Guilford, J. P., & Hoepfner, R. (1971). *The analysis of intelligence*. McGraw-Hill.

21. Harvey, P. D. (2019). Domains of cognition and their assessment. *Dialogues in Clinical Neuroscience*, 21(3), 227–237. https://doi.org/10.31887/DCNS.2019.21.3/pharvey.

22. Hebb, D. (1949). *The organization of behavior*. John Wiley and Sons.

23. Herculano-Houzel, S. (2019). Life history changes accompany increased numbers of cortical neurons: A new framework for understanding human brain evolution. *Progressive Brain Research*, 250, 179–216. https://doi.org/10.1016/bs.pbr.2019.06.001.

24. Hilgetag, C. C., & Goulas, A. (2016). Is the brain really a small-world network? *Brain Structure and Function*, 221, 2361–2366. https://doi.org/10.1007/s00429-015-1035-6.

25. Humphreys, G. F., Ralph, M. A. L., & Simons, J. S. (2021). A unifying account of angular gyrus contributions to episodic and semantic cognition. *Trends in Neurosciences*, 44(6), 452–463. https://doi.org/10.1016/j.tins.2021.01.006.

26. Ivanova, M. V., Zhong, A., Turken, A., Baldo, J. V., & Dronkers, N. F. (2021). Functional contributions of the arcuate fasciculus to language processing. *Frontiers in Human Neuroscience*, 15, 672665. https://doi.org/10.3389/fnhum.2021.672665.

27. Kang, E. K., Sohn, H. M., Han, M.-K., & Paik, N.-J. (2017). Subcortical aphasia after stroke. *Annals of Rehabilitation Medicine*, 41(5), 725–733. https://doi.org/10.5535/arm.2017.41.5.725.

28. Kwakkel, G., Veerbeek, J. M., van Wegen, E. E., & Wolf, S. L. (2015). Constraint-induced movement therapy after stroke. *The Lancet. Neurology*, 14(2), 224–234. https://doi.org/10.1016/S1474-4422(14)70160-7.

29. Lopez-Barroso, D., & de Diego-Balaguer, R. (2017). Language learning variability within the dorsal and ventral streams as a cue for compensatory mechanisms in aphasia recovery. *Frontiers in Human Neuroscience*, 11. https://doi.org/10.3389/fnhum.2017.00476.

30. McClelland, J. L., & Cleermans, A. (2009). Connectionist models James L. McClelland & Axel Cleermans. In T. Byrne, A. Cleermans, & P. Wilken (Eds.), *Oxford companion to consciousness*. Oxford University Press.

31. Menon, V. (2011). Large-scale brain networks and psychopathology: A unifying triple network model. *Trends in Cognitive Sciences*, 15(10), 483–506. https://doi.org/10.1016/j.tics.2011.08.003.

32. Ming, G.-L., & Song, H. (2011). Adult neurogenesis in the mammalian brain: Significant answers and significant questions. *Neuron*, 70(4), 687–702.

33. Moretti, R., Caruso, P., Crisman, E., & Gazzin, S. (2018). Thalamus and language: What do we know from vascular and degenerative pathologies. *Neurology India*, 66(3), 772–778.

34. National Institutes of Health. (2015). Blueprint: Human Connectome Project. https://neuroscienceblueprint.nih.gov/human-connectome/connectome-program

35. Pchitskaya, E., & Bezprozvanny, I. (2020). Dendritic spines shape analysis: Classification or clusterization? Perspective. *Frontiers in Synaptic Neuroscience*, 12. https://www.frontiersin.org/article/10.3389/fnsyn.2020.00031.

36. Penfield, W. G., & Roberts, L. (1959). *Speech and brain mechanisms*. Princeton University Press.

37. Popovic, M. A., Carnevale, N., Rozsa, B., & Zecevic, D. (2015). Electrical behaviour of dendritic spines as revealed by voltage imaging. *Nature Communications*, 6(8436). https://doi.org/10.1038/ncomms9436.

38. Purokayastha, S., Roberts, M., & Carrasco, M. (2021). Voluntary attention improves performance similarly around the visual field. *Attention, Perception, & Psychophysics*, 83, 2784–2794. https://doi.org/10.3758/s13414-021-02316-y.

39. Radanovic, M., & Almeida, V. N. (2021). Subcortical aphasia. *Current Neurology and Neuroscience Reports*, 21, 73. https://doi.org/10.1007/s11910-021-01156-5.

40. Rasch, B., & Born, J. (2013). About sleep's role in memory. *Physiological Reviews*, 93(2), 681–766. https://doi.org/10.1152/physrev.00032.2012.

41. Silva, P. R., Farias, T., Cascio, F., dos Santos, L., Peixoto, V., Crespo, E., Ayres, C., Ayres, M., Marinho, V., Bastos, V. H., Ribeiro, P., Velasques, B., Orsini, M., Fiorelli, R., de Freitas, M. R., & Teixeira, S. (2018). Neuroplasticity in visual impairments. *Neurology International*, 10(4), 7326. https://doi.org/10.4081/ni.2018.7326.

42. Sweatt, J. D. (2016). Neural plasticity and behavior—sixty years of conceptual advances. *Journal of Neurochemistry*, 139(S2), 179–199. https://doi.org/10.1111/jnc.13580.

43. Szaflarski, J., Allendorfer, J., Ball, A., Banks, C., Dietz, A., Hart, K., Lindsell, C., Martin, A., & Vannest, J. (2014). Randomized controlled trial of constraint-induced aphasia therapy in patients with chronic stroke. *Neurology*, 82(10 Supplement).

44. Taub, E., Uswatte, G., King, D. K., Morris, D., Crago, J. E., & Chatterjee, A. (2006). A placebo-controlled trial of constraint-induced movement therapy for upper extremity after stroke. *Stroke*, 37(4), 1045–1049.

45. Thiebaut de Schotten, M., Dell'Acqua, F., Valabregue, R., & Catani, M. (2012). Monkey to human comparative anatomy of the frontal lobe association tracts. *Cortex*, 48(1), 82–96.

46. Tremblay, P., & Dick, A. S. (2016). Broca and Wernicke are dead, or moving past the classic model of language neurobiology. *Brain and Language*, 162, 60–71. https://doi.org/10.1016/j.bandl.2016.08.004.

47. Van Essen, D. C., Smith, S. M., Barch, D. M., Behrens, T. E., Yacoub, E., Ugurbil, K., & WU-Minn HCP Consortium. (2013). The WU-Minn Human Connectome Project: An overview. *NeuroImage*, 80, 62–79. https://doi.org/10.1016/j.neuroimage.2013.05.041.

48. von Bartheld, C. S., Bahney, J., & Herculano-Houzel, S. (2016). The search for true numbers of neurons and glial cells in the human brain: A review of 150 years of cell counting. *Journal of Comparative Neurology*, 524(18), 3865–3895. https://doi.org/10.1002/cne.24040.

49. Voss, P., Thomas, M. E., Cisneros-Franco, J. M., & de Villers-Sidani, É. (2017). Dynamic brains and the changing rules of neuroplasticity: Implications for learning and recovery. *Frontiers in Psychology*, 8, 1657. https://doi.org/10.3389/fpsyg.2017.01657.

50. Watts, D. J., & Strogatz, S. H. (1998). Collective dynamics of "small world" networks. *Nature*, 393(6684), 440–442.

51. Wernicke, C. (1874). *Der aphasische symptomencomplex*. Cohn & Weigert.

52. Yeshurun, Y., Nguyen, M., & Hasson, U. (2021). The default mode network: Where the idiosyncratic self meets the shared social world. *Nature Reviews Neuroscience*, 22, 181–192. https://doi.org/10.1038/s41583-020-00420-w.

53. Zhang, J. (2019). Basic neural units of the brain: Neurons, synapses and action potential. *ArXiv*. https://doi.org/10.48550/arXiv.1906.01703.

54. Zhang, J., Yu, J., Bao, Y., Xie, Q., Xu, Y., Zhang, J., & Wang, P. (2017). Constraint-induced aphasia therapy in post-stroke aphasia rehabilitation: A systematic review and meta-analysis of randomized controlled trials. *PloS One*, 12(8), e0183349. https://doi.org/10.1371/journal.pone.0183349.

55. Zhang, Y., Han, K., Worth, R., & Liu, Z (2020). Connecting concepts in the brain by mapping cortical representations of semantic relations. *Nature Communications*, 11, 1877. https://doi.org/10.1038/s41467-020-15804-w.

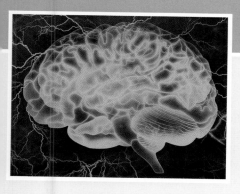

10

Adult Disorders of Language

Let the young know they will never find a more interesting, more instructive book than the patient himself.

Giorgio Baglivi

KEY TERMS

acceleration-deceleration injury
agraphia
alexia
alexia with agraphia
alexia without agraphia
altered mental status (AMS)
Alzheimer disease (AD)
amyloid plaques
aneurysm
anomic aphasia
anosognosia
aphasia
aphasic alexia
aprosodia
arteriosclerosis
arteriovenous malformation (AVM)
border zone
Broca aphasia
central (parietal-temporal) alexia
cerebrovascular accident (CVA)
circumlocution

cognitive-communicative (cognitive-linguistic) disorders
coma
conduction aphasia
confabulation
chronic traumatic encephalopathy (CTE)
deep dyslexia
delirium
dementia
denial
diffuse axonal injury (DAI)
dyslexias
encephalopathy
extinction
focal lesions
frontotemporal dementias (FTD)
glioma
global aphasia
infarction
ischemia

molecular commotion
neglect
neoplasm
neurofibrillary tangles
occlusion
phonologic alexia
posterior (occipital) alexia
primary progressive aphasia (PPA)
prosopagnosia
subcortical aphasia
surface dyslexia
thromboembolic
thrombus
transcortical aphasia
Transcortical Motor aphasia
Transcortical Sensory aphasia
transient ischemic attack (TIA)
traumatic brain injury (TBI)
unilateral inattention
vegetative states
Wernicke aphasia

Cognitive-communicative disorders were introduced in Chapter 9 and are detailed in this chapter. This introduction to the world of cognitive-communicative disorders has hopefully intrigued and fascinated you: There is a seemingly endless array of signs, symptoms, and syndromes that follow neurologic damage. The challenge to our field is to organize, refine, interpret, and draw conclusions from the confusing presentations to create and implement helpful treatment plans. What helps us perform our jobs well is a solid knowledge of anatomy and physiology of the nervous system, which will guide the diagnosis and develop the treatment plan. This chapter focuses on deficits of language, including aphasia, alexia, and agraphia, and deficits related to right hemisphere functions; deficits of cognition, including the impairments in dementia and in **traumatic brain injury (TBI)**, and the cognitive impairments secondary to Covid-19 infections.

APHASIA

Aphasia is an acquired language disorder due to brain damage, which manifests in difficulty producing or comprehending spoken or written language. Stroke is the most common cause, although many other injuries can produce aphasia. Sudden events such as TBI, or a slowly progressing illness such as a brain tumor, can result in aphasia. The American Speech-Language-Hearing Association (ASHA)[3] estimates that 1 million people are living with aphasia in the United States, yet a survey found that the vast majority of laypeople (~85%) have never heard of this diagnosis. The consequences of aphasia may be short term but are more often chronic, and they affect the individual's autonomy and quality of life.[19]

Etiology and Neuropathology of Aphasia

Aphasia results from focal damage to areas of the brain primarily responsible for the understanding and production of language. A focal lesion is different from diffuse damage to several parts of the brain. **Focal lesions** are caused by interruption in the blood flow to the area of the brain supplied by the particular arterial distribution. Because the middle cerebral artery perfuses most of the cortical language centers, it is also known as the artery of aphasia. Damage to this artery or one of its branches may produce aphasia.

Reduction of blood flow to an area is called **ischemia**. Blood carries oxygen to the brain, which is the biggest user of oxygen, consuming ~20% of the body's supply at any given time. Without an ongoing flow of oxygenated blood, the brain cannot function for long. In fact, if the brain is deprived of blood for ~30 to 180 seconds, the average person will lose consciousness; after 3 to 5 minutes irreparable brain damage or even death may result. Exceptions exist, such as interruption to blood flow in the presence of hypothermia; in this situation, the reduction in body temperature seems to have a protective effect on the brain, reducing the consequences of reduced oxygen.

When an area of the brain experiences a reduction in perfusion, and therefore oxygen, neuronal cell death or an **infarction** has occurred. If an area of the brain is infarcted, necrotic (dead) tissue remains in the affected area. Eventually, the infarcted area softens and liquefies, causing waste matter. This waste is removed, probably by astroglial action (gliosis), sometimes leaving a cavity that has the appearance of a crater in the brain with a rim of scar tissue around it formed by the astrocytes.

Several medical conditions may interrupt the vital oxygenated blood supply to the brain. These include **cerebrovascular accident (CVA)**, TBI, brain infections leading to focal abscess, vasculitis (or arteritis), and neoplasm. Trauma is discussed later in this chapter. Throughout these discussions, keep the fact in mind that TBI can result in both focal and diffuse brain damage. The following discussion of common causes of interruption to blood flow to the brain focuses on CVA and neoplasms.

Cerebrovascular Accident

The most frequent cause of interrupted blood flow is CVA, also known as stroke. Stroke is the fifth leading cause of death in persons older than 55 years, and it is increasing in younger adults and children. American Heart Association[2] statistics show that each year ~795,000 people in the United States experience new or recurrent strokes of either ischemic or hemorrhagic origin. On average, every 40 seconds someone in the United States has a stroke, and there is a stroke-related death every 4 minutes. More concerning is that aging is a risk factor for stroke; in the Western Hemisphere, improvements in medical care have made it possible for people to live longer, increasing the chance of stroke.

Stroke can result from two mechanisms of blood flow interruption and oxygen deprivation: **occlusion**, also called ischemia, or hemorrhage.

Occlusive mechanisms. In a stroke of occlusive origin, ischemia, an arterial vessel becomes occluded, reducing or stopping the flow of blood through that artery. The most common cause of arterial occlusion is a disease process known as **arteriosclerosis**, which is characterized by a thickening or hardening of the arterial wall with consequent reduction of elasticity of the vessel. This thickening may be caused by a proliferation of cells, particularly blood platelets, along the vessel wall, or abnormal fatty deposits on the artery walls. In either case, the buildup results in loss of elasticity, or fibrosis, of the vessel wall. As the deterioration of the wall increases, rigidity increases, which leads to a rise in hypertension (high blood pressure), putting the person at an even higher risk for CVA.

Current thinking is that most CVAs are embolic in origin, meaning that extraneous material in the vessel has occluded a cerebral vessel distal to its point of origin. This embolus has broken away from the vessel wall, traveling through the vessel as it branches, until it reaches a branch that is too small to allow it to continue moving with the blood flow (Fig. 10.1).

If the accumulation is exclusively composed of blood platelets, it is known as a **thrombus**, which can partially or completely occlude a vessel. This occlusion creates a reduction in blood flow and possibly a CVA, which would be thrombotic in origin. In cases where the origin of the CVA is not ascertained, the diagnosis may be called a **thromboembolic** stroke.

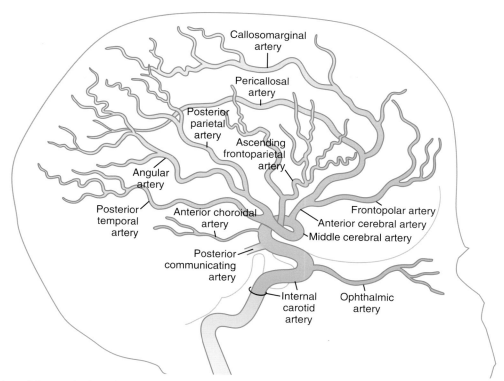

Fig. 10.1 Lateral view of the cerebral arteries detailing the branches of the anterior and middle cerebral arteries. (From Swaiman, K., Ashwal, K., Ferriero, D., et al. [2012]. *Swaiman's pediatric neurology* [5th ed.]. Saunders.)

An embolus may occur relatively fast as compared to a thrombus, where it may take minutes or weeks to clog an artery to the point of occlusion. The correlating clinical presentation may appear suddenly and increase in severity over minutes, hours, or even days. When the symptoms seem to increase, it is referred to as "stroke in evolution," and it may proceed in a stepwise fashion. The maximal deficit is referred to as a completed stroke.

Another type of CVA is called a **transient ischemic attack (TIA)**. A TIA is sometimes called a mini stroke, which is acceptable because the symptoms often mimic the effects of a completed stroke for a short time. However, with a TIA the disruption of blood flow is temporary, and the neurologic signs are transient, usually lasting less than 1 hour and resolving within 24 hours. The occurrence of a TIA usually indicates that platelet formation is underway, generally in the internal carotid artery distribution. There is a 20% chance of suffering a stroke during the first year after the TIA, and a 30% to 60% chance within 5 years. A TIA is a warning and should be taken seriously.

Hemorrhagic mechanisms. The rupture of a vessel in the brain causes a cerebral hemorrhage. Trauma to the brain often results in hemorrhage into the subarachnoid area and can cause hemorrhaging into other areas. The two most common causes of hemorrhage of a cerebral artery without trauma are rupture of an aneurysm and an arteriovenous malformation.

Cerebral aneurysm. An **aneurysm** is a focally weakened artery, where stretching of the wall leads to bulging or ballooning in one section. This bulge may eventually cause the walls to thin sufficiently that they break or hemorrhage

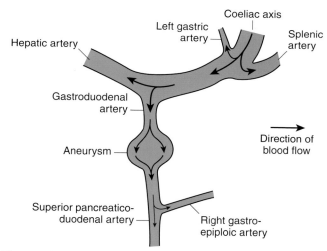

Fig. 10.2 Illustration of an aneurysm (of the gastroduodenal artery). (From Kessel, D., & Robertson, I. [2011]. *Interventional radiology* [3rd ed.]. Churchill Livingstone.)

without warning (Fig. 10.2). Points where cerebral vessels branch off or make sharp turns are most vulnerable for aneurysm development. Aneurysms tend to occur at the base of the brain in the subarachnoid space. Approximately 90% of spontaneous subarachnoid hemorrhages are thought to be due to undiagnosed aneurysms.

Many aneurysms are thought to be congenital. Small aneurysms may never rupture and remain silent throughout life. Large aneurysms may cause symptoms before rupture because they compress adjacent structures, such as cranial nerve roots.

Arteriovenous malformation. Arteriovenous malformation (AVM) is rare, estimated to occur in less than 1% of the population. An AVM is a tangle of abnormal blood vessels, occurring most commonly in the brain and spinal cord. This condition is thought to be a congenital condition and may not be detected until a seizure or a hemorrhage occurs. An aneurysm may develop from an AVM, and it can grow over time, damaging adjacent structures. With deterioration of the walls in these abnormal vessels, a hemorrhage can occur into the subarachnoid space, brain tissue, ventricles, or brainstem, depending on the location of the AVM.

Neoplasms in the Brain

A **neoplasm** is an abnormal mass of tissue, better known as a tumor. Benign tumors grow slowly and stay in one place. Malignant tumors expand, often rapidly, and once detected are treated aggressively with surgery, chemotherapy, and/or radiation. As a brain tumor spreads, it presses on adjacent structures and may invade and destroy the tissue, obstructing circulation. The abnormal growth may impact language areas directly or indirectly, causing aphasia.

Tumors are classified according to their origin, with the most common source in the brain being the neuroglia; the term **glioma** is the general name for a tumor originating on glial cells, which are the supportive tissues of the brain. Of the gliomas, astrocytomas, ependymomas, oligodendrogliomas, and tumors with mixtures of two or more cell types (fibrillary astrocytomas) are the most common primary brain tumors in adults.

Aphasia Classification

ASHA[3] classifies aphasia based on the patient's language output. If speech production is halting and effortful, the aphasia type is considered nonfluent. If the person can produce connected speech with relatively intact sentence structure but with reduced meaning, the aphasia type is called fluent. This is the classification scheme that will be used in this chapter, although there are numerous other classification schemes, some employing anatomic sites, including cortical lesions, association fiber lesions, and nonspecific lesion site aphasia. Box 10.1 summarizes the cortical-subcortical differences in aphasia.

Nonfluent or Expressive Aphasia

Nonfluent aphasia is sometimes called expressive aphasia because the patient demonstrates difficulty with verbal expression. Expressive aphasia is generally associated with anterior lesions. **Broca aphasia, transcortical motor aphasia,** and **global aphasia** are subtypes of nonfluent aphasia.

Broca aphasia. Patients with Broca aphasia are nonfluent, with greater difficulty in verbal expression than language comprehension. Verbal expression is marked by production of single words or short phrase with long pauses. Multisyllabic words may be produced syllable by syllable, with pauses between the syllables. Misarticulations are common, with distortions of consonants and vowels.

Agrammatism is common and refers to the absence of functions words, such as conjunctions, articles, and prepositions, although content words are retained, particularly nouns, verbs,

---

BOX 10.1   Localization of the Aphasias in the Central Language Mechanism

Aphasias of the Perisylvian Zone
Broca aphasia
Wernicke aphasia
Global aphasia
Conduction aphasia

Transcortical Aphasias of the Border Zone
Transcortical motor aphasia
Transcortical sensory aphasia
Mixed transcortical aphasia

Aphasias of the Subcortical Areas
Thalamic aphasia
Striatal disorders
Internal capsule disorders
Striatal or capsular disorders

Insular or capsular disorders
Data from Alexander, M. P., & Naeser, M. A. (1988). Cortical-subcortical differences in aphasia. In: F. Plum (Ed.), *Language, communication and the brain.* Raven Press.

---

and occasionally adjectives. Typically, patients string words with *and* in order to connect them. The following is an excerpt[7] from the Cookie Theft Picture Description task from the Boston Diagnostic Aphasia Examination which is shown in Fig. 10.5:

> *"mother…and…and…uh…runnin over…and floor…and…uh…two kids…"*

Written content mimics verbal output, with similar agrammatic features, and overuse of the connecting word *and.*

Comprehension of spoken language is functional, although some patients may demonstrate difficulty with syntactic relations. For example, sentences such as "It was the cat that the dog chased" present comprehension challenges to this population, while more predictable sentence structures are easily comprehended (e.g., "The dog chased the cat").

Self-monitoring is typically well preserved. Patients show awareness of their physical and communication impairments and demonstrate frustration by failed or impaired attempts. This awareness also means that they tend to cooperate more fully in rehabilitative efforts.

The lesion site in Broca aphasia was historically thought to be Broca area in the premotor cortex. However, there are numerous cases of patients with expressive aphasia and lesions that are not restricted to Broca area, although they typically include frontal lobe lesions. For this reason, the term nonfluent aphasia has become more prevalent.[30] Most lesions that cause nonfluent aphasia have cortical correlates in the frontal lobe. Descending pyramidal tracts pass below this area, which explains why most patients with nonfluent aphasia also have contralateral hemiparesis or hemiplegia.[7] Fig. 10.3 shows a computed tomography (CT) scan of a patient with a left hemisphere CVA resulting in Broca aphasia.

Transcortical motor aphasia. Transcortical motor aphasia is a nonfluent aphasia with markedly reduced verbal output, good repetition, and good auditory comprehension.

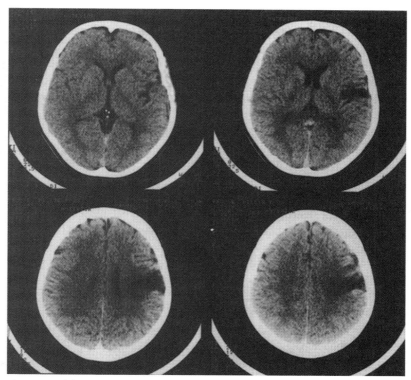

Fig. 10.3 Computed tomography scans of four horizontal slices from a patient with Broca aphasia and a right hemiparesis. Note the darkened area in the left hemisphere, which defines the infarction. (Courtesy of Howard S. Kirshner, MD, Department of Neurology, Vanderbilt University School of Medicine, Nashville, TN.)

The typical site of damage is the anterior superior frontal lobe in the dominant hemisphere, important for initiation and maintenance of purposeful activity, including speech. Patients are notably attentive, task oriented, poor conversationalists, and often overlooked because they are quiet. Right hemiparesis typically accompanies this aphasia.

This type of aphasia, like its sensory counterpart discussed under fluent aphasia, is sometimes called an isolation syndrome or border zone aphasia because the lesion spares the perisylvian language zones of the frontal and temporal lobe. However, the lesion also impairs the connection between the language zones and the rest of the brain. In this aphasia, the damage is in the **border zones** or the watershed regions surrounding the perisylvian cortex. In transcortical motor aphasia, the lesion is thought to occur close to the supplementary motor area, in the watershed region between the anterior and middle cerebral artery. In transcortical sensory aphasia, the lesion is thought to be in the watershed region between the middle and posterior cerebral arteries. In both **transcortical aphasia** types, repetition is better than expected because of the sparing of cortical language centers. The intact repetition contrasts markedly with perislyvian zone aphasia (Broca, global, Wernicke, and conduction) types, which all include a repetition deficit. Transcortical aphasias are relatively rare.

Global aphasia. As the name indicates, all language skills are impacted in global aphasia. The patient demonstrates a severe impairment of both understanding and expression of language, and may initially be mute or use repetitive, nonmeaningful vocalization. Comprehension is often reported to be better than production with global aphasia, and patients may become adept at interpreting nonverbal communication through gestures, facial expressions, and body language. Patients often use nonverbal skills to communicate with others, including facial expression, intonation, and gestures. Repetition is severely impaired, as is confrontation naming, reading, and writing. This aphasia is usually associated with a large lesion in the perisylvian area.

Fluent Aphasias. With fluent aphasia, the affected individual can produce connected speech. Sentence structure is relatively intact but lacks meaning. Fluent aphasias include Wernicke, transcortical sensory, conduction, and anomic aphasia.

Wernicke aphasia. **Wernicke aphasia**, like Broca, goes by several alternate names, including sensory aphasia, receptive aphasia, and posterior aphasia. Wernicke aphasia is typically caused by damage to the temporal lobe of the dominant hemisphere, resulting in impaired comprehension of spoken or written material. In severe cases, patients may fail to understand even simple verbal stimuli. With milder cases, patients may understand the global message but fail to comprehend specifics.

In addition to comprehension difficulties, this population typically exhibits fluent, sometimes copious verbal output that may lack relevance to topic, and which may include paraphasia/paraphasic errors and neologisms. Paraphasic errors include the substitution of one word for another, such as *watch* for *clock*, or one phoneme for the target, such as *dar* for *car*. Neologism literally means "new word." Neologistic errors are typically nonsense words substituted for the target, such as calling a shirt a "slumbop." Verbal output that contains such errors is sometimes called jargon or empty speech and is difficult for the listener to follow. The following in an excerpt from a conversation reported by Brookshire,[7] where a clinician asks the patient to describe their home (p. 195):

"Well, it's a meender place and it has two. Two of them. For dreaming and pinding after supper."

The fluent verbal output is also characterized by normal phrase length and relatively intact syntactic structure. Articulation and prosody are also typically intact.

Unlike patients with nonfluent aphasia, patients with Wernicke aphasia typically demonstrate poor awareness of their comprehension or expression difficulty. This reduced awareness creates challenges for the treating team as patients appear to be unaware of their impairments or unconcerned by them. The fluent output together with the reduced awareness can produce excessive verbal output, called press of speech or logorrhea (verbal diarrhea).

Reading and writing skills are significantly impaired. Reading comprehension is typically significantly impaired. Writing tends to mimic verbal output, with effortless and copious production but reduced content. If the patients produce paraphasic errors or neologisms in speech, then these will likely be present in their written work.

Like in Broca aphasia, the lesion site in Wernicke aphasia is now disputed. The damage in Wernicke aphasia was historically thought to be located in the posterior portion of the superior temporal gyrus of the dominant hemisphere, the auditory association area, or to Wernicke area in the sylvian fissure. However, neuroimaging studies in recent decades have demonstrated a wide distribution, including the temporal, parietal, and frontal network areas that support language comprehension. The anatomic site labeled Wernicke area has been shown to be critical for retrieval of phonologic forms used for verbal communication and memory tasks.[5,30]

What is well established in terms of the anatomic site of the lesion is that motor cortices are spared. Fluent patients are typically able to walk and use their arms normally, in contrast to nonfluent patients. However, the temporal lobe impact often affects short-term retention and recall of verbal material: Fluent patients tend to perform poorly on memory tasks, particularly as the task increases in length or complexity.[7]

Transcortical sensory aphasia. **Transcortical sensory aphasia** is characterized by fluent speech marked by paraphasic errors and neologisms. Comprehension is poor, in sharp contrast to repetition, which is surprisingly good. Reading, writing, and naming are poor.

A mixed transcortical aphasia has been described in the literature. This is a rare aphasia, characterized by severely disordered language except in repetition. Patients do not speak unless they are spoken to and answer only in repetition. The most striking feature is echolalia, the repetition of heard phrases.

Conduction aphasia. **Conduction aphasia** is characterized by intact comprehension and fluent, melodic speech. However, these patients have extraordinary difficulty on repetition tasks. The repetition difficulty increases with longer targets, such as multisyllabic words or longer phrases. Phoneme substitutions are frequent because of the inability to match acoustic information with motor plans for execution of phonemes. Reading aloud is also impaired for the same reason. Additionally, verbal output may contain literal paraphasias and pauses due to word-finding difficulty.

The lesion site was long considered to be the arcuate fasciculus, explaining the disconnection between frontal and temporal lobes and the consequent difficulty with repetition. However, more recently imaging has demonstrated cases of conduction aphasia lesions outside the arcuate fasciculus.[1] Associated characteristics vary. Some patients show a right hemiparesis and/or hemisensory loss. Patients may also show a visual field deficit, and some patients may demonstrate an ideomotor apraxia.

Anomic aphasia. Word-finding difficulty, known as anomia, is common to many types of aphasia and occurs in conditions that do not otherwise impact language. Anomia occurs in most types of dementia and is a clear diagnostic feature of Alzheimer syndrome. Anomia is often the only major language residual after recovery from aphasia of any clinical type and may remain a long-lasting problem in the recovered aphasic patient. In neurologic conditions in which the whole brain is generally affected, anomia is a common language symptom. Some of the conditions that produce anomia include encephalitis, increased intracranial pressure, subarachnoid hemorrhage, concussion, and toxic-metabolic **encephalopathy**. Clearly, anomia is not a good localizing symptom.

The term **anomic aphasia** is applied to people whose primary communication difficulty is word retrieval in both verbal and written modalities. The word retrieval difficulties lead to unusual pauses, substitutions of nonspecific words for the target, and **circumlocution** (roundabout language to describe a word). An example of circumlocution is someone who points to his wrist and says, "I wear it here" to indicate the word 'watch'.

Paraphasic errors, if present, tend to be semantic rather than phonemic. For example, the patient may use the word *mother* for *father* or *socks* for *shoes*. Careful testing may reveal subtle comprehension difficulties. Reading and writing are more variable, and word-finding difficulties are obvious in written language.

Anomic aphasia may appear as an isolated syndrome or be the final stage of recovery from other syndromes, such as Wernicke, conduction, and transcortical aphasias. In these cases, using the term 'residual aphasia' may be preferable.

As can be expected, there is no one site of lesion that correlates with anomia. In severe and isolated anomia, a possible focal lesion may be found in the left angular gyrus, frontal lobe, or inferior temporal gyrus.[7]

Subcortical and Crossed Aphasia. In the ASHA[3] model of aphasia, crossed and subcortical aphasia types are considered exceptional as they do not fit neatly within the fluent-nonfluent dichotomy or any other common classification system. Crossed aphasia occurs with a lesion to the nondominant hemisphere. **Subcortical aphasia** results from lesions below the cortex, such as the thalamus or basal ganglia an MRI of a lesion in the basal ganglia resulting in aphasia is shown in Fig. 10.7. Fig. 10.8 lists the signs and symptoms of each of the subcortical speech or language disorders that they identified. These aphasias were discussed in Chapter 9.

Primary Progressive Aphasia. Primary progressive aphasia (PPA) is not a true aphasia, but a unique group of neurodegenerative processes that target the language networks of the brain. In other words, PPA is a type of dementia that manifests initially as language difficulty, in the context of relatively preserved cognitive functions and personality.[3] Symptoms typically occur before the age of 65.

There are three recognized variants of PPA: nonfluent, semantic, and logopenic. The nonfluent PPA type is also called agrammatic; this variant is characterized by an insidious impairment of speech production, including agrammatic language output and effortful, halting speech with inconsistent errors and distortions. This PPA subtype initially resembles a nonfluent aphasia. Atrophy in the brain is predominantly present in the perisylvian cortices centered on the inferior frontal gyrus and anterior insula.

The semantic variant is characterized by impaired knowledge about words, and later objects and concepts across all sensory modalities. The semantic variant is associated with dysfunction and atrophy of the semantic appraisal network and is most severely noted in the anteromesial temporal lobe.

The logopenic variant is characterized by progressive anomia and impaired phonologic processing, and in auditory verbal memory. Atrophy and dysfunction involve the left temporoparietal cortices.[29]

Fig. 10.4 depicts a coronal magnetic resonance imaging (MRI) scan of a patient who was diagnosed with PPA, with the finding of atrophy in the left temporal lobe and the description of nonfluent speech and anomia.

There is no single treatment approach for people with PPA; however, an early and accurate diagnosis is crucial to allow patient and families to plan for the future and to access needed services. Medically, disease-modifying therapies may be developed in the near future, although none exists at this time. Skilled speech therapy has been shown to be effective in enhancing neuroplasticity. In the early stages, all PPA patients retain their capacity for learning, which can be utilized in planning treatment strategies. This ability to learn in the presence of a progressive disease suggests a degree of neuroplasticity that can be harnessed in rehabilitation.[29]

Testing and Intervention for Aphasia

Aphasia testing has had a long history in neurology and speech-language pathology. Broca reportedly tested his patients with conversational questions in addition to testing tongue movements, writing, and arithmetic. He also described their gestures. In 1926 British neurologist Henry Head (1861–1940) published the first systematic aphasia examination in English. The test was not standardized and contained some items that were difficult even for healthy people to perform. Today clinical neurologists usually assess language and aphasia disturbances as part of the mental status examination of higher cerebral functions, which is part of the traditional neurologic examination. The mental status examination assesses major functions of the total nervous system and lateralizes and localizes dysfunction when it is present.

The language functions tested by the neurologist are found in Table 10.1.[24] An example of a bedside examination of speech

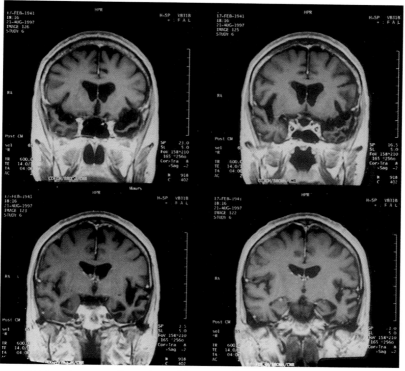

Fig. 10.4 Coronal magnetic resonance imaging scan of a patient with progressive, nonfluent aphasia. Note the marked atrophy of the left temporal lobe, which is easiest to see in a coronal projection. The temporal lobe atrophy and his symptoms of slow speech and anomia, which were progressive in nature, are consistent with the descriptions of the logopenic variant of primary progressive aphasia. (Reprinted from Bradley, W. G., Daroff, R. B., Fenichel, G. M., & Marsden, C. D. [Eds.]. [2000]. *Neurology in clinical practice* [3rd ed., vol. I]. Butterworth-Heinemann.)

TABLE 10.1	Language Functions of Major Classic Aphasias				
	Spontaneous Speech	**Comprehension**	**Repetition**	**Reading**	**Writing**
Broca	Nonfluent	+	−	±	−
Wernicke	Fluent	−	−	−	Paragraphic
Conduction	Fluent	+	−	+	−
Global	Mute	−	−	−	−
Anomic	Disorder of word recall	+	+	+	+
Transcortical motor	Nonfluent	+	+	+	−
Transcortical sensory	Fluent	−	+	+	−
Mixed transcortical (isolation of speech area)	Nonfluent	−	+	−	Paragraphic

+, Relatively intact; −, impaired; ±, variable.
Developed by Howard S. Kirshner, MD, Department of Neurology, Vanderbilt University School of Medicine, Nashville, TN.

and language designed for the clinical neurologist is found in Appendix C.

SLPs and psychologists have been more concerned about developing aphasia tests that precisely measure language behavior under standardized conditions than about providing tests that predict and confirm possible lesions or verify the validity of classic models of neurologic language mechanisms. Testing is performed to assist in discharge and treatment planning. Direct intervention for the language deficits may be provided on an individual or group basis, and literature is growing on treatment techniques.

Role of the SLP

The SLP is perhaps the most critical member of the rehabilitation team for the person with a significantly limiting aphasia. Numerous books, articles, websites, and treatment programs are devoted to language therapy with patients with aphasia. An attempt to describe treatment methods would not do justice to this vast amount of literature and is not the purpose of this text. Research on innovative treatments involving constraint-induced aphasia therapy, transcranial magnetic stimulation or direct current stimulation, and group communication therapy[9] is helping clinicians combine or replace more traditional evidence-based treatment methods with these newer methodologies to enhance recovery of language skills. The SLP should be well versed and dedicated to evidence-based medical and behavioral treatments and, as a member of the rehabilitation team, know something about pharmacologic intervention as well.

Pharmacology in Aphasia

The main purpose of pharmacologic intervention in post-stroke aphasia is to improve and facilitate neuroplasticity. However, evidence for pharmacologic stimulation of neuroplasticity is limited. Part of the problem is the lack of animal models for pharmaceutical studies, as animals cannot express aphasic deficits. An additional problem in this line of research is the nature of the problem: Language is not centered in one brain locus. Different areas of the brain interconnect with each other to facilitate language. Even the dual-stream model

cannot totally explain this connection (explored more fully in Chapter 9). This model states that the dorsal pathway, running from the posterosuperior temporal to the inferior frontal cortices, is responsible for phonologic processing; while the ventral pathway, running from the temporal lobe to the basal occipitotemporal cortex and with anterior connections, helps with semantic processing.

Despite little evidence, pharmacologic intervention now centers on the neurochemical foundations for communication. Dopamine released from the brainstem helps with speech generation and may regulate the laryngeal cortical representation as well as other components. Thus, the dopaminergic system is considered to help innervate the frontal-parietal network, regulate syntactic language processing, and regulate pragmatic aspects of language functions.

One pharmaceutical agent that increases acetylcholine, donepezil, has shown promise in improving cognitive functions in Alzheimer disease patients and has been considered in treating patients with aphasia. A well-prepared, randomized controlled trial showed good improvement of language functions while the aphasic patients were taking this medication, but these positive effects disappeared once medications were stopped, suggesting that the advantages of donepezil are not associated with neural reorganization. Other agents have been studied, such as amphetamines, which have dopamine and norepinephrine reuptake inhibition, and have demonstrated some efficaciousness for people with aphasia, and the nootropic agent memantine, which has stimulant effects. In all cases, intervention was more efficacious when combined with speech therapy, particularly constraint-induced intensive therapy. Although no consensus has been reached to date, pharmaceutical therapy is likely a useful adjunct to rehabilitative speech therapy.[9]

ASSOCIATED CENTRAL DISTURBANCES

Neurolinguistic disorders sometimes co-occur with language-based impairments, although they sometimes occur in isolation. These disorders are referred to as associated central disturbances because the site of the lesion is within the areas described under central language mechanism, but these are not properly classified as aphasic disturbances. The accompanying central disturbances include apraxia, agnosia, alexia, and agraphia. Apraxia is discussed in Chapter 6 because it is a motor speech disorder; agnosia is discussed in Chapter 5 as part of the discussion on the various sensory systems. Alexia and agraphia are briefly reviewed here.

Alexia (Acquired Dyslexia)

Alexia is difficulty with comprehension of the written or printed word as the result of a cerebral lesion. Alexia is an acquired reading disorder, in contrast to **dyslexia**, an innate or constitutional difficulty with reading ability. Some authors refer to alexia as acquired dyslexia to differentiate these from the congenital disorder. The classic term word blindness is rarely used in neurology or speech pathology. When used, it implies difficulty in reading words, although letter recognition is more intact.

In 1980, a distinction was made between central neurogenic dyslexia and peripheral dyslexia. In central dyslexia, a language impairment impacts reading. In peripheral dyslexia, difficulty processing the visual stimulus impairs reading. Central alexias include alexia with agraphia, and phonological, surface, and deep dyslexias. Peripheral alexias include **alexia without agraphia** (pure alexia), neglect dyslexia, attentional dyslexia, and aphasia alexia.[11] Table 10.2 summarizes these disorders and their lesion site.

Peripheral alexias

In peripheral dyslexia, a visual deficit causes reading difficulty rather than a language disturbance.

Alexia without agraphia

Alexia without agraphia is also known as **posterior alexia** or **occipital alexia**. The cardinal feature of this uncommon syndrome is loss of the ability to read printed material but retained ability to write both spontaneously and to dictation. This is a dramatic disorder where a patient may write lengthy meaningful messages, but then be unable to read it. Another clinical feature is difficulty understanding words spelled aloud.

Patients usually can regain some reading ability, but reading usually remains quite effortful. The writing seen in the syndrome is not entirely normal, but retained writing capacity is impressive compared with the minimal reading ability. Often, the patient writes better to dictation or spontaneously than when copying. Right homonymous hemianopsia is usually present. Other language functions generally are intact.

This alexia occurs suddenly as the result of a left posterior cerebral artery occlusion in a right-handed person. Dejerine[16] attributed this syndrome to a combination of two impairments. First, the left hemisphere is deprived of visual input by the posterior lesion. Second, visual information from the right hemisphere is disconnected from left hemisphere structures important for word recognition, typically ascribed to the angular gyrus. In other words, because the left visual cortex was damaged, all visual information was perceived by the right hemisphere; because of the callosal lesion,

TABLE 10.2	**Alexia and Agraphia**
Associated Central Disturbance	**Description of Disturbance**
Agraphia	A disorder of writing caused by cerebral injury; lesion in the left frontal or parietal lobe or in the complex pathways necessary for writing
Alexia	A disorder of reading caused by cerebral injury
Types of Alexia	Characterizing Features
PERIPHERAL ALEXIAS	
Alexia without agraphia	Able to write but has difficulty reading
Neglect alexia	Omits parts of single words
Attentional dyslexia	Single-word reading is intact; letters migrate in longer strings
Aphasic alexia	Lesions are the same as in the major aphasias
CENTRAL ALEXIAS	
Alexia with agraphia	Total reading impairment; limited writing
Phonological dyslexia	Errors on nonsense and low-frequency words
Surface dyslexia	Impaired reading of irregularly spelled words
Deep dyslexia	Semantic substitutions during reading tasks

information could not be transferred to the left, eloquent, hemisphere. The intact angular gyrus synthesizes visual and auditory information necessary in both reading and writing; in this syndrome, this gyrus is now disconnected from all visual input. Because the lobule and its connections with the language area is intact, the patient is able to write normally. The reading impairment in the context of relatively preserved writing gives this syndrome the name pure alexia.

Neglect dyslexia. This disorder often co-occurs with left spatial neglect. In this type of alexia, there is a failure to identify the initial portion of a letter string. Lexical understanding is typically preserved and helps the patient correct misread words. For example, the word *blend* may be read without the initial *b* when it is presented alone. In a sentence, however, the intact lexical system helps the reader correct the error. In right neglect alexia, the final part of a word may be omitted, so the person may read *planet* as *plan*. Again, context is helpful, and the patient is typically able to rectify the word.

Attentional dyslexia. In this syndrome, single-word reading is preserved but, in a string, letters migrate to neighboring words, hindering reading. Patients with attentional dyslexia may even demonstrate difficulty identifying letters within words even though the words are read correctly. This type of dyslexia is sometimes noted in Alzheimer disease and other neurodegenerative diseases.

Central Alexias

These alexias are associated with a language disturbance.

Alexia with agraphia. Also known as **central alexia** or **parietal-temporal alexia**, **alexia with agraphia** typically occurs with a lesion in or near the angular gyrus at the posterior end of the sylvian fissure. This damage isolates the visual cortex from language centers in the temporal and frontal lobes. Written information presented visually cannot be communicated to these language centers, and the patient is unable to read orally or silently and is unable to write.

Alexia with agraphia is classically described as an almost total reading disorder, with limited writing ability, only minimal aphasia, and acalculia (acquired difficulty with calculations). Patients cannot identify words spelled aloud, which does not happen in alexia without agraphia. Patients exhibiting alexia with agraphia can copy printed material much better than they can write spontaneously or to dictation, which also is different from the presentation in alexia without agraphia.

Alexia with agraphia is seen in many aphasia syndromes and rarely occurs in isolation. Sometimes called **aphasic alexia**, the reading and writing difficulties that coexist with other communication disturbances are sometimes targeted later in therapy because the other aphasic symptoms are more prominent. The aphasia type is more fluent, not surprising as the lesion is posterior. Gerstmann syndrome is sometimes present. This syndrome is defined when agnosia for the fingers, acalculia, right-left disorientation, agraphia, and alexia are all present. A right homonymous visual field defect frequently is reported but not consistently present.

Phonologic dyslexia

Phonologic alexia is characterized by an inability to read nonsense words, with some difficulty noted with low-frequency words. Errors often are visual errors. These patients are assumed to be impaired in the ability to use letter-to-sound conversion rules of the language. Lesions occur in the perisylvian cortex, including the supramarginal and angular gyri, and are typically smaller than in other alexias.

Surface dyslexia. **Surface dyslexia** is distinguished by poor ability words with irregular or exceptional print-to-sound correspondence. Words such as *colonel* and *yacht* are not bound by print-to-sound rules and present significant difficulties for patients with surface dyslexia. These patients tend to read regular words correctly, as well as nonsense words that follow grapheme-to-phoneme conversion rules, such as *blape*. Most patients with this impairment also demonstrate semantic difficulty on nonreading tasks. Etiology is typically a left hemisphere stroke involving the temporal lobe.[11]

Deep dyslexia. **Deep dyslexia** is identified by the presence of semantic errors in reading aloud. Reading is marked by errors that are related in meaning for the target, such as saying "child" for "girl" or "quiet" for "listen." Visual errors can occur, such as misreading "skate" as "scale," and morphologic errors, such as reading "governor" for "government."

Deep dyslexia implies that the dyslexic reader goes directly to the semantic value of a word from its printed form without appreciating the sound of the word. Deep dyslexia has also been called phonemic, syntactic, or semantic dyslexia.

Agraphia

Writing is a complex learned motor act that involves a conversion of oral language symbols into written symbols. The language symbols to be written are assumed to originate in the posterior language areas in the dominant hemisphere of the brain. These oral symbols are translated into visual symbols in the inferior parietal lobe. The linguistic message is then sent forward to the frontal lobe for motor processing. Lesions in any of these language areas or pathways may produce the writing disorder called **agraphia**. The most common type of agraphia is secondary to aphasia and known as aphasic agraphia. Agraphia also may be seen in the absence of aphasia.

COGNITIVE-COMMUNICATION IMPAIRMENTS RELATED TO RIGHT HEMISPHERE DAMAGE

Brain injuries or diseases that involve the right hemisphere, or those with more diffuse damage, can produce a different type of language disorder than that seen with focal left hemisphere damage. The cognitive communicative impairments following a right (nondominant) hemisphere injury do not follow the same patterns seen in left (dominant) hemisphere injury.

The right hemisphere is equally vulnerable to the effects of reduced perfusion, meaning that the same conditions that were discussed relative to the left hemisphere can also occur in the nondominant hemisphere, including CVA, focal trauma, and neoplasms, among others.

With right hemisphere lesions, a broad spectrum of deficits is possible, depending on the site of damage and the extent of the lesion. The most dramatic deficits are neglect, denial, inattention, denial, visual and spatial perceptual disorders, and constructional disturbances. When communication is affected, it is not because of a language impairment but due to extralinguistic impairments impacting communication, such as prosodic deficits or difficulty with interpretation of humor and metaphors. Attention difficulties also exert an adverse effect on communication in this population.

Box 10.2 lists some nonlinguistic and extralinguistic deficits that may be discovered in a careful diagnostic examination of a patient with a right hemisphere lesion, and they are briefly discussed next. The list of deficits is only representative; it cannot be exhaustive, as great variability exists in the type and severity of symptoms in this population.

Neglect and Denial

Neglect, also known as **unilateral inattention**, is a syndrome in which a patient fails to recognize one side of the body and the environmental space surrounding that side. The neglected side is typically free of paresis or paralysis, and visual fields

BOX 10.2 Signs and Symptoms of Nonlinguistic and Extralinguistic Deficits

Nonlinguistic Deficits

Difficulty in recognizing and using significant contextual cues

Difficulty integrating these significant cues into an overall pattern

Extralinguistic Deficits

Distinguishing significant from irrelevant information

Integration and interpretation of contextual information

Inhibiting impulsive responses

Grasping figurative and implied meaning

Topic maintenance and efficiency of expression

Appreciation of the communicative situation and listener needs

Recognizing and/or producing emotional responses

Modified from Myers, P. S. (1999). *Right hemisphere damage*. Singular Publishing Group.

are typically intact. Nevertheless, patients may shave half their face, wear only one sleeve of their shirt, or eat half the food on their plate. Even worse, they may injure themselves on the neglected side without recognizing the effects of the injury, such as bumping into door frames or cutting themselves with a knife.

The exact neurologic locus of the neglect syndrome with right hemisphere lesions is not exactly known. Chronic parietal lobe damage shows a high correlation with the syndrome. Neurologic testing for unilateral inattention is conducted through double simultaneous stimulation, in which the sensory modalities of touch, hearing, and sight are tested. Visual testing involves having the patient fixate on a point on the neurologic examiner's face. The examiner moves the fingers into both the right and left peripheral visual fields, and the patient reports where the fingers are seen. **Extinction** is present when the patient suppresses stimuli from one side. Extinction may occur in all modalities or in only a single modality. When extinction is elicited, the degree of inattention can be assessed by increasing the strength of the stimulus on the inattentive side.

Many patients develop a dramatic **denial** of their neurologic illness; the denial may range from mild to severe and is usually associated with neglect. An example of severe denial is the patient's lack of recognition of a hemiplegia. The condition was documented by Russian neurologist Joseph Babinski (1857–1932); his patient had a left-sided hemiplegia and left-sided sensory loss, although the patient appeared completely unaware of the neurologic deficit. If the patient's hemiplegic arm was placed on the bed and he was asked to raise his hand, the patient would lift the physician's arm aloft. If he were asked to grasp his left arm with his nonparalyzed right arm, he would grasp the physician's arm instead of his own. Asked to move his paralyzed arm even though his arm was completely hemiplegic, the patient would emphatically say that he could move his arm. Babinski used the term **anosognosia** to describe this unawareness. The term is sometimes used to describe other denial symptoms, but it may be most apt in this context.

Prosopagnosia

Prosopagnosia refers to the inability to recognize familiar faces and their expressions. The patient may recognize individuals by voice or other physical features rather than face recognition.

Although some authors report prosopagnosia following anterior temporal lesions, there is no current consensus. Bilateral lesions, fusiform gyrus (at the base of the temporal and occipital lobes) lesions, white matter lesions around the fusiform gyrus, and the inferior longitudinal fasciculus have all been reported to cause prosopagnosia. It is likely that a variety of lesions can cause prosopagnosia, which reflects the widely distributed networks involved in face processing. In the case of unilateral lesions, these are far more likely to be right hemisphere based.[10]

Visual-Perceptual and Construction Deficits

Right hemisphere lesions are associated with deficits in meaningful interpretation and recall of complex visual structures. Deficits in the perception and recall of letters, words, and numbers may produce problems in reading. With construction deficits, patients may not be able to copy simple figures or to draw a simple figure, such as a daisy, from memory.

Prosodic Deficits

A common impairment following right hemisphere syndrome is known as **aprosodia**. Prosody, among other things, conveys appropriate emotional affect. Prosody also carries pragmatic information, allowing a listener to discriminate among questions, statements, and explanations. When normal stress or emphasis is disturbed in a sentence, conveying new information becomes difficult.

Patients with aprosodia or dysprosodia are often unable to provide variations in their voices and they speak in a flattened emotional tone. Linguistic prosody aids meaning; for example, the difference between convict (verb) and convict (noun) is largely dependent on prosody. Affective prosody conveys attitude. For example, in the sentence "Oh yes, I am fine", the intention may be sincere or sarcastic; prosody would indicate the intent. Patients with aprosodia may fail to grasp these subtle differences or fail to convey them in their verbalizations. Affective aprosodia is typically the result of right hemisphere damage.

A partial list of nonlinguistic and extralinguistic deficits is in Box 10.2, showing why some patients present with communication disorders that are subtle in nature but which may be devastating in social relationships.

DEMENTIA

Dementia is defined as any disorder producing a decline in cognition significant enough to interfere with independent, daily functioning. Dementia interrupts a person's occupational, domestic, and social functioning.[18] Dementia is an acquired, persisting syndrome rather than one disease. There are many causes of dementia, including neurologic, psychiatric, and medical conditions. Many diseases can also contribute to an existing dementia, thus exacerbating the manifestations.

Some dementia types are more common in the older population, while others appear in younger populations.

The incidence and prevalence of dementia are difficult to determine because studies differ vastly depending on how dementia is defined and what population is studied. Where there is consensus, however, is that the incidence of dementia is rising rapidly, with an increasing percentage of the population being affected. This is especially true because most forms of dementia are found in persons older than 65 years, and the number of elderly people in the population is greater than ever before and is expected to rise. The World Health Organization (WHO) estimates 55 million people with dementia living worldwide currently, and an approximate 10 million new cases per year.[31] It is good to remember that although dementia affects mainly older people, it is not an inevitable consequence of aging. Additionally, some conditions target mainly younger people.

Classification of Dementias

Dementia can be broadly classified into two categories: neurodegenerative (irreversible) and nonneurodegenerative (reversible). This categorization is imperfect. Patients often have diseases that can be categorized differently from the dementia itself. For example, CVA is nondegenerative, but multiple CVAs can and do result in dementia.[18] Dementia may also be classified by site of anatomy; this is the classification used in this section, and the dementias will be presented by site: cortical, subcortical, or mixed.

Cortical Dementias

As the name indicates, these are dementias that target cortical zones. Foremost among the cortical dementias is **Alzheimer disease (AD)**. This dementia is the most common neurodegenerative dementia from middle age to the elderly. AD has a prevalence of 5% in people over 65 years of age, rising to 30% in those above age 85. AD begins slowly and insidiously, with progressive memory decline, and progresses to include behavioral, visuospatial, and language deficits. Mean survival rate after onset of AD is 10 to 12 years. The stages and their characteristics are summarized in Table 10.3.

Frontotemporal dementias (FTD) are a group of neurodegenerative dementias targeting the frontal and parietal lobes selectively. The hallmark of FTD is a gradual progressive decline in behavior and/or language. Onset is at a relatively young age, with an average age of onset between 55 and 60 years. Pick disease falls in this group of dementias.

The distinguishing difference between FTD and AD is that patients with FTD retain important features of memory, keep track of day-to-day events, and are fairly well oriented in time and space, unlike patients with AD.

Neuropathology of the cortical dementias. The neuropathology of AD shows the presence of **neurofibrillary tangles** and **amyloid plaques** in the cytoplasm of nerve cells. These plaques, which begin in the walls of small blood vessels, are thought to result from defective enzymes that cause abnormal production of beta-amyloid protein. The tangles are associated with an abnormal tau protein production and are made

TABLE 10.3	Clinical Features of the Stages of Alzheimer's Dementia
Stage	**Characteristics**
Stage I: Mild	Memory for new learning is defective, and remote recall is mildly impaired. Language shows word retrieval problems and some difficulty understanding humor, analogies, and complex implications. The patient may be vague and may not initiate conversation when appropriate. The patient may also show indifference, anxiety, and irritability.
Stage II: Middle	Memory for recent and remote events is more severely affected, and language shows vocabulary diminishment. The patient repeats ideas, forgets topics, has difficulty thinking of words in a category, loses sensitivity to conversational partners, and rarely corrects mistakes. Comprehension is reduced, and language may rely on jargon and paraphasias. The patient becomes increasingly indifferent, irritable, and restless.
Stage III: Late	Memory is severely impaired, as are all intellectual functions. Language is rarely used meaningfully, and some patients are mute or echolalic. Motor function is compromised by limb rigidity and flexion posture.

up of clumps of these microtubules. These aberrant formations are more pronounced in the inferior temporal lobe, which has connections with the hippocampus, and they accumulate in the amygdala and in the posterior association regions of the cortex. The presence of abnormal proteins in the brain is also linked with FTD.

Cortical dementia shows extensive loss of pyramidal neurons in all parts of the brain, corresponding with a loss of motor function, and a loss of up to 50% of cholinergic neurons. Microscopic examination of the brain tissue of persons with AD also shows neuritic plaques, which are remains of degenerated nerve fibers.

Subcortical and Mixed Dementias. Subcortical dementias may accompany extrapyramidal syndromes, such as in Parkinson disease and Huntington chorea, depression, white matter diseases such as multiple sclerosis and AIDS-related encephalopathy, and some vascular diseases causing lacunar states. With subcortical dementias, cognition slowly and progressively deteriorates. Forgetfulness and alterations of affect are noted. Memory is affected but is often aided by cues and structure. In terms of mood, the person may appear depressed or apathetic with decreased motivation. The cognitive impairment has been described as one of dilapidation. Patients appear unable to synthesize and manipulate information to produce sequential steps to solve a complex problem, although they may correctly perform individual steps. The neurologic examination of these patients is abnormal, with motor, posture, tone, and speech problems noted.

Role of the SLP

The SLP is usually called on to help identify subtle language disorders that may signal intellectual deterioration because language is highly sensitive to even mild changes in brain function. The purpose of the assessment by the SLP may be to assist in making the differential diagnosis by trying to determine whether true aphasia, apraxia, or amnesia is present without language involvement. In addition, the SLP helps the patient and family understand the diagnosis and establish compensations both for the present deficits and for expected future ones. If communication is expected to decline, such as in cases of PPA or FTD, the clinician's role is to also suggest ways that family and other caregivers might improve communication with the patient, including training caregivers in facilitating and maintaining communication for as long as possible.

ALTERED MENTAL STATUS

Altered mental status (AMS) refers to a group of clinical symptoms, rather than a specific diagnosis, and it is a common reason for emergency room visits. AMS may be due to cognitive problems, arousal disorders, or decreased levels of consciousness. Patients often manifest vague symptoms, which creates challenges for diagnosticians. Severity ranges from confusional states, often called delirium, to coma. AMS can also develop while a patient is hospitalized, called ICU (intensive care unit) delirium.

Several conditions produce confusion, including metabolic imbalance, adverse drug reactions, and alcohol and drug withdrawal. AMS is not typically the result of focal brain lesions; widespread cortical and subcortical neuronal dysfunction generally is present. Confusion symptoms are also seen during the period of posttraumatic amnesia in traumatic head injury.

Symptomatic language impairment is often noted in AMS, with language disturbances a secondary symptom of the confusion. While vocabulary and syntax are generally normal, language is largely irrelevant and confabulatory in nature.

Confabulation is the verbal or written expression of fictitious experiences, generally filling a gap in memory. For example, a patient may relate in detail the time they last worked with their SLP when in fact they have never met. Confabulation is less marked in the presence of aphasia because it requires that the language areas be relatively intact. Confabulation is more often associated with generalized cerebral deficit or dysfunction rather than focal lesions. Some instances in which focal lesions are associated with confabulation are in the Wernicke-Korsakoff amnestic syndrome and in ruptured aneurysms of the anterior communicating artery.

Delirium

Delirium is defined as acute fluctuating consciousness, with sudden confusion developing rapidly and fluctuating during the day. Patients with delirium demonstrate inattention, disorganized thinking (incoherence), and perceptual disturbances, such as visual hallucinations. Delirium can co-occur with other medical conditions, such as dementia or high fever, and it is dangerous if unrecognized and untreated. There are two manifestations of delirium: hyperactive and hypoactive. In the hyperactive state, patients demonstrate agitation or even aggressiveness. In the hypoactive state, patients may appear drowsy and be slow to respond. The hypoactive condition is more dangerous as the delirium may not be detected early enough for appropriate medical management.

Coma

Coma is a state of unconsciousness in which a person cannot be awakened. Patients in a coma do not respond to tactile, visual, or auditory stimuli, and they do not respond to painful stimulus. Coma can occur as a response to severe TBI or hypoglycemia in diabetic patients. Damage to cortical tissue and/or to the reticular activating system in the brainstem are considered as neurologic bases for coma.

Vegetative States

Vegetative states are disorders of consciousness in which patients who sustain severe brain damage are in a state of partial arousal rather than true awareness. In vegetative states, the patient may have complex reflexes, be able to open the eyes and yawn, and may move away from noxious stimuli, such as a bad smell or a pinprick on the skin. However, patients have no awareness of themselves or their environment. Neurologically, there is significant dysfunction in the cerebral hemispheres, while the brainstem and diencephalic structures remain functional. The latter structures are what account for the motor responses of these patients. After 4 weeks in a vegetative state, the diagnosis is amended to persistent vegetative state. The prognosis for patients with these presentations is typically bleak.

TRAUMATIC BRAIN INJURY

TBI is caused by a sudden injury that damages the brain. TBI can occur with a strike to the head or with an injury that penetrates the skull. TBI is the leading cause of morbidity and mortality in the world due to its high incidence and long-term sequelae.[26] TBI is sometimes called the silent epidemic because it is a growing public health concern, contributing significantly to the rates of death and disability. A WHO review initiative found that 69 million people worldwide experience TBI each year, with most cases in the mild to moderate severity levels.[17]

The risk for a TBI is higher for men than for women, and higher for certain ages. Between the ages of 0 and 4 years, TBI is typically caused by falls. Between ages 15 and 19 years, the beginning driving years, TBI is typically caused by car accidents. In older people, falls are the primary cause of TBI. The primary causes of TBI for nonmilitary situations are falls, motor vehicle accidents, and assaults. For military personnel in war zones, blast injuries are the leading cause of TBI. The direct medical costs and the indirect costs in loss of productivity are estimated to be in the billions.

Knowledge about the deficits resulting from TBI has greatly increased over the years, as have the number of rehabilitation programs and treatment methods specific to TBI. TBI is clearly another cause of cognitive-communicative or cognitive-linguistic disorders.

Neuropathology of Injury

TBI can be the result of a closed head injury or a penetrating wound. A closed head injury leaves the skull intact, but the delicate brain tissues are injured by the uncontrolled movement from the impact. Examples of closed head injuries include motor vehicle accidents or falls where the head strikes a pavement. In a closed head injury, the typical mechanism is an acceleration-deceleration injury. In a car accident, the vehicle is providing the acceleration; in a fall, the acceleration is caused by the movement of the fall. The deceleration is the sudden stoppage of the movement. Because of the laws of physics, the hard object (the skull) will move faster than the softer object. This speed difference means that the brain will still be moving as the skull stops abruptly upon hitting the windshield or the ground. The brain tissue then will hit the inner walls of the skull, causing discrete focal lesions as well as more widespread lesions due to bruising. The locus of the strike to the head is known as coup damage. Contusions (bruising) may also occur opposite the point of direct impact. Damage sustained at the site opposite the point of impact is called contrecoup damage.

If the injury is not linear, as can happen in a car accident, it could result in a rotational injury, which includes a diffuse axonal injury (DAI). In this type of injury, the brain not only hits at the coup and countercoup points, it also rotates within the skull. This rotation induces more numerous contusions of the brain. If the rotation is severe enough, axons may shear and break off, causing the DAI. The diffuse brain injury is the result of several factors, one of those being molecular commotion. The molecular structure of the brain is disrupted as the impact force causes acceleration, rotation, compression, and expansion of the brain within the skull. Another factor causing devastating diffuse injury occurs as the brain tissues are compressed, torn apart, and sheared on the bony prominences of the skull, resulting in the breakages of axons. This breakage of axons triggers processes within the neural tissue, such as breakage of the microtubules and destabilization of the cytoskeleton. Fluid may collect in the axon at the various points of disruption causing swelling at those points giving it a beaded appearance.[26] If sufficient localized swelling is not contained, it also may cause axon to rupture, a process called secondary axotomy. DAI can result in permanent microscopic alterations of white and gray matter.

DAI, even severe DAI, may occur without skull fracture or cortical contusion. This accounts for the fact that CT scans in the emergency department may show no abnormality. In nonhuman primate models, DAI has been produced just on rapid acceleration of the head with no impact as well as in cases of mild brain injury in which the nonhuman primate had only transitory alterations in the level of consciousness (e.g., in sports such as football and in blast-related TBI).

More secondary problems can occur for people with closed head injury and DAI. Secondary mechanisms occur as a result of the initial direct forces, such as ischemia, hypoxia, edema, hemorrhage, brain shift, and raised intracranial pressure (ICP). Medical and surgical efforts in the emergency department are often targeted at treating or preventing secondary injury to improve the prognosis. Such procedures may include a blood transfusion, placing the patient in a drug-induced coma, performing a craniotomy, or removing a part of the skull to allow for brain tissue to expand without additional trauma due to the ICP.

Closed head injuries are the most common type of brain injury, occurring with or without loss of consciousness; if loss of consciousness occurs, it is often a signal of a more profound injury. Penetrating head wounds are less common although no less concerning. A penetrating wound occurs when the skull is penetrated, and the dura mater is breached. This type of injury occurs with projectiles from gunshots or shrapnel. As can be expected, these injuries carry a high mortality rate. Damage in the brain is along the path of the penetrating object and is considered focal brain damage. This damage disrupts brain networks and can carry foreign material into the brain, leading to infections.

Neurobehavioral Effects

The neurobehavioral sequelae of moderate to severe TBI are usually divided into two classes: focal deficits and diffuse deficits. Focal deficits may be manifested as a specific language deficit (aphasia, alexia, agraphia, etc.) or as a paralysis of specific muscles or muscle groups. Disorders such as mutism, dysarthria, palilalia, voice disorder, hearing loss, and visual or auditory perceptual dysfunction may be considered focal deficits. If present, they are complicating factors in rehabilitation efforts, and their specific treatment may be enormously complicated by the presence of diffuse deficits. Diffuse deficits are more common and are most often manifested as cognitive disorganization. The cognitive processes of attention, perception, memory, learning, organization, reasoning, problem solving, and judgment are often affected. These aspects of cognition and the possible effects of their disruption on behavior and language are outlined in Table 10.4.

Blast Injuries

Another population at extreme risk for TBI is military personnel who are in combat areas in which the use of explosives (bombs, grenades, land mines, mortar/artillery shells) is commonplace. While the use of body armor has allowed soldiers to survive some blasts, evidence suggests that exposure to the blast can produce neurological consequences. In fact, brain injury has become known as the signature wound of the wars in the Middle East, with roughly half the soldiers who were exposed to explosives suffering the results of neurotrauma as a consequence. Blast-induced traumatic brain injury (bTBI) is not only a significant military health concern, it also affects civilians, and the effects range from mild symptoms to fatal outcomes.

The mechanism of injury has become well documented. The injury results from the complex pressure wave generated

TABLE 10.4 Cognitive Impairment after Traumatic Brain Injury: Effect on Behavior and Language

Aspect of Cognition	Effect on Behavior	Effect on Language
Attention Holding objects, events, words, or thoughts in consciousness	Short attention span; distractible, weak concentration	Decreased auditory comprehension, confused or inappropriate language, poor reading comprehension, poor topic maintenance
Perception Recognizing features and relations among features	Weak perception of relevant features; possible specific deficits (including field neglect); poor judgment based on visual or auditory cues; stimulus bound (i.e., focus on part of the whole); spatial disorganization	Difficulty in reading and writing, poor comprehension of facial and intonation cues
Memory and Learning Encoding: recognizing, interpreting, and formulating information, including language, into an internal code (knowledge base, personal interests, and goals affect what is coded) Storage: retaining information over time Retrieval: transferring information from long-term memory to consciousness	Memory problems, inability or inefficiency in learning new material	Difficulty following multistep directions, word-finding problems, difficulty with reading comprehension and spelling, poor integration of new and old information; language may be fragmented, lacking logic, order, specificity, and precision; difficulty with math also seen
Organizing Processes Analyzing, classifying, integrating, sequencing, and identifying relevant features of objects and events; comparing for similarities or differences; integrating into organized descriptions, higher level categories, and sequenced events	Poor organization of tasks and time; difficulty setting and maintaining goals; poor problem solving, self-direction, self-confidence, and social judgment	Disorganized language (verbal and written), difficulty discerning main ideas and integrating them into broader themes, poor conversational skills (may get lost in details), difficulty outlining material for study, difficulty with math
Reasoning Considering evidence and drawing inferences or conclusions; involves flexible exploration of possibilities (divergent thinking) and use of past experience	Concrete, impulsive, and reactionary; may be easily swayed; vulnerable to propaganda; difficulty discerning cause and effect and consequences of behavior; poor social judgment	Difficulty understanding and expressing abstract concepts; socially inappropriate, lack of tact; difficulty using language to persuade, understand humor, learn academic subjects, and follow complex conversations
Problem Solving and Judgment Problem solving: ideally involves identifying goals, considering relevant information, exploring possible solutions, and selecting the best solutions Judgment: deciding to act or not to act based on consideration of relevant factors, including prediction of consequences	Impulsive, uses trial-and-error approach, difficulty predicting consequences of behavior, shallow reasoning; poor safety and social judgment, inflexible thinking, poor self-direction, poor use of compensatory strategies	Difficulty understanding and expressing steps in problem solving to get a particular outcome; difficulty in math and higher academic tasks, socially inappropriate behavior, lack of tact, difficulty in understanding explanations for behavior

Modified from Szekeres, S. F., Ylvisaker, M., & Holland, A. L. (1985/1998). Cognitive rehabilitation therapy: A framework for intervention. In M. Ylvisaker (Ed.), *Traumatic brain injury rehabilitation: Children and adolescents* (2nd ed.). Butterworth-Heinemann.

by the blast. This pressure results from an instant rise in the atmospheric pressure around the body that is much higher than tolerated by humans. It is called a blast overpressurization wave. This is followed rapidly by blast-underpressurization, which creates a relative vacuum effect. These extreme pressure differences result in both stress and shear wave forces as the waves hit the body of anyone near the blast.[6,32]

There are four basic mechanisms of injury to the persons around the blast[8]:

- Primary blast injury—the explosion itself resulting in the overpressurization wave. It dissipates quickly, causing the most injury to those closest to the explosion.
- Secondary blast injury—the injury caused by energized fragments, perhaps resulting in penetrating brain injuries.

- Tertiary blast injury—the injury resulting from being thrown from the area of the blast.
- Quaternary blast injury—results from significant blood loss or from inhalation of toxic gases.

Exposure to bTBI results in physical, psychological, and cognitive symptoms, and is collectively referred to as post-concussive syndrome. Physical symptoms include headache and alterations in sleep patterns. Psychological symptoms include mood changes and post-traumatic stress syndrome (PTSD). Cognitively, patients commonly present with retrograde amnesia, executive function difficulties, confusion, and difficulty with attention and with memory.[32] In one study comparing victims of primary blast injury with a group injured through blunt force trauma found blast injury resulted in greater hypometabolism in the right superior parietal region. These patients showed significantly greater difficulty on measures of attentional control, possibly indicating involvement of the parietal-frontal attentional network.[25]

Mild Traumatic Brain Injury

A mild TBI or concussion may produce symptoms immediately, but in other cases, symptoms appear hours or even days after the injury. These symptoms are not limited to cognitive-communicative functions; they also include several physical and social-emotional symptoms. Cognitive-communicative changes include difficulty with attention and concentration, cognitive speed, mental fogginess, and memory problems, although other difficulties can also be reported. Physical symptoms include light sensitivity, dizziness, reduced stamina, headaches, and visual changes. Social-emotional symptoms include sleep disorders, anxiety, irritability, and depression.[8]

It is estimated that many people who experience a mild TBI do not seek medical care, even if they are exhibiting symptoms. Most people recover well from mild TBI, but roughly a quarter will develop long-term deficits, particularly if treatment is not sought. This consequence affects the older population disproportionally because a TBI can place the person at higher risk for the development of Alzheimer or Parkinson disease.[20]

A further consideration is that repeat mild TBIs may result in cumulative damage. Such effects are seen in many sports, especially football, although other sports certainly put the athlete at risk for concussion or brain injury due to repetitive blows to the head. Repeat traumas can result in chronic traumatic encephalopathy, discussed next.

Chronic Traumatic Encephalopathy

A neuropathologic condition known as **chronic traumatic encephalopathy (CTE)** has been linked to repetitive instances of mild TBI. Historically, late-life behavioral changes in boxers were described with the term "punch drunk"; later, in 1937, dementia pugilistica was used to designate the symptoms of cognitive, motor, and behavioral changes seen in boxers.[28] Further study of brain injury, particularly as related to sports injuries, showed that the disease was not limited to only the sport of boxing. Case studies also began to be reported

of nonathletes who experienced repetitive brain injury from different causes (e.g., domestic abuse, head-banging behavior, injury during seizure activity) who later began to exhibit the described symptoms. Traumatic encephalopathy was introduced in the mid-20th century.

Descriptions of symptoms of CTE include a wide spectrum of changes in behavior, cognition, and motor skill. Problems with attention, memory, and executive function are noted in most cases. The pathology of CTE was seen through autopsy studies, which showed a distinctive pattern of progressive brain atrophy with accumulation of tau neurofibrillary and glial tangles, microvascular pathology, neuroinflammation, and degeneration of white matter, among other pathologic changes.[12,14,15] The location and distribution of the tau deposits help distinguish CTE from other well-known neurodegenerative disorders such as Alzheimer and Parkinson diseases.[14] In CTE the tau tangles tend to form in an irregular distribution pattern in the frontal and temporal areas of the cortex, clustered in dense patches in the depths of the sulci and in the more superficial layers of the cortex. Also important was the finding that beta-amyloid deposits, which are a hallmark sign of Alzheimer disease, were observed in fewer than half of the brains of persons with CTE.

Role of the SLP

In any patient with any degree of cognitive-communicative deficit after a TBI, the SLP is a critical part of a rehabilitation team. Although the involvement with the patients with mild TBI may be brief (but important), the most successful rehabilitation of patients with moderate to severe TBI is known to be intensive and long term in nature. Much of what is done to overcome the resulting deficits in attention, memory, reasoning, and problem solving, which are the basis of the difficulty in communication, involves training the individual to self-monitor the use of strategies that enable adaptation of the external and internal environment to compensate for weaknesses. Follow-up with patients who have had success in vocational and social life after TBI has shown that the ability to incorporate these strategies and adapt them to new challenges seems to be key.

Assessment and Treatment

Although evaluation measures have been developed for the cognitive-communicative impairment in TBI, testing must extend beyond these batteries. Often, the patient's description of difficulties in daily life or in work is helpful for a more accurate diagnosis. The SLP must attempt to determine which, and to what degree, cognitive processes underlying language performance are disrupted and whether the language impairment has a true aphasic component. An example of a TBI battery was compiled by Parrish et al.,[27] for evaluation of cognitive communication problems of returning combat veterans with mild TBI. This protocol consisted of a rating scale, selected portions of the Woodcock-Johnson III, the Functional Assessment of Verbal Reasoning and Executive Strategies (FAVRES), and the Attention Process Training Test, as well as informal measures of conversation collected while the patients were in a group situation.

COGNITIVE-COMMUNICATIVE DIFFICULTIES FOLLOWING COVID-19 INFECTIONS

Covid-19 is caused by a severe acute respiratory virus (SARS-CoV-2), but it also affects multiple systems besides the respiratory. Patients have reported neurologic symptoms, with an estimated 85% of severe infections resulting in neurologic symptoms. There is accumulating evidence for neural damage in some individuals. In fact, imaging has demonstrated loss of gray matter in multiple regions, particularly in the left hemisphere, and postmortem investigation found ischemic lesions and neuroinflammation in the CNS.[21]

Cognitive problems are some of the most prevalent symptoms in long Covid, the chronic phase following recovery from the respiratory infection. Long Covid is estimated to affect between 10% and 25% of Covid patients. The cognitive symptoms are often described as "brain fog."[4] Researchers have focused on the cognitive domains impaired by the infection that causes this brain fog. In one study, 181 patients recovering from this infection were tested on memory, language, and executive functioning domains. A consistent pattern of memory deficits was found, with verbal memory the most affected domain. Interestingly, findings included a slower response time on verbal memory tasks in addition to a reduced accuracy on such tasks when compared with the control group that had not experienced Covid.[21]

Other researchers[4] found dysexecutive symptoms in their samples, including executive functioning and naming difficulties, in addition to the processing speed and memory impairments. These cognitive effects were more disastrous to populations with preexisting cognitive difficulties, including those suffering from multiple scleroisis,[22] people with neurodegenerative diseases,[23] and the elderly.

Significant cognitive impairment has even been reported in asymptomatic and mild cases of this infection, and for up to 7 months after the infection. Given the significant impact of Covid-19 on cognition, it is not surprising that there was an associated impact on functionality and quality of life. There are numerous reports of increased economic, health, and social burdens in people following Covid-19 infections. These reports indicate an urgent need to study cognitive impacts of this illness and so develop appropriate therapies and assistance.[13]

SYNOPSIS OF CLINICAL INFORMATION AND APPLICATIONS FOR THE SLP

- Aphasia is an acquired disorder of language caused by focal brain damage that can affect any of the four modalities: listening, speaking, reading, and writing.
- The most common etiology of aphasia is CVA, or stroke, which occurs when the arterial distribution to a part or all of the perisylvian language cortex is interrupted. This interruption by a stroke is caused by occlusion of an artery or by hemorrhage resulting from arteriovenous malformation, aneurysm, or trauma.
- Aphasia may also be found after focal lesion caused by trauma, abscess from brain infection, or brain tumor.
- Brain tumors, which primarily arise from neuroglia, are classified according to their origin. Tumors are also graded from I to IV according to the tumor's tendency to spread.
- The most popular aphasia classification system is the Boston classification, which includes Broca, Wernicke, conduction, global, anomic, transcortical motor, transcortical sensory, and mixed transcortical aphasias. Each type has a characteristic profile relative to comprehension, fluency, repetition, reading, and writing.
- The aphasias classified well by the Boston system are also relatively consistent with the site of the lesion, although many questions still exist concerning the traditional localization, especially in conduction aphasia. Anomic aphasia does not localize damage well because storage and retrieval of words seem to be widely diffused in the brain.
- Subcortical damage to parts of the basal ganglia, thalamus, and internal capsule has been found to result in particular patterns of communication difficulty consistent with aphasia.
- The SLP is a critical member of the rehabilitation team for persons with aphasia, providing the most complete evaluation and setting treatment goals and plans.

- Some advances have been made in the use of pharmacologic treatment in aphasia, but the drugs studied have always been found to be most effective when combined with behavioral treatment provided by speech pathology.
- Central disturbances associated with aphasia are agnosia, apraxia, alexia, and agraphia. Alexia is a disorder of reading imposed on literate individuals after brain damage. The classic aphasias have associated reading deficits. Two other classifications exist: alexia without agraphia and alexia with agraphia. Psycholinguistic classifications of reading deficits also have been made: deep dyslexia, surface dyslexia, and phonologic alexia.
- Agraphia is a deficit in producing written language.
- Cognitive-communicative disorders are communication disorders related to damage to the nondominant hemisphere or diffuse brain damage. Communication deficits associated with right hemisphere damage, dementia, and TBI are classified as cognitive-communicative disorders.
- The communication deficit associated with right hemisphere damage is primarily related to extralinguistic deficits rather than the true linguistic deficits such as problems with word retrieval, syntax, comprehension, reading, and writing. Attention has a major effect on the communicative effectiveness of these patients.
- Patients with right hemisphere damage have difficulty with distinguishing relevancy, integrating and interpreting context cues, inhibiting impulsive responses, maintaining topic maintenance and efficient expression, grasping figurative language, and producing and responding to emotional responses.

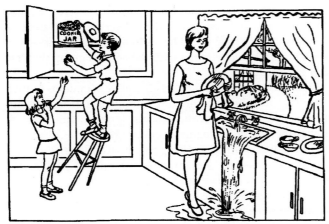

Fig. 10.5 Connected-speech elicitation picture (commonly referred to as the cookie theft picture) from the Boston Diagnostic Aphasia Examination. (Reprinted from Goodglass, H., Kaplan, E., & Barresi, B. [2001]. *The assessment of aphasia and related disorders* [3rd ed.]. Lippincott, Williams & Wilkins.)

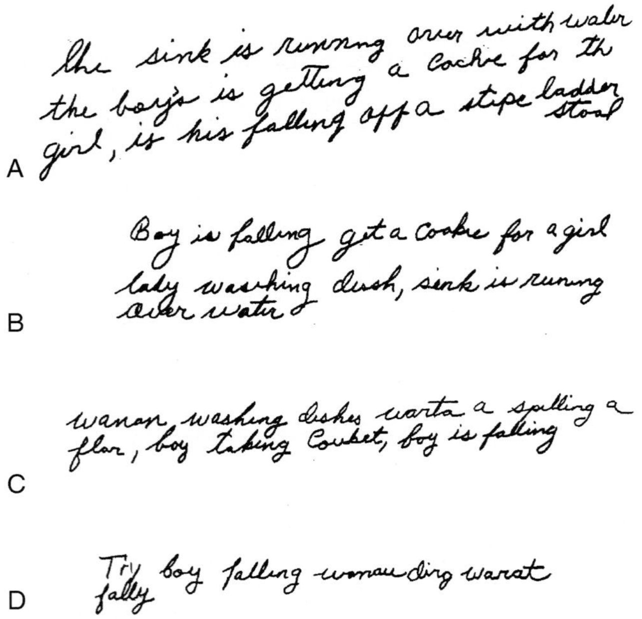

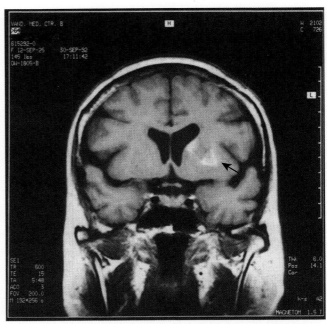

Fig. 10.7 Magnetic resonance imaging scan showing a lesion in the head of the caudate, anterior putamen, and anterior limb of the internal capsule (black arrowhead) resulting in a mild subcortical aphasia characterized by hesitant speech and anomia. The patient showed good recovery after a period of speech therapy. (Courtesy of Howard S. Kirshner, MD, Department of Neurology, Vanderbilt University School of Medicine, Nashville, TN.)

Fig. 10.6 Writing samples from four administrations of the paragraph writing subtest of the Boston Diagnostic Aphasia Exam describing the cookie theft picture (see Fig. 10.5). Samples (A) and (B) were done 2 months apart, ~2 years after the first symptoms of difficulty with speech were first noted by the patient. Sample (C) was done 1 year after (B) and sample (D) 1 year after (C).

Subcortical Aphasia

Striatal Lesions	Striatal and Internal Capsule Lesions
No aphasia Dysarthria possible Hypophonia	No definite aphasia Dysarthria possible

Internal Capsule Lesions	Insular and External Capsule lesions

No aphasia
Left dysarthria possible
Right affective dysprosody
	Fluent aphasia
	Anomia
	Paraphasias in
	  repetition
	  oral reading
	  spontaneous speech
	No dysarthria

Fig. 10.8 The signs and symptoms of language and speech disorders associated with subcortical lesions. (Modified from Alexander, M. P., & Naeser, M. A. [1988]. Cortical-subcortical differences in aphasia. In F. Plum [Ed.], Language, communication and the brain. New York: Raven Press.)

CASE STUDY

A 61-year-old man noticed a stutter and difficulty expressing himself soon after a stressful situation. His dysfluency became more obvious over the next 2 years, and his wife began to notice that he had difficulty with auditory comprehension as well. Audiometric testing revealed only a mild bilateral high-frequency hearing loss. Evaluation at this 2-year mark found normal performance on bedside neurologic examination of memory, calculations, general information, and copying of geometric figures. Speech was described as hesitant with occasional literal and verbal paraphasic errors and a marked tendency to add extra syllables to words (palilalia). Comprehension testing found him needing extra repetitions to perform even one-step commands presented verbally, but he could readily follow complex written commands. On the Boston Diagnostic Aphasia examination (Fig. 10.5) he had some difficulty with reading but only at the complex paragraph level. Writing was hesitant and contained numerous spelling errors (Fig. 10.6A). Repeat evaluations were done over the next 2 years, showing a pattern of progressive deterioration of auditory comprehension, speech intelligibility, and writing. Reading comprehension was slower to deteriorate, but by 4 years after onset he could comprehend only some single words written to aid communication. His wife reported mild forgetfulness at home, and he showed impaired visual memory and learning on neuropsychologic testing. He remained well groomed and socially appropriate with recognition of examiners who worked with him.

Questions for Consideration

1. This patient is an example of what condition discussed in this chapter?
2. CT scans of this patient showed generalized cortical atrophy and ventricular enlargement. If more definitive imaging such as MRI had been available, what would it likely have shown as the focus of the atrophy?
3. The long-term retention of the ability to copy geometric figures and draw a clock would speak to the intactness of which part of the brain?

REFERENCES

1. Acharya, A. B., & Maani, C. V. (2022). *Conduction aphasia.* StatPearls Publishing. PMID 30725691.
2. Akhoundi, F. H., Sahraian, M. A., & Moghadasi, A. N. (2020). Neuropsychiatric and cognitive effects of the COVID-19 outbreak on multiple sclerosis patients. *Multiple Sclerosis and Related Disorders, 41,* 102164. https://doi.org/10.1016/j.msard.2020.102164.
3. American Heart Association. (2022). Heart disease and stroke statistics update fact sheet. https://www.heart.org/-/media/PHD-Files-2/Science-News/2/2022-Heart-and-Stroke-Stat-Update/2022-Stat-Update-At-a-Glance.pdf.
4. American Speech-Language-Hearing Association. (n.d.). Classification of aphasia. https://www.asha.org/siteassets/practice-portal/aphasia/common-classifications-of-aphasia.pdf.
5. Becker, J. H., Lin, J. J., Doernberg, M., Stone, K., Navis, A., Festa, J. R., & Wisnivesky, J. P. (2021). Assessment of cognitive function in patients after COVID-19 infection. *JAMA Network Open, 4*(10), e2130645. https://doi.org/10.1001/jamanetworkopen.2021.30645.
6. Binder, J. R. (2017). Current controversies on Wernicke's area and its role in language. *Current Neurology and Neuroscience Reports, 17,* 58. https://doi.org/10.1007/s11910-017-0764-8.
7. BrainLine. (2010). Blast injuries and the brain. *Brainline.* http://www.brainlinemilitary.org/content/2010/12/blast-injuries-and-the-brain.html.
8. Brookshire, R. H. (2015). *Introduction to neurogenic communication disorders* (8th ed.). Elsevier.
9. Centers for Disease Control and Prevention. (2022). Traumatic brain injury and concussion. https://www.cdc.gov/traumaticbraininjury/concussion/symptoms.html.
10. Cichon, N., Wlodarczyk, L., Saluk-Bijak, J., Bijak, M., Redlicka, J., Gorniak, L., & Miller, E. (2021). Novel advances to post-stroke aphasia pharmacology and rehabilitation. *Journal of Clinical Medicine, 10*(17), 3778. https://doi.org/10.3390/jcm10173778.
11. Corrow, S. L., Dalrymple, K. A., & Barton, J. J. (2016). Prosopagnosia: Current perspectives. *Eye and Brain, 8,* 165–175. https://doi.org/10.2147/EB.S92838.
12. Coslett, H. B., & Turkeltaub, P. (2016). Acquired dyslexia. *Neurobiology of language.* Academic Press. https://doi.org/10.1016/B978-0-12-407794-2.00063-8.
13. Coughlin, J. M., Wang, Y., Munro, C. A., Ma, S., Yue, C., Chen, S., Airan, R., Kim, P. K., Adams, A. V., Garcia, C., Higgs, C., Sair, H. I., Sawa, A., Smith, G., Lyketsos, C. G., Caffo, B., Kassiou, M., Guilarte, T. R., Pomper, M. G. Neuroinflammation and brain atrophy in former NFL players: An in vivo multimodal imaging pilot study. Neurobiol Dis. 2015 Feb;74:58–65. doi: 10.1016/j.nbd.2014.10.019. Epub 2014 Nov 7. PMID: 25447235; PMCID: PMC4411636.
14. Crivelli, L., Palmer, K., Calandri, I., Guekht, A., Beghi, E., Carroll, W., Frontera, J., García-Azorín, D., Westenberg, E., & Winkler, A. S., et al. (2022). Changes in cognitive functioning after COVID-19: A systematic review and meta-analysis. *Alzheimer's & Dementia, 18*(5), 1047–1066. https://doi.org/10.1002/alz.12644.
15. Daneshvar, D. H., Goldstein, L. E., Kiernan, P. T., Stein, T. D., & McKee, A. C. (2015). Post-traumatic neurodegeneration and chronic traumatic encephalopathy. *Molecular and Cellular Neurosciences, 66(Part B),* 81–90.
16. Dejerine, J. (1891). Sur un cas de cécité verbale avec agraphie suivi d'autopsie. *Mémoires de la Société de Biologie, 3,* 197–201.
17. Dewan, M. C., Rattani, A., Gupta, S., Baticulon, R. E., Hung, Y.-C., Punchak, M., Agrawal, A., Adeleye, A. O., Shrime, M. G., Rubiano, A. M., Rosenfeld, J. V., & Park, K. B. (2018). Estimating the global incidence of traumatic brain injury. *Journal of Neurosurgery, 130*(4), 1080–1097.
18. Fischer, B. L., Parsons, M., Durgerian, S., Reece, C., Mourany, L., Lowe, M. J., Beall, E. B., Koenig, K. A., Jones, S. E., Newsome, M. R., Scheibel, R. S., Wilde, E. A., Troyanskaya, M., Merkley, T. L., Walker, M., Levin, H. S., & Rao, S. M. (2014). Neural activation during response inhibition differentiates blast from mechanical causes of mild to moderate traumatic brain injury. *Journal of Neurotrauma, 31*(2), 169–179.
19. Gale, S. A., Acar, D., & Daffner, K. R. (2018). Dementia. *American Journal of Medicine, 131*(10), 1161–1169. https://doi.org/10.1016/j.amjmed.2018.01.022.
20. Galletta, E. E., & Barrett, A. M. (2014). Impairment and functional interventions for aphasia: Having it all. *Current Physical Medicine and Rehabilitation Reports, 2*(2), 114–120. https://doi.org/10.1007/s40141-014-0050-5.

21. Gardner, R. C., & Yaffe, K. (2015). Epidemiology of mild traumatic brain injury and neurodegenerative disease. *Molecular and Cellular Neuroscience, 66*, 75–80.

22. Guo, P., Ballesteros, A. B., Yeung, S. P., Liu, R., Saha, A., Curtis, L., Kaser, M., Haggard, M. P., & Cheke, L. G. (2022). COVCOG 2: Cognitive and memory deficits in long COVID: A second publication from the COVID and cognition study. *Frontiers in Aging Neuroscience, 14*. https://doi.org/10.3389/fnagi.2022.804937.

23. Hicks, R. R., Fertig, S. J., Desrocher, R. E., Koroshetz, W. J., & Pancrazio, J. J. (2010). Neurological effects of blast injury. *Journal of Trauma: Injury, Infection, and Critical Care, 68*(5),1257–1263. https://doi.org/10.1097/TA.0b013e3181d8956d.

24. Iodice, F., Cassano, V., & Rossini, P. M. (2021). Direct and indirect neurological, cognitive, and behavioral effects of COVID-19 on the healthy elderly, mild-cognitive-impairment, and Alzheimer's disease populations. *Neurological Sciences, 42*(2), 455–465. https://doi.org/10.1007/s10072-020-04902-8.

25. Kirshner, H. S. (1995). *Handbook of neurological speech and language disorders.* Marcel Dekker.

26. Mendez, M. F., Owens, E. M., Reza Berenji, G., Peppers, D. C., Liang, L.-J., & Licht, E. A. (2013). Mild traumatic brain injury from primary blast vs. blunt forces: Post-concussion consequences and functional neuroimaging. *NeuroRehabilitation, 32*(2), 397–407.

27. Najem, D., Rennie, K., Ribecco-Lutkiewicz, M., Ly, D., Haukenfrers, J., Liu, Q., Nzau, M., Fraser, D. D., & Bani-Yaghoub, M. (2018). Traumatic brain injury: Classification, models, and markers. *Biochemistry and Cell Biology, 96*(4), 391–406. https://doi.org/10.1139/bcb-2016-0160.

28. Parrish, C., Roth, C., Roberts, B., & Davie, G. (2009). Assessment of cognitive-communicative disorders of mild traumatic brain injury sustained in combat. *Perspectives on Neurophysiology and Neurogenic Speech and Language Disorders, 19*(2), 47–57. https://doi.org/10.1044/nnsld19.2.47.

29. Riley, D. O., Robbins, C. A., Cantu, R. C., & Stern, R. A. (2015). Chronic traumatic encephalopathy: Contributions from the Boston University Center for the study of traumatic encephalopathy. *Brain Injury, 29*(2), 154–163.

30. Ruksenaite, J., Volkmer, A., & Jiang, J. (2021). Primary progressive aphasia: Toward a pathophysiological synthesis. *Current Neurology and Neuroscience Reports, 21*, 7. https://doi.org/10.1007/s11910-021-01097-z.

31. Tremblay, P., & Dick, A. S. (2016). Broca and Wernicke are dead, or moving past the classic model of language neurobiology. *Brain & Language, 162*, 60–71. https://doi.org/10.1016/j.bandl.2016.08.004.

32. World Health Organization. (2021). Dementia. https://www.who.int/news-room/fact-sheets/detail/dementia.

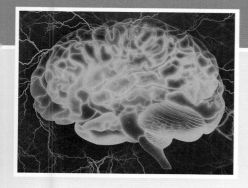

11

Pediatrics: The Developing Brain

An examination of infant behavior is an examination of the central nervous system.

Arnold Gesell and Catherine S. Amatruda, Developmental Diagnosis, 1947

CHAPTER OUTLINE

KEY TERMS

allocortex
apoptosis
asymmetric tonic neck reflex
  (ATNR)
bite reflex
cortex
ectoderm
embryo
fetal period
forebrain (prosencephalon)
gag reflex
growth cone

hindbrain (rhombencephalon)
induction
mesocortex
mesoderm
midbrain (mesencephalon)
mitosis
Moro reflex
neocortex
neural plate
neural tube
neuroprogenitor cells
notochord

obligatory
primary neurulation
rooting reflex
secondary neurulation
spinal dysraphism
suck reflex
supine
swallowing reflex
synaptic stabilization
teratology
tongue reflex
vesicles

INTRODUCTION

This text is unlike many in neuroanatomy in that it starts the student studying the anatomy of the brain by learning the brain structure, function, and disorders using adult models. This approach was used initially and continues into the seventh edition for two reasons. First, many students come into the study of speech-language pathology or audiology knowing little about the brain and sometimes little about the anatomy of the rest of the body. As you can certainly agree by now, the number of terms that must be mastered in neuroanatomy is intimidating, and then one must try to understand how all those parts work together to produce movement, sensation, emotion, and thought. The study of embryology throws one immediately into learning how a structure was formed but not necessarily what it does and how it is related to the other structures developing simultaneously. This text is organized so that the student with little knowledge can learn the structures and their location and function and the relationship to others first and then learn how they evolved after conception.

The second reason this approach was used is that students assigned to study this depth of material are adults at least 18 years of age. As adults, we are much more familiar with the movement patterns and cognitive processes of a more mature nervous system than we are of the system we have just or several years ago left behind—that of the young child. Thus, it may be much easier to identify with the examples of various functions and, perhaps, effects of injury on function.

Your particular instructor may choose to have you do this part of the text first rather than following the organization of the text; this, of course, is also fine and is in fact fairly typical. At whatever point you are when you are studying the next part of the text, may you find the miracle of the development of this complex nervous system of ours fascinating!

DEVELOPMENT OF THE NERVOUS SYSTEM

The embryologic development of the nervous system is an intriguing sequence of events occurring over a brief period. The spinal cord and brain (with the exception of the cerebellum) reach development of their full number of neurons by the 25th week of gestation. This includes the billions of cells of the cerebral cortex, both the neurons, and the neuroglial cells.

Dendrites of the neuronal cells begin to develop a few months before birth but are quite primitive in the newborn. In the first year of life dendritic processes develop on each cortical neuron to establish the startling number of connections each nerve cell makes with other neurons. The average number of connections that a single cell will make is within a range of 1000 to 10,000.

Early Development

During the second week after conception, the blastocyst that has been formed from **mitosis** of the zygote is embedded in the uterus. As this process takes place, the inner cell mass changes and produces a thick, two-layered plate called the embryonic disk. At the beginning of the third week, this mass is referred to as the **embryo**, with the embryonic period lasting through the eighth week. Many embryologists divide the embryonic period into 23 stages called Carnegie stages, but this depth of detail is beyond the scope of this chapter. The ninth week after fertilization until term (or 38 weeks after the last normal menstrual period) is the **fetal period**.

During the embryonic period, three primary germ layers that give rise to the tissues and organs begin to form at the beginning of the third week. These are the **ectoderm, mesoderm**, and endoderm. The mesoderm gives rise to muscle, connective tissues, cartilage, bone, and blood vessels, whereas the endoderm forms the linings of the digestive and respiratory tracts. The embryonic ectoderm gives rise to the epidermis and the nervous system. From these few dozen cells of the ectoderm of an almost infinitesimal weight comes the approximately 800-g (1.75-pound) brain of the child at birth. Most, although not all, of the neuron cells will complete their cell division before birth.[1]

Also during the third week a cellular rod called the **notochord** develops. The notochord defines the primitive axis of the embryo and gives it some rigidity. The vertebral column segments will form from the mesoderm around the notochord. Important to embryonic development is a function known as **induction**, essentially meaning that the proper development of one structure of the nervous system is dependent on the proper development of its neighbors. The notochord is important in induction as it directs the overlying ectoderm to thicken and form the **neural plate**. The neural plate eventually gives rise to the central nervous system (CNS).

On day 18 of development the neural plate begins folding in along its axis to form a neural groove with neural folds along each side. These folds move together and begin to fuse, with fusion occurring first in the middle and then progressing cranially and caudally. Closure at the cranial end is more rapid than at the caudal end. This fusing of the neural folds forms the **neural tube** (Fig. 11.1), which then separates from the surface ectoderm. The closure of the neural tube is complete by the end of the fourth week.

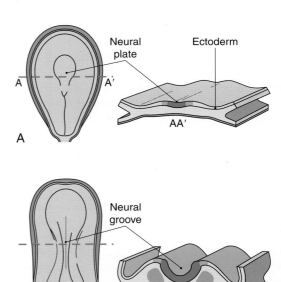

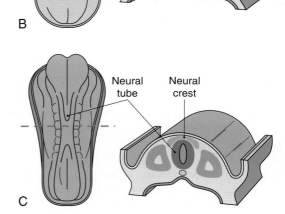

Fig. 11.1 Early development of the human nervous system. Drawings on the left are external views; cross sections are shown on the right. (A) Neural cells develop from ectoderm (skin-to-be) cells to form the neural plate. (B) The plate folds in to form the neural groove. (C) Further folding inwards forms the neural tube. (From Stokes, M. [2012]. *Physical management in neurological rehabilitation* [3rd ed.]. Mosby Ltd.)

When the neural tube is formed, three layers that consist of four zones appear for a brief period. These zones give rise eventually to important adult derivatives. The zones and eventual derivatives are as follows[2]:

- Ventricular zone (VZ): first to appear; contains rapidly dividing neuroprogenitor cells. At least three classes of these cells have been found in the human VZ:
  - Radial glial cells, expressing only glial markers
  - Multipotent precursor cells coexpressing glial and neuronal markers
  - Committed neuronal precursor cells
- Marginal zone (MZ): contains few cell bodies; mostly consists of processes of the cells making up the VZ and eventually invaded by axons from the intermediate zone. Becomes layer 1 of the adult cortex.
- Intermediate zone (IZ): latest to appear and formed between the VZ and MZ; contains immature postmitotic cells migrated from the VZ. Some of their processes will find their way to the MZ.
- Subventricular zone: forms between the VZ and IZ and contains progenitor cells that do not migrate further. They eventually become the macroglial cells of the CNS and some specialized cells of the brainstem and forebrain.

As the neural tube is rising from the ectoderm, the mesodermal layer of the embryo is forming longitudinal columns that soon divide into paired cubelike structures called somites (see Fig. 11.5 later). Eventually 42 to 44 pairs of somites develop. They form distinct surface elevations on the embryo. These somites differentiate into muscle, bone, and connective tissues (i.e., nonneural tissue).

A cross section of the developing embryo (see Fig. 11.1) shows another activity occurring as the neural folds fuse during the fourth week of development. Some of the neuroectodermal cells that lie along the crest of the neural folds break away from the other cells and migrate to the sides of the neural tube. These cells form the neural crest. The neural crest soon separates into two parts that migrate to the right and left dorsolateral aspects of the tube, where they will give rise to various important structures in the peripheral nervous system and to the ganglia of the autonomic nervous system. The dorsal root ganglia of the spinal nerves are derived from the neural crest, as are parts of the ganglia of cranial nerves V, VII, IX, and X. In addition to these ganglion cells, the neural crest also is responsible for Schwann cells and cells forming the meninges of the brain and spinal cord.

At the beginning of the fourth week, the embryo is almost straight, and temporary openings called neuropores appear at the cranial and caudal ends of the tube. These openings close by the end of the fourth week, and a longitudinal folding at the head (midbrain flexure) and the tail (cervical flexure) areas occurs, giving the embryo a characteristic C-shaped curve. Also during this time, four brachial or pharyngeal arches develop in the head area. Primary derivatives of the first arch are the bones of the jaw and the muscles of mastication. The second, third, and fourth arches primarily give rise to the muscles and cartilages of the face, larynx, and pharynx. Fig. 11.2 shows a 5-week-old embryo depicting some of these structures.

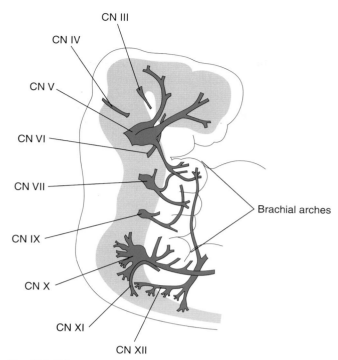

Fig. 11.2 Schematic drawing of a 5-week-old embryo shows distribution of most of the cranial nerves, especially those supplying the pharyngeal arches. (From Moore, K. L., Persaud, T. V. N., & Torchia, M. G. [2016]. *The developing human: Clinically oriented embryology* [10th ed.]. Elsevier.)

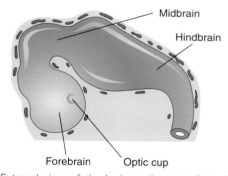

Fig. 11.3 External view of the brain at the end of the fifth week. Primitive spinal cord can be seen inferior to the hindbrain. (From Moore, K. L., Persaud, T. V. N., & Torchia, M. G. [2016]. *The developing human: Clinically oriented embryology* [10th ed.]. Elsevier.)

As the cranial and caudal ends of the neural tube begin to become more differentiated, cells from the neuroectoderm called **neuroprogenitor cells** begin to flourish. They migrate and differentiate to form specific areas of the brain. By the end of the fourth week of development, the neural tube is closed. After closure, an enlarged rostral region develops containing three subdivisions of the brain. The portion of the neural tube cranial to the fourth pair of somites develops into the brain. A narrow region caudal to the fourth pair of somites develops into the primitive spinal cord (Fig. 11.3).

How the neural tube develops into the mature CNS is regulated by a process called neurulation. **Primary neurulation** is the process that forms the brain and the spinal cord through the lumbar vertebrae. **Secondary neurulation** is the process by which the caudal neural tube (and eventually the caudal neural plate) gives rise to the sacral and coccygeal vertebrae. Problems with neural development during the primary or secondary neurulation process lead to dysraphic defects (defects of fusion). A condition called anencephaly can result from a defect of primary neurulation. With this there is a failure of the anterior neural tube closure. This results in facial deformities and an unformed brain with the skull perhaps not present. A birth defect related to a defect of secondary neurulation may occur in spinal cord embryologic development and is still commonly known as spina bifida, though the more acceptable current medical terminology for these conditions is **spinal dysraphism**.[3] In this condition the posterior neural tube fails to completely close, resulting in a cleft of the lower spinal cord. The condition falls into two main categories: open and closed dysraphic defects. Closed dysraphism is referred to in older and some contemporary literature as spina bifida occult. However, the tissue abnormality is rarely unsuspected or occult since there are typically signs on the outer skin surface such as dimples, discolored patches, hairy tufts or there is an obvious subcutaneous mass.[4] Two primary manifestations of open spinal dysraphism are illustrated in Fig. 11.4. The majority of children born with a myelomeningocele will also have hydrocephalus and/or a Chiari II malformation.[5] These conditions especially, as well as environmental factors or other CNS insults, can result in neurocognitive deficits in addition to the motor impairment in these children.

EMBRYOLOGY OF THE PERIPHERAL NERVOUS SYSTEM

Embryologic development of the neural tube forms the cells that arise from the lateral edge of the neural plate, detach, and move laterally to the neural tube forming what is called the neural crest. The neural crest gives rise to most of the peripheral nervous system and to a number of other structures. This early development of the nervous system is illustrated in Fig. 11.1.

The peripheral nervous system also arises from specialized epidermal cells called placodes that are found in the developing head region of the embryo. These cells join neural crest cells, and together placodes and neural crest cells form the ganglia of cranial nerves V, VII, VIII, IX, and X (Fig. 11.5). The neural and nonneural elements of the peripheral nervous system derived during this developmental period are summarized in Box 11.1.

SPINAL CORD

The spinal cord develops from caudal portions of the neural tube. The neural canal of this region becomes the central canal of the spinal cord. Neuroblasts that give rise to the spinal cord neurons are produced between weeks 4 and 20 of development by a proliferation in the ventricular layer lining the neural canal. These cells migrate peripherally to form four longitudinal plates. These plates will become the gray matter of the spinal cord. Within this gray matter a pair of anteriorly located cell masses, which constitute the basal plate, and a pair of posteriorly located masses, which constitute the alar plate, will form. The basal plate develops

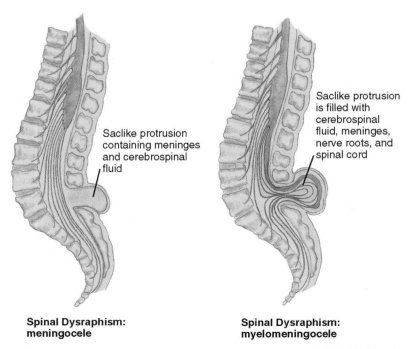

Saclike protrusion containing meninges and cerebrospinal fluid

Saclike protrusion is filled with cerebrospinal fluid, meninges, nerve roots, and spinal cord

Spinal Dysraphism: meningocele

Spinal Dysraphism: myelomeningocele

Fig. 11.4 Primary manifestations of open spinal dysraphism: meningocele and myelomeningocele. (Modified from James, S., & Ashwill, J. [2013]. *Nursing care of children* [4th ed.]. Saunders.)

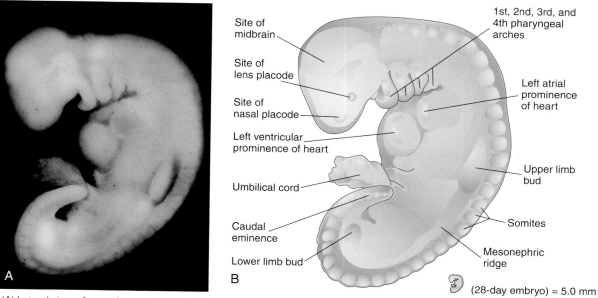

Fig. 11.5 (A) Lateral view of an embryo at ~28 days. The rostral and caudal neuropores are closed, and somites are clearly visible. (B) Drawing indicating the structures shown in (A). The embryo has a characteristic C-shaped curvature, four pharyngeal arches, and upper and lower limb buds. (A, From Nishimura, H., Semba, R., Tanimura, T., & Tanaka, O. [1977]. *Prenatal development of the human with special reference to craniofacial structures: An atlas.* National Institutes of Health.)

BOX 11.1 Peripheral Nervous System Elements Derived from the Neural Crest

Neural Elements
Neurons of:
- Posterior root ganglia
- Paravertebral (sympathetic chain) ganglia
- Prevertebral (preaortic) ganglia
- Enteric ganglia
- Parasympathetic ganglia of cranial nerves VII, IX, and X
- Sensory ganglia of cranial nerves V, VII, VIII, IX, and X

Nonneural Elements
- Schwann cells
- Melanocytes (forming melanin for the skin)
- Odontoblasts (forming dentine underlying tooth enamel)
- Satellite cells of peripheral ganglia
- Cartilage of the pharyngeal arches
- Ciliary and papillary muscles
- Cells of the adrenal medulla
- Pia and arachnoid of the meninges
- Some of the sensory cells in these ganglia arise from placodes

into the anterior, or ventral, horn of the spinal cord, and the alar plate becomes the posterior, or dorsal, horn of the spinal cord (Fig. 11.6).

The lateral walls of the developing spinal cord thicken differentially into zones. The MZ gradually becomes the white matter of the cord as axons grow into it. A shallow groove, called the sulcus limitans, develops on the lateral walls of the developing cord. This groove divides the dorsal lamina, or alar plate, from the ventral lamina, or basal plate. The alar plate or dorsal part of the spinal cord is later associated with afferent (sensory) functions and the basal plate or ventral part of the spinal cord with efferent (motor) functions.

Until the third month of development, the spinal cord extends the entire length of the developing vertebral column. At this time the dorsal (sensory) and ventral (motor) roots of the spinal cord extend laterally from the spinal cord and unite in the intervertebral foramina to form the spinal nerves. The vertebral column elongates at a more rapid rate than the spinal cord, thus making the spinal cord shorter than the vertebral column. At birth the end of the cord, called the conus medullaris, is located at the level of the third lumbar vertebra. In the adult it is located approximately between the first and second lumbar vertebrae. As the differential growth of the two structures takes place, the nerve roots located between the conus medullaris and the intervertebral foramina elongate. The lumbar, sacral, and coccygeal nerve roots are directed downward at an angle to reach their targeted exit point at the associated vertebral foramina. This elongated bundle of nerve fibers is known as the cauda equina (horse's tail).

EMBRYOLOGY OF THE CENTRAL NERVOUS SYSTEM

Development of the Meninges
Embryologically, the meninges develop from the neural crest and the mesoderm, which eventually develop into the CNS. Both the neural crest and the mesoderm form the primitive meninges.

Development of the Ventricles
The development of the ventricle system illustrates brain growth from the neural crest and neural tube. By about the

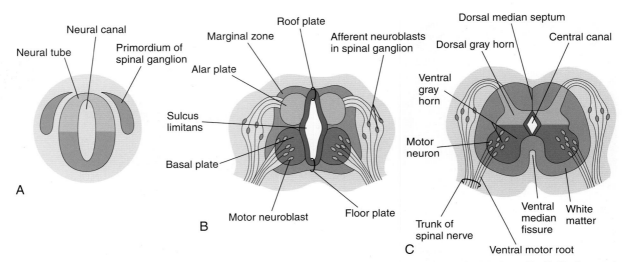

Fig. 11.6 Development of the spinal cord. (A) Transverse section of the neural tube of an embryo of ~23 days. (B, C) Similar sections at 6 and 9 weeks, respectively. (From Moore, K. L., Persaud. T. V. N., & Torchia, M. G. [2016]. *The developing human: Clinically oriented embryology* [10th ed.]. Elsevier.)

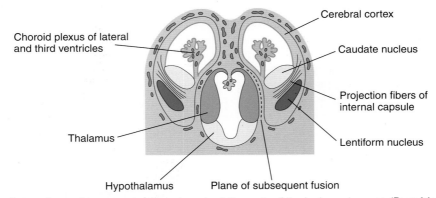

Fig. 11.7 At 11–12 weeks of gestation, rudimentary structure of nearly all the parts of the brain are present. (From Moore, K. L., Persaud, T. V. N., & Torchia, M. G. [2016]. *The developing human: Clinically oriented embryology* [10th ed.]. Elsevier.)

third week of development, the nervous system consists of a tube that is closed at both ends and is somewhat hook shaped. The cavity of this canal, the neural tube, eventually gives rise to the ventricles of the adult brain and the central canal of the spinal cord.

Embryology of Cortical and Subcortical Structures

During the fourth week of gestation the neural folds expand and fuse to form three primary brain **vesicles**. These are the **hindbrain**, or **rhombencephalon**; **midbrain**, or **mesencephalon**; and **forebrain**, or **prosencephalon**. The central canal of the neural tube dilates into a rudimentary ventricular system, and in the thin roof of the ventricles the choroid plexus develops to produce cerebrospinal fluid. By about the sixth week of development these divisions have further divided, and significant brain development can be noted. The rhombencephalon divides into the myelencephalon, which later becomes the medulla oblongata, and the metencephalon, which is the future pons and cerebellum. The midbrain or mesencephalon does not divide. The prosencephalon divides into the diencephalon and the telencephalon. The diencephalon later

becomes the thalamic complex and the third ventricle. The optic cup, which eventually becomes the optic nerve and retina, also rises from the diencephalon division.

At approximately the third month of development the telencephalon divides into three parts. All the structures of the brain are present, though in quite immature versions, by the end of the third month of gestation (Fig. 11.7). The rhinencephalon will contain the olfactory lobes. The second division, the striatal area, is the site of groups of neuronal cell bodies called the basal ganglia or basal nuclei. Only in higher vertebrate and human development does the third division of the telencephalon take place. This division is the suprastriatal structure called the neopallium. This is what is seen as the cerebral hemispheres, called the **cortex**. Fig. 11.8 outlines the primary brain vesicles and the ensuing derivational pattern.

The smooth surface of the hemispheres begins to convolute at ~20 weeks of gestation, and by week 24 gyri and sulci gradually appear. The first sulcus to appear is the lateral sulcus with its floor, the insula, gradually covered by further development and enfolding. This folding in of the cortical tissue allows this outer layer of neurons to increase greatly,

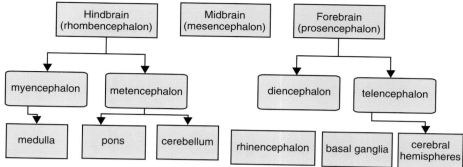

Fig. 11.8 Derivatives of the three primary brain vesicles.

eventually reaching an approximate dimension of 2300 cm² without the brain becoming too large for the skull.

We have discussed previously the fact that the cerebral cortex and some subcortical areas are stratified into layers. The cortex begins to stratify into layers, and at approximately 6 months of gestation the demarcation of the cortex into layers or lamina is present. The **allocortex**, or archicortex, which is found primarily in the limbic system, is composed for the most part of three layers. The **mesocortex** is found as transition cortex between the archicortex and the neocortex. The mesocortex contains three to six layers and is found in regions such as the insula and the cingulate gyrus. The **neocortex**, or isocortex, of the cerebral hemispheres is composed of six layers. All six layers can be microscopically differentiated early in development, but the final differentiation of the outer three layers is not complete until middle childhood.

NEURONAL MIGRATION IN THE CEREBRAL CORTEX

As all cells in the developing embryo do, neurons migrate from their place of "birth" to where they will eventually function as part of a system. During the formation of the neural tube, neuroprogenitor cells or neuroblasts have begun DNA replication and mitosis, arising in the VZ at the surface of the lateral ventricles. As cells divide and multiply, they cluster at the ventricular surface, thickening the walls of the tube. As they undergo their last division, they start to migrate away from the ventricular surface. At least two types of progenitor cells are active: neuroblasts, which will become neurons; and glioblasts, which will generate astrocytes, oligodendrocytes, and radial glial cells. The embryo will typically produce almost twice as many neurons as will eventually be found in the mature brain. Depending on the area of the brain in question, between 15% and 50% of these neurons will be eliminated through genetically programmed cell death, or **apoptosis**. The activation of this cellular process in which enzymes break down proteins causing DNA fragmentation and eventual cell death occurs naturally in many areas of the developing brain; most programmed cell disappearance/death seems to take place approximately between weeks 28 and 41 gestation.

Neurons in complex vertebrate nervous systems migrate somewhat differently than in simpler nervous systems. The specific mechanisms of this neural migration are not yet totally understood, and the complex details of the processes that are understood are beyond the scope of this text. The primary modes of migration as presented by Nadarajah et al.,[6] are briefly summarized here. The student who wishes to explore this further is directed to this article and to the work of Cooper.[7]

Development of the stratification of the cortex is an inside-out pattern of development. Neurons that start migrating first go the shortest distance, and the later ones migrate through the earlier ones. We previously mentioned zones created in the neural tube. In corticogenesis with the migration of neurons, plates are also created, with the preplate, subplate, and cortical plate most often mentioned.

Nadarajah et al.,[6] used time-lapsed photography to study the movement of neurons as they position themselves in the developing neocortex. They affirmed two distinct modes of migration for pyramidal neurons, which are excitatory projection neurons:

- Somal translocation: This mode appears to be the prevalent migratory method of early born cortical neurons. All of the immature neurons are bipolar with a leading process radially oriented toward the pial surface, while the other process remains attached initially to the VZ surface. In somal (or perikaryal) translocation, the neuroblasts detach from the VZ. Through a process called nucleokinesis the soma (cell body that contains the nucleus) is transported from the ventricular surface to the pial surface. Nucleokinesis involves a caging of the nucleus by microtubules and the centrosome of the cell. The alternating elongation and contraction of the microtubules move the nucleus and the cell outward to the pial surface.
- Glia-guided locomotion: Fig. 11.9 shows the embryologic development of the layers of the cortex as they are formed by glia-guided locomotion. In the very early stages, as outlined earlier, the cerebral new growth is relatively thin, and this kind of guidance is not typical. However, as the cerebral vesicles begin to thicken, neurons migrate primarily by traveling along processes of radial glia that seem to form a scaffolding for them to be guided along. The formation of the cortex of the cerebellum is formed in

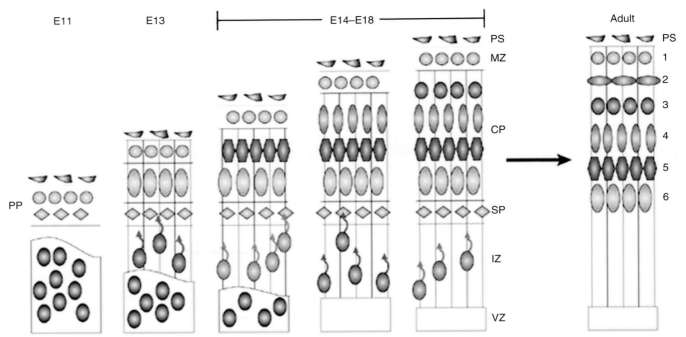

Fig. 11.9 Key developmental stages of development of the neocortex of the radial component of the formation of the neocortex of a mouse brain. The mouse brain is used extensively in research on brain development, as its embryology is similar to human development. This embryologic time period here represents around 6–18 weeks in human gestation. Migration along radial glia is shown as vertical bars. E = Embryologic day. At E11 the preplate *(PP)* is established by a postmitotic wave of neurons that has migrated from the ventricular zone *(VZ)* to the pial surface *(PS)*. By E13 a second postmitotic neuronal wave has migrated through the intermediate zone and split the PP into the marginal zone *(MZ)* and subplate *(SP)*, creating the cortical plate *(CP)*. During E14–E18, subsequent waves of neurons expand the CP in an inside-out fashion, as each wave of neurons passes its predecessors to settle underneath the MZ. In adulthood, the SP degenerates, leaving behind the six-layered neocortex. (From Gupta, A., Tsai, L.-H., & Wynshaw-Boris, A. [2002]. Life is a journey: A genetic look at neocortical development. *Nature Reviews Genetics, 3*(5), 342–355.)

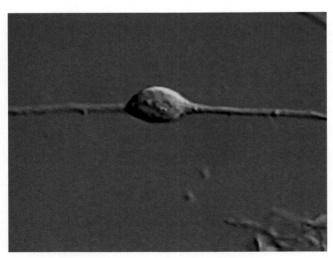

Fig. 11.10 A granular neuron cell of the cerebellar cortex migrating and guided along a radial glial process. (From Gasser, U. E., & Hatten, M. E. [1990]. Central nervous system neurons migrate on astroglial fibers from heterotypic brain regions in vitro. *Proceedings of the National Academy of Sciences, 87*(12), 4543–4537.)

similar manner. Fig. 11.10 is a frame from a movie made at Hatten Laboratories using high-contrast optics.[8] This frame pictures a granule neuron of the cerebellar cortex migrating through glia guidance (https://www.youtube.com/watch?v=ZRF-gKZHINk&ab_channel=BaoBui). In glia-guided migration, the nucleus will remain in the posterior part of the cell. An adhesion junction forms beneath the nucleus, and a leading process of the cell radiates out toward the direction of migration. The neuron moves by release and reformation of the adhesion junction, moving it along the glia scaffolding it is traveling along.

Neuronal Migration Disorders

Despite the complexity of the chemical guidance and signaling involved in the migration of neurons to their proper placement for normal brain function, most children are born with the appropriate migratory pattern and timing having occurred during development. However, abnormal neuronal migration does occur during brain and nervous system development and results in a category of birth defects called neuronal migration disorders (NMDs). When neurons do not end up where they belong, structural abnormalities including missing or malformed parts of the brain may occur. Such disorders as schizencephaly, polymicrogyria, pachygyria, microgyria, micropolygyria, neuronal heterotopias, agenesis of the corpus callosum, and agenesis of the cranial nerves are found in the literature as disorders of NMDs. Disorders with the suffix *-gyria* are migration disorders that have resulted in changes in the number and structure of the infolding of the cortex of the brain or the cerebellum. Pachygyria refers to a condition in which the gyri are described as broad and flat in appearance and few in number. With polymicrogyria there are too many gyri, and they are smaller than normal with shallow sulci. Heterotopia literally means "out of place," and neuronal heterotopia refers to clumps of neurons discovered to be located in the wrong place in the brain. As you may imagine, any of the disorders found in this group may impact speech-language development.

Making Connections

After making their way to the targeted region of the neocortex, the young neurons must establish connections with other neurons and become integrated into neural networks. To do this they develop an axon and also dendrites. The dendrites will eventually form dense arbors of connections near the vicinity of the cell body. Dendritic spines develop and become the site of many of the synaptic contacts onto dendrites. These spines form at different rates in different parts of the brain with the maximal rate occurring at about 6 months after birth.[8]

The axon of each neuron cell contains on its tip a structure called a **growth cone**. It is from the site of the growth cone that the axon elongates and extends out into the surrounding neural tissue, guided by tropic factors or molecules that send it toward a particular target. Also influencing the axon are trophic factors, which help maintain its metabolism. The axon may branch, and each branch will also contain a growth cone. Some branches established will not ever become innervating connections. On those that do, the growth cone becomes a presynaptic terminal, and the target neuron membrane begins to express the necessary postsynaptic mechanisms, such as neurotransmitter receptors and second messenger molecules. Although many synaptic connections will be made during this period of development, many are later lost or they are replaced by other connections. For **synaptic stabilization** to take place there must be (1) signal generation by a presynaptic cell, possibly the neurotransmitter required by the adult synapse; (2) a means for the postsynaptic cell to respond to the signal; and (3) a retrograde signal from the postsynaptic cell to the presynaptic cell to tell it which contacts should remain in maturity.[9] There is competition for synaptic space, and the advantage in the developing brain especially is given to the contact used most frequently.

Critical Periods

The study of abnormal embryonic development is called **teratology**. Teratogens are defined as any environmental factor that can cause complications during pregnancy or produce a permanent abnormality in structure or function, restriction of growth, or death of the embryo or fetus.[10] Teratogens can also cause complications of pregnancy, including spontaneous abortion, miscarriage, or preterm labor. Environmental factors include medications, drugs, maternal conditions, and chemicals. Several factors determine whether an environmental agent will have an effect on a developing embryo. A fundamental concept of teratology is that certain stages of embryologic development are more vulnerable to teratogens than other stages. The most critical period for the growth of a particular organ is the period of most rapid cell division for that particular tissue or organ. Thus, the critical period varies depending on the organ of concern. For brain development, the most critical period is from 3 to 16 weeks. Major anomalies occur during the third and fourth week as the neural tube and the neural crest form. The fetal period is also quite susceptible to teratogens, such as alcohol, and future cognitive development may be affected, resulting in some degree of intellectual disability. When labeling an agent or condition as a teratogen, the chemical or physical nature of the agent as well as other factors have to be taken into consideration. Factors such as the route, length, and dose of exposure, the developmental stage at which the exposure occurs, the genetic susceptibility of the mother and embryo or fetus, and the presence and nature of concurrent exposures have been taken into consideration in research and in development of standards of practice for medical practitioners managing pregnancies. Table 11.1 lists some environmental teratogenic agents or conditions that are known to cause CNS deficits given the appropriate timing and condition of exposure or occurrence during brain development.

Primitive Reflexes of the Newborn

The speech-language pathologist (SLP), especially when working in public schools or centers primarily with a young child population, must understand the primitive reflex profile to discern whether dysarthria, primitive reflexes, or other speech-language or cognitive problems exist in a child. An understanding of the primitive reflex patterns of infants helps the SLP understand the development of these reflexes into more permanent movement patterns. Furthermore, the SLP also learns how primitive communication patterns such as cooing (as related to the emergence of reflex patterns and then more advanced movement patterns) and random sound productions of the newborn infant lead to speech sound development.

EXAMINATION OF PRIMITIVE REFLEXES

The neurologic examination of the newborn with suspected cerebral damage has in recent years relied heavily on the concept of a primitive reflex profile. Primitive and postural reflexes follow an orderly sequence of appearance and disappearance, beginning in the fetal period and extending through the first years of life. The reflexes are mediated at a subcortical level. First described by Rudolph Magnus (1873–1927), who received a Nobel Prize for his efforts, these reflexes can help determine degrees of prematurity or suggest neurologic dysfunction. If a normal reflex pattern does not appear on schedule, or if a reflex pattern persists beyond the age at which it normally disappears, the newborn or infant is considered at risk for cerebral injury or other neurologic involvement. Some pediatric neurologists assert that neurologic abnormalities at birth predict a diagnosis of minimal cerebral dysfunction at later ages, but others have found a limited association between neonatal abnormalities and neurologic signs, particularly at 1 year and beyond. It should be

TABLE 11.1 Agents or Conditions that Can Be Teratogenic to Central Nervous System Development

Agent or Condition	Additional Consideration
Radiation	
Infectious agents	
Chickenpox (varicella)	During first 20 wk
Rubella	
Toxoplasmosis	
Agent Orange	
Thermodisruptions	
Hyperthermia	Body temperature $\geq 102\,°F$
Hypothermia	Body temperature $\leq 95\,°F$
Exposure to toxic metals	
Lead	$>20\,\mu g/dL$
Mercury	$>3\,\mu g/dL$
Lithium	Avoid during first trimester; no breast feeding if taking lithium
Chemical exposure	
Polychlorinated biphenyls	Exposure to airborne level of $>0.0001\,mg/m^3$
Toluene	Exposure to $>375\,mg/m^3$ $>8\,hr/day$
Maternal conditions	
Diabetes	
Iodine deficiency	
Maternal phenylketonuria	
Folic acid deficiency	
Maternal habits/intake	
Alcohol abuse	Best practice is to abstain throughout pregnancy
Tobacco (nicotine)	
Marijuana	
Cocaine	
Lysergic acid diethylamide	
Thalidomide	
Warfarin	
Angiotensin-converting enzyme inhibitors	
Statins	
Isotretinoin (Accutane, Retin A)	

Data from Gilbert-Barness, E. (2010). Teratogenic causes of malformation. *Annals of Clinical and Laboratory Science, 40*(2), 99–114.

TABLE 11.2 Primitive and Postural Infantile Reflexes of the First Year

Reflex	Response
Asymmetric tonic neck reflex	Infant extends limbs on chin and flexes on occiput side when turning head
Symmetric tonic neck reflex	Infant extends arms and flexes legs with head extension
Step reflex	Infant simulates a walking motion when held underneath the arms, leaning forward slightly, with feet allowed to touch a hard flat surface
Tonic labyrinthine reflex	Infant may retract shoulder and extend neck and trunk with neck flexion; tongue thrust reflex may occur
Segmental rolling reflex	Infant may roll trunk and pelvis segmentally with rotation of head or legs
Galant reflex	Infant arches body when skin of back is stimulated near vertebral column
Moro reflex	Infant may adduce arm and move it upward, followed by arm flexion and leg extension and flexion
Babinski (plantar) reflex	Infant's big toe extends up and back while the other four toes fan out when the sole of the foot is stroked from the heel toward the ball of the foot

BOX 11.2 Primitive Postural and Oral Reflexes Most Commonly Tested in Early Childhood Exams

- Rooting
- Suck
- Asymmetric tonic neck reflex
- Moro
- Grasp
- Step

Despite questions about the reliability of prediction for a diagnosis of minimal neurologic abnormality, the careful evaluation of early primitive reflexes and later-evolving postural reflexes provides a basis for diagnosis and therapy of disturbed motor function. Examination can usually provide a locomotor prognosis, indicating when and how a child with cerebral palsy will walk. Table 11.2 summarizes the primitive and postural reflexes of the first year. A physician or other medical practitioner such as a physical therapist may need to test all of these reflexes in an infant for whom an initial reflex exam has found signs of developmental problems. For most infant wellness exams, there are six primitive reflexes that are typically covered in a screening (Box 11.2). Although the SLP may be more interested in the neurologic status of oral and pharyngeal reflexes, an understanding of at least these primitive and postural

noted, however, that there is a growing body of research into the relationship between neuromotor delay/impairment in children and language and learning disorders.[11] The finding of neuromotor delay/impairment often includes a finding of persistent primitive reflexes.

reflexes is essential in the assessment of the neurologic maturity of a child suspected of cerebral injury.

A notable lack of consensus exists on the definition of the stimulus and response in the widely tested primitive reflexes. In addition, no agreement has been reached on how the responses change with time and growth. Six reflexes are reviewed in this chapter. They are commonly assessed by neurologists and pediatricians and are typical of the first year of life, with the peak development at approximately 6 months. Testing during this peak time avoids assessing the transitory neurologic signs of the newborn but is sufficiently early to allow a neurologic diagnosis before 1 year of age. These six reflexes also appear to be predictive of later motor function in the child. There are several sources online for training medical professionals in eliciting these and other neonatal reflexes (e.g., https://www.youtube.com/watch?v=rHYk1sYsge0&ab_channel=RegisteredNurseRN), and the student is encouraged to look at these as a part of the study of child development.

Stepping Reflex

The stepping reflex appears early in development and may disappear a few weeks after birth unless trained.[12] This reflex is considered one of the precursors to locomotion by walking. It is elicited by holding the child upright with feet touching a solid flat surface. When the reflex is present, a stepping (or walking/dancing) movement of the child's legs is seen. The reflex typically disappears by 2 weeks without practice/training.

Grasp Reflex

The grasp reflex delights all meeting an infant for the first time. This reflex is elicited simply by stroking the palm of the infant's hand with the reflex resulting in the child's fingers closing in a grasp. The reflex usually will disappear between 4 and 6 months.

Asymmetric Tonic Neck Reflex

The **asymmetric tonic neck reflex** (**ATNR**) probably is the most widely known of the early body reflexes. The reflex was shown to be universally present in the healthy infant by child development specialist Arnold Gesell (1880–1961). When **supine**, the healthy child may lie with the head turned to one side. The extremities on that side (the chin side) are extended, with a corresponding flexion of the contralateral extremities on the opposite (occiput) side. This position is described as the fencer's position (Fig. 11.11).

To test for the presence of the reflex, the child is placed in a supine position. Observations are made of active head turning and subsequent movement of the extremities. The head is then passively turned through an arc of 180 degrees to each side. This maneuver is repeated five times on each side. Consistent changes in muscle tone in the extremities generally define the presence of the reflex. A clearly positive response is visible extension of extremities on the chin side and flexion on the occiput side when the head is passively turned. If extension of the extremities on the chin side and flexion on the occiput side last more than 30 seconds, the response may be called **obligatory**.

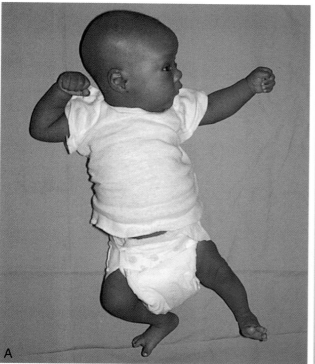
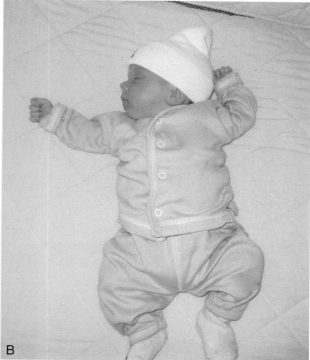

Fig. 11.11 (A, B) Asymmetric tonic neck reflex. Flexion of the arm and leg on the occipital side with extension of the arm on the chin side, creating the fencer's position. (Modifed from Chaves-Gnecco, D., & Feldman, H. M. [2018]. Developmental/behavioral pediatrics. In B. J. Zitelli, S. C. McIntire, & A. J. Nowalk [eds.], *Atlas of pediatric physical diagnosis* [7th ed., pp. 71–100]. Elsevier.)

If the response is found beyond the eighth or ninth month, it is indicative of possible cerebral damage and poor motor development and suggests that the cortical control of upper motor neurons is not on schedule and that motor behavior is still controlled at subcortical levels. Obligatory tonic neck reflexes persisting into the second year and beyond usually are incompatible with independent standing and walking; they may disappear later, however, and the child may learn to walk alone. The ATNR may be seen in various types of cerebral palsy, predicting brain injury, but it is not useful for distinguishing between spastic and dyskinetic types. This reflex suggests brain injury only and is in no way completely diagnostic for cerebral palsy or its subtypes. The ATNR can reemerge after a catastrophe such as cardiac arrest and may be present in progressive disease. It has little or no effect on the development of speech and shows little relation to the oral and pharyngeal reflexes.

Moro Reflex

The **Moro reflex** (also known as the startle reflex), along with the ATNR, is one of the best-known and best-studied reflexes of child neurology. It is present in almost all newborns except for small premature babies. With sudden but gentle head lowering, a rapid and symmetric abduction and upward movement of the arms occurs. The hands open, and gradual adduction and flexion of the arms occur. The lower limbs also show extension and then flexion. The Moro usually reaches a peak at 2 months and diminishes by 4 months. A persistent reflex has been associated with cerebral palsy and intellectual disability.

To test for the Moro reflex, the child is held in the examiner's arms, well supported at the head, trunk, and legs. The examiner gently but suddenly lowers the child's head and body in a dropping motion.

The most significant aspect of the stimulus is the quality of suddenness. Primitive and postural reflexes sometimes reinforce more circumscribed reflexes, but no evidence exists that the primitive Moro reflex tends to reinforce oral and pharyngeal reflexes in children with cerebral palsy. The persisting Moro reflex is much less valuable to the neurologist as a sign of cerebral injury than is the ATNR.

In summary, persisting infantile primitive and postural reflexes have been a classic sign of CNS dysfunction. In particular, they have been extremely useful in the early diagnosis of cerebral palsy. Infantile reflex behavior also has been incorporated in motor treatment programs for children with cerebral palsy. An important fact for the SLP is that the primitive and postural body reflexes, with some exceptions, appear to have limited influence on oral and pharyngeal reflexes. Although these neonatal and early reflexes are important in assessing delayed development of motor function before age 12 to 18 months, they are of only limited use in the pediatric neurologic examination for the older child. The more conventional neurologic signs of altered muscle tone and abnormal muscle stretch and superficial reflexes, as well as the results of objective neurodiagnostic tests, are of equal value in making a diagnosis for the examining pediatric neurologist.

Oral and Pharyngeal Reflexes

Over the past half century, study of the normal infant reflexes and their relation to brain disease has promoted SLPs and others interested in the management of cerebral palsy to consider another set of reflexes—the oral and pharyngeal reflexes. Table 11.3 summarizes the major oral reflexes. Some speech specialists have assumed that abnormal oral and pharyngeal reflexes play a significant role in the speech development of the child with cerebral palsy who is dysarthric or is likely to develop dysarthria with the onset of speech. Absent or persisting reflexes, they argue, are predictive of dysarthria. Neurologists are more likely to argue that when the oral and pharyngeal reflexes are integrated into a spontaneous feeding pattern, they become more diagnostically and prognostically significant in neurologic disease. Similarly, SLPs are beginning to question whether the isolated artificially elicited reflexes of the first few months of life have as much diagnostic and prognostic importance in speech performance as do the dysphagic symptoms commonly seen in many children with cerebral palsy.

The type, number, and reliability of abnormal oral and pharyngeal reflexes found in those with cerebral palsy vary from study to study. Research strongly suggests that little or no correlation exists between the presence and number of abnormal oral and pharyngeal reflexes and the severity of dysarthria in cerebral palsy, as defined by a measure of articulation proficiency. In fact, the dysphagic symptoms—disordered biting, sucking, swallowing, and chewing—are slightly better predictors of articulation proficiency than is an elicited set of neonatal oral and pharyngeal automatisms. The correlation, however, between speech impairment and dysphagic symptoms is not particularly strong. This limited relation

TABLE 11.3	Infantile Oral Reflexes		
Reflex	**Stimulus**	**Age of Appearance**	**Age of Disappearance**
Rooting	Perioral face region is touched	Birth	3–6 mo
Suck	Nipple in mouth	Birth	6–12 mo
Swallowing	Bolus of food in pharynx	Birth	Persists
Tongue	Tongue or lips being touched	Birth	12–18 mo
Bite	Pressure on gums	Birth	9–12 mo
Gag	Tongue or pharynx being touched	Birth	Persists

between speech and dysphagia strongly implies that motor control for speech and the feeding reflexes may be mediated at different levels in the nervous system. Evidence indicates that the feeding reflexes are mediated at the brainstem level and that voluntary speech is controlled at the cortical, subcortical, and cerebellar levels, with the prime voluntary pathways for speech being the corticobulbar fibers. Brainstem reflex pathways apparently subserve only vegetative and reflex functions and are inactive during the execution of normal speech. Therefore, early motor speech gestures are probably not directly related to the development of motor reactions in feeding during infancy and childhood, even though some of the motor coordination and refinements in speech acquisition are analogous to some of the biting and chewing gestures in feeding.

Even though early oral motor behavior in feeding may only have a limited resemblance to actual motor patterns for speech, management programs to improve muscle function and coordination in eating have been initiated as a possible prophylactic measure for future dysarthria. The assumption of these programs is that any improvement in motor activity of the oral musculature gained through feeding therapy might conceivably result in improvement in speech performance because the parallel activities of speech and feeding have muscles in common. At the very least, feeding therapy is likely to make eating faster and easier. This, of course, is an important consideration in the total management of the child with a neurologically based disorder, one that should not be overlooked by SLPs and neurologists. Direct motor training of the muscles during speech, rather than feeding training, appears to be the most effective method for improving the dysarthria because cortically mediated speech activities drive the muscles at a more rapid and coordinated rate than do brainstem-mediated feeding activities.

Despite the controversy about oral reflexes and speech in diagnosis, management, and prognosis, a description of six commonly tested oral pharyngeal reflexes is offered for the SLP who wants to consider this aspect of disturbed oral motor functions in the cerebrally injured infant or child. In the typical infantile oral motor evaluation, eliciting each of these infantile automatisms artificially one by one is best to determine whether they are absent or abnormally persisting. Next, the spontaneous functions of mastication and deglutition in the feeding act should be assessed to determine how these neonatal reflex behaviors have become integrated into a more complex and voluntary oral-pharyngeal pattern of feeding. Infantile mastication and deglutition use the six cranial nerves (V, VII, IX, X, XI, XII) important for future speech, so evaluation of early feeding allows valuable cranial nerve assessment for the child who is too immature to cooperate in standard cranial nerve testing.

Rooting Reflex

If the perioral facial region is touched, two responses in combination make up the **rooting reflex**. The side-to-side head-turning reflex usually is elicited by gently tapping on the corners of the mouth or cheek. The response is the head

alternately turning toward and away from the stimulus, ending with the lips brushing the stimulus. Occasionally, the response occurs without the stimulus when the infant is hungry.

This activity usually precedes any actual suck. The side-to-side head-turning response is present in the term baby and premature infant. The reflex usually disappears by 1 month of age and is replaced by the direct head-turning response, a simple movement of the head toward the source of stimulation. The source is grasped with the lips and sucked. In the direct head-turning response, if the stimulus is applied to the corners of the mouth, the bottom lip usually lowers, and the head and tongue orient toward the stimulus. The direct head-turning response is established at 1 month and disappears by the end of the sixth month of life. Persistence beyond 1 year may suggest cerebral injury, and asymmetry of response indicates damage to one side of the brain or facial injury. The cranial nerves involved in the reflex are V, VII, XI, and XII. The reflex is mediated by the pons, medulla, and cervical spinal cord.

Suck Reflex

If a finger or nipple is placed in the infant's mouth, bursts of suck behavior occur interspersed with periods of rest. The **suck reflex** is integrated at birth but does not start until about week 32 of pregnancy, becoming fully integrated at around week 36. This accounts for the weak or immature sucking pattern often seen in premature infants. Babies also have a hand-to-mouth reflex, which often results in sucking on the hands or fingers. This may be seen in utero as well. In full-term infants, the sucking action develops more purpose within 2 or 3 months, and jaw activity is incorporated into the pattern. Involuntary suck may disappear between 6 months and 1 year. Persistent suck beyond gestational age of 1 year suggests brain injury. The reverse, the inability to suck, may also be an early sign of cerebral injury. The cranial nerves involved in sucking are V, VII, IX, and XII. The reflex is mediated at the pons and medulla.

Swallowing Reflex

The **swallowing reflex** develops after the suck reflex is integrated into a total feeding pattern. Suck activities produce saliva, which accumulates in the reflexogenic area of the pharynx. The swallowing reflex is triggered, and swallowing may be observed by visible upward movement of the hyoid bone and thyroid cartilage of the larynx. The upward movement of the thyroid cartilage of the larynx may also be palpated during the swallow. Separating suck and swallowing is sometimes difficult because a swallow may precede a suck or follow a first or second swallow. The act of deglutition involves muscles of the mouth, tongue, palate, and pharynx and depends on a highly coordinated movement pattern. Cranial nerves V, VII, IX, X, and XII are involved in the act of swallowing. An immature swallow with tongue thrusting is sometimes seen until approximately 18 months of age. A mature swallow is present afterward. The reflex is mediated at the level of the brainstem in the medullary reticular formation. Disturbances in swallowing are frequent manifestations of neurologic deficits in the infant and child, and they comprise the most important sign of neurologic disorder among the feeding reflexes.

Tongue Reflex

The **tongue reflex** may be considered part of a suckle-swallow reaction in which the tongue thrusts between the lips. If lips or tongue are touched, cranial nerve XII predominates. Excessive thrusts beyond 18 months are abnormal. This reflex is mediated at the medulla.

Bite Reflex

Moderate pressure on the gums elicits jaw closure and a bite response. The **bite reflex** is present at birth; in the normal infant it disappears by 9 to 12 months, when it is replaced by a more mature chewing pattern. The reflex may be exaggerated in the brain-injured child and may interfere with feeding and dental care. Its persistence inhibits the lateral jaw movements of chewing seen in the spontaneous mastication pattern. A weak response is seen with brainstem lesions, and corticobulbar lesions exaggerate the response. Cranial nerve V innervates the reflex, which is mediated at the low midbrain and pons.

Gag Reflex

A stimulus applied to the posterior half of the infant tongue or on the posterior wall of the pharynx causes rapid velopharyngeal closure. This primary action is accompanied by mouth opening, head extension, and depression of the floor of the mouth with elevation of the larynx and diaphragm. This **gag reflex** is present at birth and continues throughout life. The gag serves as a protective mechanism for the esophagus. Brain-damaged children often show a hyperactive gag. In the severely motor-involved child, the gag may be difficult to elicit. In the ataxic child, the gag is sometimes hypoactive. Cranial nerves IX and X innervate the gag, and the reflex is mediated at the level of the pons and medulla.

SYNOPSIS OF CLINICAL INFORMATION AND APPLICATIONS FOR THE SLP

- During the second week after conception, the embryonic disk embeds in the uterus; it is referred to as the embryo from the third to the eighth week and beginning at the ninth week is called the fetus.
- During embryologic development of the brain, the ectoderm becomes the epidermis and nervous system.
- During embryologic development of the brain, the mesoderm becomes the muscles, connective tissues, cartilage, bone, and blood vessels.
- During embryologic development of the brain, the endoderm becomes the linings of digestive and respiratory tracts.
- The ectoderm thickens and forms a neural plate that gives rise to the CNS.
- Neural folds fuse to form the neural tube, which separates from the ectoderm.
- Four zones are briefly formed within the lining of the neural tube. Important adult derivatives will develop from these zones.
- The neural tube closes by the fourth week, regulated by a process called neurulation.
- The neural crest is formed from the sides of the neural tube to eventually form parts of the peripheral and autonomic nervous systems, including spinal nerves, cranial nerves, Schwann cells, and cells that form the meninges of the brain and spinal cord.
- The neural folds expand and fuse to form the three primary vesicles: rhombencephalon, mesencephalon, and prosencephalon. Further divisions take place with the exception of the mesencephalon.
- At 20 weeks of gestation, the brain begins to convolute from a smooth surface.
- At 24 weeks of gestation, the gyri and sulci are formed.
- The neural crest and mesoderm are primitive meninges.
- Cortical neuroprogenitor cells replicate their DNA and divide in the ventricles and migrate in an inside-out pattern to various parts of the pial surface of the neocortex; this migration results in the stratification of the cortex.
- The two primary means of neural migration are somal translocation and guidance along the processes of radial glia.
- Young neurons send out an axon with a growth cone on the tip. Dendritic processes also extend from the neurons. The axon's growth cones are guided by tropic molecules to particular targets, synapsing on spines of dendrites, establishing early cortical networks.
- Teratology is the study of abnormal embryonic development.
- Teratogens are environmental agents or conditions that may induce developmental interruptions after exposure to the mother.
- Genetic factors affecting development include chromosomal abnormalities.
- Environmental teratogens may include drugs, infections, medications, and chemicals.
- The most critical period for growth of a particular organ is the period of most rapid cell division; critical periods vary depending on the organ.
- The critical period for brain development is from 3 to 16 weeks of gestation.
- Major problems may occur during the third or fourth week as the neural tube and neural crest form.
- Major infantile reflexes in the developing child are the grasp reflex, asymmetric tonic neck reflex, symmetric tonic neck reflex, stepping reflex, tonic labyrinthine reflex, segmental rolling reflex, Galant reflex, and the Moro reflex. The four most frequently assessed in a pediatric well-child exam of the neonate are the grasp, stepping, asymmetric tonic neck, and Moro reflexes.
- Oral reflexes in the developing child that appear at birth include rooting, suck, swallowing, tongue, bite, and gag; the gag reflex persists throughout life, but the others usually disappear by 6 to 18 months of age.
- Swallowing is controlled by the integration of functions of central nerves V, VII, IX, X, and XII; it requires coordination but not in a form as intricate as speech.

REFERENCES

1. Brumbach, A., & Goffman, L. (2014). Interaction of language processing and motor skill in children with specific language impairment. *Journal of Speech, Language, and Hearing Research*, *57*(1), 158–171. https://www.ncbi.nlm.nih.gov/pmc/articles/PMC4004610/.

2. Corbin, J. G., Gaiano, N., Juliano, S. L., Poluch, S., Stancik, E., & Haydar, T. F. (2008). Regulation of neural progenitor cell development in the nervous system. *Journal of Neurochemistry*, *106*(6), 2272–2287.

3. Cooper, J. A. (2013). Cell biology in neuroscience: Mechanisms of cell migration in the nervous system. *Journal of Cell Biology*, *202*(5), 725–734.

4. Dewolf, A. H., Sylos Labini, F., Ivanenko, Y., & Lacquaniti, F. (2021). Development of locomotor-related movements in early infancy. *Frontiers in Cellular Neuroscience*, *14*, 623759. https://doi.org/10.3389/fncel.2020.623759.

5. Edmondson, J. C., & Hatten, M. E. (1987). Glial-guided neuron migration in vitro: A high-resolution time-lapse video microscopic study. *The Journal of Neuroscience*, *7*(6), 1928–1934.

6. Gilbert-Barness, E. (2010). Teratogenic causes of malformation. *Annals of Clinical and Laboratory Science*, *40*(2), 99–114.

7. Haines, D. E., & Mihailoff, G. A. (2018). *Fundamental neuroscience for basic and clinical applications* (5th ed.). Elsevier.

8. Nadarajah, B., Alifragis, P., Wong, R. O., & Parnavelas, J. G. (2003). Neural migration in the developing cerebral cortex: Observations based on real-time imaging. *Cerebral Cortex*, *13*(6), 607–611.

9. Preston, R. (2020). Musculoskeletal disorders. In D. H. Chestnut (Ed.), *Chestnut's obstetric anesthesia: Principles and practice* (6th ed., pp. 1139–1159). Elsevier.

10. Tantibanchachai, C. (2014). Teratogens. *Embryo Project Encyclopedia*. http://embryo.asu.edu/handle/10776/7510.

11. Tortori-Donati, P., Rossi, A., & Cama, A. (2000). Spinal dysraphism: A review of neuroradiological features with embryological correlations and proposal for a new classification. *Neuroradiology*, *42*(7), 471–491.

12. Wilson, P., & Stewart, J. (2020). Meningomyelocele (spina bifida). In R. M. Kliegman et al. (Eds.), *Nelson textbook of pediatrics*. (21st ed., pp 3409–3410). Elsevier.

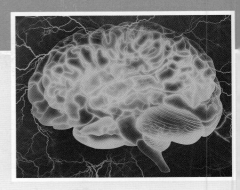

12

Pediatric Clinical Speech Syndromes

When I was born I was so surprised, I didn't talk for a year and a half.

Gracie Allen

KEY TERMS

anarthria
anoxia
ataxic cerebral palsy
athetoid cerebral palsy
cerebral palsy
childhood apraxia of speech (CAS)
deglutition

developmental dysarthria
developmental motor speech disorder
Duchenne dystrophy
jaw reflex
mastication
modified feeding

monoplegia
muscular dystrophy
prematurity
pseudohypertrophic
spastic cerebral palsy
topologic involvement
triplegia

RELATION OF REFLEXES, BRAIN DEVELOPMENT, AND SPEECH DEVELOPMENT

The development and progression of the reflexes presented in the preceding chapter help the speech-language pathologist (SLP) understand the way early speech and language development occurs in progression after reflexes are in place and as they mature. Once many of the reflexes are extinguished as the child's brain develops, pleasure sounds, cooing, babbling, and eventually phonemic development occur, as previously discussed. Neurolinguistic theory postulates that the developing brain ontogenetically allows the child to form the eventual sounds that comprise that individual's phonemic system. This is attributable to brainstem development and other relevant neurologic systems (central nervous system and peripheral nervous system).

Reflexes develop first, and a delayed or persistent reflex should trigger a red flag to the SLP that the development of phonemes may be interrupted and subsequently the morphemic and perhaps pragmatic systems for that child.

Assessing Mastication and Deglutition

In the infant or child at risk for neurologic injury, the clinical evaluation of neural control of the oral and pharyngeal activities involved in chewing and swallowing allows the SLP to estimate the motor potential of those muscles, which ultimately fall under the control of higher nervous centers devoted to the production of speech. The fact that speech and feeding are mediated at different levels within the nervous system implies that evaluation of chewing and swallowing predicts future muscle activity in speech in only a limited manner. Only gross estimates of muscle potential for speech can likely be derived from any nonspeech examination because of the semiautonomous control of the muscles for the dual function.

In addition to gross estimation of muscle function in mastication and deglutition, however, the infantile oral motor examination of the cranial nerves for speech permits the SLP and neurologist to observe signs of possible neurologic disorder that may not be readily apparent in other motor behaviors. **Mastication** and **deglutition**, as relatively complex motor behaviors in the repertoire of infant motor activity, are highly sensitive to neurologic dysfunction. Dysphagia may be an early and even sometimes isolated sign of brain injury. This kind of examination, being somewhat enjoyable to an infant or child (with the exception of those hypersensitive to oral touch), may be a way to begin to assess the child's motor control for speech if the child is uncooperative for more traditional speech evaluation techniques. SLPs are also becoming highly valued for their expertise in helping evaluate the child whose feeding/swallowing ability is questioned. We often can help rule out a neurologic disorder in a child who has sensitivity or behavioral issues manifested in problems with oral intake.

Modified Feeding

Examination of chewing and swallowing is best accomplished through the technique of **modified feeding**. In the preverbal child, this technique can replace the more traditional procedures of the adult speech cranial nerve test, which requires a level of maturity not yet developed in the infant and very young child. By selectively placing small morsels of solid food in different locations in the oral cavity of the child, an examiner can judge the integrity of the bulbar muscles and the brainstem neural pathways innervating these muscles. Healthy children from birth to 36 months respond well to the technique, which may also be used with motor-handicapped children with oral motor involvement well beyond 3 years of age. In the healthy child, spontaneous feeding emerges from the neonatal oral and pharyngeal reflexes and reaches its full maturity at approximately age 3 years. Experiences with solid foods provide a gradual refinement and integration of movements of the lips, tongue, palate, and pharynx for chewing and swallowing.

When testing the infant or motor-handicapped child without sitting balance, the child should be placed in a chair in which the body and head can be well supported (e.g., a tumble-form chair) or in the primary caregiver's or clinician's lap in a well-supported position. In the child with some sitting balance, placement in a relaxed sitting position with adequate head support is preferred. See Chapter 7 for a summary of the cranial nerves.

Cranial nerve VII. Placement of a small food bolus on the lower lip in midline and observation of the child's oral reaction to it provide evidence of the ability to use the muscles of the lip and lower face purposefully. Pursing the lips during rooting and sucking indicates intact facial movement. Lack of a smiling response may suggest severe bilateral facial muscle involvement. The healthy baby smiles to a human face at 2 to 4 months of age. A sober expression and sluggish grin must be carefully evaluated as possible neurologic signs of a bilateral corticobulbar system involvement ultimately affecting the paired nerves of cranial nerve VII. An asymmetric smile with a unilateral flattening of the nasal fold on one side of the face may be associated with unilateral paresis. This sign is not as obvious in the infant and young child as it is in the adult. Lack of lip tonicity may be present, and lip seal may not be maintained. In typically developing children, drooling typically disappears due to maturity of oral-motor control, thus many children with neurologic impairment may experience poor control of saliva with drooling well past age 2 years. This may result from poor lip seal or weakness/discoordination of other oral structures in the oral phase of swallowing or dysphagia due to difficulty in the oral and pharyngeal stage due to hyper- or hypotonicity, poor coordination, or difficulty with head and neck muscle control.

Cranial nerve XII. The child with cerebral injury often is unable to shape, point, and protrude the tongue in retrieving food from the lower lip by licking. The lack of tongue protrusion is common in both spastic and athetoid children. In the brain-injured infant, the tongue often will not cup, even during crying. Neither will the tongue thin, nor will the tip elevate with precision. This inability to produce any fine tongue movements suggests motor involvement of both the intrinsic and the extrinsic tongue musculature.

Unilateral or bilateral atrophy of the tongue may be seen in young children, and this loss of muscle bulk suggests lower motor neuron disease. However, fasciculations are rarely seen in the tongue muscles of infants.

Excessive tongue thrust, sometimes called the tongue reflex, is common in children with severe brain damage. It is particularly common in athetosis, and it may be associated with orthodontic problems and excessive drooling. In addition, occasional wavelike involuntary movements are seen in the body of the tongue, mimicking the involuntary movements of the limbs and trunk in extrapyramidal athetosis.

Cranial nerve V. When confronted with a small food bolus on the lips or tongue, the young child begins the total act of deglutition by initiating voluntary mastication. The aim of the evaluation at this point is to determine whether the bolus of food can be pulverized and whether the particles of food can be selectively manipulated to be transported to the back of the oral cavity. With a large food bolus, the tongue is usually elevated, so the bolus is placed between the tongue surface and the anterior hard palate and crushed. Smaller boluses of food are crushed between the hard palate and tongue, and the tongue directly begins a wavelike, peristaltic movement, carrying the food to the pharynx. If the food bolus is large, the tongue often acts in a whiplike fashion to propel the food laterally between the molars for grinding and pulverization. Observation of the vigorous tongue actions confirms the integrity of the neural control of the tongue. Disorders involving neurologic integrity of the tongue and jaw innervation often limit cerebrally damaged children to eating only diced or liquefied food.

Adequate biting and vigorous anterior-posterior movements of the mandible plus lateral grinding action of the jaws assure the SLP that cranial nerve V innervation is intact and that muscles innervated from the pons are functional. On the other hand, an exaggerated and too-powerful bite may be a manifestation of an abnormal **jaw reflex** (also known as the masseter reflex), suggesting an upper motor neuron lesion above the level of the pons. In older children with brain damage, a firm tap on the lower jaw may elicit a clonus, suggesting a hyperactive jaw reflex. If the lower jaw deviates to one side on opening or during mastication, pterygoid muscle weakness may be present on the side of deviation. In athetosis the jaw may become a major articulator, producing the motor power for elevating a poorly controlled tongue in achieving tongue tip-alveolar ridge contact and other tongue-elevation gestures.

Integration of cranial nerves V, VII, IX, X, and XII. When the food bolus is well masticated, the final involuntary stage of deglutition is initiated. The nasopharynx is closed by the muscles of the soft palate and the pharyngeal constrictors. Cranial nerves IX and X produce this closure. Saliva or the food bolus is pushed through the palatal fauces into the pharynx and onto the esophagus in a peristaltic wave. Muscles of the soft palate, the pharyngeal constrictors, and muscles of the tongue and larynx work in intricate coordination to propel the food bolus to the esophagus. In one sense, swallowing becomes the ultimate integration of the nervous mechanisms to be used later in motor expression of speech.

Speech, however, requires more intricate coordination of muscles than chewing and swallowing. This fine coordination is accomplished through increasing cortical and cerebellar control of the pontine and bulbar muscles. Certain other complex motor adjustments are seen in speech but are not seen in chewing or swallowing. As an example, the grooved fricative /s/ requires finer motor control than is seen in mastication. To produce an adequate /s/, a central groove in the tip and blade of the tongue must be formed, with the sides of the tongue firmly anchored between the lateral dentition. This specific tongue configuration, common to speech, is not seen in brainstem-mediated functions. Intricate coordination of intrinsic and extrinsic tongue muscles is needed for the grooved fricatives. These fine motor configurations are not present in feeding. Thus, assessment of mastication and deglutition in a preverbal child suspected of neurologic impairment is most appropriate, but when speech emerges, the evaluation should be based on the motor control for phonemes, syllables, words, and sentences assessed in the traditional articulation test format and on the results of a standard oral examination that includes assessment of the speech cranial nerves (see Chapter 7).

The actions of the cranial nerves for speech and the corticobulbar system, which activate the cranial nerve nuclei, can be assessed in infancy through observation of chewing and swallowing. All the nervous action of the bulbar muscles is integrated into the single act of feeding in infancy.

Motor Speech Disorders in Pediatric Populations

Alteration or interruption to development of the motor control areas and pathways in utero or early cerebral injury to speech mechanisms of the developing brain results in conditions classified as motor speech disorders. Included in a classification of the motor speech disorders are the dysarthrias, anarthria, and childhood apraxia of speech. Dysarthria in the pediatric population is a speech disorder resulting from damage to the immature nervous system; it is characterized by weakness, paralysis, and/or incoordination of the speech musculature. **Anarthria** refers to a complete lack of speech as a result of profound paralysis, weakness, and/or incoordination of the speech musculature. The diagnosis usually implies that useful speech will not develop because of the severity of the oral motor involvement. **Childhood apraxia of speech (CAS)** is an impaired ability to execute the appropriate movements of speech voluntarily in the absence of paralysis, weakness, and incoordination of the speech muscles. CAS is sometimes referred to as developmental apraxia of speech or verbal dyspraxia, but that may be misleading because children with correctly identified CAS will not outgrow the speech impairment without treatment as "developmental" may imply.[1]

Dysarthria in regard to children implies a neurologic or neurogenic speech deficit caused by a dysfunction of the motor control centers of the developing central and/or peripheral nervous systems. Disturbances are in the areas of strength, speed, steadiness, coordination, precision, tone, and range of motion or movement in the speech muscles. Apraxia is considered a motor planning disorder of speech, whereas dysarthria is associated with a partial disturbance of the speech mechanism involving motor movements. Anarthria usually is associated with a total lack of speech as a result of severe to profound motor disturbances.

Certain types of pediatric dysarthrias have been well studied; other types have received less attention in the speech pathology literature. The dysarthrias found in the various forms of cerebral palsy, for instance, have been extensively studied for many years, whereas research on the dysarthrias of childhood muscular dystrophy is much less common. The speech signs commonly observed in the dysarthrias are reviewed in Table 12.1.

TABLE 12.1 **Dysarthrias of Cerebral Palsy**	
Disorder	**Speech Signs**
Spastic dysarthria	Bilateral corticobulbar involvement; dysphagia; articulation disorder; hypernasality; slowed rate; loudness, pitch, and vocal quality disturbances; slow, stiff, and abrupt movements; increased muscle tone; muscle rigidity
Dyskinetic dysarthria	Athetosis (usually); dysphagia; hypernasality; articulation disorders; prevocalizations; loudness, pitch, and vocal quality disturbances; involuntary and often uncontrolled movements; often slow and writhing movements
Ataxic dysarthria	Articulation and prosodic disorders; unequal stress, loudness, and pitch; speech has an explosive, scanning quality
Mixed dysarthria	Often a combination of spastic and dyskinetic dysarthrias

Table 12.2 shows the major differences between dysarthria and apraxia from the point of muscle movements and range of motion as seen in many childhood motor disturbances such as cerebral palsy.

Cerebral Palsy

Dysarthria is most commonly seen in children diagnosed as having **cerebral palsy**, a neurologic condition caused by injury to the immature brain and characterized by a nonprogressive disturbance of the motor system. Many associated problems often are seen, such as intellectual disability, hearing and visual impairments, and perceptual problems produced by the infantile cerebral injury. Cerebral palsy is considered a major developmental disability with incidence being roughly two to three persons per 1000 live births. Prevalence data from the National Health Interview Study of the years 2015 to 2017 found a prevalence of 0.3%.[7]

Cerebral palsy has been variously classified, but most experts currently accept three major categories of clinical motor disorders: spasticity, dyskinesia, and ataxia. By far, the most common type of dyskinesia is athetosis.

Table 12.3 presents a classification of the forms of cerebral palsy. As in adult disorders, spasticity implies a lesion in the pyramidal system, dyskinesia implies a lesion in the basal ganglia, and ataxia denotes a lesion in the cerebellar system. However, syndromes are often not as clear-cut in the child as they are in the adult. Many children with cerebral palsy show a mixed picture. For instance, a child whose clinical picture is primarily dyskinetic, with typical slow, writhing movements of the limbs, grimaces of the face, and involuntary movements of the tongue and muscles of respiration, may also display hypertonic muscles and the upturning toe of the classic Babinski sign. The structural closeness of the neural pathways in the relatively small infant brain no doubt produces such mixed clinical pictures.

TABLE 12.2 Differences between Apraxia and Dysarthria

Apraxia	Dysarthria
Sound substitutions not on the target sound	Sound distortions usually related to the target sound
Inconsistent errors; motor planning	Inconsistent speech sound substitutions from coordination problems
Often vocal or nonvocal groping behaviors	Groping for sound production precision is not noted verbally or nonverbally
Motor planning and execution difficulties	Motor disturbances causing distortions and not planning difficulties

TABLE 12.3 Classification of Cerebral Palsy

Type/Lesion Area	Function	Subdivisions	Clinical Signs	Limb Involvement
Spastic Pyramidal tract	Skilled movements of limbs and digits Innervation of motor neurons for flexor movements of the limbs	Corticospinal tract Corticobulbar tract	Interrupts motor information of the brainstem and spinal cord Weakness or paralysis of various muscles	Paraplegia (lower extremities vs. upper extremities), diplegia (lower extremities more than upper extremities)
			Upper motor neuron lesions	Quadriplegia (lower and upper extremities); hemiparesis (left or right side of body) or monoplegia (only one lower extremity)
Dyskinetic Basal ganglia	Refer to Table 2.1 for the basal ganglia system Related to motor speech functioning Automatic execution of learned motor movements	Preferred term is basal ganglia-related pathways and subcortical nuclei	Either akinesia or lack of movements or dyskinesia or involuntary excessive movements; breathiness, roughness, hoarseness, tremor; exaggerated jaw movements; lip retrusion	Upper extremity, lower extremity, neck, and trunk involvement
Ataxic Cerebellum	Coordination of movements of the upper and lower extremities as well as at all stages of speech production; sensory input from larynx and articulators and speech processing	Inferior peduncle Middle peduncle Superior peduncle	Ataxia Sometimes diplegia	Upper extremities Lower extremities Trunk

Children with cerebral palsy may also be classified according to **topologic involvement**. Common topologic pictures are hemiplegia, diplegia, and quadriplegia (see Table 12.3). **Monoplegia**, **triplegia**, and paraplegia occasionally are seen. Children may also be classified by etiology. Common causes are **prematurity**, **anoxia**, kernicterus, birth trauma, and infection. Approximately 1 to 2 of every 1000 schoolchildren have some form of cerebral palsy. Of the three major types, spasticity is the most prevalent, dyskinetic is next, and ataxia is the least common.[34] Box 12.1 summarizes the major causes of cerebral palsy in children.

Dysarthria is a major problem in the population and effects functional communication in over 50% of children with cerebral palsy.[33] Dysarthria may be complicated in some children by intellectual disability, hearing loss, and perceptual disorders. Despite complicating factors, the two major dysarthrias—spastic dysarthria and dyskinetic dysarthria of athetosis—in cerebral palsy can be differentiated. Spasticity and athetosis cannot be identified by articulatory errors alone; however, when vocal and prosodic features are incorporated into perceptual judgments of speech, the two clinical types become distinct, just as spastic and hyperkinetic types are distinct among adult dysarthrias.[17]

Spastic Cerebral Palsy

Spastic cerebral palsy is characterized by hypertonic reflexes. With this type of reflex, when a muscle contracts, the opposing muscle stretches abnormally, thus excessively increasing muscle tone. That muscle group becomes rigid; movement

---

BOX 12.1   Causes of Cerebral Palsy

Prenatal brain damage may result from:
- Impaired migration of new brain cells with the following risk factors:
  - Maternal infection (e.g., cytomegalovirus, HIV, meningitis, toxoplasmosis, rubella)
  - Toxins
  - Drugs
  - Radiation exposure
- Prematurity and low birthweight with the following risk factors:
  - Low-grade infection of mother's urinary-genital tract
  - Alcohol and drug abuse, cigarette smoking
  - Poor maternal nutrition
  - Multiple fetuses
- Trauma to mother

Perinatal brain damage may result from:
- Increased pressure on brain during delivery
- Impaired circulation to the fetal brain
- Poor respiration
- Low birthweight

Postnatal brain damage may result from:
- Physical trauma
- Infection
- Respiratory distress
- Cerebrovascular disorders

---

therefore becomes extremely difficult. These muscle movements have been described in the literature as laborious, jerky, and unusually slow. These children often exhibit infantile patterns of the rooting reflex that involve the tongue, lips, and mandible.

Spastic hemiplegia usually is caused by damage to the corticospinal tract, with the possibility of corticobulbar involvement. Cranial nerve XII, the hypoglossal nerve, usually is also involved, with the tongue showing contralateral deviation from the affected side on protrusion. Dysarthric speech and dysphagia may resolve after a brief period, but phonologic development is often delayed, and language and cognitive disturbances may also accompany.

Spastic diplegia usually involves all four extremities, but the lower extremities display more involvement than the upper extremities, differentiating it from quadriplegia. Marked hypertonicity with flexion and extreme adduction of the hips in diplegia often results in scissoring or crossing of the legs during walking, producing a scissors gait, a widely known clinical sign of child spasticity. These children sometimes also display toe walking because of hamstring and Achilles tendon involvement. Children with diplegia often display mild dysarthria with articulatory involvement only, but others with more severe dysarthric signs often display respiratory, laryngeal, palatal, and pharyngeal impairments in addition to articulation problems. Some dysphagia and drooling may also be present.

Spastic quadriplegia usually displays equal involvement of both upper and lower extremities with severe involvement of the legs and arms and floppiness of the neck. In this condition both the corticospinal and corticobulbar tracts are affected. These children also display major problems with respiration, articulation, and laryngeal movements as well as compromised palatal and pharyngeal musculature. This type of spastic cerebral palsy usually has the highest incidence of intellectual disability or developmental delay.

Dyskinetic Cerebral Palsy

The most common of the dyskinetic syndromes of cerebral palsy is **athetoid cerebral palsy**. It is much less common than spastic cerebral palsy. Love[29] reported that ~5% of the total cerebral palsy population of children would be considered "pure" athetoid, whereas 10% would be diagnosed as dystonic athetosis.

Slower motor development and hypotonia are the first signs of motor difficulties in athetoid children. Sitting balance is either delayed or not developed at all. One of the most prevalent signs is the absence of the Moro and the tonic neck reflexes.

In certain cases hypertonic athetosis progresses to a mixed type, usually spastic athetoid. In general, all four limbs are involved; a different presentation is rare. Speech problems usually are present along with swallowing difficulties and drooling. Severely affected motor movements of the upper and lower extremities usually correlate to the severity of the speech disorder present.

Ataxic Cerebral Palsy

Love[29] reported that **ataxic cerebral palsy** is the most uncommon of the cerebral palsy syndromes. Dyssynergia that translates into incoordination of the upper and lower extremities typically is present. The most identifying sign is a staggering, somewhat lurching wide gait pattern. Muscles are hypotonic, and gait does not seem to have directional control. Ataxic cerebral palsy usually involves damage to the cerebellum. The feedforward motor commands initiated by the cerebellum may be interrupted or poorly sequenced causing the increased reliance on sensory feedback for speaking. This delay in motor processing may result in slowed speech with abnormal pauses and disruptions in speech rhythm.[37]

Table 12.4 summarizes the major differences among spastic, athetoid, and ataxic cerebral palsy, including characteristics and areas of damage to the brain.

Worster-Drought Syndrome or Congenital Suprabulbar Paresis

This disorder is a rare type of cerebral palsy resulting in an isolated paresis or weakness of the oral musculature, often without major motor signs in the trunk or extremities. Described by neurologist Worster-Drought, this condition usually affects the corticobulbar fibers that innervate cranial nerves X (vagus) and XII (hypoglossus).[18] The muscles of the lips, pharynx, palate, and tongue are involved to varying degrees with dysarthria marked by misarticulations and hypernasality. The individual may have a history of dysphagia, and drooling and laryngeal involvement are occasionally seen.

Muscular Dystrophy

Next to cerebral palsy, **muscular dystrophy** is the childhood neurologic disorder most likely to present a dysarthria. The most common type of muscular dystrophy is the pseudohypertrophic type, also called **Duchenne dystrophy**, which is associated with a sex-linked recessive gene, occurs primarily in males, and usually is manifest by the third year of life. During early development, motor milestones are often delayed, and a retrospective study using parent report found that language milestones were also frequently delayed.[14] These early delays in language milestones were found to be associated with later cognitive impairments. Duchenne muscular dystrophy is marked by a characteristic progression of muscle weakness starting in the pelvis and trunk and eventually involving all the striated muscles, including those of the speech mechanism. The visceral muscles usually are spared. Enlargement of the calf muscles and occasionally other muscle groups accounts for the term **pseudohypertrophic**. Infiltration of fat and connective tissue produces the pseudohypertrophic effect.

In the later stages of the disease a flaccid dysarthria may appear, marked by articulation disorder and voice quality disturbances. Often, the articulation disorder is mild, with only one or two phonemes in error. Dystrophic patients show reduced oral breath pressure and vocal intensity. They do not sustain phonation as well as healthy children do, and they show serious involvement of the muscles of speech. Rate of tongue movement and strength of the tongue are poor. Retracting and pursing the lips as well as pointing and narrowing the tongue are noticeably disordered actions, and phonemes requiring tongue and lip elevation often are in error. A broadening and flattening of the tongue is sometimes seen in advanced cases. Respiratory and laryngeal muscles are also weakened, affecting respiratory and phonatory performance. Despite weakness, labial phonemes generally are produced more accurately than are tongue-tip consonants. Box 12.2 presents the speech and physical signs in the **developmental dysarthria** of pseudohypertrophic muscular dystrophy.

TABLE 12.4 Differences among Spastic, Athetoid, and Ataxic Cerebral Palsy

Type	Characteristics	Damage Area(s)
Spastic	Spasticity: hypertonic Rigidity Stretch reflex Slow movements; laborious Presence of infantile reflexes	Pyramidal tract
Athetoid	Involuntary writhing movements	Extrapyramidal tract
	Uncoordinated volitional movements	Basal ganglia tracts
Ataxic	Poor balance	Cerebellum
	Poor direction control in gait	
	Rate dysfunction in gait	

Adapted from Owens, R. E., Metz, D. E., & Haas, A. (2003). *Introduction to communication disorders: A lifespan perspective* (2nd ed.). Allyn and Bacon.

BOX 12.2 Developmental Dysarthria in Pseudohypertrophic Muscular Dystrophy

Speech Signs (Flaccid Dysarthria)
Articulation disorder
Reduced vocal intensity
Respiratory weakness
Articulator weakness
Broad, flattened tongue

Physical Signs
Onset: 3–4 yr
Proximal weakness
Pseudohypertrophic calf muscles
Proximal atrophy
Hyporeflexia, except ankles
Intellectual disability (one-third of cases)

CHILDHOOD APRAXIA OF SPEECH

The following definition of CAS was adopted by the American Speech-Language-Hearing Association (ASHA) in 2007[1]:

CAS is a neurologic childhood (pediatric) speech sound disorder in which the precision and consistency of movements underlying speech are impaired in the absence of neuromuscular deficits (e.g., abnormal reflexes, abnormal tone). CAS may occur as a result of known neurologic impairment, in association with complex neurobehavioral disorders of known or unknown origin, or as an idiopathic neurogenic speech sound disorder. The core impairment in planning and/or programming spatiotemporal parameters of movement sequences results in errors in speech sound production and prosody.

It has been difficult to establish incidence and prevalence of CAS because we do not as yet have clear diagnostic criteria nor do we have adequate standardized test procedures for establishing its presence.[30] Data gleaned by SLPs' review of reports of over 12,000 children referred for speech disorders in a large metropolitan area estimated 3.4% to 4.3% of the children referred were given a diagnosis of CAS.[15] Given the known comorbidities in children with CAS, it is likely that the higher incidence estimate is closer to the true number of children with CAS.

Pathophysiology

This **developmental motor speech disorder** can be congenital or acquired; it occurs in children with known neurologic etiologies such as intrauterine stroke, infections, or trauma and may occur as part of a complex neurobehavioral disorder such as those caused by genetic or metabolic disorders. Because comorbidities frequently accompany CAS, it is often difficult to separate from the other disorders present. Idiopathic cases in which no associated neurologic disorder or injury can be easily identified are not uncommon, however.

The *FOXP2* Gene

A genetic basis for CAS has been investigated with particular emphasis on the study of the KE family in London. Research on 30 members of four generations of this family found that almost half the members of the family had a significant communication impairment.[24] The disorder was first presented as a grammar-specific disorder, but more in-depth research later revealed a severe articulatory deficit (thought to be apraxia of speech) as well as deficits in other linguistic areas and, in some members, intellect.[42] Orofacial apraxia was also found in some members. Genetic studies of this family pointed to mutations in the *FOXP2* gene on chromosome 7. There are other studies of children and family members with a speech sound disorder diagnosed in some members as CAS where a syndrome was also present in which a gene mutation on another chromosome was identified. Research on children with galactosemia, a metabolic disorder affecting the body's processing of sugar, found an incidence of CAS in 63% of the 24 cases studied.[39]

Genetic alteration of the *FOXP2* gene either through disruption during development or through copy or structural variants has since been linked to a number of speech-language disorders. CAS is known to be the core phenotype of a *FOXP2*-related speech-language disorder.[31] The type of alteration will determine whether the disorder will involve only speech and language or more global developmental and/or behavioral disorders will accompany it. Genomic sequencing studies using large cohorts of affected individuals with speech-language disorders have lagged behind the study of other disorders due in part to the lack of consistency in diagnosis and in clinical practice, particularly in language disorders but also in speech disorders such as CAS.[16]

Neuroimaging Studies

Despite progress, neither the etiology nor the neurophysiology of CAS has been confirmed. However, the advent of better access to safe neuroimaging studies as well as the use of event-related potentials has provided some interesting insight into neurophysiology. Liégeois et al.,[27] used functional magnetic resonance imaging (fMRI) to study the affected and unaffected members of the KE family. Tasks used were repetition and covert and overt verb generation. Imaging found more posterior and extensively bilateral activation in all generation tasks. In trying to ascertain differences in brain structure related specifically to CAS, however, the studies of the KE family members were confounded by the presence of linguistic and cognitive deficits in many of the affected members.

Kadis et al.,[26] analyzed cortical thickness from MRI for seven regions of interest in 14 children identified with idiopathic CAS who were receiving speech therapy for the disorder and age-matched control subjects. The only consistent difference in gray matter volume was found in the left supramarginal gyrus. No significant differences were found for the typical motor-speech programming areas nor for the superior temporal gyrus, which is an area found to show differences in gray matter volume bilaterally in children with speech sound disorders not related to CAS.[2]

Yet another neurophysiologic approach was taken by a group at Haskins Laboratory.[36] This study involved children with CAS and a matched control group performing a picture-naming task. The pictures were varied by complexity of structure with monosyllabic and multisyllabic words used. Evoked-related potentials were recorded while the children performed these naming tasks. Group differences were found that the authors hypothesize supported both prespeech phonologic processing and motor planning. The subjects with CAS showed reduced amplitude over the right hemisphere before speaking multisyllabic words compared with monosyllabic words. The time window of this reduction was thought to be consistent with phonologic encoding. The group with CAS also was found to show a later time onset of movement both in the stimulus locked and response locked conditions, regardless of the complexity of the stimulus. This suggested differences in phonetic processing (motor planning/programming). As the authors point out, this study is primarily descriptive. It does lend support to what clinicians have always suspected—that neurobiologic differences do exist in children with CAS; clinically, they appear to physiologically require a longer time to prepare for speech production.

Fiori et al.,[20] used a connectome analysis approach to their research on neuroanatomic correlates of CAS, hypothesizing that altered structural connectivity in white matter inter- and intrahemispheric pathways would be found in children with CAS when compared with typically developing children. Using diffusion tensor imaging, fractional anisotrophy measures were used to compare connectivity patterns of 17 children with idiopathic CAS with 10 age-matched typically developing controls. Recall from Chapter 3 that fractional anisotrophy (FA) is one of the factors considered in studying the white matter tracts of the brain and is a measure of the variability in directionality of fibers in white matter tracts. Following the determination of the FA for each subject studied, the relationship between FA and scores on speech and language measures was then investigated. The researchers hypothesized that reduced FA in areas involved in speech and language would be found in children with CAS, implying impairment in the microstructure of white matter tracts in the brain. The statistical approach used for analysis would allow for identification of clusters or subnetworks. The microscopically altered white matter identified by reduced FA was, as expected, found in children with CAS but not in the 10 control subjects. Three subnetworks with altered FA were identified and consistent with previous research,[26] two components were intrahemispheric but in both hemispheres, and one component was interhemispheric. The three subnetwork areas with reduced FA were (1) intrahemispheric connections between seven nodes in the left hemisphere, including connections of frontotemporal regions and postcentral gyrus; (2) intra- and interhemispheric connections between eight nodes, including intrahemispheric connections between left middle frontal gyrus and right parietal and occipital gyrus (also including interhemispheric connections between the left occipital gyrus and right cerebellum and interhemispheric connections between the right supplementary motor area and left frontal gyrus); and (3) two right intrahemispheric connections between three nodes, including connections between the angular gyrus, superior temporal gyrus, and inferior occipital gyrus. Once the reduced FA was identified, data from the speech-language assessments were studied for any relationship or correlation. The speech-language assessment done on each child included parental report on medical and early vocal behavior history and speech-language developmental milestones, evaluation of verbal and nonverbal oral-motor skills, phonetic inventory, presence and consistency of phonologic errors, expressive grammar, and receptive/expressive vocabulary. Analysis of the correlation between the measures of FA of all the significant connections and clinical testing scores found significant correlations in a number of connections. In subnetwork 1, low FA in connections involving the superior frontal and middle temporal correlated with low performance in oral-motor skills. A correlation between low FA in the inferior frontal and middle temporal gyrus connections and slow diadochokinessis, poor expressive grammar, and poor lexical production was found to be significant. For subnetwork 2, low FA for the interhemispheric connection between the right superior occipital gyrus and the left precuneus correlated with slow diadochokinetic rate. No significant correlations were supported for the low FA in subnetwork 3 connections. Results of this investigation add support to previous studies on neuroanatomic correlates for CAS. They note previous studies also suggesting the likelihood of a bihemispheric involvement in CAS and the fairly consistent finding that the superior and middle temporal gyri are important for phonemic discrimination. The indictment of the cerebellum and inferior frontal gyrus connections is also in keeping with previous evidence from neuroanatomic studies on speech disorders.

Future Directions

The possibilities for further exploration to identify the developmental and neuroanatomic differences found in children with CAS and to extend that knowledge to better assessment and treatment methodology look promising. The advent of better neuroimaging technology and significant advancements in research in genetics have resulted in renewed interest and dedication to early identification and early treatment of many childhood speech-language disorders, including apraxia of speech.

Assessment and Treatment

The disordered movements of the articulators in CAS frequently result in a serious phonologic problem in the school-age child. If an apraxic disorder of the oral muscles is present in the preschool years, it may well delay the development of speech and language, and the language developmental milestones of one-word utterances, two-word combinations, and three-word sentences may be disrupted. Although a clear-cut syndrome has not yet emerged despite considerable clinical research on the topic, it is now a fairly well-accepted clinical diagnosis, though accurate assessment methodology with secure sensitivity and specificity has not yet been established.

The differential diagnosis of CAS has and continues to challenge the SLP. The treatment methods that may progress the child with CAS may differ significantly from the treatment methodology used with children with articulation disorders or phonologic disorders. It is important to try to diagnose a true case of CAS as early as possible so that targeted treatment methods can be begun. A number of studies have tried to identify characteristics that would differentiate speech apraxia from other speech production disorders. Checklists have also been formulated to help identify characteristics associated with CAS, and these have been used by many clinicians with varying success. The 2007 technical report by ASHA on CAS[1] reviewed the literature on behavioral markers for CAS available at that time, finding considerable variability in subjects used and overlap with markers often present in children with speech disorders but no oral-motor involvement. The two measures that appeared to show the most sensitivity were maximal performance for multisyllabic word production and prosody.

Strand et al.,[41] targeted the even more difficult problem of identifying motor speech impairment in younger children or in children with little verbal ability. The DEMSS (Dynamic Evaluation of Motor Speech Skill) was supported as a reliable and valid test for this purpose with the probability of correct classification based only on the DEMSS total score being greater than 90%. The dynamic aspect of the test requires assessment of the child's ability to directly imitate simple phonetic content and syllable structure while cuing is provided. Vowel accuracy, total accuracy, prosody, and consistency are the measures taken for the total.

Despite increased interest in accurate diagnosis and effective treatment, research publications continue to lack rigorous standards and quality, with replication sadly lacking. A systematic review of research on differential diagnosis of CAS and other speech disorders failed to find any studies that met the American Academy of Neurology's criteria set for a Class 1 diagnostic article. Fifteen studies available at that time did provide contributions to diagnostic criteria that might be used by clinicians for best practice.[32]

In 2017, a series of careful investigations aimed at finding a single-sign behavioral marker of CAS resulted in technical reports and articles on the clinical utility of the pause marker for identification and differentiation of CAS.[39,40] The findings of this series showed good validity, sensitivity, and specificity when inappropriate pauses were identified in speaking samples using both perceptual tasks and acoustic instrumentation. However, this methodology has not been further elucidated for routine clinical use. Preston et al.,[35] caution against the notion of a single diagnostic task or assessment instrument at this point in time, noting that multiple aspects of speech production (e.g., voicing errors, lexical stress, syllable deletions) may be needed particularly to inform the clinician about the best path for treatment of a motor-based speech impairment.

Although new research has come forth regarding signs and symptoms of CAS, a review of the current literature suggests that the differentiating features listed in Box 12.3 continue to be the ones that have gained the most consensus. It remains the case, however, that the clinical research at this point in time on the signs and symptoms that would identify the presence of CAS in children under the age of 3 years is sorely lacking. This recommendation of ASHA regarding assessment of children under age 3 years in whom CAS is suspected should likely be adopted in clinical practice: "Until such resources are available, differential diagnosis of CAS in very young children and in the context of neurological and complex neurobehavioral disorders may require provisional diagnostic classifications, such as CAS cannot be ruled out, signs are consistent with CAS, or suspected to have CAS."[1]

BOX 12.3   Features of Speech Behavior that May Help Differentiate CAS from Other Disorders

- Inconsistent errors on consonants and vowels in repeated productions of syllables and words[a]
- Lengthened and disrupted coarticulatory transitions between sounds and syllables
- Inappropriate prosody, especially at the word and phrase level
- Poor accuracy of movements[b]
- Poor accuracy of vowel production
- Slow diadochokinetic rate[c]

[a]American Speech-Language-Hearing Association[1]
[b]Strand et al.[42]
[c]Murray et al.[32]

Treatment of CAS is beyond the scope of this text. New treatment methodologies are being studied and presented in the clinical literature of our profession on an accelerated basis. The astute clinician will carefully research this literature for evidence-based practice methods and will perhaps contribute to the literature from personal clinical research and practice.

In summary, CAS is still controversial. Many researchers do not agree on symptomatology, causes, assessment, treatment procedures, or even operational definition. Our evidence base is increasing, but further study into this disorder is needed before agreement is reached on how best to identify and treat it.

OTHER DISORDERS OF SPEECH PRODUCTION

Articulation and Phonologic Disorders

As children mature and develop from the basic oral reflex stage to more sound or articulatory development, some simply become delayed in phonologic and/or articulatory development without a neurologic motor speech component. Articulation disorders have their roots in the phonetic (sound) development that children progress through as their oral motor skills mature. These children currently are referred to as having phonologic processing disorders. Phonologic disorders have their basis in the study of phonology from a linguistic point of view. These children, now served in clinics, do not necessarily have a motor speech component that must be addressed either linguistically or neurolinguistically.

Salient differences exist between children with an articulation disorder and those with a phonologic disorder. Much is distinguished by phonetic versus phonemic errors. Phonetically, this child struggles with speech sound form and development, but phonemically the child displays problems with language-based functions of phonemes.[33] This becomes a matter of sound formation (articulation disorder) versus phonemic function (phonologic disorder). Because motor speech delay or impairment is not present, children with articulation disorders display disturbances in the neurologic processes of sound development, and children with phonologic disorders represent an impairment of the phonemic system within the language. Articulation disorders are phonetic in nature, whereas phonologic disorders are phonemic.[3]

Locke,[28] of the University of Sheffield in England, offers a theory of neurolinguistic development to explain how an infant develops from simply recognizing faces and voices to learning parents' or caregiver's voice characteristics. Locke explains "the first phase is indexical and affective" (p. 266), in which the infant is strongly oriented to a person's face and voice. The infant's second phase is "primarily affective and social . . . whereby its function is to collect utterances for social purposes" (p. 266) regulated by the right hemisphere. The third phase facilitates discovery and is ultimately responsible for the child's development of speech and language rule usage. The fourth and last phase is integrative in nature. This underlies Locke's idea that "children who are delayed in the second phase have too little stored utterance material to activate their analytic mechanism at the optimum (neurolinguistic) moment and when sufficient words are learned, the capability has already begun to decline" (p. 266). This could explain, from a neurolinguistic viewpoint, the delay in speech development in infants and young children. Finally, Locke suggested "the resulting neurolinguistic resources, not being specialized for phonological operations, are minimally adequate but not optimal for development of spoken language" (p. 266). Table 12.5 outlines Locke's system, including the neurolinguistic components of speech development and language capacity.

A delay in neurolinguistic development can lead to speech delays and phonologic disorders. Children develop through periodic phases, as described in Table 12.5, and if an interruption (e.g., cerebral palsy, muscular dystrophy) or delay (e.g., intellectual disability, autism) occurs, speech development would either be absent or significantly altered.

Disorders of Fluency

The World Health Organization defines stuttering as "speech that is characterized by the frequent repetitions or prolongations of sounds, syllables or words, or by frequent hesitations or pauses that disrupt the rhythmic flow of speech."[19] Many people who stutter also exhibit secondary symptoms such as facial grimaces, extremity movements, or eye blinks. Fluency disorders or stuttering has a prevalence of ~5% during early childhood.

Many children, however, recover spontaneously, leaving a prevalence across the general population of around 1%.[44]

The various theories about what causes disorders of fluency and how best to treat them in children who do not naturally develop fluent speech will be taught as you progress through your curriculum. Stuttering has been researched extensively by SLPs; there have always been questions about possible neurologic differences that could account for some or all of the symptomology, which, of course, can vary greatly between individuals. It is only recently that our field has had access to imaging and other techniques that can begin to answer that question. Neuroimaging studies are rapidly adding knowledge about brain structure and function in adults and children with fluency disorders. They suggest that subtle functional brain differences do exist, perhaps leading to the eventual discovery of a neurologic basis for stuttering.[38]

Findings from Neuroimaging Studies

Table 12.6 lists a few selected neuroimaging studies, all done on adults, and briefly summarizes the findings. As you will see, the findings vary. A limitation of most studies on adult stutterers is that it is difficult to ascertain whether the brain activity or connections discovered are related to the etiology of the disorder or are related to compensatory mechanisms that the person has developed to deal with the disfluencies. Few studies have been done on children, and there is a critical need for this type of research to pinpoint the etiology of developmental stuttering and, perhaps one day, successfully treat it early enough to prevent persistence into adulthood. There have been a few studies on school-age children and adolescents that do support anatomic differences in basal ganglia structures,[10] the putamen,[4] and the caudate nucleus.[21] Finally, in the largest pediatric neuroimaging study of stuttering to that date, Chang et al.,[11] used FA to look at differences in white matter development in 3- to 10-year-olds (47 children who stutter [CWS] and 42 children with no stuttering [CWNS]). Lower FA values indicate poor organization of the white matter tracts in these areas with more crossing of bundles of fibers rather than coherent tracts to and from the connecting areas. It could also imply poor myelination of the fibers or poor integrity of the membranes of the cells. Studies of FA during the developmental periods of childhood and adolescence typically show increases related to development as well as to skill acquisition and training.

TABLE 12.5	**Phases and Processing Systems and Neurolinguistic Correlates**		
Age of Onset	Developmental Phases and Systems	Neurolinguistic and Neurocognitive Mechanisms	Linguistic Domain
0–3 mo	Vocal learning	Specializing in social understanding	Prosody and sound segment development
5–7 mo	Utterance acquisition	Specializing in social understanding	Stereotypic utterances
20–37 mo	Analysis and computational	Grammatical analysis skills	Phonology, morphology, and syntax
3+ yr	Integration and elaboration	Social understanding and grammatical analysis	Automatic operations and expanded lexicon and sound development

Modified from Locke, J. (1997). A theory of neurolinguistic development. *Brain and Language, 58*(2), 265–326.

TABLE 12.6   Selected Neuroimaging Studies on Adults Who Stutter

Author (Year)	Summary of Findings from Neuroimaging
Chang et al. (2009)[9]	Reduced activation during speech perception and planning in frontal and temporoparietal areas; increased activation during speech production in right superior temporal gyrus, bilateral Heschl gyrus, insula, bilateral precentral, supplemental motor area, and the putamen
Xuan et al. (2012)[43]	Study of brain activity during resting state: altered brain activity compared with controls in areas involved in motor, language, auditory, and cognitive processing; altered functional connections between areas as well
Ingham et al. (2012)[25]	Stuttering frequency across two tasks correlated with cortical-striatal-thalamic circuit activity; primarily highlights the variability found in functional imaging studies
Connally et al. (2013)[13]	Study of white matter tracts: reduced integrity in the three cerebellar peduncles as well as the left angular gyrus; greater connectivity in the corticobulbar tract

In this study using FA to look at stuttering, significant decreases in FA were found in CWS with the lowest values found in the left hemisphere white matter underlying large parts of the sensorimotor cortical regions (inferior frontal gyrus, premotor cortex, motor cortex, middle and superior temporal gyri, and inferior parietal areas). These areas are along the superior longitudinal fasciculus. Decreased FA in CWS was also noted in the left cerebellum and brainstem and the entire length of the corpus callosum. Though smaller than those in the left hemisphere, right-sided decreases were found in part of the inferior frontal gyrus (BA 44), the middle and superior temporal gyri, and the supramarginal gyrus. The authors posit that these lower FA values indicating white matter structural differences in CWS suggest "deficits in long-range connectivity that support efficient sensorimotor and interhemispheric integration and cortical-subcortical interaction for skilled movement control" (p. 704) and "underlie precise timing of movement" (p. 708).

External Timing Effect. As you will learn in your later study of treatment of stuttering, external timing aids (such as pacing techniques, metronome, etc.) often induce fluency in persons who stutter. Because of this, there has been interest in the neuroanatomic support for the brain's internal timing mechanisms as well as what parts of the brain may be most responsive to external timing cues. Etchell's[19] research on a group of adult stutterers suggested that internal timing differences account for disfluent speech and that the basal ganglia and supplementary motor connections are involved in this deficient timing. The involvement of the cerebellum and the right inferior frontal gyrus as well as the left premotor cortex was proposed by Etchell et al.,[19] as possible primary neural

structures that use external timing cues to provide compensation when there are internal timing deficits in the controlling neural network. Frankford et al.,[22] used fMRI to further study modulation of brain activation and connectivity patterns with external timing mechanisms ("overt isochronously pacing") used in a sentence reading task performed by both adults who stuttered (AWS) and adults who did not stutter (ANS). In designing this study researchers also sought to control for a previously ignored issue in studying the rhythm effect in stuttering: the fact that the pacing of speech slows the rate of speaking as well as overlaying a rhythm. It is also well known that slowing the speaking rate often improves fluency in people who stutter. Study design included a combination of training and analytic procedures to separate out the effects of rate on the findings of the study. Complex and detailed anatomic information on the findings, implications, and limitations of this study can be found in the article. The authors provided a general conclusion from the overall imaging and analysis of primary activation areas and connectivity patterns related to the effect of rhythmic timing overlay on fluency. They found, as has been demonstrated many times, that external pacing of speech significantly reduces the number of disfluencies and in some cases normalized speaking. In regard to activation and connectivity, they found the primary connectivity changes to be within the cerebellum and between the cerebellum and the prefrontal cortex; this study supports the previous findings that, with external timing, there occurs activation of compensatory timing systems and suggests possible modulation of feedback control and attentional systems within the brain circuitry.

Future Directions. As noted earlier, there is high interest in the use of neuroimaging techniques to identify brain differences and the evolution of these differences in children who develop onset of stuttering and who persist in stuttering often despite intervention. A primary site of exciting and careful research is the Speech Neurophysiology Lab at the University of Michigan (https://chang.lab.medicine.umich.edu/publications). Though certainly not the only research lab investigating stuttering, research from investigators here have contributed to the growing body of knowledge suggesting functional brain activity, connectivity, and structural differences in people who stutter. Research has found differences in gray matter volume variation, energy metabolism,[6] cortical thickness in specific regions, and white matter integrity of connections through the arcuate fasciculus and the corpus callosum,[12] gyrification,[23] cortico-basal ganglia-thalamo-cortical loop involvement in speech,[8] and genetic makeup.[5]

Many ways of seeing into the windows of the brains of adults and now children have been made available with the advances in neuroimaging techniques, making them less and less invasive. It is now up to the researchers and clinicians to continue to design studies that will help us learn more about which brain structures are responsible for promoting fluent speech and when and why they are most vulnerable to disruption. We may then be able to prevent developmental stuttering from occurring or at least treat it so that the disorder of fluency does not follow the child into adulthood.

SYNOPSIS OF CLINICAL INFORMATION AND APPLICATIONS FOR THE SLP

- Oral reflexes in the developing child that appear at birth include rooting, suckling, swallowing, tongue, bite, and gag; the gag reflex persists throughout life, but the others usually disappear by 6 to 18 months of age.
- Swallowing is controlled by the integration of functions of central nerves V, VII, IX, X, and XII; it requires coordination but not in a form as intricate as speech.
- Early cerebral injury of the speech mechanisms in the infant brain results in motor speech and/or swallowing disorders.
- The speech production disorders associated with brain injury include developmental dysarthria, anarthria, and apraxia of speech.
- Developmental dysarthria is characterized by weakness, paralysis, and incoordination of the speech musculature.
- Developmental anarthria is characterized by a lack of speech as a result of profound paralysis, weakness, or incoordination of the speech muscles.
- Dysarthria is characterized by a disturbance in the motor control centers of the developing brain.
- Disturbances include strength, speech, steadiness, coordination, precision, tone, and range of motion.
- Dysarthrias can be categorized as spastic, dyskinetic, ataxic, or mixed.
- Spastic dysarthria is characterized by bilateral corticobulbar involvement, increased muscle tone, slowed rate, and loudness.
- Dyskinetic dysarthria is characterized by athetosis, dysphagia, hypernasality, articulation disorder, and vocal quality disturbance.
- Ataxic dysarthria is characterized by unequal stress, articulation and prosodic disorder, disturbance of balance, and an awkward gait.
- Cerebral palsy can be subdivided into three major categories: spasticity, dyskinesia, and ataxia.
- Approximately 75% to 85% of children with cerebral palsy have dysarthria to some extent.
- Other complications of cerebral palsy include intellectual disability and hearing loss.
- Spastic cerebral palsy is characterized by hemiplegia, paraplegia, diplegia, and quadriplegia of upper and lower extremities.
- Athetoid cerebral palsy is the most common of the dyskinesias of cerebral palsy and is characterized by hypotonia and the absence of the Moro and tonic neck reflexes.
- Ataxic cerebral palsy is the most uncommon of all cerebral palsy syndromes and is characterized by disturbed balance, lurching gait, hypotonic muscles, and damage to the cerebellum.
- Next to cerebral palsy, muscular dystrophy is the most likely condition to display dysarthria. Flaccid dysarthria may appear with an articulation problem, reduced vocal intensity, respiratory weakness, and a broad and flattened tongue; one-third of the cases include intellectual disability.
- CAS is a disorder affecting the precision and consistency of movements underlying speech production.
- CAS can be related to a neurologic or neurobehavioral disorder but also may be idiopathic.
- Mutation of the *FOXP2* gene on chromosome 7 is thought to be associated with speech impairment similar to CAS. Other genetic mutations have been found to be a possible source as well.
- Neuroanatomic differences in children with idiopathic CAS are suspected and have been identified in a few studies. No consistent etiology has been identified. Poor feedforward control and differences in phonetic processing have been supported by research.
- Neurolinguistics is concerned with the underlying process of communication, including phonology, morphology, syntax, semantics, and pragmatics in regard to various aspects of brain function.
- Locke offers an explanation of the neurolinguistic components underlying speech-language development.
- Stuttering or disorder of fluency has a prevalence of ~5% in early childhood and ~1% in the general population.
- Neuroimaging studies have become more prevalent in the past few years in the study of adults and children with developmental stuttering. Studies suggest disorganized white matter connections underlying sensorimotor areas in the left hemisphere and less so in the right hemisphere. Differences in basal ganglia and supplementary motor area, cerebellar structures and processing loops, gray matter volume, and gyrification have been found, with deficits in internal timing mechanisms proposed.

CASE STUDY

H. T., a 10-year-old boy, was brought to the emergency department by his parents. H. T. was home alone with his younger sister after his parents went out with friends. After putting his sister to bed, H. T. found liquor bottles in the wet bar of the family room and some beer in the refrigerator. He consumed a fifth of vodka and two bottles of beer within 5 hours. His parents came home and found him passed out on the kitchen floor. They called 911, and H. T. was rushed to the hospital. His blood alcohol level was four times the legal limit set for an adult. The medical team revived him, and he was admitted to the hospital. A few hours later H. T. began to have several severe grand mal seizures. Seizure activity was intermittent for almost 6 hours. MRI was completed at this time. Several areas of diffuse damage appeared on the image, but the radiologist could not deter-

mine whether any particular parts of the CNS were affected. Imaging was ordered to be repeated. The next morning the house neurologist on call and the physical and speech therapists were summoned out of concern for the patient. H. T. was disoriented ×3 and had to be prompted to answer questions. Speech was slurred, with intermittent loudness and softness in voice output, reminding the staff of the drunken state he was in when brought to the emergency department. Physical therapy provided minimal assistance to have H. T. walk across the room. Gait was wide and unsteady. Both fine and gross motor skills were tremulous and unbalanced. Alternating motion rates were slow and deliberate, and H. T. often stopped and started again several times. Many phonemic errors were noted. Social Services was consulted, and history indicated that this has

continued

continued

happened several times before, but this was the first time that H. T. passed out and had seizures, according to the parents.

Questions for Consideration
1. The speech symptoms, gait, and other behaviors appear to be reminiscent of which type of dysarthria?
   Flaccid
   Ataxic
   Spastic
   Mixed
2. What primary area of the CNS do you think was affected in this child?
3. Will this damage resolve as in the past, or will it be more permanent this time?

REFERENCES

1. American Speech-Language-Hearing Association. (2007). Ad Hoc Committee on Childhood Apraxia of Speech. *ASHA*. http://www.asha.org/policy/PS2007-00277/.

2. American Speech-Language-Hearing Association. (n.d.). Childhood apraxia of speech (practice portal). *ASHA*. www.asha.org/Practice-Portal/Clinical-Topics/Childhood-Apraxia-of-Speech/.

3. Bauman-Waengler, J. (2004). *Articulatory and phonological impairments: A clinical focus*. Allyn and Bacon.

4. Beal, D. S., Gracco, V. L., Brettschneider J., Kroll, R. M., & De Nil, L. F. (2013). A voxel-based morphometry (VBM) analysis of regional grey and white matter volume abnormalities within the speech production network of children who stutter. *Cortex*, *49*(8), 2151–2161.

5. Benito-Aragón, C., Gonzalez-Sarmiento, R., Liddell, T., Diez, I., d'Oleire Uquillas, F., Ortiz-Terán, L., Bueichekú, E., Chow, H. M., Chang, S.-E., & Sepulcre, J. (2020). Neurofilament-lysosomal genetic intersections in the cortical network of stuttering. *Progress in Neurobiology*, *184*, 101718. https://doi.org/10.1016/j.pneurobio.2019.101718.

6. Boley, N., Patil, S., Garnett, E. O., Li, H., Chugani, D. C., Chang, S.-E., & Chow, H. M. (2021). Association between gray matter volume variations and energy utilization in the brain: Implications for developmental stuttering. *Journal of Speech, Language, and Hearing Research*, *64*(6S), 2317–2324. https://doi.org/10.1044/2020_JSLHR-20-00325.

7. Centers for Disease Control and Prevention. (2022). Data and statistics for cerebral palsy. *National Center on Birth Defects and Developmental Disabilities*. https://www.cdc.gov/ncbddd/cp/data.html.

8. Chang, S. E., & Guenther, F. H. (2020). Involvement of the cortico-basal ganglia-thalamo-cortical loop in developmental stuttering. *Frontiers in Psychology*, *10*. https://doi.org/10.3389/fpsyg.2019.03088.

9. Chang, S.-E., Kenney, M. K., Loucks, T. M. J., & Ludlow, C. L. (2009). Brain activation abnormalities during speech and non-speech in stuttering speakers. *NeuroImage*, *46*(1), 201–212.

10. Chang, S.-E., & Zhu, D. C. (2013). Neural network connectivity differences in children who stutter. *Brain*, *136* (Pt 12), 3709–3726.

11. Chang, S.-E., Zhu, D. C., Choo, A. L., & Angstadt, M. (2015). White matter neuroanatomical differences in young children who stutter. *Brain*, *138* (Pt 3), 694–711.

12. Chow, H. M., Garnett, E. O., Li, H., Etchell, A., Sepulcre, J., Drayna, D., Chugani, D., & Chang, S. E. (2020). Linking lysosomal enzyme targeting genes and energy metabolism with altered gray matter volume in children with persistent stuttering. *Neurobiology of Language*, *1*(3), 365–380. https://www.mitpressjournals.org/doi/full/10.1162/nol_a_00017.

13. Connally, E. L., Ward, D., Howell, P., & Watkins, K. E. (2014). Disrupted white matter in language and motor tracts in developmental stuttering. *Brain & Language*, *131*, 25–35.

14. Cyrulnik, S. E., Fee, R. J., De Vivo, D. C., Goldstein, E., & Hinton, V. J. (2007). Delayed developmental language milestones in children with Duchenne's muscular dystrophy. *Journal of Pediatrics*, *150*(5), 474–478.

15. Delaney, A. L., & Kent, R. D. (2004). Developmental profiles of children diagnosed with apraxia of speech. Philadelphia: Poster session presented at the annual convention of the American-Speech-Language-Hearing Association.

16. den Hoed, J., & Fisher, S. E. (2020). Genetic pathways involved in human speech disorders. *Current Opinion in Genetics & Development*, *65*, 103–111. https://doi.org/10.1016/j.gde.2020.05.012.

17. Eggink, H., Kremer, D., Brouwer, O. F., Contarino, M. F., van Egmond, M. E., Elema, A., Folmer, K., van Hoorn, J. F., van de Pol, L. A., Roelfsema, V., & Tijssen, M. A. J. (2017). Spasticity, dyskinesia and ataxia in cerebral palsy: Are we sure we can differentiate them? *European Journal of Paediatric Neurology*, *21*(5), 703–706.

18. Emery, A. E. H., Emery, M., Swash, M., Mikol, J., Walusinski, O., & Goebel, H. H. (2017). *20th anniversary meeting of the Meryon Society Worcester College, Oxford. Neuromuscular Disorders*, *27*(3), 298–303.

19. Etchell, A. C., Johnson, B. W., & Sowman, P. F. 2014). Behavioral and multimodal neuroimaging evidence for a deficit in brain timing networks in stuttering: A hypothesis and theory. *Frontiers in Human Neuroscience*, *8*, 1–10.

20. Fiori, S., Guzzetta, A., Mitra, J., Pannek, K., Pasquariello, R., Cipriani, P., Tosetti, M., Cioni, G., Rose, S. E., & Chilosi, A. (2016). Neuroanatomical correlates of childhood apraxia of speech: A connectomic approach. *NeuroImage: Clinical*, *12*, 894–901. https://doi.org/10.1016/j.nicl.2016.11.003 .

21. Foundas, A. L., Mock, J. R., Cindass, R., & Corey, D. M. (2013). Atypical caudate anatomy in children who stutter. *Perceptual and Motor Skills*, *116*(2), 528–543.

22. Frankford, S. A., Heller Murray, E. S., Masapollo, M., Cai, S., Tourville, J. A., Nieto-Castañón, A., & Guenther, F. H. (2021). The neural circuitry underlying the "rhythm effect" in stuttering. *Journal of Speech, Language, and Hearing Research*, *64*(6S), 2325–2346. https://doi.org/10.1044/2021_JSLHR-20-00328.

23. Garnett, E. O., Chow, H. M., & Chang, S. E. (2019). Neuroanatomical correlates of childhood stuttering: MRI indices of white and gray matter development that differentiate

persistence versus recovery. *Journal of Speech, Language, and Hearing Research, 62*(8S), 2986–2998. https://www.ncbi.nlm.nih.gov/pmc/articles/PMC5114583/.

24. Gopnik, M., & Crago, M. B. (1991). Familial aggregation of a developmental language disorder. *Cognition, 39*(1), 1–50.

25. Ingham, R. J., Grafton, S. T., Bothe, A. K., & Ingham, J. C. (2012). Brain activity in adults who stutter: Similarities across speaking tasks and correlations with stuttering frequency and speaking rate. *Brain and Language, 122*(1), 11–24.

26. Kadis, D. S., Goshulak, D., Namasivayam, A., Pukonen, M., Kroll, R., De Nil, L. F., Pang, E. W., & Lerch, J. P. (2014). Cortical thickness in children receiving intensive therapy for idiopathic apraxia of speech. *Brain Topography, 27*, 240–247.

27. Liégeois, F., Baldeweg, T., Connelly, A., Gadian, D. G., Mishkin, M., & Vargha-Khadem, F. (2003). Language fMRI abnormalities associated with *FOXP2* gene mutation. *Nature Neuroscience, 6*, 1230–1237.

28. Locke, J. (1997). A theory of neurolinguistic development. *Brain and Language, 58*(2), 265–326.

29. Love, R. J. (2000). *Childhood motor speech disability* (2nd ed.). Allyn and Bacon.

30. McCauley, R. J., & Strand, E. A. (2008). A review of standardized tests of nonverbal oral and speech motor performance in children. *American Journal of Speech-Language Pathology, 17*(1), 81–91.

31. Morgan, A., Fisher, S. E., Scheffer, I., et al. (2017). *FOXP2*-related speech and language disorders. In M. P. Adam, H. H. Ardinger, & R. A. Pagon (Eds.), *Gene Reviews®*. University of Washington-Seattle. https://www.ncbi.nlm.nih.gov/books/NBK368474.

32. Murray, E., McCabe, P., Heard, R., & Ballard, K. J. (2015). Differential diagnosis of children with suspected childhood apraxia of speech. *Journal of Speech, Language, and Hearing Research, 58*(1), 43–60.

33. National Institute of Neurological Disorders and Stroke. (2021). Cerebral palsy: Hope through research. https://www.ninds.nih.gov/Disorders/Patient-Caregiver-Education/Hope-Through-Research/Cerebral-Palsy-Hope-Through-Research#3104_15.

34. Nordberg, A., Miniscalco, C., & Lohmander, A. (2014). Consonant production and overall speech characteristics in school-aged children with cerebral palsy and speech impairment. *International Journal of Speech-Language Pathology, 16*(4), 386–395. https://doi.org/10.3109/17549507.2014.917440.

35. Preston, J. L., Benway, N. R., Leece, M. C., & Caballero, N. F. (2021). Concurrent validity between two sound sequencing tasks used to identify childhood apraxia of speech in school-aged children. *American Journal of Speech-Language Pathology, 30*, 1580–1588.

36. Preston, J. L., Molfese, P. J., Gumkowski, N., Sorcinelli, A., Harwood, V., Irwin, J. R., & Landi, N. (2014). Neurophysiology of speech differences in childhood apraxia of speech. *Developmental Neuropsychology, 39*(5), 385–403.

37. Salman, M. S., & Tsai, P. (2016). The role of the pediatric cerebellum in motor functions, cognition, and behavior: A clinical perspective. *Neuroimaging Clinics of North America, 26*(3). 317–329.

38. Shriberg, L. D., Potter, N. L., & Strand, E. A. (2011). Prevalence and phenotype of childhood apraxia of speech in youth with galactosemia. *Journal of Speech, Language, and Hearing Research, 54*(2), 487–519. https://doi.org/10.1044/1092-4388 (2010/10-0068).

39. Shriberg, L. D., Strand, E. A., Fourakis, M., Jakielski, K. J., Hall, S. D., Karlsson, H. B., Mabie, H. L., et al. (2017). A diagnostic marker to discriminate childhood apraxia of speech from speech delay: I. Development and description of the pause marker. *Journal of Speech, Language, and Hearing Research, 60*(4), S1096–S1117. https://doi.org/10.1044/2016_JSLHR-S-15-0296.

40. Shriberg, L. D., Strand, E. A., Fourakis, M., Jakielski, K. J., Hall, S. D., Karlsson, H. B., & Wilson, D. L. (2017). A diagnostic marker to discriminate childhood apraxia of speech from speech delay: IV. The pause marker index. *Journal of Speech, Language, and Hearing Research, 60*, S1153–S1169. 317–329. https://www.ncbi.nlm.nih.gov/pmc/articles/PMC5548089/

41. Strand, E. A., McCauley, R. J., Weigand, S. D., Stoeckel, R. E., & Baas, B. S. (2013). A motor speech assessment for children with severe speech disorders: Reliability and validity evidence. *Journal of Speech, Language, and Hearing Research, 56*(2), 505–520.

42. Vargha-Khadem, F., Watkins, K., Alcock, K., Fletcher, P., & Passingham, R. (1995). Praxic and nonverbal cognitive deficits in a large family with a genetically transmitted speech and language disorder. *Proceedings of the National Academy of Sciences of the United States of America, 92*(3), 930–933.

43. Xuan, Y., Meng, C., Yang, Y., Zhu, C., Wang, L., Yan, Q., Lin, C., & Yu, C. (2012). Resting state brain activity in adults who stutter. *PLoS One, 7*(1), e30570.

44. Yari, E., & Ambrose, N. (2013). Epidemiology of stuttering: 21st century advances. *Journal of Fluency Disorders, 38*(2), 66–87.

13

Pediatric Disorders of Language

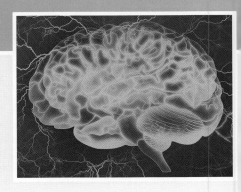

There is in every child at every stage a new miracle of vigorous unfolding.

Erik Erikson

CHAPTER OUTLINE

KEY TERMS

autism spectrum disorder (ASD)
cerebral plasticity
childhood disintegrative disorder
    (CDD)
corpus callosum
developmental language disorder
dichotic listening

DSM-5
ear advantage
intellectual disability
Landau-Kleffner syndrome (LKS)
language dominance
language lateralization
myelination

myelinogenesis
neurotrophins
pervasive developmental disorder
    (PDD)
progenitor cells
Rett syndrome

BRAIN GROWTH

Acquisition of speech and language is clearly tied to physical development and maturation in the infant and child, yet the exact nature of the interaction of growth and development with emerging speech is unknown. What is known, however, is that the course of speech and language development is a correlate of cerebral maturation and specialization. But a critical question remains: What indexes of cerebral maturation are of significance to language acquisition? Clearly critical periods occur in the maturation of the brain as well as growth gradients in different brain structures. Can these critical periods be equally applied to the stages of language acquisition?

Brain Weight

One obvious index of neurologic development is the change in gross brain weight with age. The most rapid period of brain growth is during the first 2 years of life. The brain more than triples its weight in the first 24 months. At birth, the brain is ~25% of its adult weight, and at 6 months it has reached 50% of its full weight. At 1 year, the average age at which the first word appears, the brain is 60% of its adult weight. Thus, the brain makes its most rapid growth in the first year of life. By 2.5 years, the brain has reached ~75% of its full growth, and at 5 years it is within 90% of its complete maturation. Table 13.1 illustrates this increase in brain weight. It is not until 10 years of age that the brain achieves

TABLE 13.1 Language and Brain Growth from Birth to 12 Years

Age	Language Milestones	Brain Weight (g)
Birth	Crying	335
3 mo	Cooing and crying	516
6 mo	Babbling	660
9 mo	Voicing intoned jargon	750
12 mo	Approximating first words	925
18 mo	Early naming	1024
24 mo	Making two-word combinations	1064
5 yr	Kindergarten age, sentences	1180
12 yr	Fully matured brain weight	1320

~95% of its ultimate weight. By ~12 years, or puberty, full brain weight is reached.

The late neurolinguist Eric Lenneberg (1921–1975) argued that the accelerated curve of brain growth in the first years of life matched the course of rapid early acquisition of language of the child.[25] He further claimed that primary linguistic skills were achieved by the age of 4 or 5 years and that the ability to acquire language diminished sharply after puberty, when accelerating brain growth reached a plateau.

Differential Brain Growth

Just as the total brain grows at different rates at different ages, so do its different parts, and various brain structures reach their peak growth rates at different times. For instance, brainstem divisions, such as the midbrain, pons, and medulla, grow rapidly prenatally and less rapidly postnatally. The cerebellum develops rapidly from before birth to the age of 1 year. The cerebral hemispheres, important in language development, grow rapidly early, contributing ~85% to total brain volume by the sixth fetal month.

The differential growth of the cortex of the cerebral hemispheres is of vital importance for speech and language function because the majority of neural structures for communication are integrated there. Most cortical neurons are in place at birth, but brain growth may be measured through the development of synaptic connections and myelination. One method of establishing a schedule of cortical growth gradients in cerebral maturity is to determine what cortical areas are most developed in myelination at birth. The motor area of the precentral gyrus of the frontal lobe is the first cortical area developed at birth. It is soon followed by the somatosensory area of the postcentral gyrus of the parietal lobe. Next, quite soon after birth, the primary visual receptor area of the occipital cortex matures. The primary auditory area, Heschl gyrus in the temporal lobe, matures last. The medial surface of the hemispheres shows the final development of the brain.

The cortical association areas lag behind the development of the cortical receptor areas that are present and active at birth. In fact, the major association areas devoted to speech and language mature well into the preschool years and even beyond.

The progressive development of Broca area and the development of Wernicke area are related to progressive stabilization of the phonologic system. As the phonemic motor planning system matures, the auditory association system increases its ability to process longer and more complex sequences of connected phonemes. The arcuate fasciculus connecting Broca and Wernicke areas apparently begins myelination in the first year and continues for some time afterward.

At 1 year the normal child has a vocabulary of one or more word approximations, usually names for objects that have been seen and sometimes touched. This stage of language development requires the ability to mix neural information from the auditory, somesthetic, and visual association areas. The association area of the inferior parietal lobe is where information from the temporal auditory association areas, the occipital visual association area, and the parietal association area combine to provide the neural basis for the feat of naming that the 1-year-old child displays. The rapid growth of vocabulary in the second and third years of life therefore may well be a correlate of the maturation of this significant posterior association area in the parietal lobe, which combines information from surrounding association areas. It no doubt is a master association area, rightly named by Geschwind as "the association area of association areas."[19]

The left hemisphere is destined to serve as the primary neurologic site for speech and language mechanisms in most infants, children, and adults. The left hemisphere shows early structural differences that support later **language dominance**. The sylvian fissure is longer on the left in fetal brains, and the planum temporale on the left is larger in the majority of fetal and newborn brains. Although the temporal lobe appears well differentiated from early life, Broca area is not differentiated until 18 months, and the corpus callosum is not completely myelinated until age 10 years. The inferior parietal lobe, the master association area, is not fully myelinated until adulthood, often well into the fourth decade.

Differential Brain Growth Anomaly: Agenesis of the Corpus Callosum

The corpus callosum is defined under the category of commissural fibers; that is, it interconnects corresponding structures in the left hemisphere with the right hemisphere. The largest bundle of these fibers is called the **corpus callosum** (Fig. 13.1A). Consisting of a rostrum, genu, body, and splenium, it is formed by over 190 million axons, primarily excitatory in nature, traversing from one hemisphere to the other.[32] These fibers emerge and are sculpted in developmental stages during embryonic, fetal, and postnatal periods.

Agenesis of the corpus callosum (see Fig. 13.1B) is a condition present at birth in which there is partial or complete absence of the corpus callosum. In the general population the prevalence is 0.02% to 0.5% with 2% to 3% of patients with intellectual disability affected.[23] As would be expected, abnormal pathways have been shown on imaging studies to develop in the brain. Despite the presence of abnormal organization, there has always been found a great variability in function and cognition of acallosal patients.

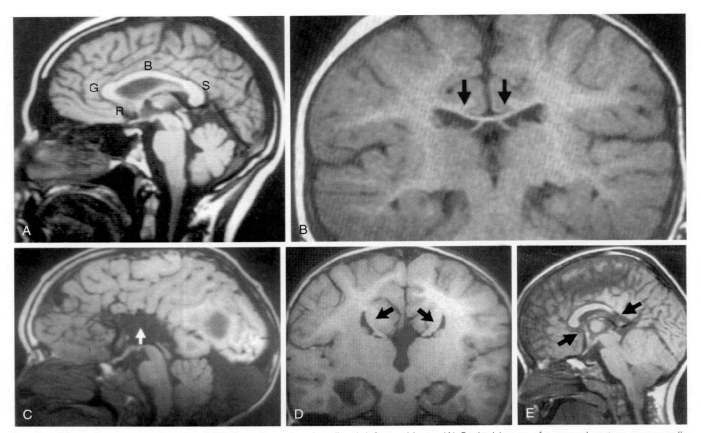

Fig. 13.1 Magnetic resonance imaging (MRI) from normal and acallosal-defect subjects. (A) Sagittal image of a normal mature corpus callosum from a 15-year-old subject (*R*, rostrum; *G*, genu; *B*, body; *S*, the splenium). (B) Coronal image of a normal corpus callosum *(black arrows)*. (C) Sagittal image showing agenesis of the corpus callosum with the medial hemispheric sulci radiating into the third ventricle *(white arrow)*. (D) Coronal image of true agenesis of the corpus callosum with Probst bundle formation *(black arrows)*. (E) Sagittal image showing a patient with Chiari II malformation and partial agenesis of the corpus callosum. The rostrum and splenium are absent *(black arrows)*. (Adapted from Kamnasaran, D. [2005]. Agenesis of the corpus callosum: Lessons from humans and mice. *Clinical and Investigative Medicine, 28*(5), 267–282.)

Until recently, this was assumed to be the result of compensatory strategies developed through mechanisms of neural plasticity. A recent study using in utero diffusion tensor imaging (DTI) provided evidence that this may not be the primary cause of the variability. Using the DTI and streamlined tractography, white matter pathway development was studied in 20 fetuses with isolated agenesis of the corpus callosum and compared with that of 20 gestation-age matched fetuses with normally developing brains.[11] After the imaging, the researchers constructed macroscopic connectomes of the pathways in different regions. The authors wanted to characterize white matter architecture before occurrence of the natural reorganization that would take place early postnatally through axon refinement and pruning and then later as a result of experience-driven changes. They found that the acallosal fetal brains showed a globally altered connectivity network already present compared with the normally developing brains. Gradually increasing connectivity strength was found in aberrant pathways running anterior-posteriorly. Less network centrality was found in dense areas of connectivity like the thalamus and cingulate cortex. These findings indicated that callosal agenesis manifests itself not only in aberrant pathways that run adjacent to the medial part of the hemispheres but also in excessive structural

connectivity that intensifies during gestation. This provides support for the likelihood that abnormal fiber development in children with callosal agenesis is more likely governed by genetically determined prenatal events than by compensatory mechanisms in later life.

The frequent observation of variability of function of these children combined with the results of the study outlined earlier demands that clinicians carefully assess each child with a diagnosis of agenesis of the corpus callosum, being careful to remember that there is not a typical developmental pattern for speech and language. There have been case studies and reports of treatments of those patients that will be helpful, but all children will serve as their own control.

A Word on Genetics

In introductory chapters of this text and in Chapter 11, we have touched upon the genetic basis of brain development in humans and the consequence of alteration/interruption to the normal genetic sequence. As the research cited earlier on callosal agenesis suggests, it is not hyperbole to state that discoveries about the genetic basis of speech and language disorders are of critical importance to medical science. This text will not attempt to discuss in any depth the confirmed or proposed genetic basis of the many syndromes or disorders in children with speech-language disorders. It is important, however, for a speech-language pathologist (SLP) to be aware that chromosomal deletion and microdeletion syndromes are now being identified very early (some in utero) in a child's life. This of course provides an excellent opportunity to initiate intervention and habilitation early in life, including feeding, speech, language, and hearing services.

It is not uncommon today for doctors to advise parents of children identified with some disorders to seek genetic testing (chromosomal analysis) for that child and counseling for themselves (or, perhaps, for an older child). Genetic testing, even limited in scope, is not a decision to be taken lightly. Parents may ask for your help in understanding why their physician may be recommending this or in understanding what genetic testing involves. Typically, the physician is suggesting this to help them understand the probability/possibility of a genetic mutation being passed down to future children in their generation and beyond. It also may confirm or suggest the diagnosis of a particular syndrome. The confirmation of a particular syndrome can lead to better individualization of medical treatment and/or therapeutic intervention for that child; in many syndromes, symptoms will likely include disorders of communication.

In a very broad sense, chromosomal anomalies may be divided into two categories of abnormality: numeric or structural. Numeric abnormalities include those with an extra chromosome (trisomy) and those with a missing chromosome (monosomy). Down syndrome results from the presence of an extra copy of chromosome 21. Turner syndrome, which affects only girls and women, results from a partial or completely missing X chromosome. Males with Klinefelter syndrome have an extra X chromosome.

Structural abnormalities include those in which there are deletions or duplications of various parts. Fragile X syndrome is the most common inherited cause of intellectual disability and results from a genetic abnormality of repetition on a particular gene on the X chromosome. Many of the abnormalities may be further categorized into deletion and microdeletion syndromes. In microdeletion, smaller segments of the chromosome are involved, typically evading identification through standard testing. More technologically advanced testing methods, such as chromosomal microarray analysis, which use fluorescent probes may be used. Table 13.2 lists some known microdeletion syndromes that can now be identified through certain genetic testing.

Box 13.1 contains an example of a report written by a geneticist after the initial counseling meeting with parents following genetic testing of their child. This kind of simplified explanation of an extremely complex procedure may be provided to your clients, and they may consult you for further counseling regarding the procedure or identified disorder.

Myelination for Language

Myelination is the process by which oligodendrocytes produce layers of myelin that wrap around axons, sheathing them and enabling more rapid signal transmission. Myelination has been considered one of the more significant indexes of brain

TABLE 13.2 Microdeletion Syndromes Identified through Genetic Analysis and Known to Impact Cognitive and Language Development

Syndrome	Chromosomal Deletion	Signs/Symptoms
Angelman syndrome	Maternal chromosome at 15Q11	Seizures, ataxia, frequent laughter, hand-flapping, severe intellectual disability
DiGeorge syndrome (velocardiofacial syndrome)	22q11.21	Cardiac anomalies, cleft palate, intellectual disability, psychiatric problems
Langer-Giedion syndrome	8q24.1	Sparse hair, bulbus nose, hearing loss, intellectual disability
Prader-Willi syndrome	Paternal chromosome at 15q11	As an infant: hypotonia, poor feeding, failure to thrive. In childhood/adolescence: obesity, small hands and feet, intellectual disability, obsessive-compulsive disorder
Smith-Magenis syndrome	17q11.2	Brachycephaly, midfacial hypoplasia, hoarse voice, short stature, intellectual disability
Williams syndrome	7q11.23	Aortic stenosis, intellectual disability, elfin facies

Modified from Merck Manual (prof. ver.). (2022). https://www.merckmanuals.com/professional/pediatrics/chromosome-and-gene-anomalies

maturation and is often a prime correlate of speech and language. Myelination allows more rapid transmission of neural information along neural fibers and is particularly critical in a cerebral nervous system dependent on several long axon connections in white matter tracts between hemispheres, lobes, and cortical and subcortical structures. **Myelinogenesis** is a cyclic process in which certain neural regions and systems appear to begin the process of laying down myelin early and others much later. In some instances the myelogenetic cycle is short and in other cases much longer. Clear differences in rate of myelogenesis exist between different pathways. Myelination of the cortical end of the auditory projections extends beyond the first year, whereas myelination of the cortical end of the visual projections is complete soon after birth. It should be understood that when considering white matter microstructure, there is no static period across human development. It is fast and dynamic during childhood through young adulthood, becomes somewhat static in middle adult years, and then accelerates again as some deterioration begins in later life.[9]

BOX 13.1   Example of a Report of Initial Genetic Counseling Meeting

REASON FOR VISIT: Genetic counseling regarding abnormal chromosome microarray (CMA) results.

HISTORY OF PRESENT ILLNESS: Patient is a 4-y.o. male who presents to my genetic counseling clinic today with his mother and father to discuss his CMA, which revealed a 6p22.3 deletion of uncertain clinical significance.

SYNOPSIS: He came to clinic today with his parents to discuss his CMA results and the option of parental testing. Beginning with basic genetics concepts, we reviewed that our bodies are made up of trillions of cells. In our cells are our chromosomes, or packages of DNA. We have 46 chromosomes, or 23 chromosome pairs. One copy comes from mom and one copy comes from dad. Because our chromosomes are fragile, sometimes our chromosomes lose material or develop extra pieces as a result of errors in the cell division process. Sometimes these extra or missing pieces do not cause any problems for our bodies, and other times they do cause problems. We discussed that on the short (p) arm of chromosome 6 at position 22.3, chromosome material is missing. The deleted region contains at least one known gene that is not currently associated with a specific phenotype. This variant is currently classified as unknown clinical significance. Parental testing may clarify the significance of this deletion. If the deletion is found to be inherited from a parent who does not have signs or symptoms similar to him, then we would be more suspicious that the change is benign (harmless). If the deletion were pathogenic (harmful), we would expect for the parent to have signs/symptoms similar to their child. If the deletion is found to be de novo (new and not inherited) in him, we would have further evidence to explore this deletion but causation would not be proven. His parents elected to pursue parental testing today. Blood was drawn and sent through our center to complete the testing.

Su et al.,[30] utilized quantitative magnetic resonance imaging (MRI) to study sequential myelination of seven regions of interest (ROIs) associated with language development in 241 neurologically intact children ranging from postnatal age of 0 to 429 weeks. Their findings showed all areas sharing the same curve of myelination. No myelination was found in any of these areas at birth with the myelinogenesis reaching maturation at about the age of 18 months and then much more slowly continuing with age progression. The higher cortical areas (Broca, Wernicke, angular gyrus) matured more slowly and later than the primary cortical areas (primary motor, visual and auditory cortex). The fibers of the arcuate fasciculus myelinized at about the same rate as the higher cortical areas until age 18 months but then laid down myelin even more slowly, especially after age 3, than did the other areas. Though the findings from imaging studies vary somewhat among the studies, most results are within similar range and show that myelination cycles can be roughly correlated with the milestones of speech and language development.

Prematurity and Dysmaturation

Prematurity or preterm birth (defined as birth <37 weeks of gestation) affected 1 of every 10 infants born in the United States in 2020, declining very slightly from 2019. The rate of preterm births continued to be about 50% higher among Black women than among White or Hispanic women. The survival rate for preterm infants has steadily increased through advances in medical care, and the survival rate for an infant born at 24 weeks was reported in 2018 to be at 60% to 65%. This increased survival rate also, unfortunately, results in a high number of developmental neurologic disorders. This is due to the occurrence of a distinctive form of cerebral white matter injury (WMI) first identified in the 1960s and termed periventricular leukomalacia (PVL) as well as neuronal axonal disease affecting cerebral white matter as well as many other brain structures such as the thalamus, cerebellum, cortex, brainstem, and basal ganglia. Taken together, this constellation of injury is referred to as the encephalopathy of prematurity. The earlier the child is born, the more severe the injury to the developing brain. Those children who are born with very low birthweight (≤1500 g [≤3.3 pounds]) are substantially at risk for disability due to this and the subsequent dysmaturational events following the initial injury related to early birth.[36] In the early 1960s a study of a large number of premature babies identified unique lesions of white matter (i.e., PVL). This white matter injury was described as consisting of coagulated necrotic tissue, an excessive number of astrocytes, and microglia activation.[15] PVL is thought to occur due to damage to premyelinating oligodendrocytes (pre-OL) cells in this immature brain. Pre-OL cells perform a midpoint function in the development of new oligodendrocytes, which can begin the process of forming myelin sheaths and eventually mature fully into myelinating oligodendrocytes.[22] Microglia and astrocytes are activated, and gliosis will develop. Secondary injury to cortical gray matter may follow with impact on axonal differentiation. The etiology of PVL has been hypothesized to be anoxia, though inflammation has also been highlighted as a possible cause of white matter damage. The impact of damage to the pre-OL cells is decreased myelination as well as axonal dysmaturation, the combination of which results in delayed or impaired cortical and thalamic development.[3]

In his 2019 topical review of dysmaturation in the premature brain, Volpe[36] provides a review of research on neuroprotective and neurorestorative interventions. In regard to neuroprotective intervention, the article lists several pharmaceutic interventions being studied at that time. Only the drug erythropoietin had been studied in detail, however, with findings showing promising ability to mitigate WMI in premature infants. Large-scale trials were still in progress. In regard to neurorestorative interventions, the author discussed the fact that the dysmaturational events that follow the initial injury of premature birth do evolve, allowing time for possible interventions other than pharmaceutic to make a significant difference in outcome. Some interventions, such as stem cells, epidermal growth factor, and microglia manipulations, had been studied only in experimental settings with all needing further study but showing some positive findings for future use. A body of clinical research on modification of environmental factors has suggested a positive effect on the development of the premature brain if they are implemented in a timely manner during the neonatal period (and sometimes beyond).[33] These interventions included optimal nutrition, including research on breast feeding, formula fortification, zinc, iron, and polyunsaturated fats. The second large category of studies included those on experiential factors, including the auditory environment, nature of the auditory input, infant's visual experience, impact of pain and stress, and the impact of parenting, parental education, and social factors. A most interesting study on parental language input in the preschool years suggests that, regardless of parent IQ and educational level, the amount and complexity of language provided for the child in the preschool years can be correlated with the rate of change in cortical thickness of language processing areas during the kindergarten through middle school years.[12] The interested student is referred to these articles and the studies referenced by the reviewers. These studies will lead to further investigation and, it is hoped, confirmation that there are effective neuroprotective and neurorestorative interventions that can enhance brain development (and, thus, speech-language development) for the premature baby.

CEREBRAL PLASTICITY

Children who have begun to develop language normally and then sustain cerebral injury, particularly to the left hemisphere, often show a loss of language skills and a significant effect on further language development, at least initially. The younger the child, however, the more quickly the language disturbance appears to resolve itself, and the child appears to become grossly normal or near normal in language function. This fact is in relatively sharp contrast to the adult who sustains left cerebral injury. In adult brains, resolution of language difficulty after focal injury to the (typically) dominant left hemisphere rarely reaches the level of normality of functioning that is possible in the child.

One explanation given for this phenomenon is that the child's brain demonstrates considerable plasticity of function in that undamaged areas are capable of assuming language function. In terms of language function, cerebral plasticity is defined as a state or stage in which specific cortical areas are not well established because of the brain's immaturity. The brain is more plastic during the most rapid periods of brain growth, and damage to the left hemisphere before the end of the first year of life is often associated with a shift of language function to the right hemisphere. By contrast, injury to the left hemisphere after this critical period is less likely to be associated with a functional reorganization of the brain. Studies from various neurosurgical centers show that approximately one-third of patients with left hemisphere damage before age 1 year continue to have language mediated exclusively by the left hemisphere. In patients in whom left hemisphere dominance for language continues even in the face of damage, it is dependent primarily on the integrity of the frontal and temporal-parietal language areas. This explanation of cerebral plasticity of language mechanisms rests on the concept of a transfer of functional areas from the left hemisphere to uncommitted areas in the right hemisphere.

The period of time in which plasticity changes occur is called the critical period. Each area of the cortex has its own critical period; therefore, a child's recovery from an injury depends on two factors: where the lesion occurred and the exact critical period for that part of the brain. This critical period has many implications for language functioning in a developing child. Axonal and synaptic developments are especially vulnerable to perinatal hypoxia, malnutrition, and even environmental toxins such as air pollution, paint, and fumes. When axonal and synaptic development are affected, this vulnerability has adverse consequences on cognitive and language development. Sensory and social deprivation studies have also shown that environmental stimuli can have a significant effect on development during the critical period. To this end, a longitudinal study done by investigators from the Family Life Project in North Carolina involved studying parental and household variables of 1112 families in relation to language development findings at age 36 months.[35] Language was measured by only the receptive language measure of the Wechsler Preschool and Primary Scale of Intelligence and the expressive tests of the Preschool Language Scale (4th ed.). Thirteen covariant variables were included, typical to study of environmental factors in child development. These included parental variables (such as parental age at first birth, income, education, employment, depression, etc.) and child variables (prenatal exposure to alcohol or drugs, number of different child care settings, geographic isolation). The research targeted interest area beyond these variables was termed "household chaos." This included factors associated with instability and disorganization. Household disorganization rating considered these 5 factors: household density, number of hours of TV watching, household preparation prior to the visits, cleanliness of the house and neighborhood noise level. The findings of the study found the chaos factor disorganization to be the most significant predictor of delayed language development, as measured in the study, during the first 3 years of life. This was over and beyond factors of socioeconomic status and parenting frequently cited. Although development of other skills was not studied nor was more rigorous measure of language development undertaken, this study continues to reinforce what neurodevelopmental literature emphasizes about a child's experiences and interactions with the sensory and cognitive environment. Environmental enrichment programs are considered to be the most effective in overcoming cognitive problems, including delays in speech-language development. The structure, focus, and attention to the child's needs provided by these preschool and early intervention programs are supported by many studies, including this one, as critical to enhancing language and other neurodevelopmental areas, especially for children from chaotic households.

Development of Language Dominance

An overriding fact of brain functioning is that the cerebral hemispheres demonstrate asymmetry and that language is dominant in one of them. Cerebral dominance appears to be a developing function because, although anatomic differences favor the temporal lobe in the left hemisphere, strong evidence suggests that language is less fixed in the immature brain. Lenneberg[25] advanced the theory that the course of **language lateralization** follows the course of cerebral maturation. He argued that lateralization is completed by puberty, based on the assumption that at birth the two hemispheres have equal potential for the development of language mechanisms, and gradual lateralization is associated with the period of major growth.

Current anatomic evidence suggests that the hemispheres may not have equal potentiality for language and that the left hemisphere is organized differently from the right, with speech mechanisms for language in the left.[20] The planum temporale is larger in adults, newborns, and fetuses (Fig. 13.2).[37]

Research comparing macroscopic aspects (width, height, length, and total volume of the area) of postmortem brains with structural patterns (neuronal density, axonal density, etc.) concluded that the asymmetry could not be explained by neuronal density or glial cell volume.[5] However, the findings pointed to axonal myelination as a possible explanation. Further support was provided by Galuske et al.,[18] who demonstrated a strong relation of asymmetry of the planum temporale to the organization of the clusters of neurons that characterize the area and the spacing of those clusters. These factors can be referred to as the intrinsic microcircuitry of the area, and area 22 of the temporal lobe is indicative of greater complexity of connections. The authors of this study concluded that this higher level of organizational complexity (increasing the area volume) could be partially attributable to use-dependent modifications that occur during development with increasing exposure to human language. As Habib and Robichon[20] point out, however, this conclusion of exposure-dependent increase in volume is incompatible with the fact that the asymmetry is present in the neonate and even the fetus. More likely, they conclude, a genetically predetermined pattern of asymmetry exists that is further reinforced under the influence of specific environmental influences.

Cerebral dominance for language has been long associated with laterality of other functions. As long ago as 1865, Jean Bouillaud (1796–1881) suggested that language dominance and handedness were related in some way. For many years the preferred hand was believed to be contralateral to the cerebral hemisphere dominant for language. This meant that the left cerebral hemisphere was dominant for language in right-handers and the right hemisphere in left-handers. Primarily through the cortical-stimulation studies of Penfield and Roberts, current thinking is that the left hemisphere is almost always language dominant in right-handers, with ~95% of this group left-brained for language. In left-handers, ~50% to 70% also show language dominance in the left hemisphere.

Hand preference is a relevant but not totally reliable index in predicting language dominance. Right-handedness is a relatively universal trait and is usually associated with other preferences in laterality. Human beings also tend to prefer one foot, eye, and ear consistently. Degrees of laterality vary. Some people are more strongly right-handed than others, but true ambidexters, those who use either hand equally well, are quite rare.

Most right-handed people demonstrate ear preference, which is considered consistent with a contralateral hemisphere laterality for language in the brain. This preference can be demonstrated through **dichotic listening** tasks, in which simultaneous auditory stimuli are presented to both ears at once. Listeners generally show a consistent lateral preference in recognition of stimuli in one ear over the other, called an **ear advantage.** Only 80% of right-handers show a distinct right ear advantage, so the relation to cerebral dominance for language is not always clear.

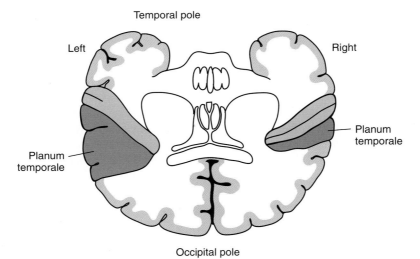

Fig. 13.2 Cerebral asymmetry in the planum temporale. Geschwind and Levitsky demonstrated a larger left planum temporale in 65 adult subjects, a larger right planum temporale in 11 subjects, and equal plana temporale in 24 subjects. The drawing shows an exposed upper surface of the temporal lobe with a cut made at the plane of the sylvian fissure. Note a large left planum lying behind the transverse gyrus of Heschl. On the right are two transverse gyri and a small planum. (Modified from Geschwind, N., & Levitsky, W. [1968]. Left-right asymmetries in temporal speech region, *Science, 161,* 186–187; Ludlow, C., & Doran-Quine, M. [Eds.]. [1979]. *The neurologic bases of language disorders in children: Methods and directions for research* [NIH Publication 79-440]. National Institutes of Health Publication.)

CHILDHOOD LANGUAGE DISORDERS

To truly understand the origin of language disorders and why a child exhibits disordered linguistic behavior, students should review the neurologic language processing structures in the central nervous system. Likewise, a review of the structures responsible for expressive language and transmitting a processed message from Wernicke area to Broca area through the association pathways will help the student understand how a message is verbalized through an intricate programming of motor speech structures that allow an individual to verbalize an idea. Many of the pediatric clients you will serve will have language disorders associated with identified medical conditions, while others will be categorized as a developmental language disorder.

Developmental Language Disorders

In the next section of this chapter we will briefly discuss developmental language disorders in children. By far, the most prevalent childhood language abnormalities are those that are developmental rather than acquired. The term **developmental language disorder** is adopted here, rather than specific language impairment (SLI), which came to the forefront in the 1980s and is still in wide use in our professional literature. In 2012 the American Speech-Language-Hearing Association (ASHA) was asked to respond to the proposal to include the diagnosis of SLI in the new edition of the *Diagnostic and Statistical Manual of Mental Disorders, Fifth Edition* (**DSM-5**). Although the decision was not without controversy, ASHA recommended that the diagnosis not be included, citing debate over the robustness and validity of diagnostic criteria. ASHA maintained that SLI was primarily used in research rather than widely used in clinical settings. Therefore, SLI is not in the DSM-5. Language disorder is listed under communication disorders with the criteria described as "persistent difficulties in the acquisition and use of language across modalities (i.e., spoken, written, sign language, or other) due to deficits in comprehension or production," and "language abilities that are 'substantially and quantifiably' below age expectations."[2]

Historically, SLI had been defined as a language disorder that delays the mastery of language skills in children who have no hearing loss or other developmental delays.[28] Other definitions also may have included "no evidence of lack of opportunity" as a criterion. In 2017[8] child language researchers and clinicians from the United States, Australia, and Great Britain made a compelling argument for the use of *language disorder* rather than SLI. They included in their overall term two subgroups: (1) children who would qualify for a diagnosis of language disorder associated with X and (2) children who would qualify for a diagnosis of developmental language disorder (DLD). Group 1 should include those confirmed to have a biomedical condition that could affect their language development, such as Down syndrome, intellectual disability, or sensorineural hearing loss. Children in the DLD category are those whose language difficulties are not associated with

developmental or acquired medical conditions but may have co-occurring, but not causative, impairments in areas such as attention, speech, emotional problems, literacy, executive function, etc. DLD by this definition does not require a significant gap between verbal and nonverbal ability since children with nonverbal IQ scores above the level of intellectual disability could be diagnosed with a DLD.

Because this question of terminology and inclusionary criteria has not yet been totally agreed upon for clinical or research use at the time of this writing, the research cited here is primarily on children who were diagnosed with SLI as well as DLD. Other terms found in the literature that may refer to the same disorder are *language delay*, *language impairment*, or *developmental dysphasia* (particularly in Australia and Great Britain). According to the National Institute on Deafness and Other Communication Disorders, developmental language disorder affects 7% to 8% of kindergarten children and its effects can persist into adulthood.

The familial nature of developmental language disorders has been documented, although with much variation in study design and criteria for disorder. Increased frequency of language impairment in persons with first-degree relatives affected has been found in these studies.[31] This finding has been strengthened by twin studies showing increased concordance in monozygotic twins compared with dizygotic twins, strongly suggesting genetic influence. Genetic variability related to both autism and language impairment was one of the principal interests of a large study published in 2014.[9] The study identified two novel chromosome locations: 15q23-26 and 16p12. Further study found 15q to be specific to oral language impairment.

Neural Basis of Developmental Language Disorders

A search of the literature regarding any neurologic basis for language disorders that appears to be developmental or not strongly related to an identifiable accompanying disorder reveals few studies. This is perhaps because of the complexity of language development itself, with the importance of genetic and environmental factors acknowledged and well accepted. With the advent of neuroimaging techniques safe for use with children, there have been studies of brain function attempted in the past few years, but little consistency has been found. Liégeois et al.,[26] summarized selected studies in a 2014 review. For this study, the authors reviewed more than 2000 abstracts and articles published between 2008 and 2013. Criteria excluded duplicate studies, studies with children with brain injury, studies with no imaging, and studies in which MRI data included no quantitative analysis. The level of evidence for the five studies used was classified as Level III-2 (a concurrent study with comparative controls) by the Australian classification criteria. Their report noted the variability of inclusion criteria and diagnoses in these studies, with one study using adults identified with language impairment as children and continuing to score low on language assessments. Structural imaging studies were included in four of the five studies. Three of these four focused on children. Even in such a small number of subjects there was great variability with studies of gray matter finding increase in some temporal lobe areas in some subjects while another found decrease. Study of subcortical structures such as the caudate nucleus found similar contrary results. Studies of white matter using fractional anisotropy (FA) also found contradictory results in different subjects. Two functional imaging studies on subjects with language disorder were reviewed with both finding hypoactivation of the posterior superior temporal gyrus. In the summary of findings the authors caution that, given the heterogeneity of the studies, any consistency found must be considered speculative, but there was converging evidence suggesting possible neural correlates for language disorder. These were:

- Morphologic reductions in the superior temporal gyrus and sulcus in either hemisphere, suggesting a role for intact auditory processing during typical language development
- Reduced activity in the left posterior superior temporal gyrus, consistent with the morphologic reductions, again suggesting abnormal auditory processing as a factor in poor language development
- Reduction in FA in the superior longitudinal fasciculus

The primary summary of the findings of this review study stated that cortical and subcortical anomalies had been found in a wide network supporting language function with little consistency across studies except in the superior temporal gyri.

Neurotrophic factors have been briefly mentioned in this text in Chapters 2 and 4. These brain chemicals belong to a family of secreted proteins called **neurotrophins** and to a class of proteins known as growth factors. As such, they promote the survival of neurons by preventing cells from initiating programmed cell death as well as stimulating a targeted differentiation of **progenitor cells** resulting in the formation of neurons. A group of Turkish researchers[7] was able to look at serum levels of four different neurotrophic factors in blood samples taken from 43 children (ages 18–60 months) diagnosed with language disorders and compare the levels with 43 age-matched control subjects with normal language development. After accounting for confounding influences such as developmental level and psychiatric symptoms, a regression analysis found a significant relationship between the presence of a language disorder and low levels of brain-derived neurotrophic factor (BDNF) as well as neurotrophin-3 (NF-3) levels. Though, as the authors point out, this study has limitations and needs replication and expansion, the finding of significantly lower levels of circulating BDNF and NF-3—brain chemicals that are critical for normal nerve formation, axon growth, and synaptogenesis—in children with idiopathic language disorders is important. It certainly suggests that there is value in continuing to investigate and identify the neurologic basis of these disorders with the goal of one day identifying very early the likelihood of their occurrence and either preventing it or intervening in the preverbal time period of development.

Language Impairment in Children with Intellectual Disability

Cognitive deficits limit language development, and the linguistic skills of the developmentally delayed child are generally poorer than those of the cognitively normal child of equivalent chronologic age. Language development in the majority of developmentally delayed children proceeds on a slower but normal course until early adolescence, when development reaches a plateau. Some have argued that, as in other children, their language development is paced by cerebral maturation. The lack of development of adequate speech and language in **intellectual disability** often serves as one of the earliest and most sensitive signs of an abnormality in development of the nervous system for the pediatric neurologist and SLP. Table 13.3 outlines the major language characteristics of children with developmental delay.

Language delay and generalized intellectual disability have various causes. Neurologic factors delay or arrest myelinization (maturation), which would inevitably cause brain tissue to remain undeveloped. Certain biologic factors, such as

TABLE 13.3 Language Characteristics of Developmentally Delayed Children

Language Parameter	Characteristics
Phonology	Primitive forms
	Similar to preschoolers no matter the age of the child
Morphology	Preschool developmental characteristics
	Often uses the incorrect form of a free or bound morpheme
Syntax	Short sentence lengths
	Simple sentences lacking complexity
	Lack of clauses and compound sentence structures
Semantics	Concrete thinking; little abstract language comprehension or expression
	Lack of understanding of inferences
	Simple meanings of words noted
Pragmatics	Misunderstands gestures
	Lack of the use of gestures for getting a point across
	Poor turn taking
	Lack of asking for clarification increases miscommunications
	Usually does not initiate topics
Receptive language	Poor comprehension
	Heavily relies on context to understand information presented

Modified from Owens Jr., R. E. (2004). *Language disorders: A functional approach to assessment and intervention* (4th ed.). Allyn and Bacon.

TABLE 13.4	Causal Factors of Intellectual Disability/Developmental Delay and the Accompanying Syndromes
Causal Factors	**Syndrome Outcomes**
Chromosomal/genetic	Fragile X
	Down syndrome
Complications of pregnancy/maternal infections	Rubella/German measles
	Syphilis
	Gonorrhea
	AIDS
Chemical/lead toxicity	Fetal alcohol syndrome
	Lead poisoning (eating lead-based paint chips is a common cause)
	Crack cocaine
Metabolic malfunctions	Phenylketonuria
	Poor maternal diet lacking vitamins and minerals
Complications of pregnancy and delivery	Skull malformation/immaturity of development
	Premature birth
	Lack of prenatal care

Data from Owens Jr., R. E., Metz, D. E., & Haas, A. (2003). *Introduction to communication disorders: A lifespan perspective* (2nd ed.; pp. 165–166). Allyn & Bacon.

genetic or chromosomal abnormalities, maternal infections in the first trimester of pregnancy, chemical or lead toxicity, metabolic malfunctions, and complications from pregnancy or delivery may also cause intellectual disability and a delay of speech-language development. Table 13.4 illustrates causes and consequent syndromes that lead to arrested cognitive and language development.

The practicing SLP or the student of speech-language pathology should keep uppermost in mind that a child with developmental delay should always be assessed for language impairment. There is an expectation that language development will mirror cognitive development. The child whose language or speech development significantly lags behind their cognitive development, given no other medical conditions that would affect language development specifically, should be diagnosed as having a language disorder with treatment provided by an SLP. As mentioned, it should not be relevant to the diagnosis whether the cognitive testing shows a verbal versus nonverbal gap, though this may be good information for the diagnostician and clinician.

Language Disorders Associated with Known Medical Conditions

Language Impairment in Children with Epilepsy

Epilepsy is a neurologic disorder in which the activity of the nerve cells is disrupted causing seizures that result in abnormal behaviors. A seizure is defined as abnormal electrical activity in the brain, with the two main types being either generalized (involving both sides of the brain) or partial (focal) beginning in one part of the brain (and perhaps spreading to generalize). The two main types of generalized seizures are grand mal and petit mal. Recurrent seizures indicate a seizure disorder or epilepsy. Epilepsy can be idiopathic, and there appears to be some genetic influence. It also is often associated with neurologic disorders of childhood such as cerebral palsy, abnormal cortical development, or hippocampal sclerosis. Brain injury often will result in the development of a seizure disorder, and infections that affect the brain can also cause the onset of epilepsy.

The abnormal surges in electrical activity that occur during seizures may disrupt neuronal connections and interfere with the development of new connections. Obviously, a seizure disorder could delay or impair language development in a child. Children with epilepsy are often diagnosed with language impairment, learning disability, and sometimes intellectual disability. About 40% of children with epilepsy have accompanying deficits in attention and may have attention-deficit/hyperactivity disorder. Language outcome is dependent on the presence of comorbidities, age of onset, success of seizure control (usually with drugs), and type and severity of the disorder.

A recent study on children with a focal seizure disorder in the left hemisphere demonstrated the presence of language difficulty and may have contributed to helping us understand normal language development. A group of children, aged 4 to 12 years, who had focal seizures of the left hemisphere were compared with a matched group of healthy children on an auditory decision task and studied with functional MRI (fMRI).[11] The researchers identified eight ROIs in the perisylvian area and performed component analyses on these. In the healthy children the analysis suggested the existence of two functional networks that could be activated and synchronized to accomplish the language task. The ventral network or stream (implying white matter connectivity) was described as consisting primarily of Brodmann areas 45 and 47 in the frontal lobe as well as anterior and middle temporal lobe areas nodes; these areas were found to be tightly synchronized during language tasks in healthy subjects. A dorsal network or stream consisted primarily of Brodmann area 44, the angular gyrus, and a middle temporal node. For the dorsal activations there was also found a tight network synchrony between inferior parietal areas in general, and inferior frontal and temporal areas (mirroring the connections of the arcuate fasciculus).

This study thus supported the functional separation of language systems in the typically developing child. In these children both networks were recruited during the experimental task. The children with focal epilepsy, however, overall showed failure to recruit the ventral network, particularly in the younger children, and this was associated with poorer language performance. The study did not find, as predicted, less functional connectivity in the children with epilepsy compared with the healthy control subjects but did find poor activation of the ventral language network or stream. This ventral network is implicated in semantic processing of sentences and semantic decision making and thus is critical for auditory processing and comprehension. At least for this study, the poor language performance on testing highlights the importance of the ventral network for normal language development and the effect of childhood epilepsy on its continued maturation.

Landau-Kleffner Syndrome

An important but rare cause of acquired language impairment is Landau-Kleffner syndrome (LKS), which is usually associated with sudden onset of difficulty with language development in children for whom the etiology initially may not be clear. The clinical picture in this group is extremely varied. The age of onset of the disorder is generally between 3 and 7 years.[17] The onset of the language disturbance lasts from a few hours or days to more than 6 months. The presence of clinical seizures is reported in only 75% to 80% of children with the syndrome. It is important in diagnosis to have the electroencephalogram (EEG) done while the child is sleeping because the seizure activity most often occurs during slow-wave sleep and may be missed with a routine EEG done on an awake child. The presence of sudden regression or slowing of language development with no known etiology should be a red flag for the presence of subclinical seizure activity, and this testing should be pursued to rule it out. LKS usually affects understanding of spoken language more than expressive, although both expressive and receptive deficits may be present. Adults who appear to have recovered well may still report some difficulty with auditory processing. A brief article by Alpern[1] in The ASHA Leader provides discussion of LKS as well as a link to a video case study for those interested in further exploration.

AUTISM SPECTRUM DISORDER

Until the DSM-5 was released in 2013,[4] the disorder called autistic disorder was just one of five disorders listed under the classification pervasive developmental disorders (PDD). This terminology had been introduced in 1980, and by the time of publication of the DSM-IV it had come to include (1) childhood disintegrative disorder (CDD), (2) Rett syndrome, (3) Asperger syndrome, (4) PDD, not otherwise specified (PDD-NOS), and (5) autism. In the DSM-5, the classification PDD had been replaced with autism spectrum disorder (ASD), subsuming under this category autism, Asperger syndrome, and PDD-NOS, collapsing them into a single diagnosis: ASD. Rett syndrome and CDD were eliminated from this classification. Rett syndrome was eliminated because many symptoms of autism found in a child diagnosed with Rett could be diagnosed with ASD, using a specifier of "with known genetic or medical condition." CDD was taken out because of the differences between it and the other spectrum disorders, especially the severity and acuity of it as well as accompanying symptoms in other systems. It is a rare but devastating disorder from which recovery is typically minimal.

Asperger syndrome was subsumed under ASD because there is little research evidence to separate a person diagnosed with Asperger from one diagnosed with high-functioning ASD. In regard to PDD-NOS, the committee found that the symptoms identified were primarily subthreshold symptoms for the diagnosis of autism and were so vague as to be used in various ways in diagnosis.

Whereas in the DSM-IV there were three subdomains with communication and social interaction being separate domains, the DSM-5 collapsed these two into one. Table 13.5 describes the two domains for ASD and the criteria under each that are recognized for the diagnosis of ASD in the DSM-5.

In 1996 the Centers for Disease Control and Prevention (CDC) began monitoring the prevalence of ASD, initiating it with study among children in metropolitan Atlanta, Georgia. In 2000 the US Congress authorized the Children's

TABLE 13.5 Domains and Domain Criteria for Autism Spectrum Disorder from the DSM-5

Persistent deficits in social communication and social interaction across multiple contexts as manifest by *at least two* of the following: Deficits in social-emotional reciprocity, which may range, for example, from abnormal social approach and failure of normal back-and-forth conversation, to reduced sharing of interests, emotions, or affect, to failure to initiate or respond Deficits in communicative behaviors used for social interaction, ranging, for example, from poorly integrated verbal and nonverbal communication, to abnormalities in eye contact and body language or deficits in understanding and use of gestures, to a total lack of facial expressions and nonverbal communication Deficits in developing, maintaining, and understanding relationships, ranging, for example, from difficulties adjusting behavior to suit various social contexts, difficulties in sharing imaginative play or in making friends, to absence of interest in peers	Restrictive, repetitive patterns of behavior, interests, or activities as manifest by *at least two* of the following, currently or historically: Stereotyped or repetitive motor movements, use of objects or speech (such as simple motor stereotypies, lining up toys or flipping plates, echolalia, idiosyncratic phrases) Insistence on sameness, inflexible adherence to routines or ritualized patterns of verbal or nonverbal behavior (such as extreme distress at small changes, difficulties with transitions, rigid thinking patterns, greeting rituals, need to take same route or eat same food every day) Highly restricted, fixated interests that are abnormal in intensity or focus (such as strong attachment to or preoccupation with unusual objects, excessively circumscribed or perseverative interests)

Modified from Kaufman, W. E. (2012). DSM-5: The new diagnostic criteria for autism spectrum disorders. *Autism Consortium.* https://www.yumpu.com/en/document/view/22806863/dsm-5-the-new-diagnostic-criteria-for-autism-spectrum-disorders.

Health Act of 2000 authorizing the establishment, through the CDC, of the Autism and Developmental Disabilities Monitoring (ADDM) Network. Since that time biennial surveillance tracking of persons diagnosed with ASD has occurred in a network of ADDM monitoring sites in 11 different states. At the time of this writing, the last full report released by the ADDM was from a 2018 study of the data from these 11 sites.[10] Two studies were reported—one surveillance study of children 8 years of age and one of children 4 years of age. The age of 8 was chosen because previous study had shown that most children with ASD had been identified by age 8. The age of 4 was chosen to study the prevalence and characteristics of children identified earlier in life as having or suspected to have ASD.

Data on 4-year-old children began to be collected in 2010, and one of the key findings of the 2018 report was that children with autism were being identified earlier in life. Children born in 2014 were 50% more likely to receive a diagnosis or a special education classification of ASD by age 4 years than were children born in 2010. Differences from earlier network data were also found regarding identification by race and median household income. Data from study of the 4-year-old children found that more Black, Hispanic, and Asian or Pacific Islander children were identified with ASD than were White children. These results were identified as new patterns because the study of 8-year-old children found no such differences. A study of the prevalence of 10 developmental disabilities done using data taken from the National Health Interview Survey of the years 2009 to 2017 was highlighted in the CDC's discussion of ASD. This study, published in *Pediatrics*,[38] using parent-report of diagnosis by a physician or other professional found nonsignificant increase for a diagnosis of stuttering (within the last 12 months) and decreased prevalence for blindness, cerebral palsy, seizures, moderate to profound hearing loss, and other developmental delay. The findings of both studies should be considered positive, suggesting that there has been progress made in these many US communities in regard to awareness, early identification, and access to services for children with ASD and other developmental disabilities.

The CDC states that the critical period for developing autism occurs before, during, or immediately after birth. It is not known what causes autism, but research studies have identified some possible risk factors (Box 13.2).

BOX 13.2 Risk Factors Associated with Autism Spectrum Disorder (ASD)

- Genetic factors
- A sibling with ASD
- Certain genetic or chromosomal conditions such as fragile X or tuberous sclerosis
- Prescription drugs valproic acid or thalidomide taken during pregnancy
- Age of parent: mother age <20 or >40; father age >50; relative risk also increases with increase in age difference between mother and father

---

Neurobiologic Research on Autism

The etiology of ASD is controversial and, as indicated, is unknown. We do know that it has a strong genetic component. In recent years, fMRI has been found to be a useful tool to study neurobiologic function of people with ASD. Dichter[13] provided a comprehensive review of fMRI findings in ASD through 2011. He found that despite the heterogeneity of persons with ASD, several common themes emerged in the studies in regard to brain function. Task-based studies have been performed addressing social perception and cognition with tasks designed around such things as face processing, theory of mind (ability to infer feeling states and/or intentions), cognitive control (go/no-go tasks, task switching, etc.), communication, and reward processing. Dichter[13] reported that fMRI findings during these types of tasks highlighted:

- Hypoactivation during social processing tasks in regions Dichter[13] defines as "nodes" in the "social brain," including the prefrontal cortex, posterior superior temporal sulcus, amygdala, and the fusiform gyrus
- Aberrant frontostriatal activation during cognitive control tasks, including the dorsal prefrontal cortex and the basal ganglia
- Anomalous mesolimbic responses to reward
- For language tasks, findings included decreased lateralization differential, decreased synchrony in brain regions processing language, decreased automaticity of language processing, and recruitment of regions not typically demonstrated to process language
- Functional connectivity studies tend to show decreased connectivity between frontal and posterotemporal regions known to participate actively in processing social-affective information. Some recent studies found both local overconnectivity and distant underconnectivity of social processing regions.

Also briefly reported on by Dichter[13] were structural MRI studies in ASD. He found reports of accelerated brain growth during early development in children with ASD and reports of large head circumference and brain volume. One longitudinal study reported a transient period of postnatal overgrowth of the brain in 70% of children with ASD before age 2; this overgrowth was not present in adolescence or adulthood. Some studies have found a link between increased white matter in the frontal lobe of children with ASD and reduced white matter later in adolescence and adulthood. This is consistent with the FA studies, which have found increased FA in brain areas associated with social processing in young children but reduced FA in adolescents and adults with ASD.

The Dichter[13] review reported that studies of functional connectivity done during a resting state (rather than task-based study) in subjects with ASD found quite contradictory results, with some highlighting reduced connectivity between areas and others finding overconnectivity in similar areas. A 2015 study of subjects with high-functioning ASD sought to explain this inconsistency.[21] Resting-state functional connectivity studies were performed for both inter- and intra-hemispheric connectivity. Adults with high-functioning ASD were compared with matched control subjects. No consistent pattern of connectivity was found in any of the ASD groups compared with control groups. Both increased and decreased connectivity was found. For interhemispheric connectivity, the magnitude of the distortion pattern correlated significantly with behavioral symptoms of ASD. The authors concluded that a neural characteristic of ASD may actually be idiosyncratic connectivity; they hypothesized that this diversity may result from the behavioral disconnection of the person with ASD from the social and environmental factors typically experienced by humans known to shape and regularize typical neural organization.

The heterogeneity of persons with autism is the most consistent aspect of the disorder, and this has been well documented by research and numerous clinical reports. One of the more consistent findings regarding the associated communication disorder is the shift or variability in brain lateralization. Floris et al.,[16] used a technique called normative modeling to attempt to help "dissect the heterogeneity in lateralization" in autism. The authors purpose was to add to scientific knowledge about gray matter stratification as a neural marker for ASD using methodology that could overcome the problem of small sample effects encountered in many studies. They used data from a cohort of 352 subjects with autism and 233 neurotypical subjects involved in the largest European multicenter study on ASD to date in 2017. From this dataset they were able to derive gray matter volume laterality values. They then were able to use normative modeling to find individual deviations from the normal pattern of brain laterality across age (subjects ranged in age from 6–30). A major finding was that both extreme left- and rightward deviations were associated with the presence of a language disorder, but only rightward deviations differentiated between persons with autism with accompanying language disorder and those who had autism but no language disorder. The authors conclude that this atypical rightward lateralization may constitute a biologic marker for the subgroup of persons with autism with language disorder. If this could be used clinically in medical diagnosis, it could be extremely useful as earlier research has suggested that onset of language prior to age 2 and level of language at ages 5 and 6 are predictive of functional outcome later in life for individuals with autism.[27]

Finally, research on the development of disturbances or disruption of neurodevelopmental pathways during embryo development should be highlighted. This is a critical area of investigation as it could lead to better identification of biomarkers for autism and other disease conditions, as well as the development of therapeutics such as pharmaceutic intervention. The explanation and in-depth study of research into signaling pathways in the brain during development is beyond the scope of this text; however, students should be aware of this research and the extraordinary promise of the information it may provide to scientists. A review article by Upadhyay et al.,[34] provides an overview of neurodevelopmental signaling mechanisms in relation to various etiologic factors known to be associated with autism. The significance of alterations to the development of the related pathways is reviewed in regard to knowledge to date at time of publication.

Although we have not identified a cause or a cure for autsim, treatment for the associated behavior, communication, and learning deficits has improved greatly in the past few years as more programs and funding for clinical research have become available. We do not know whether the true incidence of autism has increased or whether medical and allied health professionals are just better at accurately identifying the disorder (or if it is diagnosed inappropriately in a number of cases). It is becoming clear that we must continue to search for the cause(s) and identify preventative measures if possible. Because at this point we do not know how to prevent it, early identification and effective treatment are critical to improve quality of life for those affected.

PEDIATRIC TRAUMATIC BRAIN INJURY: A PUBLIC HEALTH BURDEN

According to the Brain Injury Association of America, the leading cause of death and disability in children and adolescents in the United States is traumatic brain injury (TBI). In 2018, the CDC submitted a congressional report on the management of children with TBI.[10] Data from 2012 indicated that sports and recreation-related injuries were leading causes of emergency department visits among children, with an estimated 325,000 reported that year. Data from a large survey in 2013 were cited finding that in the United States that year, there were approximately 640,000 TBI-related emergency department visits, 18,000 TBI-related hospitalizations, and 1500 TBI-related deaths among children 14 years of age and younger. In the 0- to 14-year age group, the leading cause of emergency department visits, hospitalizations, and deaths were accidental falls and being struck by or against an object. In the 15- to 24-year age group, the leading causes were motor vehicle accidents and falls. Though many in the public think of head injury as an acute problem, the data show that 61% of children with a moderate to severe TBI experience a disability as a result of the injury. Thus, pediatric TBI represents a significant public health burden in this country; SLPs are an important part of the rehabilitation-focused effort for these children.

The mechanism of TBI was discussed in Chapter 10 with the concepts of coup-contrecoup, molecular commotion, and diffuse axonal injury introduced. The same mechanisms are at work when TBI occurs to the immature brain. Examination of early literature on pediatric TBI reveals that physicians and rehabilitation professionals knew little about the actual short- or long-term effects of injury to children of different ages. Until the advent of safe imaging methods that could be used on young children, there was a dearth of research. Although the numbers of children injured each year is large, it is difficult to find large groups of children on which behavioral studies can be designed without a well-coordinated multicenter study. Because of the nature of the mechanism of injury, there is also great heterogeneity among the potential subject groups. Nevertheless, progress has been made in research on children with TBI, altering the way brain injury is treated by medical and rehabilitation professionals and paving the way for future breakthroughs in treatment.

Pathophysiology

An important advance in the study of the effects of TBI has been provided by research detailing the pathophysiology of injury to the immature brain. Different studies supported findings showing that the effect of injury was different in some respects in the developing brain than in the mature brain. A review and discussion of some of these differences[6] found discrepancies in biomechanical properties, aspects of homeostasis, and structural and functional responses to injury when TBI to the developing brain was compared with that of the mature brain. A summary of these differences is found in Box 13.3.

Although neurodegenerative changes after TBI have been well documented in adults, there has not been much study of this change in the pediatric population. A 2014 review of original research attempting to document changes in children and youth after TBI included 16 studies that fit the authors' criteria.[24] These studies, consisting of both cross-sectional and longitudinal designs, found evidence for long-term changes. Volume loss was found in selected brain regions. These included the hippocampus, amygdala, globus pallidus, thalamus, periventricular white matter, cerebellum, and brainstem. A decrease in overall brain volume was found in some studies with increased cerebrospinal fluid and ventricular space. Decreased integrity in the cellular structure of the corpus callosum was noted on DTI studies.

A comprehensive review of the pathophysiology of TBI in pediatric patients was published in 2020 by faculty in the Brain Research Center and the BrainSport Center at UCLA.[29] The principal conclusion that can be deduced from this review is that there continued to be only a small number of research studies done on this population with findings that could only be described as suggestive or promising, needing reduplication or further exploration. This is due to the heterogeneity of the population and the inherent difficulty of doing a well-controlled study on groups of children and adolescents who are injured at different times in their development and through different mechanisms of injury (motor vehicle accidents, abuse, falls, sports injuries, etc). Some of the research cited was performed in a lab using mice and had not yet been translated into research on human brains. Despite the limitations, interesting findings summarized from the studies are worth mentioning here as are the highlighted areas in which the authors suggest that future research is sorely needed. Some of the interesting findings from the summary of research reviewed include:

- The proinflammatory response to brain injury is exaggerated and lasts longer in children than in adults. This may facilitate prolonged inflammation, which can contribute to a myriad of neurologic problems in maturing brains.
- Some studies showed atypical synaptic pruning and increased synaptic density after brain injury in children. Atypical pruning has been related to neurodevelopmental disorders such as schizophrenia, autism, and epilepsy and even to long-term neurodegenerative changes such as Alzheimer disease.
- There may be effects much later such as neurodegenerative changes leading to Parkinson or Alzheimer disease. This interruption could have particular bearing on higher cognitive development if the injury occurs during adolescence when over 50% of synaptic pruning occurs in certain areas of the brain, though overall the effect of delayed or failed pruning is unclear.
- Research suggests that younger TBI victims (children and adolescents) seem to be more vulnerable to consequent social interaction deficits, anxiety, depression, and addiction disorders than adults post-TBI.
- The positive cognitive, behavioral, and immunologic changes engendered by exercise in adolescence appears to have a neuroprotective effect on response to brain injury.
- Given studies on equivalent sports, females appear to be at higher risk for mild TBI and take longer to recover. With more serious injury, however, females seem to recover better with the natural presence of increased progesterone seeming to offer some neuroprotective effects. Males and females also seem to have different symptom complaints with females noting headaches and social impairment while males complain more of balance and cognitive impairment.

Concluding the review, the authors assert the need for more research into pediatric TBI. They cited particular areas of research needed regarding the long-term effects of pituitary and hormonal dysfunction, neural inflammation, and

---

BOX 13.3 Structural and Functional Differences of the Immature Brain that Affect Recovery after Traumatic Brain Injury in Infancy

- Markedly diminished shear resistance due to the following characteristics of the developing brain:
  - Increased water content of the brain tissue
  - Capillary density
  - Cerebral blood volume
  - Reduced extent of myelination
- Reduced brain protection by the immature skull sutures and reduced calcification of the skull, increasing skull elasticity
  - Mechanical load more easily transferred to the brain tissue
  - Causes more cranial distortion and more diffuse pattern of injury

Postinjury Differences Noted in Most Immature Brains versus Adult Brains

- Increased incidence of diffuse brain swelling
- Greater compromise in vasodilation (which would result in vasoconstriction and reduced cerebral blood flow)
- Increased susceptibility to excitotoxicity
  - In developing brain, blockage of N-methyl-d-aspartate receptors induces more rapid apoptosis (programmed cell death)
- Increased dopaminergic activity, altering sensitivity of neurons to excitatory input (in animal models)

BOX 13.4   Acute and Early Postacute Predictors of Poor Outcome in Pediatric Traumatic Brain Injured Patients

- Glasgow Coma Scale score between 3 and 8
- Poor pupillary light reflex
- Hemiparesis
- Hypotension
- Subarachnoid hemorrhage
- Poor rehabilitation

Modified from Tunthanathip, T., & Oearsakul, T. (2021). Application of machine learning to predict the outcome of pediatric traumatic brain injury. *Chinese Journal of Traumatology, 24*(6), 350–355. https://doi.org/10.1016/j.cjtee.2021.06.003; Gray, M. P., Woods, D., & Hadjikoumi, I. (2012). Early access to rehabilitation for paediatric patients with traumatic brain injury. *European Journal of Trauma and Emergency Surgery, 38*(4), 423–431. https://doi.org/10.1007/s00068-012-0177-y.

metabolic dysfunction. Finally, they highlight the fact that there are markers of degeneration that are being identified in patients with TBI and state the need for long-term monitoring of the evolution of these markers in pediatric TBI patients.

Recovery in Pediatric TBI Patients

Box 13.4 lists research-based predictors of poor outcome considering primarily acute and early postacute medically based findings. SLPs who are fortunate enough to have access to medical records may find this knowledge useful in determining prognosis and intensity of treatment. You will note that "poor rehabilitation" is listed as well, however. In many settings, especially outside of trauma centers, children will not have easy access to rehabilitation specialists in the early stages of recovery or even later. Many children have little access to speech-language services until they are later enrolled in school when, as highlighted later, deficits may become obvious. It is vital that SLPs practicing in the school systems understand the deficits related to TBI and appropriate rehabilitation strategies to assist recovery of function.

It is true that the young brain has potential for recovery after injury that is much greater than the adult brain, and better recovery has always been expected from all but the most severe injuries. It had been commonly accepted that the earlier the injury, the better the recovery and that little residual deficit occurred. Studies in the 1980s and 1990s began to show that children with early TBI did appear to do well when language development and behavior were studied in their preschool years. However, when studies began to look at the learning profiles of children with early TBI once they reached the age when reading and other language-based learning skills were critical, the literature began to suggest that perhaps there were brain differences in these children that did not become evident or even suspected until higher-level cognitive-linguistic processing and attentional skills were essential to learning.

Since 1999 there have been a number of studies looking at the effect of TBI on behavior and cognitive-linguistic processing, and a few are cited here. The student using this text

will likely be able to find other studies that add knowledge to what may be happening to the young brain after TBI. It is vital that the SLP, whether serving children in medical centers, school systems, or private practice, understand the possible implications of TBI and advocate for appropriate services for these children and adolescents.

Research on Outcome

Given the increase in the population of children afflicted with TBI, it is not surprising that research targeting acute intervention, long-term outcome, and treatment method is increasing. Researchers in Australia have been particularly active in research on cognitive recovery in pediatric TBI, asking whether the developmental period when the injury occurred may significantly affect recovery and whether there is a relationship between that period and the severity of the injury in regard to residual deficits. In a longitudinal study of 149 children admitted to the Royal Children's Hospital in Melbourne with brain injury, researchers were able to follow the cognitive development through IQ testing (with the revised Wechsler Intelligence Scale for Children or, for the younger children, the Bayley Scales of Infant Development) for 10 years postinjury in children injured after age 3 and for 30 months for those injured before age 3.[3] Groups were divided by age at onset of injury: infant (age <3; $n = 27$); young (3; 0–7; 11; $n = 53$), and old (8; 0–12; 11; $n = 69$). The child's score on admission on the Pediatric Glasgow Coma Scale (GCS) was included as part of the determination of severity of injury. The Pediatric GCS is pictured in Box 13.5. These groups were divided by a categorization of severity of injury: (1) mild defined as GCS score at admission of 13 to 15, no abnormality on computed tomography (CT) or MRI, and no neurologic deficits; (2) moderate: GCS score of 9 to 12 and mass lesion or evidence of specific injury on CT or MRI; and (3) severe: GCS score of 3 to 8 and mass lesion or evidence of pathologic condition on CT or MRI.

Severe Injury Groups

For the young and old groups, the study found a definite relationship between age of injury and severity of injury in the case of severe TBI. Overall, low average IQ (full scale of 82–89) was found for children with TBI after 3 years of age, with performance related to the age of injury as age increased. Better outcomes were found for older children after severe injury. Severe TBI in children injured between ages 8 and 12 found significant increments (similar to adults) in performance in the first 12 months postinjury but then less improvement after a year postinjury. In contrast, flat recovery curves for acute period to 30 months postinjury were found for children injured between ages 3 and 7 with minimal recovery found in any domain (as measured by IQ testing).

Mild to Moderate Injury Groups

In the young and old groups, the IQ testing showed similar postinjury improvement for both mild and moderate severity. With mild TBI after age 3, mean IQs were in the average range (102–104), suggesting minimal effect on this aspect

BOX 13.5   Pediatric Glasgow Coma Scale

Sign	Pediatric Glasgow Coma Scale	Score
Eye opening	Spontaneous	4
	To sound	3
	To pain	2
	None	1
Verbal response	Age-appropriate vocalization, smile, or orientation to sound; interacts (coos, babbles); follows objects	5
	Cries, irritable	4
	Cries to pain	3
	Moans to pain	2
	None	1
Motor response	Spontaneous movements (obeys verbal command)	6
	Withdraws to touch (localizes pain)	5
	Withdraws to pain	4
	Abnormal flexion to pain (decorticate posture)	3
	Abnormal extension to pain (decerebrate posture)	2
	None	1
Best total score		**15**

The Glasgow Coma Scale is scored between 3 and 15, with 3 being the worst and 15 the best. The Pediatric Glasgow Coma Scale was validated in children age ≤2 years.
Modified from: Holmes, J. F., Palchak, M. J., MacFarlane, T., & Kuppermann, N. (2005). Performance of the pediatric Glasgow Coma Scale in children with blunt head trauma. *Academic Emergency Medicine, 12*(9), 814–819.

of recovery. Mean IQ findings for the young and old age groups with moderate severity of injury were lower but still within the average range (94–98). All showed gains above those expected in normal development during the immediate months postinjury, but then the trajectory slowed and stabilized from 12 to 30 months postinjury.

Injury in Children Younger than Age 3 Years

The children injured before age 3 years made up a smaller cohort, and cognitive development was measured with a different instrument. Thus, interpretation of the results had to be taken within a different context. They were followed for 30 months. A different, less positive pattern of recovery was suggested. Although children who sustained mild injury before age 3 continued to improve and did relatively well on the measures, children with moderate or severe brain injury during this early period of life continued to show significant decreases in global intellectual ability at all assessments (acute, 12 months postinjury, and 30 months postinjury).

Although these results need replication, the data certainly suggest that severity of injury and developmental stage when injured should be two of the factors considered significant when making decisions about follow-up for these children. Further study may elucidate whether injury during certain periods of cognitive development slows advancement and stabilization of certain skills or actually prevents growth of those skills over the long term. For those with both risk factors—moderate or severe trauma and young age—long-term clinical follow-up and monitoring, at the least, appear warranted. It is likely that these children, especially those with severe TBI, will need intervention by skilled rehabilitation professionals over a long time to promote the best outcome possible. As SLPs it is our responsibility to advocate for increased funding to meet the needs of these children, enabling the long-term rehab and careful programming and life care that many will need.[14]

WHAT ELSE?

There could be many more disorders of childhood that are associated with language delay/disorder or that place a child at risk for these. Some of those for which language characteristics could be discussed but will be left to your individual research or your professor's assignment are:

- Hearing loss
- Speech impairment
- Down syndrome
- Fetal alcohol syndrome
- Attention-deficit/hyperactivity disorder
- Dyslexia

All of these and other conditions you may encounter in your clinical work are likely to have been found or will be found to show differences in brain development, structure, or function. SLPs should be the professionals assessing the language skills of these children and designing treatment programs. This requires the knowledge you are obtaining now in your reading and coursework as well as ongoing study of the research in the speech-language pathology literature; however, it may also require study of the literature in neurology, other medical professions, imaging, psychology, rehabilitation, and education. The foundation for evidence-based assessment and treatment is widening tremendously.

Clinical Information and Applications for the SLP
- Acquisition of speech and language is clearly tied to physical development and maturation.
- The course of speech-language development is a correlate of cerebral maturation and specialization.
- An index of neurologic development is the change in gross brain weight with age.
- Brain weight triples in the first 24 months of life.
- At 10 years old, the brain achieves 95% of its ultimate weight.
- Children born with agenesis of the corpus callosum show great variability in functional and cognitive development, which may be genetically determined. All should be individually assessed for speech and language because prediction is difficult.
- Medical science is rapidly identifying genetically based developmental disorders that frequently impact speech

and language development. Structural and numeric anomalies in a person's chromosomal makeup result in syndromes due to duplication, deletion, and microdeletion errors. Genetic testing and counseling may be offered to some families on your caseload.

- Myelinogenesis is the neural process of laying down myelin along brain pathways. There are clear differences in the timing and rate of myelinogenesis during development. Most studies support a rough correlation between myelination cycles and speech-language developmental milestones.

- Advances in medicine have resulted in a significant increase in the survival rate of premature infants (prematurity = birth <37 weeks of gestation). The earlier a child is born the more likely it is that white matter injury, identified on imaging as PVL, will have occurred. The children, particularly with very low birthweight, are at much risk for disability due to the subsequent dysmaturation events. There is active research into neuroprotective measures, both pharmaceutic and environmental.

- During critical periods for language development, illness and injury may affect development, but social and environmental factors may also be significant factors in normal development. Household organization and other social areas may warrant consideration.

- Lack of or delay in speech or language development is one of the most sensitive early indicators of intellectual disability.

- The diagnosis of specific language impairment is not in the DSM-5 at ASHA's recommendation. In diagnostics, ASHA recommends that the diagnosis of language disorder be used in order not to exclude children with accompanying disorders that cannot account for the poor language development.

- Cortical and subcortical anomalies are found across many studies of children with developmental language disorders, but there is little consistency in the detailed findings except in the area of the superior temporal gyri. One promising area of research is the identification of differences in levels of particular secreted proteins, neurotrophins, and growth factors.

- Studies of children with focal left hemisphere seizures suggest tight network connectivity of a ventral stream and a dorsal stream supporting normal language development with the seizure activity interrupting activation of the ventral stream, resulting in language impairment.

- The sudden onset of language disturbance or regression without obvious etiology should be a red flag for subclinical seizure activity, possibly identifying a rare disorder called Landau-Kleffner syndrome. EEG studies should be done during sleep to best identify the seizure activity.

- The DSM-5 lists autism spectrum disorder as a category that includes autism, Asperger syndrome, and pervasive developmental disorder, not otherwise specified. Domains for communication and social interaction have been collapsed into one, and it has been determined that autism can be reliably diagnosed as early as age 2 years.

- Autism appears to have a strong genetic component. Imaging and other types of studies find much heterogeneity in this population with continued research critical to finding the cause(s). Some research on lateralization highlights the finding that children with autism and an accompanying language disorder show a rightward shift in brain lateralization compared to children with autism without a finding of language impairment. Individualized assessment and treatment is key.

- TBI occurs most often in the 0- to 4-year and 15- to 19-year age groups, with falls and motor vehicle accidents the most frequent causes of injury.

- Differences in biomechanical, structural, and functional aspects of the developing brain compared with the adult brain make prediction of outcome more difficult. One large longitudinal study in Australia found a definite relationship between severity of injury and age of onset, with younger children more vulnerable to both moderate and severe levels of injury.

- There is a need for further research on the effects of TBI in children with a critical need for study of the effect, especially on learning, of repetitive mild brain injury or concussion.

- There are many childhood conditions that likely alter brain development and cause language delay or impairment. The SLP should be aware of these and of advances in research that may suggest best practice for assessment and treatment of clients with these conditions.

CASE STUDY

B.W., a 5-year-old girl, began her kindergarten year at the local elementary school. Her teacher noted that B.W. was quite hyperactive and could not keep up with the children in her classroom during the simplest of activities. She would often sit alone because the other children were sometimes afraid of her outbursts and tantrums. The teacher noted that B.W.'s appearance seemed to be unusual, with widespread eyes and an almost blank, expressionless face most of the time. B.W. was easily distracted by noises or a new person coming into the room. She appeared to have attention difficulties and did not understand the simplest of abstract expressions. She often took things quite literally. The teacher referred her to the school psychologist. Results of testing revealed an IQ score of 72. Speech therapy evaluation further revealed poor sentence structure, often using only two- to three-word phrases; difficulty with phonics; distractibility; difficulty sharing; and throwing tantrums when she was not permitted to do what she wanted. An individual education plan was written, and B.W. was placed in the self-contained special needs classroom with 2 hours a week in speech-language therapy and 2 hours a week in the elementary learning disability classroom.

Questions for Consideration

1. On the basis of her IQ, would B.W. be classified as a developmentally delayed slow learner or as having mild to moderate intellectual disability?

2. Other than this classification, what are possible additional diagnoses that could be applied to B.W.? Would you suggest referral for any other assessments?

REFERENCES

1. Alpern, C. (2010). Identification and treatment of Landau-Kleffner syndrome. *The ASHA Leader, 15*(11), 34–35.

2. American Psychiatric Association. (2013). *Diagnostic and statistical manual of mental disorders* (5th ed.). Author.

3. Anderson, V., Catroppa, C., Morse, S., Haritou, F., & Rosenfeld, J. (2005). Functional plasticity or vulnerability after early brain injury? *Pediatrics, 116*(6), 1374–1382.

4. Autism and Developmental Disabilities Monitoring Network, Principal Investigators, Centers for Disease Control and Prevention. (2014). Prevalence of autism spectrum disorder among children aged 8 years—autism and developmental disabilities monitoring network, 11 sites, United States, 2010. *Morbidity and Mortality Weekly Report, 63*(2), 1–21.

5. Bartlett, C. W., Hou, L., Flax, J. F., Hare, A., Cheong, S. Y., Fermano, Z., Zimmerman-Bier, B., Cartwright, C., Azaro, M. A., Buyske, S., & Brzustowicz, L. M. (2014). A genome scan for loci shared by autism spectrum disorder and language impairment. *American Journal of Psychiatry, 171*(1), 72–81.

6. Bauer, R. A., & Fritz, H. (2004). Pathophysiology of traumatic injury in the developing brain: An introduction and short update. *Experimental and Toxicologic Pathology, 56*(1–2), 65–73.

7. Bilgiç, A., Ferahkaya, H., Kilinç, İ., & Energin, V. M. (2021). Serum brain-derived neurotrophic factor, glial-derived neurotrophic factor, nerve growth factor and neurotrophin-3 levels in preschool children with language disorder. *Nöro Psikiyatri Arşivi, 58*(2), 128–132. https://www.ncbi.nlm.nih.gov/pmc/articles/PMC9723830/.

8. Bishop, D. V. M., Snowling, M. J., Thompson, P. A., Greenhalgh, T., & the CATALISE-2 consortium. (2017). Phase 2 of CATALISE: A multinational and multidisciplinary Delphi consensus study of problems with language development: Terminology. *The Journal of Child Psychology and Psychiatry, 58*(10), 1068–1080.

9. Buyanova, I. S., & Arsalidou, M. (2021). Cerebral white matter myelination and relations to age, gender, and cognition: A selective review. *Frontiers in Human Neuroscience, 15*(662031), 1–22. https://doi.org/10.3389/fnhum.2021.662031.

10. Centers for Disease Control and Prevention. (2018). *Report to Congress: The management of traumatic brain injury in children.* National Center for Injury Prevention and Control; Division of Unintentional Injury Prevention.

11. Croft, L. J., Baldeweg, T., Sepeta, L., Zimmaro, L., Berl, M. M., & Gaillard, W. D. (2014). Vulnerability of the ventral language network in children with focal epilepsy. *Brain: A Journal of Neurology, 137*(8), 2245–2257.

12. Demir-Lira, Ö. E., Asaridou, S. S., Nolte, C., Small, S. L., & Goldin-Meadow, S. (2021). Parent language input prior to school forecasts change in children's language-related cortical structures during mid-adolescence. *Frontiers in Human Neuroscience, 15*(650152), 1–12. https://doi.org/10.3389/fnhum.2021.650152.

13. Dichter, G. S. (2012). Functional magnetic resonance imaging of autism spectrum disorders. *Dialogues in Clinical Neuroscience, 14*(3), 319–351.

14. eLife. (2021). Scientists identify mechanism linking traumatic brain injury to neurodegenerative disease. *ScienceDaily.* www.sciencedaily.com/releases/2021/06/210601135830.htm.

15. Elitt, C. M., & Rosenberg, P. A. (2014). The challenge of understanding cerebral white matter injury in the premature infant. *Neuroscience, 276*, 216–238. .https://doi.org/10.1016/j.neuroscience.2014.04.038

16. Floris, D. L., & Howells, H. (2018). Atypical structural and functional motor networks in autism. *Progress in Brain Research, 238*, 207–248. https://doi.org/10.1016/bs.pbr.2018.06.010.

17. Foundation Epilepsy. (2013). Landau-Kleffner syndrome. https://www.epilepsy.com/learn/types-epilepsy-syndromes/landau-kleffner-syndrome.

18. Galuske, R. A., Schlote, W., Bratzke, H., & Singer, W. (2000). Interhemispheric asymmetries of the modular structure in human temporal cortex. *Science, 289*(5486), 1946–1949.

19. Geschwind, N. (1979). Anatomical foundations of language and dominance. In C. L. Ludlow & M. E. Doran-Quine (Eds.), *The neurological basis of language in children: Methods and directions for research* (pp. 145–157). National Institutes of Health.

20. Habib, M., & Robichon, F. (2003). Structural correlates of brain asymmetry: Studies in left-handed and dyslexic individuals. In K. Hugdahl & R. J. Davidson (Eds.), *The asymmetrical brain* (pp. 681–705). MIT Press.

21. Hahamy, A., Behrmann, M., & Malach, R. (2015). The idiosyncratic brain: Distortion of spontaneous connectivity patterns in autism spectrum disorder. *Nature Neuroscience, 18*(2), 302–309.

22. Hughes, E. G., & Stockton, M. E. (2021). Premyelinating oligodendrocytes: Mechanisms underlying cell survival and integration. *Frontiers in Cell and Developmental Biology.* https://doi.org/10.3389/fcell.2021.714169.

23. Jakab, A., Kasprian, G., Schwartz, E., Gruber, G. M., Mitter, C., Prayer, D., Schöpf, V., & Langs, G. (2015). Disrupted developmental organization of the structural connectome in fetuses with corpus callosum agenesis. *NeuroImage, 111*, 277–288.

24. Keightley, M. L., Sinopoli, K. J., Davis, K. D., Mikulis, D. J., Wennberg, R., Tartaglia, M. C., Chen, J.-K., & Tator, C. H. (2014). Is there evidence for neurodegenerative change following traumatic brain injury in children and youth? A scoping review. *Frontiers in Human Neuroscience, 8*, 139. https://doi.org/10.3389/Fnhum.2014.00139.

25. Lenneberg, E. (1967). *Biological foundations of language.* Wiley.

26. Liégeois, F., Mayes, A., & Morgan, A. (2014). Neural correlates of developmental speech and language disorders: Evidence from neuroimaging. *Current Developmental Disorders Reports, 1*(3), 215–227.

27. Mayo, J., Chlebowski, C., Fein, D. A., & Eigsti, I. M. (2013). Age of first words predicts cognitive ability and adaptive skills in children with ASD. *Journal of Autism and Developmental Disorders, 43*(2), 253–264. .https://doi.org/10.1007/s10803012-1558-0

28. National Institute on Deafness and Other Communication Disorders. (2011). Developmental Language Disorder. http://www.nidcd.nih.gov/health/voice/pages/specific-language-impairment.aspx.

29. Serpa, R. O., Ferguson, L., Larson, C., Bailard, J., Cooke, S., Greco, T., & Prins, M. L. (2021). Pathophysiology of pediatric traumatic brain injury. *Frontiers in Neurology, 12*, 696510. https://doi.org/10.3389/fneur.2021.696510.

30. Su, P., Kuan, C.-C., Kaga, K., Sano, M., & Mima, K. (2008). Myelination progression in language-correlated regions in brain of normal children determined by quantitative MRI assessment. *International Journal of Pediatric Otorhinolaryngology, 72*(12), 1751–1763. https://doi.org/10.1016/j.ijporl.2008.05.017.

31. Tallal, P., Ross, R., & Curtiss, S. (1989). Familial aggregation in specific language impairment. *Journal of Speech and Hearing Disorders, 54*(2), 167–173.

32. Tomasch, J. (1954). Size, distribution, and number of fibres in the human corpus callosum. *The Anatomical Record, 119*(1), 119–135.

33. Tooley, U. A., Bassett, D. S., & Mackey, A. P. (2021). Environmental influences on the pace of brain development. *Nature Reviews Neuroscience, 22*(6), 372–384. https://doi.org/10.1038/s41583-021-00457-5.

34. Upadhyay, J., Patra, J., Tiwari, N., Salankar, N., Ansari, M. N., & Ahmad, W. (2021). Dysregulation of multiple signaling neuro-developmental pathways during embryogenesis: A possible cause of autism spectrum disorder. *Cells, 10*(4), 958–981. https://doi.org/10.3390/cells10040958.

35. Vernon-Feagans, L., Garrett-Peters, P., Willoughby, M., Mills-Koonce, R., et al. (2012). Chaos, poverty, and parenting: Predictors of early language development. *Early Childhood Research Quarterly, 27*(3), 339–351.

36. Volpe, J. J. (2019). Dysmaturation of premature brain: Importance, cellular mechanisms, and potential interventions. *Pediatric Neurology, 95*, 42–66. https://doi.org/10.1016/j.pediatrneurol.2019.02.016.

37. Wada, J. A., Clark, R., & Hamm, A. (1975). Cerebral hemispheric asymmetry in humans: Cortical speech zones in 100 adult and 100 infant brains. *Archives of Neurology, 32*(4), 239–246.

38. Zablotsky, B., Black, L. I., Maenner, M. J., Schieve, L. A., Danielson, M. L., Bitsko, R. H., Blumberg, S.J., Kogan, M. D., & Boyle, C. A. (2019). Prevalence and trends of developmental disabilities among children in the United States: 2009-2017. *Pediatrics, 144*(4), 1–11. https://doi.org/10.1542/peds.2019–0811.

Medical Conditions Related to Communication Disorders

I. Congenital Disorders
   A. *Autism spectrum disorder:* a broad range of conditions characterized by challenges with social skills, repetitive behaviors, speech, and nonverbal communication. Some cases of autism result from known genetic causes, while the cause in many other cases has yet to be identified.
   B. *Cerebral palsy:* defect of motor power and coordination related to damage of the immature brain
   C. *Congenital hydrocephalus:* condition marked by excessive accumulation of fluid, dilating the cerebral ventricles, thinning the brain, and causing a separation of cranial bones; caused by a developmental defect of the brain
   D. *Craniostenosis:* contraction of the cranial capacity or narrowing of the sutures by bony overgrowth
   E. *Down syndrome:* syndrome of intellectual disability associated with many and variable abnormalities, caused by representation of at least a critical portion of chromosome 21 three times instead of twice in some or all cells
   F. *Idiopathic intellectual disability:* intellectual disability of unknown cause
   G. *Minimal cerebral dysfunction:* syndrome of neurologic dysfunction in children usually marked by impairment of fine coordination, clumsiness, and choreiform or athetoid movements; learning disorders often associated with this diagnosis
   H. *Neurofibromatosis:* condition in which small, discrete, pigmented skin lesions develop in infancy or early childhood, followed by the development of multiple subcutaneous neurofibromas that may slowly increase in number and size over many years

II. Vascular Disorders
   A. *Cerebral embolism:* obstruction or occlusion of a vessel in the cerebrum by a transported clot or vegetation, a mass of bacteria, or other foreign material
   B. *Cerebral hemorrhage:* bleeding in the brain; a flow of blood, especially if profuse, into the substance of the cerebrum, usually in the region of the internal capsule; caused by rupture of the lenticulostriate artery
   C. *Cerebral thrombosis:* obstruction or occlusion of a vessel in the cerebrum by a fixed clot developing on the arterial wall
   D. *Pseudobulbar palsy:* muscular paralysis from bilateral upper motor neuron lesions of the cranial nerves; often accompanied by signs of dysarthria, dysphagia, and emotional lability with outbursts of uncontrolled crying and laughing
   E. *Recurrent cerebral ischemia or transient ischemic attacks:* temporary disruptions of the blood supply that produce specific neurologic signs; experienced as sudden, transient blurring of vision, weakness, numbness of one side, speech difficulty, vertigo or diplopia, or any combination
   F. *Subdural hemorrhage:* extravascularization of blood between the dural and arachnoid membranes

III. Infections
   A. *Acute anterior poliomyelitis:* inflammation of the anterior cornu of the spinal cord due to an acute infectious disease marked by fever, pains, and gastroenteric disturbances; followed by flaccid paralysis of one or more muscular groups and later by atrophy
   B. *Cerebral abscess:* intracranial abscess or abscess of the brain, specifically of the cerebrum; a collection of pus in a localized area
   C. *Covid-19 and long Covid:* viral infection caused by the SARS-CoV-2 acute respiratory virus, which caused a global pandemic beginning in early 2020. An estimated 85% of patients with severe infection reported neurologic symptoms. Long Covid is the name given to the chronic phase following recovery from the respiratory symptoms; the symptoms of long Covid often include brain fog, which could include difficulty with verbal memory, naming, executive functions, and processing speed.
   D. *Encephalitis:* inflammation of the brain
   E. *Human immunodeficiency virus (HIV):* a virus spread through contact with certain body fluids, attacking the body's T cells, which are specialized cells that help the immune system fight infection; untreated, the number of T cells is reduced to the point that opportunistic infections and diseases can occur, signaling the onset of acquired immune deficiency syndrome (AIDS)
   F. *Jakob-Creutzfeldt disease:* spastic pseudosclerosis with corticostriatospinal degeneration and subacute presenile dementia; characterized by slowly progressive dementia, myoclonic fasciculations, ataxia, and somnolence with gradual onset; usually fatal within a few months to years

G. *Meningitis:* inflammation of the membranes of the brain or spinal cord

H. *Neurosyphilis:* syphilis, an infectious venereal disease caused by a microorganism affecting the nervous system

I. *Sydenham chorea:* acute toxic or infective disorder of the nervous system, usually associated with acute rheumatism, occurring in young persons and characterized by involuntary semipurposeful but ineffective movements; movements involve the facial muscles and muscles of the neck and limbs and are intensified by voluntary effort but disappear in sleep

IV. Trauma

A. *Penetrating head injury:* open head injury, which causes altered consciousness and can produce fairly definitive and chronic aphasias

B. *Closed-head injury:* injury to the head with no injury to the skull or injury limited to an undisplaced fracture; also known as nonpenetrating head injury; can produce loss of consciousness and often produces diffuse effects

V. Tumors

A. *Astrocytomas (grades 1 and 2) and oligodendrogliomas:* less common glial cell tumors, with a better prognosis than glioblastoma multiforme; slow growing; usually treated with surgery and radiation therapy, with an average survival rate of 5 to 6 years after surgery

B. *Glioblastoma multiforme:* also known as malignant glioma or astrocytoma (grades 3 and 4), the most common primary brain tumor in adults; most frequent sites are frontal and temporal lobes, although tumors may occur anywhere in the brain; infiltrative and rapidly growing, with an average survival rate of ~1 year

C. *Meningioma:* benign tumor arising from the arachnoid cells of the brain; slow growing and usually occurring at the lateral areas and base of the brain; generally does not invade the cerebral cortex; favorable prognosis

VI. Degenerative Diseases

A. *Alzheimer disease:* progressive mental deterioration with loss of memory, especially for recent events

B. *Parkinson disease:* degenerative disease resulting from damage to the dopamine-producing nerve cells of the striatum and the substantia nigra; characterized by rest tremor, rigidity of muscles, paucity of movement, slowness of movement, limited range, limited force of contraction, and failure of gestural expression

C. *Wilson disease:* genetic metabolic disorder caused by inadequate processing of dietary intake of copper and characterized by motor symptoms, with a significant dysarthria

D. *Huntington chorea:* chronic progressive hereditary disease characterized by irregular, spasmodic, involuntary movements of the limbs or facial muscles; sometimes accompanied by dementia and dysarthria

E. *Friedreich ataxia:* hereditary disease characterized by degeneration principally of the cerebellum and dorsal half of the spinal cord; ataxic dysarthria often an accompanying sign

F. *Dystonia musculorum deformans:* hereditary disease occurring especially in children; characterized by muscular contractions producing peculiar distentions of the spine and hip and bizarre postures

G. *Multiple sclerosis:* inflammatory disease mainly involving the white matter of the central nervous system; characterized by scattered areas of demyelination causing impairment of transmission of nerve impulses; may cause a variety of symptoms, including paralysis, nystagmus, and dysarthria depending on the lesion sites

VII. Metabolic and Toxic Disorders

A. *Reye syndrome:* sudden loss of consciousness in children following the initial stage of an infection, usually resulting in death with cerebral edema (swelling) and marked fatty change in the liver and renal system; surviving children often have motor, cognitive, and speech problems

VIII. Neuromuscular Disorders

A. Progressive muscular atrophies

1. *True bulbar palsy:* disorder caused by involvement of nuclei of the last four or five cranial nerves and characterized by twitching and atrophy (of the tongue, palate, and larynx), drooling, dysarthria, dysphagia, and finally respiratory paralysis; usually a manifestation of amyotrophic lateral sclerosis

2. *Amyotrophic lateral sclerosis:* disease of the motor tracts of the lateral columns of the spinal cord causing progressive muscular atrophy, increased reflexes, fibrillary twitching, and spastic irritability of muscles

B. Muscular dystrophy

1. *Pseudohypertrophic (Duchenne) type:* type of muscular dystrophy characterized by bulky calf and forearm muscles and progressive atrophy and weakness of the thigh, hip, and back muscles and shoulder girdle; occurs in the first 3 years of life, usually in boys and rarely in girls

2. *Facioscapulohumeral type:* type of muscular dystrophy causing atrophy of the muscles of the face, shoulder, girdle, and upper arms; occurs in either sex, with onset at any age from childhood to late adult life; characterized by prolonged periods of apparent arrest

3. *Ocular myopathy:* type of muscular dystrophy affecting external ocular muscles, causing ptosis, diplopia, and occasional total external ophthalmoplegia; sometimes associated with upper facial

muscle weakness, dysphagia, and atrophy and weakness of neck, trunk, and limb muscles

C. *Myasthenia gravis:* disorder characterized by marked weakness and fatigue of muscles, especially those muscles innervated by bulbar nuclei

D. Congenital neuromuscular disorders

　1. *Möbius syndrome:* congenital disorder characterized by paresis or paralysis of both lateral rectus muscles and all face muscles; sometimes associated with other musculoskeletal anomalies

IX.　Other

A. *Delirium:* acute fluctuating consciousness, with sudden confusion developing rapidly and fluctuating during the day; dangerous if untreated, it often co-occurs with other medical conditions, such as dementia or high fever; inattention, disorganized thinking (incoherence), and perceptual disturbances are frequent symptoms; may be manifested as hyperactive and hypoactive (in hyperactive state, patients demonstrate agitation or even aggressiveness, and in hypoactive state, patients may appear drowsy and be slow to respond); the hypoactive condition is more dangerous as the delirium may not be detected early enough for appropriate medical management

B. *Epilepsy:* chronic disorder characterized by paroxysmal attacks of brain dysfunction (seizures) usually associated with some alteration of consciousness; seizures may remain confined to elementary or complex impairment of behavior or may progress to a generalized convulsion

C. *Wernicke-Korsakoff syndrome:* cerebral disorder characterized by confusion and severe impairment of memory, especially for recent events; patient compensates for memory loss by confabulation; often seen in chronic alcoholics and associated with severe nutritional deficiency

B APPENDIX

Bedside Neurologic Examination

1. Mental Status
   A. Orientation: person, place, time
   B. Memory and information
      1. Three objects at 5 min
      2. Recall of recent global event or recent holiday
   C. Language
      1. Spontaneous speech characterization
      2. Confrontation naming
      3. Auditory comprehension (commands, yes/no questions)
      4. Repetition (words, phrases)
      5. Reading (printed commands)
      6. Writing (signature, words, and sentences to dictation)
   D. Calculations
      1. Serial 7s (count by 7s to 100)
      2. Subtract $0.43 from $1.00
   E. Visuospatial ability
      1. Clock drawing
      2. Copying of figures
   F. Insight, judgment
2. Cranial Nerves
   A. I: smell
   B. II: visual fields, pupillary reactions, optic fundi
   C. III–IV: extraocular movements
   D. V: facial sensation
   E. VI: facial symmetry
   F. VII: hearing
   G. VIII and IX: articulation, palatal movement, gag reflex
   H. X: sternomastoid and trapezius strength
   I. XI: tongue movement
3. Motor Examination
   A. Bulk
   B. Spontaneous movements (fasciculations, tremor, movement disorders)
   C. Strength
      1. Evaluation of strength on right and left
         a. Deltoid
         b. Biceps
         c. Triceps
         d. Hip flexion
         e. Knee flexion
         f. Ankle dorsiflexion
         g. Ankle plantar flexion
   D. Reflexes
      1. Evaluation of reflexes on right and left
         a. Biceps
         b. Triceps
         c. Brachioradialis
         d. Ankle
         e. Plantar
         f. Jaw
   E. Stance and Romberg
   F. Gait
      1. Spontaneous gait
      2. Tandem gait
      3. Tiptoe gait
      4. Heel gait
   G. Sensory Examination
      1. Pinprick
      2. Touch
      3. Vibration
      4. Position
      5. Stereognosis, graphesthesia (cortical sensory modalities)
   H. Cerebellar
      1. Finger-nose-finger
      2. Rapid alternating hand movements
      3. Fine finger movements
      4. Heel-knee-shin

Courtesy Howard Kirshner, MD, Department of Neurology, Vanderbilt University School of Medicine, Nashville, TN.

Screening Neurologic Examination for Speech-Language Pathology

I. Mental Status
   A. *General behavior and appearance:* Is the patient normal, hyperactive, agitated, quiet, immobile? Neat, slovenly? Is the patient dressed in accordance with peers, background, and sex?
   B. *Stream of talk:* Does the patient respond to conversation normally? Is the patient's speech rapid, incessant, under great pressure? Is the patient very slow and difficult to draw into spontaneous talk? Is the patient discursive, unable to reach the conversational goal?
   C. *Mood and affective responses:* Is the patient euphoric, agitated, inappropriately cheerful, giggling? Or silent, weeping, angry? Does the patient's mood swing in a direction appropriate to the subject matter of the conversation? Is the patient emotionally labile?
   D. *Content of thought:* Does the patient have illusions, hallucinations, delusions, or misinterpretations? Is the patient preoccupied with bodily complaints, fears of cancer or disease, or other phobias? Does the patient believe that society is maliciously organized to cause difficulty?
   E. *Intellectual capacity:* Is the patient bright, average, slow, intellectually disabled, obviously demented?
   F. *Sensorium*
      1. *Consciousness:* Note whether the patient is alert, drowsy, or stuporous.
      2. *Attention span:* Note response in cerebral function test.
      3. *Orientation:* Note whether the patient can answer questions about own person, location, and time.
      4. *Memory:* Note recent and remote memory deficits disclosed during history taking.
      5. *Fund of information:* Note in history taking.
      6. *Insight, judgment, and planning:* Note in history taking.
      7. *Calculation:* Note performance on cerebral function test.

II. Speech, Language, and Voice
   A. *Dysphonia:* neuromotor difficulty in producing voice (cranial nerve X)
   B. *Dysarthria:* neuromotor disorder of articulation and voice
      1. *Labials* (cranial nerve VII)
      2. *Velars and velopharyngeal closure* (IX and X)
      3. *Linguals* (XII)
   C. *Dysphasia:* cerebral disorder of understanding and expressing language (give aphasia-screening test)
      1. *Fluent* (give screening aphasia test)
      2. *Nonfluent* (give screening aphasia test)
   D. *Dyspraxia:* cerebral disorder of articulation and prosody and/or disorder of oral movement
      1. *Dyspraxia of speech*
      2. *Oral dyspraxia*
   E. *Dementia:* cerebral disorder of language or intellectual deficit
      1. *Presenile*
      2. *Senile*
   F. *Disorganized language:* cerebral disorder of language or confusion
   G. *Dysphagia:* neuromotor disorder of swallowing (V, VII, IX, X, and XII)

III. Cranial Nerves for Speech and Hearing
   A. *Speech* (V, VII, IX, X, XI, and XII)
      1. *V:* Inspect masseter and temporalis muscle bulk; palpate masseter when the patient bites.
      2. *VII:* Evaluate forehead wrinkling, eyelid closure, mouth retraction, whistling or puffed out cheeks, wrinkled skin over neck (platysma), and labial articulation.
      3. *IX and X:* Evaluate phonation, hypernasality, swallowing, gag reflex, and palatal elevation.
      4. *XII:* Evaluate lingual articulation and midline and lateral tongue protrusion; inspect for atrophy and fasciculations.
      5. *XI:* Inspect sternocleidomastoid and trapezius contours; test strength of head movements and shoulder shrugging.
      6. Test for pathologic fatigability by requesting 100 repetitive movements (e.g., eye blinks) if the history suggests myopathic or myoneural disorder.
   B. *Hearing* (VIII)
      1. Evaluate for threshold and acuity, including adequacy of hearing for conversational speech.
      2. If history or preceding observation suggests a deficit, perform air-bone conduction audiometric screening.

IV. Motor System
   A. *Inspection*
      1. Take history, including initial appraisal of the motor system; inspect the patient for postures,

general activity level, tremors, and involuntary movements.

2. Observe the size and contour of the muscles, looking for atrophy, hypertrophy, body asymmetry, joint misalignments, fasciculations, tremors, and involuntary movements.

3. Evaluate gait, including free walking, tandem walking, and deep knee bend.

B. *Palpation*: Palpate muscles if they seem atrophic or hypertrophic or if the history suggests they may be tender or in spasm.

C. *Strength*

1. *Upper extremities*: Test biceps.

2. *Lower extremities*: Test knee flexors and foot dorsiflexors if necessary and feasible.

3. *Pattern*: Discern whether any weakness follows a distributional pattern, such as proximal-distal, right-left, or upper extremity-lower extremity.

D. *Muscle tone*: Move the patient's joints to test for spasticity, clonus, or rigidity.

E. *Muscle stretch (deep) reflexes*: Test jaw jerk (cranial nerve V afferent and efferent) as well as other muscle stretch reflexes if necessary and feasible.

F. *Cerebellar system* (gait tested previously)

1. Evaluate finger-to-nose, rebound, and alternating motion rates.

2. Carry out heel-to-knee testing.

V. Sensory Examination

A. Test superficial sensation by light touch with cotton wisp and pinprick on face.

B. Ask if the face feels numb.

C. Test superficial sensation on the tongue surface with swab stick unilaterally and bilaterally, anteriorly and posteriorly.

VI. Cerebral Function

A. When the history or antecedent examination suggests a cerebral lesion, test for finger agnosia and right-left disorientation.

B. Have the patient perform the cognitive, constructional, and performance tasks from standard aphasia or neuropsychological tests.

Data from DeMeyer, W. (1980). *Technique of the neurologic examination*. McGraw-Hill.

abducens cranial nerve VI, which supplies motor impulses to abduct the eye.

abduction movement of a body part away from the midline.

absolute refractory period the short period of membrane unresponsiveness during the passage of an action potential; another action potential cannot be generated during this time.

acceleration-deceleration injury type of injury in which the head is accelerated and then suddenly stopped (e.g., that which occurs in a motor vehicle accident).

acquired childhood aphasia language disorder in which cerebral insult halts or disturbs normal language development in a child.

action potential (AP) buildup of electrical current in the neuron.

action tremor rhythmic, oscillatory, involuntary movement affecting the outstretched upper limbs as well as other parts of the body and the voice; also known as essential tremor, heredofamilial tremor.

ADA Americans with Disabilities Act. Passed by Congress in 1990, the ADA is the law that protects the rights of people with disabilities in many areas of public life.

adduction movement of a body part toward midline.

adequate stimulus a mechanical, thermal, electrical, or chemical stimulus strong enough to change the cell membrane's potential.

adiadochokinesia inability to perform rapid, alternating muscle movements; see *dysdiadochokinesia*.

afferent traveling toward a center.

afferent fibers nerve fibers that carry information toward the cell body; often used to denote sensory fibers.

agnosia lack of sensory recognition as the result of a lesion in the sensory association areas or association pathways of the brain.

agraphia acquired disorder of writing caused by brain injury.

akinesia absence or lack of movements.

alexia acquired disturbance of reading caused by brain injury.

alexia with agraphia classic neurologic syndrome of reading disorder in which damage has occurred to the angular gyrus and the surrounding areas.

alexia without agraphia classic neurologic syndrome of reading disorder, usually caused by a left posterior cerebral artery occlusion in a right-handed person; the resulting infarct produces lesions in the splenium of the corpus callosum and the left occipital lobe.

allocortex the older, original part of the cerebral cortex.

alpha motor neurons (AMNs) neurons allowing contraction of extrafusal fibers and that have their final common path in cranial and spinal nerves.

altered mental status (AMS) a general term used to describe various disorders of mental functioning ranging from slight confusion to coma; language is typically irrelevant or confabulatory and is secondary to the cognitive symptom of confusion.

Alzheimer disease (AD) the most common type of dementia; its most striking feature is progressive deterioration of cognitive functions; language disturbance is a major symptom.

amyloid plaques axonal endings associated with pathologic deposits of extracellular beta-amyloid; found in the brain of patients with dementia of the Alzheimer type.

amyotrophic lateral sclerosis (ALS) a progressive, fatal motor neuron disease usually involving both the upper and lower motor neuron pathways; also known as Lou Gehrig disease.

analgesia loss of the sensation of pain

anarthria a severe dysarthria that prevents people from articulating speech.

anastomosis a connection between two vessels; an opening created by surgery, trauma, or pathologic condition between two spaces or organs that are normally separate.

anencephaly absence of the cranial vault at birth with the cerebral hemispheres completely absent or reduced to small masses attached to the base of the skull.

anesthesia loss of feeling or sensation.

aneurysm a sac formed by the dilation of the wall of an artery, a vein, or the heart.

angular gyrus convolution in the left parietal lobe that is critical for language processing.

anion an ion carrying a negative charge as a result of a surplus of electrons.

anomia loss of the power to name objects or recognize and recall their names.

anomic aphasia an acquired disorder of language caused by brain damage in which the primary difficulty is with word retrieval.

anosognosia An inability refusal to recognize A defect or disorder that is clinically relevant.

anoxia condition marked by the absence of oxygen supply to organs or tissue.

anterior for anatomic structures, denoting before, in front of, or the front part of.

anterior (ventral) horn cell cell in the ventral portion in an H-shaped body of gray matter in the spinal cord associated with efferent pathways.

anterior spinothalamic tract the uncrossed fibers of the spinothalamic tract, which carry sensations of light or crude touch.

anterograde transport of axons from the cell body toward the axon terminal.

aphasia acquired disorder of language caused by brain damage; may affect comprehension or expression of language in any modality (spoken, written, or gestural language).

aphasic alexia a disorder of reading caused by brain damage; the reading disorder is part of the overall aphasia syndrome (e.g., the reading disorder associated with Wernicke aphasia).

aphemia an obsolete term for loss of the power of speech.

apoptosis the death of cells occurring as a normal and controlled part of the process of growth and development.

apraxia a disorder of learned movement distinct from paralysis, weakness, and incoordination; results in a disturbance of motor planning.

apraxia of speech disorder of programming the muscles of articulation in the absence of paralysis, weakness, and incoordination.

aprosodia abnormal prosody (stress and intonation pattern in speech), usually resulting from damage to the nondominant hemisphere.

aqueduct of Sylvius small tube or outlet in the midbrain connecting the third and fourth ventricles.

arachnoid granulations these are small protrusions of the arachnoid mater into the the dura mater to return CSF to the bloodstream.

arachnoid mater a thin membranous covering (meninges) of the brain and spinal cord that lies between the dura mater and the pia mater.

arcuate fasciculus long subcortical association tract connecting posterior and anterior speech-language areas in the cerebrum.

areflexia lacking normal reflexive response to an adequate stimulus.

arteriosclerosis a chronic disease characterized by abnormal thickening and hardening of the arterial walls, with resulting loss of elasticity.

arteriovenous malformation (AVM) congenital morphologic defect resulting in an abnormal cluster of arteries directly connecting to veins; often enlarges over time and is at risk of rupture.

Asperger's syndrome a developmental disorder characterized by impaired social and occupational skills; normal language (excluding pragmatics) and cognitive development; and restricted, repetitive, and stereotyped patterns of behavior, interests, and activities; often found to show above-average performance in a narrow field against a general background of deficient functioning. This disorder is no longer in the DSM, as it has been incorporated under Autism Spectrum Disorders.

association cortex the regions of cortical tissue that conduct complex processing of inputs from primary areas.

association fiber tracts the fiber bundles that form connections between and within the association areas of the brain.

astereognosis   loss of the ability to recognize objects through touch alone; caused by brain damage.

astrocyte   a type of glial cell with numerous sheetlike processes extending from its body that are thought to provide nutrients for neurons and may have some information storage function.

asymmetrical tonic neck reflex (ATNR)   a reflex, normal in the newborn, that consists of extension of the arm and sometimes of the leg on the side to which the head is forcibly turned, with flexion of the contralateral limbs; considered abnormal if found beyond the eighth or ninth month of age in a term infant.

asymmetry   disproportion or inequality between two corresponding parts around the center of an axis.

asynergia   lack of coordination in agonistic and antagonistic muscles that manifests as a deterioration of smooth, complex movements.

asynergy   lack of coordination of agonistic and antagonistic muscles, particularly associated with cerebellar disorders.

ataxia   defect of posture and gait associated with a disorder of the nervous system; sensory ataxia, associated with dorsal column dysfunction, is distinguished from cerebellar or cerebellar pathway ataxia.

ataxic cerebral palsy   a relatively uncommon type of cerebral palsy resulting from damage to the cerebellum; characterized by hypotonic muscles and an ataxic gait pattern.

ataxic dysarthria   the motor speech disorder associated with damage to the cerebellum and/or its pathways; characterized by irregular articulatory breakdown, prosodic changes, and often a slow rate.

athetoid cerebral palsy   the most common dyskinetic type of cerebral palsy characterized by delayed motor development and involuntary, uncontrolled writhing movements.

athetosis   a neurologic disorder marked by continual, slow movements, especially of the extremities.

atopognosis   loss of the power to locate touch sensation correctly; usually caused by damage to the parietal lobe.

ATP   adenotriphosphate (ATP) is a neurotransmitter that is synthesized in the mitochondria and which is important for muscle contraction, nerve impulse transmission, and protein synthesis.

atrophy   decrease in size or wasting of a body part or tissue.

attention-deficit/hyperactivity disorder   a condition that usually becomes identifiable in children in the preschool to early childhood years (and may persist into adulthood) in which three types of behavior or primary symptoms may be identified: inattentiveness; impulsiveness with hyperactivity; or a combination of these with inattentiveness, impulsiveness, and hyperactivity prominent.

audition   hearing.

auditory agnosia   inability to recognize the significance of sounds.

auditory brainstem response (ABR)   a type of electrophysiologic audiometry in which electrical activity is evoked by brief click stimuli from the eighth cranial nerve and the brainstem; allows inference of hearing and identification of the site of lesion as the cochlea, cranial nerve VIII, or the brainstem.

autism   major developmental disability marked by disturbed stereotyped behavior and language patterns; echolalic verbal behavior is often present, as are neurologic signs.

autism spectrum disorder (ASD)   a neurodevelopmental disorder affecting social communication and pattern of behavior. In 2013, the diagnostic criteria for ASD were changed to (1) demonstration in the past or the present of deficits in social emotional reciprocity, deficits in nonverbal communication for social interaction, and deficits in developing, maintaining, and understanding relationships and (2) presence of at least two types of repetitive patterns of behavior including but not limited to stereotyped or repetitive motor movements, highly restricted fixed interests, inflexible requirement for routines, or hypo- or hyperreactivity to sensory input. Severity is rated based on the level of support the individual requires. Eliminated in the 2013 changes were the previously used subcategories such as Asperger and PDD-NOS.

autoassociator network   network used in simulations of behavior in which every unit in the network is connected to every other unit, with associations stored within a layer of neurons.

autonomic nervous system   a part of the vertebrate nervous system that innervates smooth and cardiac muscle and glandular tissues and governs involuntary actions (e.g., secretion, vasoconstriction, or peristalsis); includes the sympathetic nervous system and the parasympathetic nervous system.

axon   a straight, relatively unbranched process of a nerve cell; literally defined as the axis.

axon hillock   the specialized junction connecting the soma of a neuron to the axon and which is important in voltage changes and action potentials.

axonal regeneration   regrowth of damaged axons.

axoplasm   the protoplasm of an axon.

Babinski sign   a reflex movement; when the sole of the foot is tickled, the great toe turns upward instead of downward; normal in infancy but indicates damage to the central nervous system (as in the pyramidal tracts) when occurring later in life; also known as Babinski, Babinski reflex.

basal ganglia   subcortical structures, part of the extrapyramidal system, associated with motor control of tone and posture.

basilar membrane   this membrane is the main mechanical element of the inner ear, composed of a graded stiffness over its length,

which separates sounds into their component frequencies.

behavioral neurology   a specialty in neurology emphasizing clinical and research skills in neurodegenerative diseases and neurobehavioral syndromes.

bilateral   related to or having two sides.

bilateral innervation   supply of nerves from both sides of the body.

bilateral symmetry   movements on one side of the body that mirror movements on the opposite side.

bilingual   the ability to understand and converse in more than one language.

bipolar cell   first-order nerve cell of the retina, synapsing with the ganglion cells.

bite reflex   rapid closure of the jaw and a bite response on moderate pressure to the gums; normal in infants up to 9 to 12 months of age.

blood-brain barrier   this barrier prevents toxins and other pathogens from being released into brain tissue via the circulatory system. The barrier is composed of tight junctions around blood vessels.

border zone   the limit of the cerebral area served by either the anterior, middle, or posterior cerebral arteries.

bouton   a synaptic knob; from French, meaning "button."

brain scan   a neurodiagnostic tool using a radioisotope to detect damaged brain tissue.

brainstem   the part of the brain connecting the spinal cord to the forebrain and cerebrum; contains the medulla oblongata, pons, and mesencephalon (midbrain).

branchial   of or relating to gills or to parts of the body derived from the embryonic branchial arches and clefts.

Broca (expressive) aphasia   acquired adult language disorder characterized by nonfluent speech and language; usually accompanied by hemiplegia and an anterior lesion of the brain.

Broca area   major speech-language center in the dominant frontal lobe; important for expression of language.

callosal dysgenesis   defective development of the corpus callosum.

capsular   referring to the internal capsule.

Carl Wernicke   scientific pioneer (1848–1905) who identified an auditory speech center in the temporal lobe associated with comprehension of speech.

cation   a positively charged ion.

caudal   situated in or directly toward the hind part of the body.

caudate nucleus (CN)   this nucleus is a paired, C-shaped structure deep in the brain and close to the thalamus. The caudate nucleus is a component of the basal ganglia.

cell respiration   A chemical process in which oxygen is used to make energy from carbohydrates. This process produces ATP (Adenosine triphosphate) which may be used to produce energy to power many reactions throughout the body.

central (parietal-temporal) alexia   an acquired disorder of reading and writing caused by brain damage and usually accompanied by some degree of aphasia; also known as alexia with agraphia.

central executive network this network is one of the dominant brain networks responsible for high level cognitive tasks.

central nervous system (CNS) the brain and the spinal cord structures.

central pattern generator a term given to a cluster of neurons (afferent, interneurons, and efferent) that, when stimulated, trigger a sequenced series of physical responses. In swallowing, the medullary swallowing center, with the nucleus solitarius and the nucleus ambiguus, is thought to function as a central pattern generator.

cephalic of or relating to the head; directed toward or situated on, in, or near the head.

cerebellar hemispheres the two spherical structures comprising the cerebellum.

cerebellopontine angle located between the cerebellum and the pons and containing CSF, cranial nerves, and other tissues.

cerebellum cauliflower-shaped brain structure located just above the brainstem at the base of the skull.

cerebral palsy a disability resulting from damage to the brain before, during, or shortly after birth and outwardly manifested by muscular incoordination and often speech disturbances.

cerebral plasticity the ability of the brain to reorganize neural pathways on the basis of new learning and experiences.

cerebrospinal fluid (CSF) clear, colorless bodily fluid produced by the choroid plexuses and contained within the subarachnoid space circulating around the brain and spinal cord before being absorbed by the arachnoid villi; cushions the central nervous system and provides nutrients.

cerebrovascular accident (CVA) interruption of the blood flow to the brain as a result of occlusive (thrombotic or embolic) or hemorrhagic mechanisms; also known as stroke.

cerebrum the major portion of the brain, consisting of two hemispheres, that contains the cortex and its underlying white matter as well as the basal ganglia and other basal structures.

childhood apraxia of speech (CAS) a developmental sensorimotor speech disorder characterized by impairment of the ability to program the positioning of the articulators and the sequencing of muscle movements for volitional speech production; also known as developmental apraxia of speech.

childhood disintegrative disorder (CDD) a rare, pervasive developmental disorder on the autism spectrum in which communication and social skills develop normally until at least age 2 years (onset usually is between 3 and 4 years) followed by pronounced loss in motor, communication, and social skills.

childhood suprabulbar paresis see *Worster-Drought Syndrome.*

chorda tympani this is a component of the facial nerve VII which transmits gustatory (taste) innervation from the tongue as well as providing innervations to submandibular and sublingual glands.

chorea disorder characterized by irregular, spasmodic, involuntary movements of the limbs or facial muscles.

choreiform resembling chorea.

choroid plexus structure located in certain parts of the ventricle composed of fused ependymal and pia mater cells and associated capillaries; makes and secretes cerebrospinal fluid for circulation.

chronic traumatic encephalopathy (CTE) Chronic traumatic encephalopathy is a progressive brain condition caused by repeated blows to the head and repeated concussions. It is particularly associated with contact sports.

cingulate cortex This is a component of the cerebral cortex located medially and containing the cingulate gyrus. This structure is a component of the limbic system, important for emotional responses.

cingulate gyrus the ridge on the surface of the cerebrum located between the cingulated sulcus and the sulcus of the corpus callosum.

circle of Willis circle of arteries located at the base of the brain; serves as a vascular mechanism for collateral circulation.

circumlocution wordy and circuitous description of unrecalled terms.

clinical neurology medical discipline involving diagnosis and treatment of diseases of the nervous system.

clonus form of movement marked by contractions and relaxations of a muscle occurring in rapid succession.

cochlea the cochlea is the spiral cavity of the inner ear which contains the organ or Corti.

cochlear duct the middle chamber of the cochlea that contains the sensory end organ of hearing, the organ of Corti; also known as the scala media.

code switching in linguistics, alternating between two or more languages, dialects, or language registers in a single conversation.

cognition the mental process of knowing, which includes aspects such as awareness, perception, reasoning, memory, and judgment.

cognitive-communicative (cognitive-linguistic) disorders communication disorders resulting from the neurobehavioral sequelae of diffuse (as opposed to focal) brain damage, including deficits in information processing, attention, reasoning, and problem solving and memory.

cogwheel rigidity increased tone, equalized between agonist and antagonist muscles, with a superimposed cogwheel, ratchetlike resistance; often found in patients with Parkinson disease.

colliculi little hills or mounds within the brain; the superior and inferior colliculi are found in the midbrain.

coma a state of unconsciousness in which a person cannot be awakened and is unresponsive to visual, auditory, or tactile (even painful) stimuli.

computed tomography (CT) x-ray imaging technique in which the brain is viewed at different depths; the various views are correlated by computer to show structural lesions of the brain.

concentration gradient ratio of solute and water across a membrane.

conduction aphasia an adult language disorder in which auditory comprehension is good but exact repetition is poor; the site of the lesion producing the syndrome is in debate, but it may interrupt the arcuate fasciculus.

confabulation verbal or written expression of fictitious experiences.

confusional state acute symptoms of mental disorganization and agitation that may accompany head trauma or other medical conditions; the language is often marked by irrelevancy and confabulation.

constraint-induced therapy (CIT) a treatment method in rehabilitation in which the patient is forced to use the damaged modality to accomplish tasks normally performed with that modality (e.g., constraining the nonparalyzed left arm and requiring activities of daily living and therapy tasks to be done with the hemiparetic right arm and hand or, in constraint-induced aphasia therapy, requiring the patient to communicate verbally rather than allowing alternative communication methods or facilitation).

constructional disturbance the inability to form a construction in space because of a cerebral deficit.

contingent negative variation (CNV) a small negative potential recorded on an electroencephalogram over the front central scalp of some subjects who perform tasks requiring close attention or who have just received a warning stimulus; also known as E wave or expectancy wave.

contralateral related to the opposite side.

contralateral innervation the supply of nerve impulses from the opposite side of the body.

contralateral motor control refers to the organization where the majority of the motor impulses from each cerebral cortex innervate the opposite side of the body.

convergence the exciting of a single sensory neuron by incoming impulses from multiple other neurons.

corona radiata the corona radiata is the white matter sheet of afferent and efferent fibers that connect the cerebral cortex with the brain stem. It is so named because it resembles a radiating crown

corpus callosum the largest transversal commissure between the hemispheres; it is ~4 inches long.

corpus striatum subcortical mass of white and gray matter in front of and lateral to the thalamus in each cerebral hemisphere; is used to refer to the putamen, globus pallidus, and caudate nucleus collectively.

cortex the outer surface layer of the brain (or other organs).

corticonuclear fibers the fiber bundle pathway in each hemisphere from the motor cortex to the nuclei of the brainstem;

depending on the particular nerve, some of the fibers decussate and others travel ipsilaterally.

corticopontine tract   this tract is formed by massive projections from the cerebral cortex to the pontine nuclei.

corticospinal tract   part of the pyramidal system that descends from the cerebral cortex to different levels of the spinal cord; facilitates motor control.

cranial nerve   one of 12 pairs of nerves (fiber bundles surrounded by connective tissue) that exit the brain and pass through the skull to reach the sense organs or muscles of the head and neck with which they are associated.

declarative memory   memory for facts and events.

decussation   crossing over or intersection of parts.

deep dyslexia   an acquired reading disorder resulting from left-hemisphere brain damage and characterized by semantic errors in reading single words.

default mode network   this is a network connecting various brain regions and is most active when the person is not focused on tasks.

deglutition   the act of swallowing.

delirium   acute fluctuating consciousness, with sudden confusion developing rapidly and fluctuating during the day.

dementia   an organic mental disorder with progressive general intellectual deterioration affecting memory, judgment, and abstract thinking as well as personality changes.

dendrite   the short branching processes of a nerve cell; literally means "treelike."

dendritic spines   the spines are tiny protrusions from dendrites, important for forming contacts with neighboring neurons.

denervation   a cutting of the nerve supply by excision, incision, or blocking.

denial   following injury to the brain, some patients are noted to deny parts of their body or resulting impairments.

depolarization   loss of the difference in charge between the inside and outside of the plasma membrane of a muscle or nerve cell caused by a change in permeability and migration of sodium ions to the interior.

dermatome   the lateral wall of a somite from which the dermis is produced.

developmental anarthria   diagnosis involving complete lack of speech as a result of profound paralysis, weakness, and/or incoordination of the musculature of speech.

developmental apraxia of speech   a developmental disorder characterized by impaired ability to execute the appropriate movements of speech voluntarily in the absence of paralysis, weakness, or incoordination of the musculature of speech; also known as childhood apraxia of speech.

developmental dysarthria   speech disorder resulting from damage to the immature nervous system; characterized by weakness, paralysis, and/or incoordination of the speech musculature.

developmental dyslexia   see *dyslexia*.

developmental language disorder   congenital difficulty with the production and/or comprehension of language, ranging from mild delay to severe disorder.

developmental motor speech disorders   a group of disorders of speech production resulting from congenital weakness, paralysis, or incoordination of the speech musculature or a congenital disorder of programming the speech musculature. See *developmental dysarthria* and *childhood apraxia of speech*.

diaphragma sella   a ring-shaped fold of dura mater covering the sella turcica, in which the pituitary gland sits.

dichotic listening   test situation in which simultaneous auditory stimuli are presented to both ears at the same time; ear preference (right or left) is judged by which ear first recognizes the auditory stimulus.

diencephalon   the part of the forebrain between the cerebral hemispheres and the midbrain; includes the thalamus, hypothalamus, the third ventricle, and the epithalamus.

diffuse axonal injury (DAI)   extensive tearing of axons as a result of traumatic shearing forces that occur when the head is rapidly accelerated or decelerated, resulting in twisting or rotational force.

diffusion tensor imaging (DTI)   an MRI technique that can measure axonal organization in nervous system tissue, describing the magnitude, anistrophy, and orientation of any anistrophy.

diplegia   paralysis of corresponding parts on both sides of the body, with legs more impaired.

diplopia   double vision.

direct activation pathway   the pathway connecting the motor cortices to the peripheral neurons, serving to initiate and facilitate voluntary motor responses.

distal   away from the center of the body.

divergence   dissemination of the effect of activity of a single nerve cell through multiple synaptic connections.

dorsal   pertaining to the back; posterior.

dorsal column pathway   major sensory pathway mediating proprioception.

DSM-5   The Diagnostic and Statistical manual of Mental Disorders, 5th edition.

Duchenne dystrophy   a chronic, progressive disease beginning in early childhood that affects the shoulder and pelvic girdles, causing increasing weakness and pseudohypertrophy of the muscles followed by atrophy and the establishment of a peculiar swaying gait.

dura mater   the outermost meningeal layer covering the brain.

dysarthrias   a group of speech production disorders caused by oral-motor weakness, paralysis, or incoordination; may be congenital or acquired.

dysdiadochokinesia   the inability to perform and sustain rapid alternating movements; speech-language pathologists in particular apply this term to a motor deficit in the oral muscles; associated with cerebellar disorder syndromes; also called alternate motion rate.

dysfluency   speech marked by hesitations, prolongations, and/or repetitions that interrupt the natural prosodic flow; also refers to stuttering.

dyskinesia   disorder of movement usually associated with a lesion of the extrapyramidal system.

dyslexia   inability to read despite the ability to see and recognize letters and a history of appropriate instruction.

dysmetria   the inability to gauge the distance, speed, and power of a movement.

dysphagia   difficulty swallowing.

dysprosody   disturbance of stress, timing, and melody of speech.

dystonia   disorder in which the limbs assume distorted static postures as a result of excess tone in selected parts of the body.

ear advantage   demonstrated ear preference for certain stimuli. Dichotic listening studies have shown that verbal stimuli are more accurately reported when presented to the right ear than the left ear in persons who are left dominant for language, called right ear advantage.

ectoderm   the outermost of the three primary germ layers of an embryo.

efferent   conducting (fluid or nerve impulses) outward from a given organ or part.

efferent fibers   fibers conducting a neural impulse away from a given neuron; often refers to a motor fiber, although technically it does not necessarily refer to motor impulses.

electroencephalography (EEG)   procedure producing a graphic record of electrical activity of the brain as recorded by an electroencephalograph.

embryo   the developing human individual from the time of implantation to the end of the eighth week after conception.

encephalitis   inflammation of the brain.

encephalon   the brain.

encephalopathy   pathology of the brain.

endoderm   the innermost of the three primary germ layers of an embryo that is the source of the epithelium of the digestive tract and its derivatives and of the lower respiratory tract.

endolymph   the watery fluid in the membranous labyrinth of the ear.

enteric   relating to or affecting the intestines.

enteric nervous system   a division of the autonomic nervous system formed by neuronal plexuses in the gastrointestinal tract and directly affecting deglutition and digestion during swallowing.

ependymal cells   glial cells that compose the lining of the ventricles (the ependyma) and the choroid plexuses; cells function to help make cerebrospinal fluid.

episodic memory   includes information about recent or past events and experiences.

epithalamus small region of the diencephalon of the brain consisting of the pineal gland, habenular nuclei, and stria medullaris thalami.

equilibrium the state of being balanced.

essential tremor organic tremor not associated with any pathologic process.

esthesiometer instrument used to assess two-point discrimination for tactile sensation.

event related potentials (ERPs) very small brain voltages generated in brain structures in response to specific sensory, motor, or cognitive events or stimuli, analyzed as time-locked activity during electroencephalogram (EEG) studies.

excess and equal stress a feature noted in the speech of some persons with dysarthria, especially in ataxic dysarthria, in which normally unstressed words or syllables are stressed equally with other words with the resulting prosody sounding robotic.

excitatory postsynaptic potential (EPSP) an electrical change (depolarization) in the membrane of a postsynaptic neuron caused by the binding of an excitatory neurotransmitter from a presynaptic cell to a postsynaptic receptor, increasing the likelihood of an action potential being generated in the postsynaptic neuron.

executive functions capacities, under primary control of the prefrontal cortex, that guide complex behavior over time through planning, decision making, and response control. Common executive abilities include judgment, problem solving, decision making, planning, and pragmatics and depend on cognitive abilities such as attention, perception, memory, and language.

explosive speech loud, sudden speech attributable to damage to the nervous system.

extensor a muscle, the contraction of which tends to shorten a limb; antagonist to flexors.

exteroceptors sense receptors (as of touch, temperature, smell, vision, or hearing) excited by stimuli outside the organism.

extinction progressive reduction in strength of a conditioned response on withdrawal of the reinforcing stimulus.

extrafusal fibers these are the skeletal muscle fibers innervated by alpha motor neurons and whose contractions allow skeletal movement.

extraocular adjacent to but outside the eyeball.

extrapyramidal system the basal ganglia and its interconnections.

facilitation process of making the nerve impulses easier by repeated use of certain axons.

falx cerebelli the fold of the dura mater that separates the two cerebellar hemispheres.

falx cerebri the larger of the two folds of dura mater separating the hemispheres of the brain that lies between the cerebral hemispheres and contains the sagittal sinuses.

fasciculation involuntary contractions or twitches in a group of muscle fibers.

fasciculus a nerve fiber bundle forming a connection between groups of neurons in the central nervous system; also known as a tract.

feedback in control theory, a process in which some portion of the output signal of a system is passed (fed back) to the input; often used to control the dynamic behavior of the system.

feedforward system that reacts to changes in its environment, usually to maintain some desired state; exhibits response to a measured disturbance in a predefined way but does not handle novel stimuli.

fetal period the ninth week after conception until birth.

fissure a groove on the surface of the brain or spinal cord.

flaccid flabby, without tone.

flaccid dysarthria a classification of motor speech disorders associated with damage to the lower motor neuron or some part of the motor unit; marked by certain features depending on the part of the motor unit that is damaged.

flocculus small, irregular lobe on the undersurface of each hemisphere of the cerebellum that is linked with the corresponding side of the nodulus by a peduncle.

fluency disorders speech disorders that affect the natural prosody and flow of speech.

fluent/nonfluent a dichotomous classification of aphasic language on the basis of the type of conversational speech.

focal lesion an identifiable, circumscribed area of damage or injury.

foramen an aperture or perforation through a bone or a membranous structure.

foramina in neuroanatomy, a foramen (plural foramina) is an opening or passage in bone.

forebrain the anterior of the three primary divisions of the developing vertebrate brain or the corresponding part of the adult brain that especially includes the cerebral hemispheres, the thalamus, and the hypothalamus; in higher vertebrates, is the main control center for sensory and associative information processing, visceral functions, and voluntary motor functions; also called prosencephalon.

fractional anisotrophy a scale value measuring the degree of anistrophy in a diffusion process, often used in diffusion tensor imaging of white matter

fricatives a consonant sound produced by directing and continuing the restricted breath stream against one or more of the oral surfaces (hard palate, alveolar ridge, teeth, and/or lips); may be voiced or unvoiced. Examples include /f/, /v/, /s/, and /z/.

frontal alexia reading disorder known as the third alexia; associated with a lesion in the left frontal lobe; often accompanies a Broca's aphasia.

frontal lobe the anterior division of each cerebral hemisphere having its lower part in the anterior fossa of the skull and bordered behind by the central sulcus.

frontotemporal dementias (FTD) a syndrome complex, designated by the National Institute of Neurological Diseases and Stroke, marked by progressive deterioration in behavior and/or language with retention of important features of memory, unlike other dementias.

functional magnetic resonance imaging (fMRI) the use of magnetic resonance imaging to measure the hemodynamic response related to neural activity in the brain or spinal cord.

funiculi aggregates of fiber bundles (or tracts) in the nervous system as seen in the spinal cord; also called columns.

gag reflex reflex contraction of the muscles of the throat especially caused by stimulation (as by touch) of the pharynx.

Galant reflex a newborn reflex elicited by holding the child face down and stroking along one side of the spine; normal reaction is lateral flexion toward the stimulated side; should disappear by 9 months of age or before.

gamma-aminobutyric acid (GABA) an inhibitory neurotransmitter.

gamma motor neuron neurons innervating the muscle spindle; allow contraction of intrafusal fibers and increased sensitivity of the fibers to the muscle stretch reflex.

ganglia nerve cells with common form, function, and connections that are grouped outside the central nervous system.

gasserian ganglion the large, flattened, sensory root ganglion of the trigeminal nerve that lies within the skull and behind the orbit; also called trigeminal ganglion, semilunar ganglion.

genetics/genomics Genetics refers to the science of inheritance, such as Mendelian laws of inheritance, and is generally more focused on chromosomal regions and specific genes. Genomics plays out on the scale of entire genomes and is equally important for classic inheritance traits and so-called complex disorders.

genioglossus a fan-shaped muscle that arises from the superior mental spine; inserts on the hyoid bone and into the tongue; and advances, retracts, and depresses the tongue.

genu any structure of angular shape resembling a flexed knee.

Gerstmann syndrome a cluster of left parietal lobe lesion signs, including finger agnosia, left-right disorientation, acalculia, and agraphia; a developmental form of the syndrome has been described.

glial cells cellular elements, of which there are several types, that support and expedite the activity of the neurons; glial cells outnumber the neurons 10 to 1; also called neuroglial cells.

glioma general name for a tumor arising from the supportive tissues of the brain.

global aphasia an acquired disorder of language caused by brain damage and characterized by severe impairment of all language modalities, comprehension, verbal and gestural expression, reading, and writing.

globus pallidus (GPi) a nucleus of the basal ganglia that receives input from the caudate and the putamen and is the main output nucleus.

glottal coup a rapid, forceful closing and opening of the true vocal folds accompanied by a short, sharp vocalization; used in oral-motor examinations to assess vocal fold movement and strength informally.

Golgi tendon organs a collection of afferent fibers located in tendons or their processes that respond to tension during muscle contraction.

graceful degradation an engineering concept adopted in explanations of neural processing in which the loss of one component of a distributed processing network results in a reduced level, but not failure, of performance.

graded potential short-lived depolarizations or hyperpolarizations of an area of membrane. These changes cause local flows of current (movement of ions) that decrease with distance. When this occurs in a receptor cell, it is called a receptor potential.

gray matter the grayish substance of brain and spinal cord composed of neuronal and glial cell bodies, unmyelinated nerve fibers, and synapses.

gyrus an elevation or ridge on the surface of the cerebrum.

growth cone this is the site of axon elongation with the highest denisty of actin filaments along the axon.

helicotrema the minute opening by which the scala tympani and scala vestibuli communicate at the top of the cochlea of the ear.

hemianopsia a visual field defect of one half of the eye field.

hemiparalysis total or partial paralysis of one side of the body that results from disease of or injury to the motor centers of the brain; also called hemiplegia.

hemiplegia see *hemiparalysis*.

hemorrhage bleeding; a profuse flow of blood.

Heschl gyrus convolution of the temporal lobe that is the cortical center for hearing; runs obliquely outward and forward from the posterior part of the lateral sulcus.

hindbrain the posterior division of the three primary divisions of the developing vertebrate brain or the corresponding part of the adult brain that includes the cerebellum, pons, and medulla oblongata and that controls the autonomic functions and equilibrium; also called the rhombencephalon.

hippocampus this is a complex brain structure deep in each temporal lobe, playing a major role in learning and memory.

homeostasis the physiologic process by which the body's internal systems are maintained at equilibrium despite changes in external conditions.

homunculus caricature mapping the connections between the area of the motor or

sensory cortex and the innervated body part; literally means "little man."

Huntington chorea a progressive chorea inherited as an autosomal dominant trait characterized by choreiform movements and mental deterioration leading to dementia; accompanied by atrophy of the caudate nucleus and the loss of certain brain cells with a decrease in the level of several neurotransmitters; usually begins in middle age; also called Huntington disease.

hyoglossus extrinsic tongue muscle involved in the retraction and depression of the tongue.

hyperalgesia increased sensitivity to pain or enhanced intensity of pain sensation.

hyperesthesia unusual or pathologic sensitivity of the skin or of a particular sense to stimulation.

hyperkinesia an abnormal, involuntary increase in muscle activity.

hypernasality the perception of nasal resonance during the production of voiced sounds, particularly vowels.

hyperpolarization increased production in potential difference across a biologic membrane.

hyperreflexia a condition in which the deep tendon reflexes are exaggerated.

hypertonia extreme tension of the muscles.

hypoalgesia decreased sensitivity to pain.

hypoesthesia impaired or decreased tactile sensibility; also called hypesthesia.

hypokinesia diminished muscle movement capacity.

hypokinetic dysarthria dysarthria caused by basal ganglia disease; most commonly associated with Parkinson disease.

hyporeflexia diminished or absent reflexes.

hypothalamus portion of the brain that composes part of the third ventricle; critical to autonomic and endocrine function, including rage and aggression, regulation of body temperature, and nutrient intake; also exerts neural control over pituitary gland.

hypotonia muscle flaccidity; a decrease in normal muscle tone when passive movement is performed.

IDEA IDEA stands for Individuals with Disabilities Education Act.

ideational apraxia disorder of motor planning in which complex motor plans cannot be executed, although individual motor components of the plan can be performed.

ideomotor apraxia a motor disturbance characterized by the inability to carry out motor acts on command, but some evidence is present that these motor acts can be carried out imitatively or automatically.

IDT Interdisciplinary Team: a team made up of members from different disciplines working collaboratively toward a common purpose. SLPs are often involved as part of an IDT in educational and medical settings.

indirect activation pathway this is the pathway that connects basal ganglia and other associated nuclei, helping to prevent unwanted movements during voluntary acts.

induction in embryology, this is the process where the presence of one tissue influences the development of other tissues.

infarction refers to tissue death or necrosis due to inadequate blood supply to an affected area.

inferior situated below and closer to the feet than another part and especially another similar part of an upright body of a human being.

inhibitory postsynaptic potential (IPSP) Inhibitory postsynaptic potential (IPSP) makes a neuron less likely to generate an action potential.

innervate to supply with efferent nerve impulses.

input fibers neural elements that make synaptic connections by synapsing onto the cell body and/or onto dendrites or dendritic spines found on the dendrites.

insula a cortical region deep within the lateral sulcus linked to self awareness, interoception, pain processing, addiction, among others.

intellectual disability a developmental delay characterized by impaired learning, social adjustment, and maturational problems in all areas.

intention tremor a slow tremor of the extremities that increases on attempted voluntary movement and is observed in certain diseases of the nervous system (e.g., multiple sclerosis).

internal capsule both afferent and efferent fibers pass through the internal capsule, makign it a two-way tract for transmission to and from the cerebral cortex.

internal carotid arteries the inner branches, right and left, of the carotid artery that supply the brain, eyes, and other internal structures of the head; also called internal carotid.

internuncial functionally imposed between two or more neurons.

interoceptor a specialized nerve receptor that receives and responds to stimuli originating from within the body.

interstitial fluid extracellular fluid.

intervertebral foramina the openings between the vertebrae of the spinal cord through which the motor and sensory roots exit and unite to form the spinal nerves.

intrafusal fibers skeletal muscle fibers that serve as specialized sensory organs or proprioceptors.

intrinsic neurons (interneurons) nerve cells within the central nervous system that act as a link between sensory and motor neurons.

ipsilateral on the same side.

irritability the capacity to respond to stimuli.

ischemia insufficient blood flow to brain tissue, often leading to cell death in that area.

island of Reil part of the cerebral cortex forming the floor of the lateral fissure; also known as insula.

jaw reflex this reflex is activated when the jaw-closing muscles are suddenly stretched by a downward motion on the chin.

kernicterus a form of infantile jaundice in which a yellow pigment and degenerative lesions are found in areas of the intracranial gray matter.

lacrimal related to the tears, their secretions, and the organs concerned with them.

Landau-Kleffner syndrome (LKS) a pediatric disorder—first described in 1957 by Drs. William M. Landau and Frank R. Kleffner, who identified six children with the disorder—characterized by a gradual or sudden loss of the ability to understand and use spoken language. Abnormal electrical brain waves, documented by an electroencephalogram, are common, as are epileptic seizures; affected children often have hyperactivity; also called acquired epileptic aphasia.

language dominance the hemisphere that is the site for the major language areas and connections.

language lateralization concept that language is not exactly alike between the two hemispheres of the brain.

lateral a position farthest from the medial plane or midline of a body; related to a side.

lateral corticospinal tract through this tract, over 90% of voluntary motor fibers decussate in the brain stem and course through the spinal cord.

lateral spinothalamic tract ascending nerve fibers originating in the spinal cord and terminating in the thalamus.

L-dopa L-3,4-hydroxyphenylalanine; synthetic dopamine that crosses the blood-brain barrier; often given to Parkinson patients.

left fusiform area a region of the left posterior temporal cortex in the fusiform gyrus involved in processing of written words.

lentiform (lenticular) nucleus a component of the basal ganglia containing the globus pallidus and the putamen.

lesion an area of damage in the body.

ligand sensitive protein channels in the cell membrane that open and close in response to the presence of certain chemicals or neurotransmitters.

limb apraxia failure to perform a learned movement; may be ipsilateral or bilateral; also known as ideomotor apraxia.

limbic system interconnected nuclei in the telencephalon and diencephalon; functions include self-preservation and activities and behaviors, including emotions, sexual behaviors, memory, olfaction sensory processing; composed of the olfactory bulb, hypothalamus, amygdala, hippocampus, insular cortex, and cingulate gyrus.

localization of function a particular structure in the nervous system assigned to a specific function (e.g., Broca area is the localized area for language expression).

long-term memory the part of memory where knowledge is stored permanently and is activated when needed (usually through cues); theoretically unlimited in capacity.

Lou Gehrig disease see *amyotrophic lateral sclerosis*.

lower motor neurons (LMNs) peripheral motor neurons within the spinal cord whose axons terminate in a skeletal muscle; efferent neurons that transmit motor impulses.

magnetic resonance imaging (MRI) neuroimaging procedure in which hydrogen proteins of tissues are aligned with the magnetic field; emits a signal that is recorded in each slice (image).

magnetoencephalography (MEG) magnetic radiography depicting the intracranial fluid spaces after cerebral spinal fluid is extracted and replaced by air or gas.

magnum foramen opening in the base of the skull through which the spinal cord is continuous with the brain.

masking the drowning of a weak sound by a louder one.

mastication the chewing of food.

mechanicoreceptors sensory receptor sensitive to mechanical stimulation such as muscles and tendons, sinuses, and hair cells of the inner ear.

medial toward the midline.

medulla oblongata also known as the myelencephalon; caudal segment of the brainstem, rostral from the foramen magnum to the pons.

meninges nembranous coverings of the central nervous system developing from the neural crest and the mesoderm layer.

mesencephalon midbrain.

mesocortex transitional areas of the cerebral cortex formed at borders between true isocortex (a.k.a. neocortex) and true allocortex.

mesoderm the second germ layer apparent during the third week of development of the nervous system; forms the skin (dermis), skeleton, muscles, blood, and blood vessels.

metacognition educational process that incorporates knowledge of one's abilities, the demands of the task at hand, and the effective learning strategies needed to achieve success; may be regulated by the individual involved.

microglia type of glial cell with a primarily scavenger function.

microtubules part of an axon; help carry out the process of axon transport.

midbrain (mesencephalon) the most superior of the three structures making up the brainstem; associated structures found at the midbrain level are the tectum, inferior and superior colliculi, cerebral peduncles, and substantia nigra.

minimal cerebral dysfunction a syndrome of neurologic dysfunction in children usually marked by impairments of fine coordination, clumsiness, and choreiform or athetoid movements; often associated with learning disorders.

mitosis a type of cell division in which a single cell produces two genetically identical daughter cells; new body cells for growth and repair are produced through mitosis.

mixed dominance inconsistency in laterality of speech and related motor functions such as hand, foot, and eye dominance in some

individuals; sometimes associated with language and learning disorders.

modified feeding altered intake of food and nutrition; may include tube feedings, specialized diet plans and food consistencies, and solid and liquid restrictions.

modiolus the modiolus is a conical structure in the cochlea through which the cochlear nerve passes.

molecular commotion a state of disorganization and disruption of neuronal metabolism and excitability resulting from physical trauma to the brain.

monoloudness no variation in the loudness or volume level; static volume usually attributable to dysarthria caused by phonatory and respiratory weakness.

monopitch the use of a single pitch, resulting in a lack of pitch variations.

monoplegia paralysis of one limb.

Moro reflex infantile reflex that involves postural responses; rapid lowering of a flexed, supine head of an infant causes abduction and extension followed by flexion, of the arms.

motor association areas cortical association areas, numbered 44 to 47 in the Brodmann system, that surround the foot of the motor and premotor cortices.

motor endplate special structural enlargements of the muscle fibers at the synaptic junction.

motor fibers efferent fibers that go to the muscle and force them to contract.

motor unit a motor neuron that includes the muscle fibers it innervates.

multiple sclerosis (MS) degenerative disease of the central nervous system with no known cause; some research has linked this disease with a malfunction of the immune system; myelin degenerates but the axon remains intact; the intact axon is probably the reason for periods of remission.

multipolar cell any cell that contains more than one process (usually contains two).

muscle spindle specialized organ within a muscle; gives muscle length feedback.

muscle tone the resistance to passive movement or change of muscle length.

muscular dystrophy genetic, progressive myopathy that includes Duchenne muscular dystrophy and myotonia.

myasthenia gravis autoimmune disorder in which postsynaptic acetylcholine receptors are blocked, causing muscle weakness and fatigue.

myelin the fatty substance surrounding some axons that speeds neural transmission; the myelin-covered areas are the white matter of the brain.

myelination the process of segmental wrapping of myelin around axons; continuous myelin is interrupted by narrow gaps (nodes of Ranvier).

myelinogenesis the cyclic process of laying down of myelin on certain fiber tracts.

myoclonus rapid, asynchronous movements of the limbs.

necrose to die.

necrosis   cell death caused by local injury, such as loss of blood supply or disease; nonphysiologic processes; usually occurs in severe trauma.

neocerebellum   the newer parts of the cerebellum phylogenetically provided by the corticopontocerebellar fibers.

neocortex   theoretically, a phylogenetic division of the cerebral cortex; distinguished from the allocortex in lower animals; also called the isocortex.

neologistic jargon aphasia   a temporal lobe syndrome marked by newly coined words and unintelligible utterances.

neoplasm   tumor.

neural integration   complete and harmonious combining of components of the nervous system.

neural plate   this is a key developmental structure that serves as the basis of the nervous system in an embryo.

neural tube   embryologically, a hollow structure that gives rise to the central nervous system as the cells mature.

neurofibrillary tangles   tangles of neurofibers common in Alzheimer disease.

neurofilaments   the fine filaments seen in neurons through an electron microscope.

neurogenesis   the development of neurons from stem cell precursors.

neuroglial cells   see *glial cells*.

neurolinguistics   the study of the relation of communication and language regarding brain function; the manner in which the brain helps produce language and, in turn, communication.

neurology   a branch of science that deals with the normal as well as the diseased or disordered nervous system.

neuron   nerve cell.

neuroplasticity   the capacity of neurons to adapt to a changed environment; in some cases, neuronal areas take over function(s) of damaged neurons.

neuroprogenitor cells   these cells are the progenitors of most of the glial and neuronal cells in the CNS.

neurotransmitter   the substance released from an axonal terminal of a presynaptic neuron once the neuron is excited; travels across the synaptic cleft to excite or inhibit the targeted cell; examples are norepinephrine, acetylcholine, or dopamine.

neurotrophins   these are receptors that regulate development, maintenance, and function of the nervous system.

Noam Chomsky   20th-century linguist who postulated the theory of language controversy as innate vs. learned.

nociceptor   a receptor for pain that is stimulated by tissue damage.

Norman Geschwind   early-20th-century pioneer in behavioral neurology.

notochord   a cylindric group of cells on the dorsal aspect of an embryo; the center of the development of the axial skeleton.

nucleolus   located inside the nucleus, the nucleolus is where the ribosomal RNA genes are transcribed.

nucleus accumbens   located in the basal forebrain, the nucelus accumbens is considered to be the neural interface between motivation and action.

nucleus solitarius   located in the medulla oblongata, this is a paired structure with far reaching impact on the homeostatic system of the body.

nystagmus   rhythmical horizontal, rotary, or vertical oscillation of the eyeballs.

obligatory   without an alternative path.

occipital lobe   the posterior portion of each hemisphere that forms the posterior-lateral surface of the brain; location of visual cortex; area involved with vision.

olfaction   the sense of smell.

oligodendrocyte   type of glial cell that produces myelin for neurons in the central nervous system.

optic chiasm   the structure located on the floor of the third ventricle composed of crossing optic nerve fibers from the medial (nasal) half of each retina.

optic disk   the head of the optic nerve.

oral apraxia   buccofacial apraxia; inability to program nonspeech oral movements.

organ of Corti   lies against the basilar membrane in the cochlea; contains special sensory receptors for hearing consisting of hair cells and other support cells.

orthograde transneuronal atrophy   process involving the large-scale death of neurons in the central nervous system in response to injury to white matter.

osmotic force   the energy needed to maintain adequate body fluids and set and maintain the proper balance between the volumes of extracellular and intracellular fluids.

palilalia   repeating a word or phrase with increasing rapidity as a result of neurologic damage.

palpate   to examine by feeling and pressing with the palms of the hands and fingers.

parahippocampal gyrus   between the collateral sulcus and the hippocampal sulcus on the inferior surface of each hemisphere; above the cingulated gyrus and below the lingual gyrus.

paralimbic areas   associative areas of the cortex containing structures that form an uninterrupted girdle around the medial and basal aspects of the cerebral hemispheres; areas include the caudal orbitofrontal cortex, insula, temporal pole, parahippocampal gyrus (proper), and cingulate complex.

paralysis   loss of voluntary muscular function.

paraphasia   the substitution of words or sounds in words in such a way as to decrease intelligibility or obscure meaning.

paraplegia   paralysis of both lower extremities and, generally, the lower trunk.

parasympathetic division   pertaining to that division of the autonomic nervous system concerned with the maintenance of the body; its fibers arise from the brain and the sacral part of the spinal cord.

parasympathetic nuclei   part of the autonomic nervous system; preganglionic fibers leave the central nervous system with cranial nerves III, VII, IX, and X and the first three sacral nerves; postganglionic fibers are in the heart, smooth muscles, and glands of the neck and head and the viscera in the thorax, abdomen, and pelvis regions; most of the fibers are in the vagus nerve tract.

paresis   partial paralysis; weakness.

paresthesia   abnormal sensation of burning, tingling, or numbness.

parietal lobe   upper and central portion of each hemisphere between the frontal and occipital lobes and above the temporal lobe.

parkinsonism   a disorder that manifests the symptoms of Parkinson disease.

Parkinson's disease   a slow, progressive disease characterized by the degeneration of the substantia nigra within the basal ganglia, causing a gradual decrease of the neurotransmitter dopamine; characterized by resting tremor of the hands and feet, hypokinetic dysarthria, and a masklike facial expression.

pathologic tremor   a tremor caused by the structural and functional manifestations of a disease.

pattern-associator network   network used in simulations of behavior that allows transformation of a pattern of activity across its input units into a pattern of activity across its output units.

peduncles   very large mass (like a stalk) of nerve fibers connecting two structures in the nervous system.

perikaryon   the cytoplasmic matrix surrounding a cell body in a neuron.

perilymph   fluid contained in the bony labyrinth of the inner ear.

peripheral nervous system (PNS)   cranial and spinal nerves and their branches.

peristriate cortex   part of the occipital lobe that receives fibers from the optic radiation; the primary receiving area for vision.

perisylvian cortex   an area on the lateral wall of the dominant hemisphere for language that includes the major centers and pathways for language reception and production; see *perisylvian zone*.

perisylvian zone   the cortex surrounding the sylvian fissure in the dominant temporal lobe; site where the major neurologic components for understanding and producing language are found (e.g., Broca area, Wernicke area, the supramarginal and angular gyri).

pervasive developmental disorder (PDD)   a disorder characterized by an impairment in the development of social interaction and social pragmatic skills as well as verbal or nonverbal communication skills and the possibility of stereotyped behaviors and interests. This disorder is no longer in the DSM, as it has been incorporated under autism spectrum disorders.

phasic tone   rapid contraction to a high-intensity stretch (or change in muscle length) assessed by testing tendon reflexes.

phoneme   smallest meaningful unit of sound.

phonologic alexia   the inability to read nonsense words, especially low-frequency words; errors are usually visual errors.

photoreceptors   nerve end organs stimulated by light, as in the rods and cones of the retina.

phrenic nerves   nerves arising from the cervical spinal cord that supply the diaphragm.

pia mater   the innermost layer of the meninges that is vascular in nature.

Pick's disease   a rare and progressive and degenerative form of dementia characterized by cortical atrophy in the frontal and temporal lobes.

Pierre Paul Broca   French physician (1824–1880); localized language areas from two patients who had sustained language and motor speech losses; postulated for the first time that the left hemisphere contained the language center.

plasticity   the concept that in the immature brain some functional areas are not established and that unestablished areas may assume any one of a variety of functions.

plosives   a class of consonant speech sounds that require a complete closure of the vocal tract followed by a quick release of air and/or acoustic sound energy; they are /p/, /b/, /t/, /d/, /k/, and /g/.

pons   the part of the brainstem that lies between the medulla and the midbrain.

positive support reflex   reflex that is necessary for erect posture; when the balls of the feet (bounced on a flat surface) are stimulated, a contraction of opposing muscle groups fixes the joints of the lower extremities to bear weight.

positron emission tomography (PET)   imaging technique that visualizes the functioning brain by showing its activity through blood flow and glucose metabolism.

posterior   directed to or situated in the back; opposite is anterior; also referred to as dorsal.

posterior (occipital) alexia   see *alexia without agraphia*.

postganglionic   pertaining to nerve fibers in the autonomic nervous system that exit the ganglion.

postsynaptic terminal (receptor membrane)   what is distal to or beyond a synapse.

postural tone   the resistance striated muscles and tendons offer when stretched by a sustained, low-intensity force by a person or gravity; the recoil capability of the striated muscles and the tendons once they are fully extended by a sustained force.

potential   a relative amount of voltage in an electrical field.

pragmatic communication disorder   see *social (pragmatic) communication disorder*.

praxis   the normal performance of a motor act.

prefontal cortex   the part of the cerebral cortex that covers the anterior frontal lobe, this region is important in regulating complex cognitive skills, personality expression, and executive functions.

preganglionic   pertaining to nerve fibers in the autonomic nervous system whose cell body is within the central nervous system (brainstem or spinal cord) with its axon extending peripherally to synapse on postganglionic neurons in the autonomic ganglia.

prematurity   a state of being born after fewer than 37 weeks of gestation (birthweight is no longer considered a critical criterion).

premotor   involved in the selection of appropriate motor plans for voluntary movement, the premotor cortex is situated just anterior to the motor strip.

premotor area   area in the frontal lobe in front of the premotor cortex and inferior to the prefrontal cortex; responsible for sensory guidance of movement and control of proximal and trunk muscles.

presynaptic inhibition   inhibitory control of afferent muscle spindles before the synapse occurs.

presynaptic terminal   what is anterior to or before a synapse.

primary auditory receptor cortex   found in the temporal lobe; also known as Heschl's gyrus (areas 41 and 42).

primary cortical areas   primary areas of the cortex are dedicated to one type of sensory processing. The visual cortex and the sensory strip are examples of primary cortical areas.

primary motor projection cortex   composed mostly of precentral gyrus; voluntary control of skeletal muscles on the contralateral side of the body contained in the frontal lobe; also called the motor strip.

primary neurulation   a process in which the neural tube forms from the neural plate.

primary olfactory cortex   areas responsible for smell, consisting of anterior olfactory nucleus, olfactory tubercle, piriform cortex, and cortical amygdaloid nucleus; only sensory fibers that do not pass through the thalamus.

primary progressive aphasia (PPA)   a type of frontotemporal dementia resulting from a slowly progressive neurodegenerative process that attacks the brain's language network initially, manifesting as difficulty with language in the context of relatively preserved cognition and personality.

primary somatosensory cortex   areas 1, 2, and 3 on the postcentral gyrus; a primary receptor of general bodily sensation; thalamic radiations carry sensory data from the skin, muscles, tendons, and joints.

primary visual receptor cortex   area 17 in the occipital lobe along the calcarine fissure; receives fibers from the optic tract; also known as the striate area.

procedural memory   stores information from rule-based skills and is accessed through learned behaviors; also known as implicit memory.

progenitor cells   biologic cells that descend from stem cells and then further differentiate to create specialized cell types associated with a particular tissue type or organ.

projection neurons   the axons that originate outside the telencephalon (thalamocortical fibers) projecting to the cerebral cortex and those that arise from cerebral cortex cells (corticospinal, corticopontine, and corticothalamic) and project to other downward targeted areas.

prone   lying face down.

proprioception   perception mediated by proprioceptors.

proprioceptors   sensory nerve endings that send information regarding body movement and body positioning.

prosencephalon   see *forebrain*.

prosopagnosia   a visual agnosia characterized by the inability to recognize the faces of other people or one's own face in a mirror; associated with agnosia for color, objects, and place.

proximal   toward the midline or center of the body.

pseudobulbar (supranuclear bulbar) palsy   muscular paralysis from bilateral upper motor neuron lesions of the cranial nerves often accompanied by dysarthria, dysphagia, and emotional lability, such as outbursts of laughing or crying.

pseudohypertrophic   increase in the size of an organ or part not caused by an increase in size or number of the specific functional elements; rather, is caused by an increase in some other fatty or fibrous tissue.

pseudounipolar cell   sensory neurons in the peripheral nervous system that contain a longer dendrite and a smaller axon that connect to the spinal cord.

ptosis   drooping of the eyelid as a result of neurologic damage (paralysis).

putamen   a part of the lenticular nucleus; a structure of the basal ganglia.

pyramidal system   controls voluntary movement of the muscles for speech and all other voluntary muscles; consists of the corticospinal tract, corticobulbar tract, and the corticopontine tract.

quadriplegia   paralysis of all four limbs.

radiograph   see *x-ray*.

reasoning   the process of evaluating information to come to a conclusion.

reflex arc   a pathway leading from the receptor of a sensory stimulus to the motor response; the response is known as an automatic reflex action.

reflexes   subconscious automatic stimulus response mechanisms; in human beings, reflexes are basic defense mechanisms to sensory stimulation.

regional cerebral blood flow (rCBF)   a neuroimaging technique to study somatosensory pathways.

Reissner's membrane   a thin anterior wall of the cochlear duct that separates it from the scala vestibuli.

relative refractory period   momentary state of reduced irritation after a neural response.

rest tremor   a tremor that occurs when the limb is relaxed and supported, as in Parkinson disease.

resting potential   the difference in potential across the membrane of a cell at rest.

reticular formation a complex network of brainstem nuceli and neurons that serve as relay centers to coordinate functions necessary for survival.

reticulospinal tract nerve fibers that extend from the reticular formation in the brainstem to the spinal cord, contributing to functional contralateral muscle tone; helps with extensor and flexor muscle movements.

retrograde moving against the direction of flow.

retrograde transneuronal degeneration pathologic changes that occur across the axon and cell body of neurons as a result of an axonal lesion.

Rett syndrome a pervasive developmental disorder that affects cerebral gray matter; occurs in females and presents at birth; characterized by autistic behaviors, ataxic movements, and seizures.

rhombencephalon see *hindbrain.*

Romberg test a test in which the patient stands with feet together while the examiner notes the amount of body sway with the patient's eyes open and closed; also known as the body sway test.

rooting reflex a newborn reflex in which a touch to the infant's cheek or upper or lower lip causes the infant to turn toward that stimulus.

rostral toward the nasal or oral regions; superior in relation to the spinal cord and anterior in relation to the brain.

rubrospinal tracts fibers from the red nucleus to the spinal cord.

salience network a collection of brain regions that are active during tasks requiring attention.

saltatory transmission the type of neuronal transmission in myelinated fibers compared with the slow transmission in unmyelinated fibers.

scalae fluid-filled columns that surround the modiolus, the hollow core of the cochlea.

scanning speech related to ataxic dysarthria; quite slow, with syllable-by-syllable pausing.

Schwann cells form and maintain myelin in the peripheral nervous system.

secondary association areas sites in which elaboration of sensation occurs; considered as extensions of the primary sensory receptor areas; also known as sensory association areas or unimodal association areas.

secondary neurulation process in which the caudal neural tube gives rise to the sacral and coccygeal levels of the spinal cord; begins at approximately 3 weeks of gestation.

secretomotor stimulating secretion.

segmental rolling reflex the reflex noted when an infant rolls the trunk and pelvis segmentally with rotation of the head or legs.

selective engagement neural process in which certain neural networks are utilized for optimizing a task while others are limited in participation; primarily manifested in attention with principal cortical area involved thought to be the dorsolateral prefrontal cortex.

selectivity in neural transmission, the process through which excitatory and inhibitory influences allow only certain neural impulses to be transmitted at the level of the synapse.

sensory fibers also known as afferent fibers; carry information to the central nervous system about sensations of touch, pain, temperature, and vibrations.

sensory memory a transient representation of the sensory input of an environment. Sensory information is stored just long enough to be transient to short term memory.

septa a dividing structure, a wall.

servomechanism control system a control device for maintaining the operation of another system.

short-term memory temporary and limited in capacity; related to working memory (the active processing to hold the information); must be continuously acted on through rehearsal or imaging or information stored here will be lost over time.

Shy Drager syndrome condition of unknown etiology characterized by hypotension, constipation, urinary urgency, parkinsonian symptoms, cerebellar incoordination, muscle fasciculations, and leg tremors.

single-photon emission tomography (SPECT) imaging modality that uses the mechanism of the computed tomography scan but instead of detecting x-rays, it detects single photons emitted from an external tracer; radioactive compounds that emit gamma rays are injected into the subject; can scan metabolism and blood flow in the brain.

social (pragmatic) communication disorder as of 2013, a new diagnostic category in the DSM (*Diagnostic and Statistical Manual of Mental Disorders*) applied to persons with deficits in social use of language who do not demonstrate restricted interests or repetitive behaviors associated with ASD.

sodium-potassium pump related to the physiology of neurons; an ion pump that removes intracellular sodium and concentrates intracellular potassium.

solely special sensory A A specialized organ devoted to processing one sensory input.

soma a neuronal cell body; also called the perikaryon.

somatic pertaining to the structure of the body wall (muscles, skin, and mucous membranes).

somatosensory relating to sensating occuring anywhere in the system.

somesthetic pertaining to the senses of pain, temperature, taction, vibration, and position.

somites mesodermal tissue that develops into the axial skeleton, dermis, and skeletal muscles.

spasmodic dysphonia chronic phonation disorder of unknown etiology characterized by a strained voice quality with voice arrests caused by laryngeal adductor spasm; symptoms may occur in some movement disorders.

spastic cerebral palsy congenital condition with hypertonia, hyperreflexia, and clasp-knife reflex, increased tone, and bilateral central nervous system damage.

spastic dysarthria strain-strangle, harsh voice quality; imprecise articulation, and hypernasality caused by upper motor neuron bilateral pathology; affects phonation, articulation, respiration, and resonance.

spasticity syndrome of hypertonus with exaggeration of stretch reflexes as a result of certain neural lesions.

spatial summation achieving an action potential involving input from multiple cells of different areas of input, usually from the dendrite.

specific language impairment (SLI) a subset condition of children with developmental receptive/expressive language disorders; possible organic involvement; language disorder must not be attributable to a more generalized condition such as hearing loss, autism, or acquired neurologic damage.

speech-language pathology the study of the diagnosis, treatment, and prevention of communication disorders, including articulation, phonology, voice, fluency, expressive and receptive language, and related disorders.

speech pathology see *speech-language pathology.*

spina bifida congenital defect of the spinal cord or the vertebral column.

spinal dysraphism an umbrella term for a number of conditions present at birth that affect the spine, spinal cord, or nerve roots.

spinal peripheral nerves mixed nerves (both sensory and motor) connected to the spinal cord.

spinocerebellar pathway consists of the dorsal and ventral tracts; arise from the posterior and medial gray matter of the spinal cord; dorsal ascends ipsilaterally but the ventral crosses in the cord; both terminate in the cerebellum and allow proprioceptive impulses from all parts of the body to be integrated in the cerebellum.

spiral ganglion a cluster of nerve bodies in the dorsal root of a spinal nerve forming a nodule-like structure.

splenium the thickened posterior part of the corpus callosum.

split brain a condition in which the corpus callosum has been surgically divided so no information transfers between hemispheres.

stereocilia hair cell processes bent by movement.

stereognosis recognition of objects through nonvisual and tactile stimulation.

striate cortex primary visual cortex.

striatum a compnent of the basal ganglia necessary for voluntary movement control and composed of the caudate, putamen, and ventral striatum.

styloglossus the smallest of the styloid muscles arising from the anterior and lateral surfaces of the styloid process; aids in tongue retraction and swallowing.

subarachnoid space a space between the dura and pia mater layers filled with cerebrospinal fluid.

subcortical aphasia aphasia associated with either thalamic or basal ganglia lesions (subcortical structures).

subdural space region below the dura mater.

sublingual region below or under the tongue.

substantia nigra (SN) a mass of gray matter extending from the upper border of the pons into the subthalamus.

subthalamic nucleus (STN) considered part of the basal ganglia, the STN is located within the diencephalon and close to the midbrain.

subthalamus region composed of subcortical structures of the basal ganglia located below the thalamus.

suck reflex infant reflex that occurs when a finger is placed in the infant's mouth and bouts of sucking behavior occur; integrated at birth and develops into jaw movements after 2 to 3 months.

sulcus groove on the surface of the brain or spinal cord; also known as fissures.

summation the product of the neural impulses acting on a given synapse.

superior upper; opposite of inferior or lower.

supine lying on the back.

supplementary (secondary) motor area motor area discovered by Wilder G. Penfield located on the ventral surface of the precentral and postcentral gyri; primary function is controlling sequential movements.

supramarginal gyrus convolution in the inferior parietal lobe surrounding the posterior end of the sylvian fissure.

surface dyslexia type of dyslexia distinguished by poor ability to use grapheme-to-phoneme conversion rules.

swallowing reflex developed after the sucking reflex is integrated into feeding; sucking produces saliva that accumulates in the pharynx, triggering the reflex; may be observed by visible upward movement of the hyoid bone and thyroid cartilage of the larynx.

Sydenham chorea involuntary movement disorder following infection; usually occurs in children and adolescents.

symmetrical tonic neck reflex analogous to the asymmetrical tonic reflex but the head is manipulated in flexion and extension in midline rather than turned laterally; the normal execution of this reflex is an extension of the arms and flexion of the legs if the head is extended in midline.

sympathetic division that division of the autonomic nervous system concerned with preparing the body for fight or flight; its neurons arise in the thoracic and upper lumbar segments of the spinal cord.

synapse a juncture or connection; the functional contact of one neuron with another.

synaptic cleft the intervening space before and after a synapse.

synaptic stabilization this is the dynamic process of strengthening and maintaining active synappses through increased use.

synergy the cooperative action of muscles.

tardive dyskinesia uncontrolled involuntary movements of the face and tongue; often caused by excessive or long-term treatment with neuroleptic medications.

tectal (collicular) pathway projects to the superior colliculi in the brainstem and the thalamus and out to many regions of the cortex; substantially involved in the ability to orient toward and follow a visual stimuli.

tectorial membrane gelatinous covering of the organ of Corti in the auditory system.

tectum roof of the midbrain; location of the superior and inferior colliculi.

temporal lobe bounded superiorly by the lateral fissure and posteriorly by the occipital lobe; the center for auditory processing in the brain.

temporal summation the additive effect of successive stimuli on one nerve, which collectively can generate a response when the individual stimuli could not.

temporal visual cortex part of the visual association cortex located within the middle and inferior temporal areas.

tentorium cerebelli one of two dural folds in the dura mater that helps stabilize the brain.

teratology the study of abnormal embryology.

thalamic reticular nucleus a layer of cells enveloping the ventral thalamus whose axons are sent back into the thalamus rather than to the cortex; either facilitates or inhibits transmission of other impulses to the cortex.

thalamocortical circuit this is the main route of communication between the eye and the cerebral cortex.

thalamus two oval nodes located at the base of the cerebrum; serves as a relay station for all sensory stimulation; consists of gray matter.

thromboembolic a stroke causes by a blood clot (thrombus) that forms a blockage to an artery supplying blood to the brain.

thrombus A stationary blood clot along the wall of a blood vessel.

tinnitus ringing or buzzing sound heard in the ear.

tongue reflex typically a part of the suckle-swallow reaction in which the tongue thrusts between the lips; mediated at the medulla; usually disappears by 12 to 18 months of age.

tonic labyrinthine reflex (TLR) associated with changes in tone as a result of changes in head position affecting the orientation of the labyrinths of the inner ear.

tonotopic pertaining to the spatial arrangement in the auditory system determining where different sound frequencies are perceived, transmitted, or received.

topologic involvement relation of an anatomic structure to a specific body part or area.

transcortical aphasia several types of language disturbances whose causes are lesions outside the perisylvian area; repetition is always preserved.

transcranial magnetic stimulation (TMS) a noninvasive method of exciting neurons in the brain; uses weak electric current induced in the brain tissue by rapidly changing magnetic fields.

transient ischemic attack (TIA) a reversible neurologic defect (focal) lasting up to 24 hours; may indicate a risk for a stroke; may be caused by an embolism or obstruction of an artery.

transitory related to or marked by a transition; not permanent.

traumatic brain injury (TBI) diffuse brain damage that may be caused by an external force (e.g., closed-head injury from a car accident) or a penetrating force (e.g., open-head injury from a bullet wound).

tremor a purposeless involuntary movement that is oscillatory and rhythmic.

trigeminal ganglia on the sensory root of cranial nerve V in a cleft within the dura mater; gives off ophthalmic and maxillary nerves and is part of the mandibular nerve branch.

triplegia paralysis of an upper and a lower extremity and of the face or of both extremities on one side and one on the other.

uncus the hooked extremity of the hippocampal gyrus.

unilateral initiated from or affecting structures on only one side of the body.

unilateral inattention a subtle form of neglect syndrome characterized by the failure to recognize a side of the body and the space around it.

unilateral innervation indicating that the nerve supply to a particular structure comes from only one side of the body (may be ipsilateral or contralateral), as opposed to bilateral innervation, in which nerve fibers are distributed from both sides of the body.

unilateral upper motor neuron dysarthria a motor speech disorder primarily caused by unilateral damage to the upper motor neurons that carry impulses to the cranial nerves that innervate the speech musculature; the most affected speech parameter is articulation.

upper motor neurons (UMNs) nerves connecting cortical motor areas with cranial and spinal nerves; composed of the direct activation pathway (DAP) and the indirect activation pathway (IAP), the DAP functions for direct voluntary and skilled movements, whereas the IAP functions to control posture, tone, and movements that support voluntary movements.

vegetative states disorders of consciousness in which patients who sustain severe brain damage are in a state of partial arousal rather than true awareness, perhaps demonstrating complex reflexes, eye opening, yawning, response to noxious stimuli but failing to show awareness of themselves or the environment. Persistent vegetative state is the diagnosis after a period of 4 weeks with no change.

venous sinuses a group of sinuses in the dura that drain venous blood circulating from the cranial cavity, returning deoxygenated blood to the heart.

ventral   toward the belly or abdomen; opposite of dorsal.

ventricular system   cavities that contain cerebrospinal fluid produced by the choroid plexus located in each ventricle; the system consists of lateral ventricles and a third and fourth ventricle; connected by foramen and the aqueduct of Sylvius; found in the deepest areas of the brain.

vertebral artery   supplies the brainstem and cerebellum; from the anterior and posterior spinal arteries to the spinal cord and a branch called the posterior inferior cerebellar artery.

vesicle   a blister or bladder; the intracellular bladder is believed to be filled with neurotransmitter substances.

vestibulospinal tracts   nerve fiber tracts that mediate cerebellar and vestibular influences on the spinal cord; facilitate reflexes and control muscle tone.

videofluoroscopy   also known as a Modified Barium Swallow (MBS), this is a radiologic test which helps visualize the oral, laryngeal, and pharyngeal structures during a swallow.

visual agnosia   the inability to recognize objects by sight, usually caused by damage to the visual association area of the central nervous system.

volitional   voluntary.

Wernicke (receptive) aphasia   an acquired adult language disorder characterized by impaired comprehension and fluent, paraphasic language; the patient is free of hemiplegia, and the lesion usually is in the temporal lobe.

Wernicke area   a major speech-language center in the dominant temporal lobe; important for comprehension of language.

white matter   substance of the brain and spinal cord consisting of myelinated fibers and containing no neuronal cell bodies or synapses; in a freshly sectioned brain it glistens white because of the high content of lipid-rich myelin; also called the fimbria.

Worster-Drought Syndrome   a disorder characterized by isolated paralysis or weakness of the oral musculature without major weakness in the trunk or extremities.

working memory   the small amount of information that can be manipulated during the execution of a task.

x-ray   radiograph; film produced by radiographic imaging.

INDEX

Note: Page numbers followed by "*b*," "*t*," and "*f*" refer to boxes, tables, and figures, respectively.

A

Abducens, 120
Abduction, cranial nerves and, 120, 120*f*
Abductor spasmodic dysphonia, 146
Absolute refractory period, 69–70
Acalculia, 19
Acceleration-deceleration injury, 188
Acetylcholine, 72, 105, 139
Acoustic neuroma, 123
Acoustic-vestibular nerve (cranial nerve VIII), 123–124
Action potential, 69–70, 70*f*, 71*f*
Action tremor, 109, 110*b*
Adductor spasmodic dysphonia, 146
Adenosine triphosphate (ATP), 11
Adequate stimulus, 69
Adiadochokinesia, 113
Afferent fibers, 37–38, 41
Afferent pathways, of central auditory system, 83*f*
Agnosias, 24
  auditory, 81*t*, 84
  defined, 80
  Gerstmann syndrome, 81*t*
  parietal lobe and, 51
  Sigmund Freud and, 3
  tactile, 81*t*, 88
  types of, 81*t*
  visual, 81*t*, 91–92
Agraphia, 183*t*, 184
Akathisia, 110, 110*b*
Akinesia, 108
Alar plate, 198–199
Alcohol, 229
Alexia, 183–184, 183*t*
  with agraphia, 19, 184
  without agraphia, 183
Allocortex, 25, 201. *See also* Neocortex
Alpha motor neuron (AMN), 103–105, 104*f*
Altered mental status (AMS), 187
Alzheimer's disease, 186, 186*t*
American Sign Language, 10
American Speech-Language-Hearing Association (ASHA), 1, 231
Americans with Disabilities Act (ADA), 1
Amygdala, 26, 41
Amyloid plaques, 186
Amyotrophic lateral sclerosis (ALS), 139–140, 140*b*
Analgesia, 87
Anarthria, 212
  developmental, 212
Anastomosis, 64
Anesthesia, 20, 87
Aneurysm, 177, 177*f*
Angular gyrus, 19, 163*t*, 164

Anion, 66
Anisotropic, defined, 56
Annulospiral endings, 105
Anomia, 19, 180
Anomic aphasia, 180
Anosognosia, 185
Ansa cervicalis, 127
Anterior, defined, 4–5
Anterior (ventral) horn cells, 37
Anterior lobe, 110, 111*f*
Anterior spinothalamic tract, 85–86, 85*f*
Anterograde degeneration, 76
Anterograde transport, 13, 64, 65*f*
Aphasias, 3, 176–182 *see also* specific aphasias
  Broca's, 17
  cerebrovascular accident and, 176–178
  classification of, 178–181
  conduction, 22
  etiology of, 176–178, 177*f*
  intervention for, 181–182
  language functions of, 182*t*
  localization of, 178*b*
  neoplasms and, 178
  neuropathology of, 176–178, 177*f*
  nonfluent/expressive, 178–181
  pharmacology in, 182
  speech-language pathologist and, 182
  subcortical, 165
  testing and intervention for, 181–182
  testing for, 181–182
  Wernicke's, 19
Aphasic agraphia, 184
Aphasic alexia, 183*t*, 184
Aphemia, 150
Apoptosis, 201
Apraxia of speech (AOS), 96, 115*b*, 149*b*, 149*t*, 150–151
  childhood, 216–218
  developmental, 212
Apraxias, 96, 149–151, 149*b* *see also* specific apraxias
  dysarthria *vs.*, 213*t*
  Hugo Liepmann and, 3
  types of, 149, 149*t*
Aprosodia, 185
Aqueduct of Sylvius, 43
Arachnoid granulations, 42–43
Arachnoid mater, 41–42, 46*f*
Arachnoid villus, 42–43, 45*f*
Archicortex, 25, 201. *See also* Allocortex; Neocortex
Arcuate fasciculus, 22, 22*f*, 23*t*, 163–164, 163*t*
Areflexia, 102
Arterial spin labeling (ASL), 58*b*
Arteriosclerosis, 176

Arteriovenous malformation (AVM), 178
Articulation
  and ataxic dysarthria, 141
  and chorea, 145
  and flaccid dysarthria, 138
  and multiple sclerosis, 147
  and parkinsonism, 143
  and Shy-Drager syndrome, 148
  and spasmodic dysphonia, 146
  and spastic dysarthria, 137
Articulation disorders, 218–219
ASD. *See* Autism spectrum disorder (ASD)
Asomatognosia, 51
Asperger's syndrome, 234
Associated central disturbances, 182–184
Association cortices, 24–25
  categories of, 24–25, 25*b*
  sensory, 80
Association fibers, 21–23, 22*f*, 23*t*
Association fiber tracts, 3
Associative memory, 169
Astereognosis, 88
Astrocytes, 13, 14*b*
Asymmetric tonic neck reflex (ATNR), 205–206, 205*f*
Asymmetry, 2
Asynergia, 111
Asynergy, 111
Ataxia, 112, 112*t*
Ataxic cerebral palsy, 215, 215*t*
Ataxic dysarthria, 30, 113, 140–141, 148*b*
Athetoid cerebral palsy, 214, 215*t*
Athetosis, 109, 110*b*, 142*b*, 145–146
Atopognosis, 87
Atrophy, 102
Attention, 167, 168*b*
  traumatic brain injury and, 189*t*
Attentional dyslexia, 183–184
Attention-deficit/hyperactivity disorder, 239
Audition, 80–81
Auditory agnosias, 81*t*, 84
Auditory association cortices, 80
Auditory brainstem responses (ABRs), 57, 84
Auditory nerve (cranial nerve VIII), 81, 83
Auditory sentence processing, neurocognitive model of, 162*f*
Auditory system, lesions of, 84
Autism, 234
Autism spectrum disorder (ASD), 234–236, 234*t*, 235*b*
Autonomic nervous system, 15, 40–41
Axon, 12, 64, 65*f*
Axonal regeneration, 76–77
Axonal transport, 64, 65*f*
Axon hillock, 12–13, 64
Axon terminals (boutons), 13, 64